Primary Care

of the

Older Adult

A Multidisciplinary Approach

Second Edition

Primary Care
of the
Older Adult

A Multidisciplinary Approach

Mary M. Burke, RN, DNSc, GNP, ANP

Gerontologic Nursing Consultant
Washington, DC

Joy A. Laramie, MSN, CNP

Geriatrics
Veterans Affairs Medical Center
Washington, DC

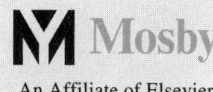

Mosby

An Affiliate of Elsevier

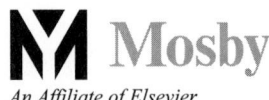

An Affiliate of Elsevier

11830 Westline Industrial Drive
St. Louis, Missouri 63146

Primary Care of the Older Adult

NOTICE

Nursing is an ever-changing field. Standard safety precautions must be followed, but as new
research and clinical experience broaden our knowledge, changes in treatment and drug therapy
may become necessary or appropriate. Readers are advised to check the most current product information provided by the manufacturer of each drug to be administered to verify the recommended
dose, the method and duration of administration, and contraindications. It is the responsibility of
the licensed prescriber, relying on experience and knowledge of the patient, to determine dosages
and the best treatment for each individual patient. Neither the publisher nor the author assumes
any liability for any injury and/or damage to persons or property arising from this publication.

Previous edition copyrighted 2000

Library of Congress Cataloging-in-Publication Data
   Primary care of the older adult: a multidisciplinary approach / [edited by] Mary M.
  Burke, Joy A. Laramie.– 2nd ed.
    p. cm.
   Includes bibliographical references and index.
   ISBN-13: 978-0-323-02395-5   ISBN-10: 0-323-02395-9 (pbk.)
    1. Aged–Medical care. 2. Primary care (Medicine) I. Burke, Mary M. II. Laramie, Joy A.
  [DNLM: 1. Primary Health Care–Aged.]
  RC952.P695 2004
  618.97–dc22
                        2003058071

Executive Publisher: Barbara Cullen
Senior Developmental Editor: Victoria Bruno
Publishing Services Manager: Catherine Jackson
Senior Project Manager: Jeff Patterson
Designer: Teresa McBryan Breckwoldt

ISBN-13: 978-0-323-02395-5
ISBN-10: 0-323-02395-9

Printed in the United States of America

Last digit is the print number: 9 8 7 6 5 4 3

To Frank,
spouse extraordinaire, who provided patience,
humor, and support throughout the two editions of this text.
Mary M. Burke

To my wonderful family:
my touchstones, my serenity, and my delight;
and
to Jamie, my soul mate.
Joy A. Laramie

Contributors

Charles Cefalu, MD, MS
Professor and Chief of Geriatric Medicine
LSUHSC/Medical Center of Louisiana
Department of Family Medicine
New Orleans, Louisiana

CONTRIBUTORS TO THE FIRST EDITION

Thomas Berryman, DPM
Podiatrist
Advanced Footcare Practice
East Stroudsburg, Pennsylvania

Cleo A. Boulter, MSN, RN
Vice President, PPS
Centennial HealthCare
Atlanta, Georgia

Janice T. Brown, RN, MSN, GNP-C, ANP-C
Instructor
Georgetown University Medical School
Washington, DC

Elizabeth Burgraff, RN, C, MS
Family Nurse Practitioner
St. Elizabeth's Medical Center
Boston, Massachusetts

Georges Catinis, MD
Assistant Professor
Gastroenterology and Transplant Hepatology
Louisiana State University
New Orleans, Louisiana

Charles Cefalu, MD, MS
Professor and Chief of Geriatric Medicine
LSUHSC/Medical Center of Louisiana
Department of Family Medicine
New Orleans, Louisiana

Mary Corcoran, OTR, PhD
Associate Research Professor
George Washington University
Washington, DC

Jill C. Cunningham, MSN, CANP
Adult Nurse Practitioner
Georgetown University Medical Center
Orthopaedics and Rheumatology
Washington, DC

Mary T. Delaney, RN, PhD
Senior Lecturer, College of Nursing
Wayne State University
Detroit, Michigan

Vaunette P. Fay, RN-CS, GNP, FNP, PhD
Associate Professor, School of Nursing
University of Texas—Houston Health Science Center
Houston, Texas

Janet Feldman, RN, PhD
Vice President
Qualatas Associates
Downers Grove, Illinois

Kathleen French, MSN, MPH, CRNP, CDE
Family Nurse Practitioner
20th Medical Group
Shaw Air Force Base, South Carolina

Kimberly H. Groner, MSN, CANP
Adult Nurse Practitioner—Rheumatology
Georgetown University Medical Center
Washington, DC

Mary Marmoll Jirovec, RN, BSN, MSN,
PhD, FAAN
Associate Professor
Wayne State University
Detroit, Michigan

Sr. Mary Paul McLaughlin, BS, MSN, CNP
Gerontologic Nurse Practitioner
St. Gertrude Monastery
Ridgely, Maryland

M. Eletta Morse, RN, BA, MSN, CRNP
Nurse Practitioner
FutureCare, Inc.
Glen Burnie, Maryland

Cheryl B. Moxley, BS, BBA, RD
Clinical Nutrition Specialist
Washington Hospital Center
Washington, DC

Carine M. Nassar, MS, RD, LD, CNSD
Senior Clinical Nutrition Specialist
Washington Hospital Center
Washington, DC

Christina M. Puchalski, MD, MS
Assistant Professor of Medicine and Geriatrics
George Washington University Medical Center
Washington, DC

Karen Reilly, ScD
Associate
Abt Associates
Cambridge, Massachusetts

Verna E. Reynolds, MD, CMD
Medical Director/Physician
Sentara Life Care
Norfolk, Virginia

Anita Rothwell, MSN
Nurse Practitioner
Kaiser Permanente
Kensington, Maryland

David A. Sayles, MD
Director, Division of Geriatric Psychiatry
George Washington University Medical Center
Washington, DC

Mohamad Sidani, MD, MS
Assistant Professor, School of Medicine
Department of Family Medicine
Louisiana State University Health Sciences
New Orleans, Louisiana

Eleanor Stewart, MD
Assistant Director of Geriatric Medicine
Providence Hospital
Washington, DC

Carol Taylor, CSFN, RN, MSN, PhD
Director, Center for Clinical Bioethics
Assistant Professor of Nursing
Georgetown University
Washington, DC

Kevin Young, MPH, LPT
Physical Therapist
Health Care Financing Administration
Baltimore, Maryland;
Maryland Orthopedics
Endicott City, Maryland

Preface

As editors to the second edition of *Primary Care of the Older Adult,* we reaffirmed our guiding premise that primary care of the older adult should be a multidisciplinary endeavor. The often complicated care of the older person requires the expertise of a variety of disciplines and obligates an approach that addresses the physical, psychological, and social aspects of care. Primary care providers are often not fortunate enough to have all members of the interdisciplinary team available, and for this reason there is a need for basic knowledge of each discipline to develop an appropriate and successful plan for the care of the older patient.

Additions to this second edition include discussion in Chapter 1, Comprehensive Geriatric Assessment and Health Maintenance Screening, of the issue of HIV/AIDS in the older adult and the special considerations for screening and care of this illness, which is often forgotten in the discussion of older adults. Chapter 4, Cancer: Risk Assessment and Screening, aims to assist the primary care provider with the often uncertain role of screening for cancer in the older adult who may not necessarily benefit from aggressive diagnostic and treatment interventions. Chapter 8, Oral Health, provides information regarding the assessment and prevention of oral health issues, a topic often overlooked in the primary care literature. Chapter 20, Genitourinary/Male: Benign Prostatic Hyperplasia and Erectile Dysfunction, includes a discussion of the assessment and treatment of erectile dysfunction. Information regarding severe acute respiratory syndrome (SARS) is included in Chapter 10. These topics have been included to provide the primary care provider with updated information on current issues.

The book is divided into four units. Unit 1, Health Maintenance, includes four chapters of basic knowledge in health assessment, health promotion, and disease prevention. Unit 2, Clinical Management, focuses on frequently experienced illnesses and conditions in the older adult and on bringing together fundamental knowledge and practical experience-based information for the practicing primary care provider. Unit 3, Vulnerabilities, comprises five chapters that capture the art of care by addressing common conditions and scenarios that every provider will encounter when providing care to older adults. The final section is Unit 4, Foundations of Care. Many times these chapters are found at the beginning of a textbook and, while there is no intention to minimize the importance of this information, the emphasis is on clinical practice. Our hope is that after practitioners and students have found the answers to their clinical questions, they will find the information in this final unit to be helpful and thought provoking.

This book has been written to help the primary care provider confidently and efficiently treat, educate, and support his or her older patient. It is intended for practicing primary care providers who wish to have an available reference with updated information and interventions. It is also useful for students who have completed foundational courses and are in clinical rotations in primary care settings with an older population. The material in the book is presented as succinctly as possible and includes relevant and timely content for primary care practitioners. The content focus is on conditions, problems, and illnesses that primary care providers encounter when treating older adult patients.

The authors hope that this book will not only improve the quality of care provided to the older patients but will also encourage students and practitioners to pursue research that will answer some of the perplexing questions that will always remain a critical aspect of primary care of older adults.

We have tried to convey our deep concern for the dignity, personal integrity, and autonomy of each older adult patient whom we serve. All of us, as primary care providers, have a responsibility to meet the needs of the patient over and above the needs of the health care organization in which we function.

Acknowledgments

An endeavor such as this requires the support, encouragement, and inspiration of many people. Most notably we acknowledge our colleagues, faculty members, students, and patients, past, present, and future, who are the core motivation for advancing knowledge and improving delivery of care.

We owe much to the contributors of the first edition, and we have listed their names and the positions that they held at that time within the frontmatter to acknowledge our debt to their expertise. We are responsible for the revision of their work with the exception of the Clinical Pharmacology chapter and the new chapters, which were authored by Joy Laramie. We would like to extend a special thanks to Charles Cefalu. He is a leader in multidisciplinary care of older adults; his chapter on Clinical Pharmacology in this edition and the first edition has added depth and breadth to the book. He is a valued colleague.

We owe a great deal to the representatives of the publishing company: Barbara Cullen, Executive Publisher; Victoria Bruno, Senior Developmental Editor; and Jeff Patterson, Senior Project Manager. Barbara Cullen was instrumental in enticing us to do the second edition and for that we are grateful. Victoria Bruno has been a personable supporter throughout this undertaking from the very beginning and deserves special kudos for keeping us on track and managing all the intricacies of this arduous process. Our thanks also go to Jeff Patterson for his speedy response to any request and for the outstanding job of shepherding this book to full production—Thank you.

We would like to make special mention of Mary Walsh—mentor, friend, and co-author. She is deeply missed.

A special acknowledgment goes to those we love as family, since nothing is possible without the unconditional love we receive from those with whom we share our lives.

Mary M. Burke
Joy A. Laramie

Contents

Unit 4 **Foundations of Care, 629**

Appendixes

Introduction to the Text

The health care delivery system in the United States strives to provide two fundamental rights: the right to access to care and the right to quality in services delivered. The current United States health care delivery system is not perfect, but this fact should never seriously impede health care professionals in the continuous pursuit of providing optimal care to their older patients.

Older adults are an extremely diverse population in abilities, life experiences, social resources, and ethnicity. Widely held generalizations and stereotypical images of older adults threaten the primary care provider's ability to conduct appropriate interviews and objective assessments. It is the responsibility of each person working with older adults to introspectively review these negative views of older people and work diligently to view each person as unique.

All older people have multiple talents and virtues. The primary provider needs to always be aware of the strengths of an older person and not view him or her as a failing organ system. Many times family members, friends, or paid caregivers will be important informants regarding the daily life and condition of the older patient. It is wise to ask the older person's permission before questions are asked of these supportive people. Dignity is many times closely related to autonomy. To be treated with dignity and kindness is a treasured commodity, but it is also a human right, and it is the responsibility of the practitioner to ensure that the right is respected.

Theories of aging reflect the complexities of the process, but none are comprehensive. Theories that attempt to explain only the physiologic changes that occur during the aging process include genetic theories, cellular theories, and organ system theories (autoimmune). Other physiologic concepts of aging that are proposed are nutrient deprivation, lipofuscin, wear and tear theory, and crosslinking theory. Psychologic theories abound and include disengagement theory, activity theory, life course theory, and continuity theory. None of these theories or constructs can claim sufficient evidence to account for aging effects that are experienced by older people. The majority of theorists and practitioners agree that with advanced age come factors such as increased vulnerability, increased susceptibility to disease, decrease in vitality, and slowed response to and recovery from stress.

Biologic principles that are paramount for understanding the diversity of older people are as follows:

1. Older people age at different rates from one another; chronologic age is not always a reflection of physiologic age.
2. Within each older person, organ systems age at different rates; a person with severe congestive heart failure may write a great symphony, thereby exhibiting a high level of cognitive function.

Generalizations concerning typical pain syndrome such as chest pain in myocardial infarction do not hold for most older adults. A symptom as benign as slight confusion in a frail older adult may well be the alarm for an impeding infarction. Pneumonia often will not present with any fever, and the x-ray results may be negative. The primary care provider must always be alert and respond to a patient or family member who reports, "I don't know what it is, but something is wrong."

The common comorbidities of age cloud the diagnostic process. The process of diagnosing is also made difficult by iatrogenic complexities of adverse response to treatments. It is well known that older people are at increased risk for complications related to multiple drug use. Every primary care visit should include a review of all prescription and over-the-counter drug use. Many times a symptom that is the result of one drug is treated by adding another drug to the regimen. A potassium supplement may be added because of a diuretic; an H_2 blocker may be added because of a nonsteroidal antiinflammatory drug, a laxative may be added because of the constipation from a calcium channel blocker. There is no easy and universal solution to this problem, but the first step is to recognize the existence of problems associated with multiple drug use and then work toward a solution.

There is a never-ending influx of new and redesigned old drugs that are marketed extensively to primary care providers, with nurse practitioners as a new and expanding customer. New drugs play an important role in many fields of health care when used appropriately, but there should be a note of caution when considering a newly marketed drug for use in the older population because of the increased risk for adverse drug reactions.

1

Comprehensive Geriatric Assessment and Health Maintenance Screening

The traditional problem-focused medical assessment is often ineffectual in assessing the multiple, complex needs of the older patient. A practitioner who attempts to identify or focus on one specific diagnosis will often fail to recognize the real issue that prompted the patient to seek medical attention—the influence of the "diagnosis" on his or her daily functioning. The recognition of the complex medical, social, and mental health problems and resulting functional disabilities of many frail older persons has led to the development of a multidimensional, interdisciplinary approach to the evaluation of this population.

The Comprehensive Geriatric Assessment (CGA) is often viewed as the procedure that defines geriatric care. CGA helps providers diagnose and prioritize problems and develop short- and long-term plans for prevention, treatment, and rehabilitation strategies that emphasize improving or maintaining patient function, reducing unnecessary use of health care resources, and prolonging survival of older patients. Improvement in function, rather than a cure for disability, is often the goal of comprehensive geriatric assessment. Function may be influenced by biologic, psychologic, and social issues experienced by the individual. Findings such as multiple chronic medical problems, depression, cognitive impairment, or lack of adequate social supports or financial assets, either alone or in combination, will significantly influence an older person's ability to carry out daily functions. Activity limitation due to chronic health conditions is common among noninstitutionalized older persons and increases substantially with age. In 1998 about 29% of persons 65 to 74 years of age reported an activity limitation compared with 47% of persons 75 years of age and over. Some 10% of noninstitutionalized persons 75 years of age and over reported needing help with personal care needs such as bathing, dressing, and eating, and 21% reported needing assistance with routine needs such as household chores and shopping (U.S. Preventive Services Task Force, 1996). By incorporating multidisciplinary perspectives into a systematic assessment, CGA evaluates the whole patient.

1

The process of CGA begins following identification of the patient in need—most commonly an older person who has experienced deteriorations in health and function. Patients most likely to benefit include the following:

- Persons over 75 years of age
- Persons with mild to moderate disabilities
- Persons who may be at risk of nursing home placement
- Persons with a poor social network

Age may be irrelevant if a person is coping with functional impairments and/or such "geriatric syndromes" as immobility, incontinence, use of multiple or inappropriate medications, cognitive impairment, weight loss, or depression or if the older person has been recently discharged from a hospital, is recently widowed, or is living alone. Therefore a chronically ill 50 year old with no family supports may be a more appropriate candidate for CGA than a healthy, active 75 year old with a strong social support system.

Assessment Environment

CGA exists as a continuum and therefore may occur in a variety of settings. The first reports of geriatric assessment programs came from a British geriatrician named Marjory Warren who created specialized geriatric assessment units during the 1930s (Williams, 1983). Depending on the individual patient's level of disability, cognition, access to transportation, and social supports, CGA may occur in the hospital, nursing facility, outpatient clinic, or home. Each of these sites presents challenges and benefits to performing the CGA. For example, in a hospital setting one has the benefit of time (the duration of the hospitalization) and, usually, opportunities to gain information from family members and friends who visit. However, because the patient is sick, the hospital setting does not offer the opportunity to assess him or her at baseline. In a nursing facility, many of the same benefits and challenges as in the inpatient setting may be found. One benefit, however, is the Minimum Data Set (MDS) (see Appendix A). The MDS is an exhaustive assessment tool required for every patient in the long-term setting that is completed mostly by the nursing staff and provides information regarding medical diagnoses, disabilities, and level of functioning; it is updated regularly. This is an important and underused tool in the comprehensive assessment of a patient in this setting.

The outpatient clinic setting is probably where most CGAs take place. This setting can be a challenging one in which to fully assess the functional capabilities of the older person. Pressures of tight schedules, tight space, and looming productivity reports are not conducive to the investment of the time and skill required for a thorough comprehensive assessment. In addition, most clinic settings are not designed with the older person in mind. Although laws that require handicapped accessibility have brought about major improvements, issues such as inappropriate lighting, sound, office design, and decor may still create challenges for the older person trying to access his or her health care provider. Poor sound barriers between examination rooms or background music may make it difficult for the person with a hearing impairment to understand what the examiner in the same room is saying. Poor lighting that casts shadows or solid colors and vertical lines in the decor may hinder depth perception. A desk in front of a sunny window may cause the person with macular degeneration to see only an outline of the person to whom he or she is speaking.

Although some of these issues may be out of the practitioner's control, some simple techniques may help overcome some of these barriers. Sitting close to and directly in front of the patient and speaking in low and even tones can help accommodate communication with persons with visual or hearing impairment. A portable amplifying device for persons without a hearing aid can be invaluable in facilitating communication with the hearing-impaired person. Appointments for older persons may be scheduled at a time when the office is less crowded, hectic, and overwhelming for the frail older patient and should routinely be of longer duration than the standard 10- or 15-minute follow-up appointment.

The average time spent per new patient in outpatient geriatric assessment units in one study was 2.7 hours (Gudmundsson and Carnes, 1996). Fortunately, the assessment of the older person can occur over several visits, with the initial visit focused on any urgent concerns and needs. The gathering of information from a new patient is often facilitated by mailing a preappointment questionnaire to the patient's home to be completed and brought in to the first appointment. The use of such a questionnaire, however, does not negate the need for discussing the information with the patient in the office. The use of a problem list that is updated at each visit offers an efficient way to track a patient's often multiple medical issues. It may be designed to include not only diagnoses, but also a medication list, advance directive information, and health screening information for quick reference at each visit. Although CGA is ideally performed by a multidisciplinary team, in reality the assessment may be performed by the primary health care provider alone. Nurse practitioners have the distinct advantage of a biopsychosocial background in approaching patients of all ages and therefore are well equipped to perform the comprehensive assessment of the frail older person.

The home is the ideal setting for CGA, allowing observation of the actual living situation, barriers, and resources with which the patient lives. Unfortunately, practitioners who have the time and desire to make home visits are rare.

Use of Assessment Tools

Many standardized tools are available to facilitate assessment of various aspects of functioning, many of which have been in use for several years and are therefore widely known and accepted. These tools are an important first step in the gathering of information regarding a person's biologic, psychologic, and social functional abilities. They provide fairly objective and standardized means for health care professionals to communicate findings. They can save time, facilitate the process of assessment, and improve accuracy and reliability; and they are particularly helpful in screening for problems that often go unsuspected, even after clinical examination. However, the person administering the instrument must have a working knowledge of its proper application to protect the reliability and validity of the test. Abnormal results on screening tools alone do not provide a diagnosis but rather indicate the need for further evaluation. One caveat is that assessment instruments are important for data collection, but relying too heavily on numeric scores can oversimplify a situation and shift attention away from the individual patient and his or her functional abilities within the patient's particular situation (Gudmundsson and Carnes, 1996).

Values/Culture

One cannot approach the assessment of the biopsychosocial issues that affect function without gleaning an appreciation of the individual's values. In this context, value goes beyond defining what the individual considers to be important in his or her life; it involves determining what traits, roles, and activities a person feels identifies himself or herself to the world and what gives that person meaning in his or her life. These values are developed over the course of a lifetime and are influenced by family, culture, religion, and life experiences. The primary care provider cannot develop a plan to meet the needs of an individual until he or she understands what the priorities and goals of the individual are. This requires actively seeking, acknowledging, and respecting this information.

As the U.S. population ages, it is becoming more diverse in terms of culture and ethnicity. In 2000, an estimated 84% of people 65 years of age and older were non-Hispanic white, 8% were non-Hispanic black, 2% were non-Hispanic Asian and Pacific Islander, and less than 1% were non-Hispanic American Indian and Alaska Native. Hispanic persons are estimated to make up 6% of the older population. By 2050, the percentage of the older population that is non-Hispanic white is expected to decline from 84% to 64%. Hispanic persons are projected to account for 16% of the older population; 12% of the population is projected to be non-Hispanic black; and 7% of the population is projected to be non-Hispanic Asian and Pacific Islander. Figure 1-1 illustrates the changing racial and ethnic composition of the United States (U.S. Census Bureau, 2000).

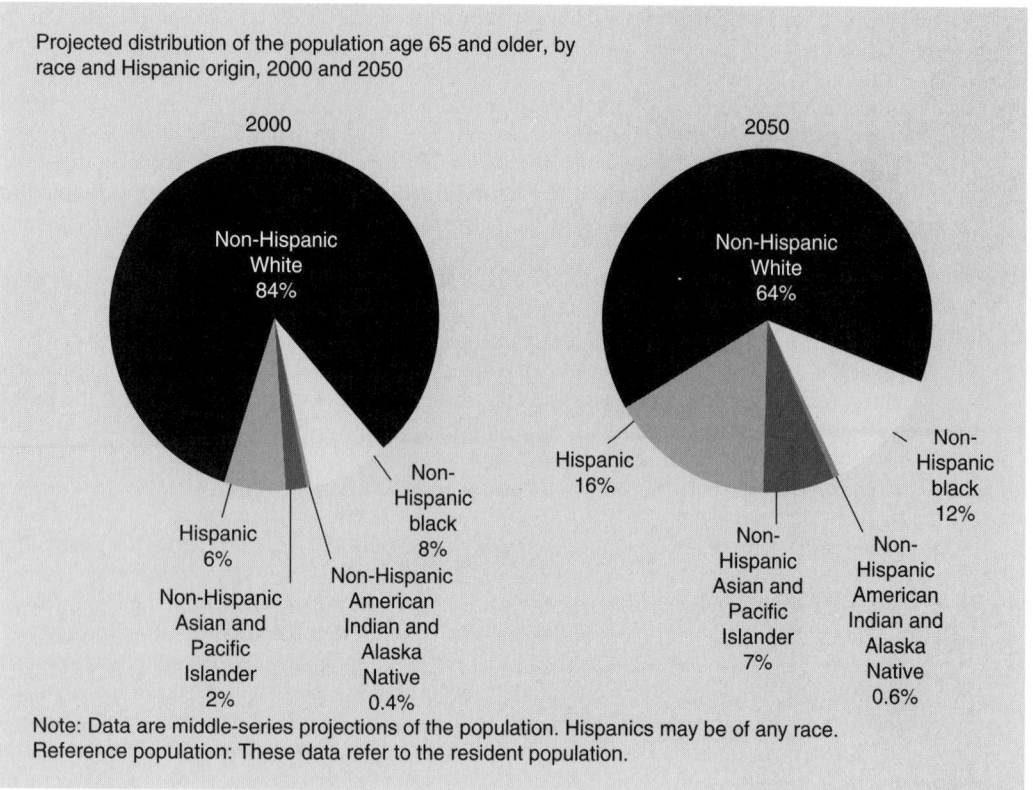

Projected distribution of the population age 65 and older, by race and Hispanic origin, 2000 and 2050

2000

Non-Hispanic White 84%

Hispanic 6%

Non-Hispanic Asian and Pacific Islander 2%

Non-Hispanic American Indian and Alaska Native 0.4%

Non-Hispanic black 8%

2050

Non-Hispanic White 64%

Hispanic 16%

Non-Hispanic Asian and Pacific Islander 7%

Non-Hispanic American Indian and Alaska Native 0.6%

Non-Hispanic black 12%

Note: Data are middle-series projections of the population. Hispanics may be of any race. Reference population: These data refer to the resident population.

Figure 1-1   Racial and ethnic composition. (From U.S. Census Bureau: Population Projections of the United States by Age, Sex, Race, Hispanic Origin, and Nativity: 1999-2100, January 2000. Available at www.census.gov/population. Accessed March 2003.)

The cultural background of an individual will influence not only the practitioner's assessment and teaching regarding language, diet, and disease risks, but will also necessitate consideration of other issues that may influence functional status, either negatively or positively. The great diversity in economic status within and among ethnic origins, as well as the patient's status regarding health insurance, necessitates consideration of a patient's ability to pay for a diagnostic test, treatment, or service that the practitioner may order. On the other hand, many black, Hispanic, Asian-American, and Native American older adults have been found to benefit from higher rates of co-residence with adult children and from social support from their extended families. Although this situation may exist out of necessity for economic survival, the availability of family members in the household or in close proximity can be a great support to ethnic and minority older adults who have few other resources.

Another important cultural consideration is the individual's feelings regarding effective and desirable practices and outcomes of health care. Cultures may use traditional American medicine in conjunction with faith healing or other traditional practices. The practitioner may be unaware of other practices unless the patient is asked. These beliefs must be recognized and respected if the maximum benefit for the patient is to be achieved. Education regarding medicine and diet may need to be tailored to the cultural beliefs and values of each individual patient. The primary care provider must recognize and respect an individual's cultural viewpoints and discover effective methods to provide health care and teaching in a manner that will be acceptable to the individual patient. As with all patients, the practitioner must ascertain that instructions are understood. The practitioner should not assume that a polite nod indicates understanding of what has been said. The patient or family member should be asked to repeat or explain instructions given. If a language barrier exists, a translator should be found.

Religious considerations play an important role in the assessment of most older individuals, whether or not they are of a culturally diverse group. Practices associated with and attitudes toward diet, medications, family roles, and decisions regarding health care may be dictated by one's religious beliefs. Again, the practitioner must learn to provide care to patients with respect for and consideration of these firmly held beliefs.

Advance Directives

Decisions regarding health care may result in any one of many different outcomes. Each individual holds his or her own beliefs concerning what constitutes a desirable, or "quality," outcome. A health care provider cannot assist a patient or family to make decisions that will work toward the desired outcome unless he or she has taken the time to ascertain what the goals of the patient or family are. This process is known as advance care planning. The following are examples of patients who require advance care planning:

- A patient with end-stage congestive heart failure desires no "heroic measures" to prolong her life, and her only desire is to see her grandson graduate from college, even if the possibility exists that she may not survive the long trip.
- A healthy 60-year-old man has no medical problems, takes no medication, and jogs 3 miles a day. Last year he watched his father die after months on a ventilator and vows never to allow that to happen to himself.
- A frail older man wishes only to have a peaceful death in his own home with his family by his side and does not care to undergo aggressive medical evaluations that may prolong his life by a few months.
- A healthy and active 90-year-old woman is looking forward to celebrating her 100th birthday, as did her mother and grandmother before her.

Each of these individuals will require a different approach to his or her care if the goals are to be met, but chances are that, without the help of their health care provider, none of them will succeed.

Although advance care planning is especially relevant for persons facing life-threatening illnesses, predicting when a previously healthy person may suffer an acute, life-threatening event is impossible. Thus the health care provider should discuss preferences regarding health care and desired outcomes with everyone. The best time to initiate these discussions is during a routine visit when a patient is healthy, but decisions should be reviewed and updated at regular intervals throughout the provider's relationship with the patient and family.

Although a critical aspect of advance care planning is the provider's knowledge of the patient's and family's values and goals, two documents have traditionally been used in the advance care planning process to guide patients and provide written documentation regarding their wishes. The living will is a document that allows a patient to specify preferences for health care in a variety of hypothetic situations. However, most of these scenarios are described in the setting of terminal illness or persistent vegetative state. This situation may not apply for all patients who wish to execute these documents. Therefore conversations regarding advance directives need to be centered on the conceivable medical possibilities that may arise within the patient's current situation.

The other document commonly used is the durable power of attorney (DPOA) for health. This is a legal document that requires legal assistance and is specifically designed to allow a person to designate a proxy to make decisions regarding health care on his or her behalf in the event of incapacitation. The person designated must understand the patient's values and wishes so that appropriate decisions are made on behalf of the patient.

Often the health care provider and family can clearly determine that the patient is not able to participate in the decision-making process (e.g., the patient with advanced dementia). However, sometimes the patient's ability to make decisions may not be clear. In these situations the provider must formally assess the patient's capacity to make decisions regarding his or her own health care. Every health care decision does not require the same degree of decision-making capacity to make an appropriate decision. An individual may be capable of performing some tasks adequately (i.e., have the capacity to make some decisions) but not others. This "decision-specific capacity" assumes that an individual has or lacks capacity for a particular decision at a particular time and under a particular set of circumstances. The determination that a patient has sufficient decision-making capacity to consent to or refuse a particular treatment is based on observation of a specific set of abilities (Mezey, Mitty, and Ramsey, 1997):

- The patient understands that he or she has the right to make a choice.
- The patient understands the medical situation, prognosis, risks, benefits, and consequences of treatment (or no treatment).
- The patient can communicate the decision.
- The patient's decision is stable and consistent over a period of time.

For example, a patient who has had a stroke that has left him aphasic may understand the choices, but if he is not able to communicate his wishes verbally, in writing, or in any other fashion, he is not able to participate in the decision-making process.

The requirements for who may perform the capacity assessment (i.e., one physician vs. a physician *and* a psychiatrist) vary between states. The nurse practitioner can play an important role in this process. All documentation of a patient's ability, or lack thereof, to communicate meaningfully may be taken into account. If a patient is certified as lacking capacity, the documentation should include the following:

- The cause and nature of the mental incapacity
- The extent of the incapacity
- The probable duration of the incapacity

The mental status of a patient with a delirium due to a pneumonia will most likely clear on treatment of the underlying infection, and his or her capacity to make health care decisions must be reevaluated following treatment. However, a patient with moderate to advanced Alzheimer's disease can be expected to have a permanent incapacity due to the progressive course of the disease process.

If a patient who has been certified as lacking capacity has previously executed a DPOA for health, the person appointed becomes the decision maker for the patient. If no DPOA has been identified, the authority to make decisions goes to one of the following (order of priority varies somewhat from state to state):

- Court-appointed guardian/conservator (if none of the following is available)
- Spouse
- Adult child
- Parent
- Adult sibling
- Nearest living adult relative

Advance care planning and execution of a DPOA can spare the patient, family, and provider a great deal of anxiety and grief. The primary care provider, whether a physician or a nurse practitioner, must be comfortable in addressing these issues. It is one of the most valuable services providers can offer their patients.

Biopsychosocial Assessment
MEDICAL ASSESSMENT

Figure 1-2 illustrates the approach to the comprehensive geriatric assessment. The individual's values influence his or her individual biopsychosocial traits, which in turn interact to determine his or her functional ability, which is the "target" of the comprehensive assessment.

All of the areas of assessment must be approached with consideration for the current or planned living situation, be it independent in a home or apartment, assisted living, or long-term care. The

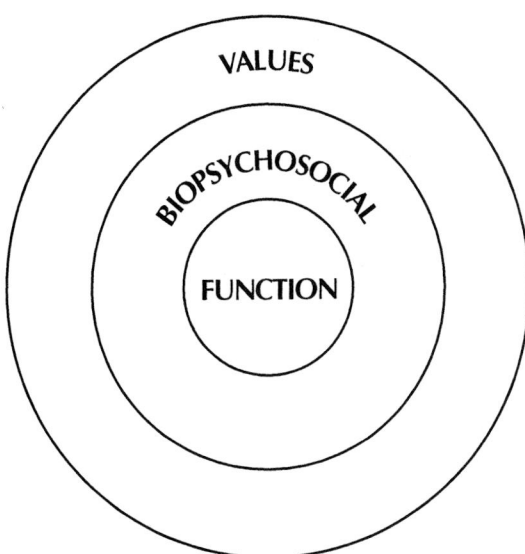

Figure 1-2   Approach to comprehensive geriatric assessment.

assessment, diagnosis, and plan for a patient in a long-term care facility will probably differ greatly from an individual living independently in the community because the presentation of disease, differential diagnoses, availability of resources, and goals of care will probably vary significantly among various settings. The biologic component of the assessment includes such issues as the medical history and physical examination, current status regarding presence or absence of disease states, risk behaviors, preventive health practices, nutrition, and medication use. Other important aspects to be evaluated are nutritional status, the presence of pain (which may influence function and quality of life), and the potential for or actual existence of abuse or neglect by caregivers (all of which will be covered in later chapters).

The assessment begins with the first contact with the patient. Did the patient call to schedule an appointment himself or herself? Was the patient able to communicate his or her needs on the phone and indicate understanding of information given to him or her such as date and time of appointment and location of office? Or did a family member make the call? The physical examination begins on the first visualization of the patient. Did the patient walk into the office independently? Is he or she able to follow instructions such as, "Follow me to the examination room," or "Step up on the scale"? If not, is it because of hearing impairment, cognitive impairment, or physical disability? Do you observe an intention tremor when you shake the patient's hand in greeting? Is the patient in the long-term care setting bedridden or ambulatory? The health care provider does not derive information solely by formal examination and assessment; even a social encounter can reveal volumes about a patient's functional abilities.

The approach to assessment of the various organ systems and disease processes is addressed in later chapters. However, a few "pearls" of assessment should be routine (in any setting) and therefore are worth mentioning separately:

1. Patients or families should always be asked to "brown bag" (i.e., bring in) the bottles of *all* medications the patient is taking, including over-the-counter medications and herbal/natural products, to *each* visit. The medication list in the chart may not always be reliable; medications may have been stopped or started by the patient or other health care providers.

2. Blood pressure and pulse should always be measured in the lying, sitting, and standing positions to determine the presence of orthostatic hypotension, an often overlooked cause of frequent falls.

3. Weight should be checked and recorded at each visit, with drops or increases addressed appropriately.
4. Hearing aids should always be removed and inspected, and the ear canals should be inspected for cerumen to ensure optimal hearing function.
5. An oral examination must always be performed to assess dentition and oral mucosa. Dentures must also be assessed for fit and then removed and inspected for rough edges that may irritate or injure the oral mucosa.
6. Abdominal examinations should always include a digital rectal examination. Although testing for fecal occult blood may not always be appropriate, examination of the prostate and assessment for the presence of impacted stool almost always is.
7. The musculoskeletal examination should not only cover assessment of muscle strength and range of motion but should include a thorough assessment of the feet; the presence of ulcers or painful calluses, excessively long toenails, and inappropriate footwear can all influence ambulatory status.
8. Whether an assessment is comprehensive or focused will depend on the presenting complaint of the patient. The health care provider should keep in mind the following "pearls" in assessment of an acute problem:
   a. Infection may present as vague changes from baseline rather than fever and localizing symptoms. A change in appetite, recurrent falls, or a nurse's or family member's report that a patient "just isn't himself" warrants investigation.
   b. The three most common sites of infection, especially in the long-term care setting, are denoted by the mnemonic *PUS*: *P*neumonia, *U*rine, *S*kin.
   c. Providers should have a low threshold of suspicion for fractures when presented with a limb that is swollen or painful.

Although screening and preventive care recommendations vary somewhat between professional health organizations, they still offer some guidance in determining issues to be addressed. Table 1-1 outlines recommendations by organization. Although 85 years of age has been proposed as a general cutoff range beyond which conventional screening tests are unlikely to be of continued benefit (Goldberg and Chavin, 1997), the health care provider must consider these recommendations in the context of the individual patient's current health status, ability to participate in the screening process, potential for benefit from screening and treatment of a particular disease, and goals of care. Immunization status is one area that is almost always appropriate to address. Persons of all ages should receive the tetanus-diphtheria (Td) vaccine every 10 years. Some individuals, especially women who have not served in the military, may have never received the vaccine and will need the primary series of three toxoid doses over 6 to 12 months. Patients with pressure ulcers are an often overlooked population of persons for whom Td vaccine is especially important. Annual influenza vaccination, usually given in October, is a vital preventive measure against the "flu" in all settings. The vaccine is important not only for older persons who may be susceptible to developing pneumonia following a case of the flu, but also for persons such as health care workers and frequent visitors to the long-term care or other care delivery setting who may bring the virus into the facility. The American College of Physicians recommends the pneumococcal vaccine for all adults after 65 years of age; persons who received the vaccine before age 65 should be reimmunized at 65 if more than 6 years have passed since the initial vaccine (Goldberg and Chavin, 1997). Persons for whom hospice-type care is desired may decline to receive the pneumococcal vaccine, preferring instead comfort-oriented symptom management and acceptance of death as a potential outcome of an infection. This may only be challenged if serious concern exists regarding the potential for pneumonia epidemic within a facility. Other preventive measures such as aspirin therapy, estrogen replacement, and vitamin and mineral supplementation are covered in other chapters.

Polypharmacy is a common and potentially critical issue in the care of older persons. Many of these patients see several health care providers simultaneously (e.g., primary physician, cardiolo-

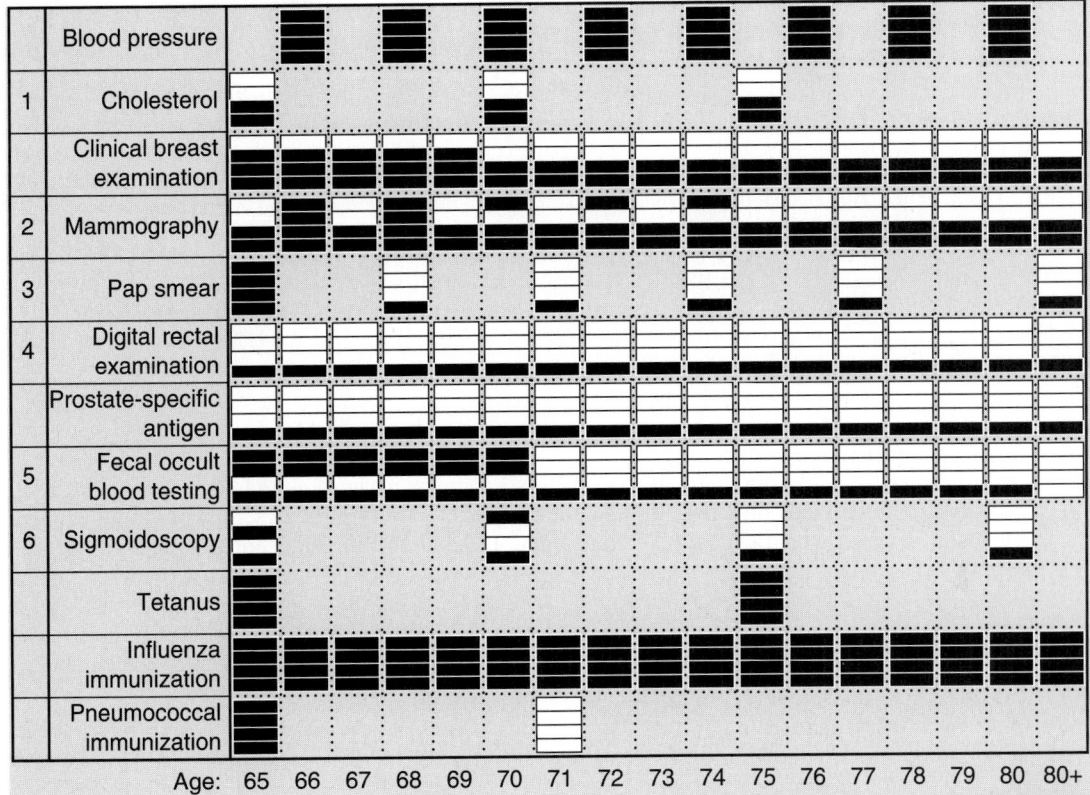

		Age: 65 66 67 68 69 70 71 72 73 74 75 76 77 78 79 80 80+
	Blood pressure	
1	Cholesterol	
	Clinical breast examination	
2	Mammography	
3	Pap smear	
4	Digital rectal examination	
	Prostate-specific antigen	
5	Fecal occult blood testing	
6	Sigmoidoscopy	
	Tetanus	
	Influenza immunization	
	Pneumococcal immunization	

Key:

American College of Physicians	ACP
US Preventive Services Task Force, 1996	USPSTF
American Academy of Family Practice	AAFP
Other Professional Organizations*	OTHER

This table shows selected, age-specific preventive care services recommended by professional health organizations, which should be offered to persons who do not have a family history, symptoms, signs, or other diseases that place them at increased risk for preventable conditions. All authorities stress the importance of assessing each person's unique risks in order to tailor preventive care.

ACP, USPSTF, and AAFP emphasize that all adults should be routinely counseled about tobacco use, nutrition, exercise, substance abuse, injury prevention, sensory loss, and dental care.

1. The USPSTF finds insufficient evidence for or against screening over 65 years of age but does recommend screening healthy individuals between 65 and 75 years of age *with* coronary heart disease risk factors such as smoking, hypertension, and diabetes. The ACP concurs but advises against screening after 75 years of age.
2. The AGS recommends discontinuation at 85 years of age; the ACP recommends 75 years of age. The USPSTF states that benefit may exist for women over 70 years of age since there is a high burden of suffering and lack of evidence for differences in the test characteristics for mammography in older women. AAFP and ACS recommend annual screening with no definitive age to discontinue screening.
3. ACP, AAFP, and USPSTF recommend no further Papanicolaou smears for women over 65 years of age who have had consistently normal smears in the previous decade.
4. The AAFP, ACP and USPSTF report that the digital rectal examination is not a good screening tool for either colorectal or prostate cancer. However, the ACS recommends this procedure; the USPSTF states that there is insufficient evidence to recommend for or against DRE.

Continued

TABLE 1-1	Screening and Preventive Care Recommendations for Asymptomatic, Low-Risk Older Adults—cont'd

5. USPSTF and ACS recommend annual screening after 50 years of age with no recommended discontinuation date. The AAFP recommendations are under review. The ACP recommends fecal occult blood testing for those who decline invasive screening.
6. ACP recommends sigmoidoscopy, colonoscopy, or air-contrast barium enema every 10 years for those between 50 and 70 years of age. The USPSTF recommends sigmoidoscopy but does not recommend an interval for screening. Guidelines are under review by the AAFP.

*Includes the Advisory Committee on Immunization Practices; National Cholesterol Education Program Panel on Detection, Evaluation, and Treatment of High Blood Cholesterol in Adults; Joint National Committee on Detection, Evaluation, and Treatment of High Blood Pressure; American Cancer Society; and American Geriatrics Society.

Modified from Hayward RSA et al: Preventive care guidelines: 1991, *Ann Intern Med* 114(9):761–762, 1991. Modified with permission. The American College of Physicians is not responsible for the accuracy of the adaptation.

gist, orthopedist, endocrinologist, and psychiatrist) and may never think to inform each of the treatments and medications prescribed by the others. This can lead to the prescribing of multiple medications, some of which may not be compatible. In addition, the confusion caused by trade and generic drug names may lead a person to take two forms of the same medication without even being aware of it. For this reason, the "brown bag" method for maintaining an updated medication list is recommended. The old adage in geriatric medicine of "Start low, go slow" is still sage; health care providers should introduce new medications at the lowest possible dose and titrate up cautiously.

HIV Screening

While human immunodeficiency virus (HIV) infection affects primarily young adults, it is occurring with increasing frequency in middle-age and older individuals. About 10% of all HIV infections—more than 55,000 cases—have been reported in persons 50 years of age and older, and 1% to 2% of cases occur in persons over 65 years of age (Woolery, 1997). Screening and counseling regarding HIV and other sexually transmitted diseases should therefore not be overlooked in the older population. Practitioners should assess risk factors for HIV infection in all patients by obtaining a careful sexual history and inquiring about drug use. Counseling and testing for HIV should be offered to all persons at increased risk for infection (U.S. Preventive Services Task Force, 1996):
- Those seeking treatment for sexually transmitted diseases
- Men who have had sex with men since 1975
- Past or present drug users
- Persons who have exchanged sex for money or drugs and their sex partners
- Women and men whose past or present sex partners were HIV-infected, bisexual, or injection drug users
- Persons with a history of transfusion between 1978 and 1985

NUTRITIONAL ASSESSMENT

Nutritional assessment requires special attention to the individual's cultural and ethnic background. The following nutritional assessment questions take into account cultural issues:
1. What is the meaning of food and eating to the patient?
2. What does the patient typically eat during:
   a. A typical day?
   b. Special events such as secular or religious holidays?
3. How does the patient define food (e.g., unless rice is served, many from India do not consider the ingestion of food to be a meal)?

4. What is the timing and sequence of meals?
5. With whom does the patient usually eat (alone, with a spouse)?
6. What does the patient believe comprises a "healthy" vs. "unhealthy" diet? Any hot/cold or yin/yang beliefs?
7. From what sources does the patient obtain food items (e.g., ethnic grocery store, home garden, restaurant)? Who usually does the grocery shopping?
8. How are foods prepared (type of preparation; cooking oils used; length of time foods are cooked; amount and type of seasoning added before, during, or after preparation)?
9. Has the patient chosen a particular nutritional practice such as vegetarianism or abstinence from alcoholic beverages?
10. Do religious beliefs and practices influence the patient's diet or eating habits (e.g., amount, type, preparations, or designation of acceptable food items or combinations)?

Because the consumption of alcohol can affect so many different aspects of health, accurately ascertaining a patient's alcohol intake is important. "Occasionally" or "socially" may mean different things to different people. Determining the actual intake (i.e., 3 beers or 5 ounces of liquor) in an average week or month, as well as the average amount in a single episode, is also important. A patient who drinks only "on weekends" may actually be drinking alcohol continuously from Friday night through Sunday evening. A patient who only drinks "once a month" may actually drink close to an entire case of beer or a liter of whiskey in one evening. This phenomenon, known as "binge-drinking," is not a benign "social" intake of alcohol, and unless patients and family members are specifically asked, this information may not be revealed. One of the quickest and most effective oral screening tools for problematic alcohol intake is the CAGE (Mayfield, McLeod, and Hall, 1974):

- Have you ever felt you could *C*ut down on your drinking?
- Have people *A*nnoyed you by criticizing your drinking?
- Have you ever felt bad or *G*uilty about your drinking?
- Have you ever had a drink first thing in the morning (an *E*ye-opener) to steady your nerves or get rid of a hangover?

If at least two of the questions are answered affirmatively, the probability of alcoholism is high. Further investigation is also needed if only one of the questions is answered affirmatively. See Chapter 28 for an older-age–specific alcohol questionnaire.

PSYCHOLOGIC ASSESSMENT

Cognitive Assessment

Unlike the physical examination in which one may learn a great deal from an informal social encounter, evaluation of cognitive status often requires formal focused assessment. Highly developed social graces or advanced education may easily cover the signs of an early cognitive impairment. A superficial and genial conversation will probably not reveal an underlying disorientation to time and place or a deficit in short-term memory. The most extensively used tool for assessment of mental status in geriatrics is the Folstein Mini-Mental State Examination (MMSE) (Figure 1-3). The score is reported as the patient's score/the highest possible score (e.g., 24/30). (A question may be omitted for some reason, thereby decreasing the highest possible score.) The MMSE takes approximately 10 to 15 minutes to administer, and each section of the tool assesses a different aspect of cognitive function: orientation, registration, attention and calculation, recall, and language. A score of 25/30 and above is generally considered to reflect only minimal cognitive impairment, whereas a patient with mid- to late-stage Alzheimer's disease may score 15/30 and below. Factors such as level of education, language barrier, and physical disabilities may affect performance.

Another tool for the assessment of cognitive function and "executive function" (e.g., planning and sequencing) is the "clock test" in which a patient is asked to draw a clock, put the numbers on it, and then draw hands indicating the time 11:15. The clock drawing is scored from 10 to 1 in the following manner:

10 to 6: Drawing of clock face with circle and numbers is generally intact

---

MMSE Sample Items

Orientation to Time
  "What is the date?"

Registration
  "Listen carefully, I am going to say three words. You say them back after I stop.
  Ready? Here they are . . .
  HOUSE (pause), CAR (pause), LAKE (pause). Now repeat those words back to
  me."
  [Repeat up to 5 times, but score only the first trial.]

Naming
  "What is this?" [Point to a pencil or pen.]

Reading
  "Please read this and do what it says." [Show examinee the words on the stimulus form.]

CLOSE YOUR EYES

Figure 1-3   MMSE Sample Items. (Reproduced with special permission of the Publisher, Psychological Assessment Resources, Inc., 16204 North Florida Avenue, Lutz, Florida 33549, from the Mini Mental State Examination, by Marshal Folstein and Susan Folstein, Copyright 1975, 1988, 2001 by Mini Mental LLC, Inc. Published 2001 by Psychological Assessment Resources, Inc. Further reproduction is prohibited without permission of PAR, Inc. The MMSE can be purchased from PAR, Inc. by calling [800] 331-8378 or [813] 968-3003.)

10: Hands are in correct position.
 9: Placement of the hands has slight errors.
 8: Placement of hour and minute hands has more noticeable errors.
 7: Placement of hands is significantly off course.
 6: Clock hands are inappropriately used (e.g., use of digital display/circling of numbers).
 5 to1: Drawing of clock face with circle and numbers is NOT intact.
 5: Numbers are crowded at one end of the clock or numbers are reversed.
 4: Number sequence is further distorted; the integrity of the clock face is now gone (e.g., numbers are missing or placed outside the boundaries of the clock face).
 3: The numbers and clock face are no longer obviously connected in the drawing; hands are not present.
 2: The drawing reveals some evidence of instructions being received but only a vague representation of a clock.
 1: Either no attempt or an uninterpretable effort is made.

Affective Assessment

Depression is probably the most common example of the nonspecific and atypical presentation of illness in older adults. Nonspecific physical complaints such as fatigue, weight loss, diffuse pain, memory or sleep disturbance, and constipation may represent a variety of treatable *physical* illnesses as well as depression. Frequently depression and physical illness coexist in older adult patients. Therefore treatable depressions are often overlooked in patients with physical illness and treatable physical illnesses are often not optimally managed in patients diagnosed as having depression (Goldberg and Chavin, 1997). The rate of suicide is higher among older adult males than any other segment of the population. A variety of biologic, physical, psychologic, and social factors predispose older adults to depression, which is discussed further in a later chapter. However, some useful screening tools can be used to assess the presence of depression in older adults. The most commonly used is the short form of the Geriatric Depression Scale (GDS) developed by Yesavage and Brink (Figure 1-4). A score between 5 and 9 suggests depression, whereas scores above 9 gen-

Geriatric Depression Scale

Choose the best answer for how you felt over the past week.

1. Are you basically satisfied with your life?		yes/no
2. Have you dropped many of your activities and interests?		yes/no
3. Do you feel that your life is empty?		yes/no
4. Do you often get bored?		yes/no
5. Are you in good spirits most of the time?		yes/no
6. Are you afraid that something bad is going to happen to you?		yes/no
7. Do you feel happy most of the time?		yes/no
8. Do you often feel helpless?		yes/no
9. Do you prefer to stay home rather than go out and do new things?		yes/no
10. Do you feel you have more problems with memory than most?		yes/no
11. Do you think it is wonderful to be alive now?		yes/no
12. Do you feel pretty worthless the way you are now?		yes/no
13. Do you feel full of energy?		yes/no
14. Do you feel that your situation is hopeless?		yes/no
15. Do you think that most people are better off than you are?		yes/no

This is the scoring for the scale. One point for each of these answers. Cut-off: normal (0-5), above 5 suggests depression.

1. no	6. yes	11. no
2. yes	7. no	12. yes
3. yes	8. yes	13. no
4. yes	9. yes	14. yes
5. no	10. yes	15. yes

Figure 1-4 Geriatric Depression Scale (short form). (From Sheikh JI, Yesavage JA: Geriatric depression scale: recent evidence and development of a shorter version, *Clin Gerontol* 5:165-172, 1986.)

erally indicate depression. Another helpful tool in screening for depression is the mnemonic SIGE-CAPS (Shua-Haim et al, 1997):

S: Changes in *Sleep* patterns or *Sexual* activities
I: Loss of *Interest* in activities
G: Feelings of *Guilt* or remorse
E: Lack of *Energy*
C: Difficulty *Concentrating*
A: Change in *Appetite* (increased or decreased)
P: *Psychomotor* agitation or retardation
S: Thoughts of *Suicide*

The Yale Task Force on Geriatric Assessment also found that the single question, "Do you often feel sad or depressed?" had approximately the same sensitivity and specificity as the GDS. Therefore even if time does not allow for administration of an entire screening tool, assessing for the presence of this important treatable problem is still possible.

SOCIAL ASSESSMENT

Social Supports

The availability and quality of social resources, such as family or other social support, housing, and income, are key ingredients of social function that can greatly influence overall functional capacity. This becomes especially important for patients who depend on the help of others to maintain an independent living situation. The relationship between social function and health becomes evident when one examines the use of health services by older adults. Studies have shown that, regardless of marital status, older adults who live with others are less likely to use health services than those who live alone (Yoshikawa, Cobbs, and Brummel-Smith, 1993). Assessment of the social supports of a family caregiver who may be providing full-time care to an older adult parent or relative is equally important. Family caregivers are a precious resource who bear many physical, emotional, and often financial burdens; it is in the best interest of the patient that they be supported in every way possible. The simple question, "Are you feeling overwhelmed?" can be critical. Caregiver stress can lead not only to illness and frustration for the caregiver but can progress to abuse and neglect of a vulnerable older adult.

An older adult patient's support system may not be a "traditional" one, yet it is no less important or valuable. An older adult living in his or her home may rely on neighbors, church members, or a building maintenance worker for assistance, support, and friendly conversation. The Older Adults Resources and Services (OARS) Social Resource Scale (Box 1-1) developed at Duke University extracts data about family structure, patterns of friendship and visiting, availability of a confidant, satisfaction with the degree of social interaction, and availability of a helper in the event of illness or disability. The results are rated using a six-point scale ranging from "excellent social resources" to "totally socially impaired." Different questions are used for patients who live in institutions (italicized). A shorter screening tool, the Family APGAR, assesses the family's *A*daptation, *P*artnership, *G*rowth, *A*ffection, and *R*esolve (Box 1-2). A score of less than 3 suggests a highly dysfunctional family, and a score of 4 to 6 suggests a moderately dysfunctional family. When assessing the social support system, the assessor should ask if the patient or family has received (or is receiving) services from any community resources such as social work, case management, or home health.

The asexual image of aging and the older adult has ancient origins reinforced by culture, ignorance, religion, families, and peers through the centuries. Sexuality, sensuality, and intimacy among older persons have been acknowledged more recently. The practitioner should not assume that simply because a person is older and may be single, divorced, or widowed, that he or she is not in a significant intimate relationship (nor, for that matter, should one assume that all older adult patients are heterosexual). The Duke Center for the Study of Aging and Human Development found that earlier interest, frequency, and enjoyment of sexual expression were reliable indicators of active sexuality in later years. Furthermore, any decline with age appeared related to death or illness of a partner rather than lack of interest. This also applies to patients living in their own homes. Sexual desires and needs do not evaporate on institutionalization. See Box 1-3 for a list of questions useful in assessing sexuality concerns in older adults.

ENVIRONMENTAL ASSESSMENT

An older adult patient's functional ability may be significantly helped or hindered by his or her living environment. An individual with limited mobility in a wheelchair may be far more dependent in a small, poorly lit, cluttered apartment than in the wide, well-lit hallways of a care facility. While the environment of a hospital, assisted living, or long-term care facility may be somewhat predictable, the practitioner should still consider these environments with the individual's particular needs and limitations in mind. A patient with chronic obstructive pulmonary disease who must

Box 1-1
OARS Social Resource Scale

Now I'd like to ask you some questions about your family and friends.

Are you single, married, widowed, divorced, or separated?

1 Single	3 Widowed	5 Separated
2 Married	4 Divorced	___ Not answered

If "2," ask following
Does your spouse live here also?
1 Yes
0 No
___ *Not answered*
Who lives with you?
(Check "yes" or "no" for each of the following.)

Yes	No	
_____	_____	No one
_____	_____	Husband or wife
_____	_____	Children
_____	_____	Grandchildren
_____	_____	Parents
_____	_____	Grandparents
_____	_____	Brothers and sisters
_____	_____	Other relatives (does not include inlaws covered in the above categories)
_____	_____	Friends
_____	_____	Nonrelated paid help (includes free room)
_____	_____	Others (specify)

In the past year about how often did you leave here to visit your family and/or friends for weekends or holidays or to go on shopping trips or outings?
1 Once a week or more
2 One to three times a month
3 Less than once a month or only on holidays
4 Never
___ *Not answered*
How many people do you know well enough to visit with in their homes?
3 Five or more
2 Three to four
1 One to two
0 None
___ Not answered

About how many times did you talk to someone—friends, relatives, or others—on the telephone in the past week (either you called them or they called you)? (If subject has no phone, question still applies.)
3 Once a day or more
2 Twice
1 Once
0 Not at all
___ Not answered
How many times during the past week did you spend some time with someone who does not live with you, that is, you went to see them, or they came to visit you, or you went out to do things together?
How many times in the past week did you visit with someone, either with people who live here or people who visited you here?
2 Two to six
1 Once
0 Not at all
___ *Not answered*
Do you have someone you can trust and confide in?
1 Yes
0 No
___ Not answered
Do you find yourself feeling lonely quite often, sometimes, or almost never?
0 Quite often
1 Sometimes
2 Almost never
___ Not answered
Do you see your relatives and friends as often as you want to or not?
1 As often as wants to
0 Not as often as wants to
___ Not answered
Is there someone *(outside this place)* who would give you any help at all if you were sick or disabled, for example, your husband/wife, a member of your family, or a friend?
1 Yes
0 No one willing and able to help
___ Not answered

Modified from Duke University Center for the Study of Aging and Human Developments. *OARS multidimensional functional assessment: questionnaire* Durham, NC, 1988, Duke University.

Continued

Box 1-1

OARS Social Resource Scale—cont'd

If "yes," ask A and B

A. Is there someone *(outside this place)* who would take care of you as long as needed, or only for a short time, or only someone who would help you now and then (taking you to the doctor or fixing lunch occasionally)?

  3 Someone who would take care of subject indefinitely (as long as needed)

  2 Someone who would take care of subject for a short time (a few weeks to 6 months)

  1 Someone who would help subject now and then (e.g., taking him or her to the doctor or fixing lunch)

  ___ Not answered

B. Who is this person?

  Name _____

  Relationship _____

Rating scale

Rate the current social resources of the person being evaluated along the six-point scale presented below. Circle the *one* number that best describes the person's present circumstances.

1. *Excellent social resources:* Social relationships are very satisfying and extensive; at least one person would take care of him or her indefinitely.

2. *Good social resources:* Social relationships are fairly satisfying and adequate and at least one person would take care of him or her indefinitely, *or*

  Social relationships are very satisfying and extensive, and only short-term help is available.

3. *Mildly socially impaired:* Social relationships are unsatisfactory, of poor quality, and few, but at least one person would take care of him or her indefinitely, *or*

  Social relationships are fairly satisfactory and adequate, and only short-term help is available.

4. *Moderately socially impaired:* Social relationships are unsatisfactory, of poor quality, and few, and only short-term care is available, *or*

  Social relationships are at least adequate or satisfactory, but help would only be available now and then.

5. *Severely socially impaired:* Social relationships are unsatisfactory, of poor quality, and few, and help would be available only now and then, *or*

  Social relationships are at least satisfactory or adequate, but help is not available even now and then.

6. *Totally socially impaired:* Social relationships are unsatisfactory, of poor quality, and few, and help is not available even now and then.

Box 1-2

Family APGAR

1. I am satisfied that I can turn to my family (friends) for help when something is troubling me. *(adaptation)*

2. I am satisfied with the way my family (friends) talks over things with me and shares problems with me. *(partnership)*

3. I am satisfied that my family (friends) accepts and supports my wishes to take on new activities or directions. *(growth)*

4. I am satisfied with the way my family *(friends)* expresses affection and responds to my emotions, such as anger, sorrow, or love. *(affection)*

5. I am satisfied with the way my family (friends) and I share time together. *(resolve)*

  Scoring:

  Statements are answered *always* (2 points), *some of the time* (1 point), *hardly ever* (0 points).

Reprinted with permission from Appleton & Lange. From Smilkstein G, Ashworth C, Montano D: Validity and reliability of the Family APGAR as a test of family function, *J Fam Pract* 15:303-311, 1982.

Box 1-3
Suggested Questions for Assessing Sexual Concerns

Sexual Satisfaction

- Have you experienced any changes in your sexual relationships lately?
- To what do you attribute this change?
- What types of sexual activities have you usually enjoyed the most, including things such as hugging, kissing, sleeping together, intercourse, masturbation, and so on?
- Do you or your partner take any prescription medications? What are they? How often do you take them? Have you experienced any changes in your level of energy since you started them? What about overall feelings of well-being? Any changes in sexual desire or activity?

For Men

- Have you noticed any changes in the intensity of your ejaculations, orgasms, or ability to attain or maintain an erection?
- Have you ever had orgasms without ejaculations?
- Has your level of enjoyment from sexual relations altered as a result of these changes?
- Have you ever had any problems with urethral discharge or urination?

For Women

- Have you ever experienced any vaginal soreness or irritation after sexual intercourse? How long does it last? Any problems with urgency or with burning on urination after intercourse? Have you experienced abdominal contractions or back pain after intercourse?
- Have you had any problems with vaginal discharge or itching?
- Have any of these problems interfered with your sexual pleasure?
- Have you or your partner experienced any changes in your health status recently? How have these changes affected your sexual relationship?

Alterations in Self-perception

- How has growing older changed your lifestyle or things you enjoy doing?
- How has the change in your health or your partner's health altered your lifestyle or goals?
- How do you rate your general health?
- On a scale of 1 to 10, how would you describe your satisfaction with your life?
- On a scale of 1 to 10, how would you describe your satisfaction with your sexual relationships?

Relationships with Others

- Have you ever discussed sexual topics with your spouse, friends, family, or health care professional?
- With whom do you talk when you have problems of any kind or just want someone to talk to?

Environment

- With whom do you live?
- Do you have a chance for privacy? To be alone? To talk with others privately if you want to?

From Burke M, Sherman S: Sexuality. In Burke M, Walsh M: *Gerontologic nursing,* St Louis, 1997, Mosby.

travel down a long hallway to reach the elevator to the dining room may find the trip too difficult and miss meals and social interaction.

The assessment of a frail older adult patient's environment becomes especially important when he or she is living in his or her own home. Safety factors to be assessed are identified in Box 1-4. The Home Safety Checklist developed by the National Safety Council is a thorough instrument used to identify fall hazards in the home (see Chapter 19). Although the tool is long and may be too time

---

Box 1-4

Environmental Assessment

1. Poorly lighted stairwells, halls, or bathrooms
2. Stairs with weak or absent banisters
3. Absence of grab bars near bathtub
4. Glare in hallways
5. Absence of a working smoke alarm
6. Wet floors and/or waxed floors
7. Poorly placed extension cords
8. Throw rugs
9. Clutter
10. Inappropriate footwear and long clothing
11. High beds
12. Improper use of walking aids
13. Restraints and protective devices

From Burke MM, Walsh MB: *Gerontologic nursing: wholistic care of the older adult,* ed 2, St Louis, 1997, Mosby.

---

consuming to administer during a visit, it may be included in the previsit questionnaire for the patient and family to complete before the visit. It may then be reviewed by the practitioner at the time of the appointment. After identification, hazards should be eliminated or reduced. One point is allowed for every NO answer. A score of 1 to 7 is excellent, 8 to 14 is good, and 15 or higher is hazardous. Although some of this information may be obtained from the patient, family, or friends, the value of a home visit cannot be overstated. If the provider is not able to do this himself or herself, a visit by a home care agency may be arranged.

ECONOMIC ASSESSMENT

In 1998, 11% of people 65 years of age and over lived in poverty (Federal Interagency Forum on Aging-Related Statistics, 2002). The primary source of income for older adults is social security, although several other sources are available: property, pensions, personal savings, investments, earnings, and a variety of financial assets (Figure 1-5). However, most persons do not benefit from all or even many of these resources.

Many providers are not comfortable discussing economic issues with patients and will instead rely on the expertise of a social worker to explore these matters. However, the provider must be aware of a patient's or family's ability to pay for treatments prescribed. Some basic information may help the provider make choices and recommendations for patients that are within their means. A simple question such as, "Do you usually have money available to cover the 'little extras' that come up?" will open the door to discussing available finances and provide at least basic information that will be important for the provider to consider. The type of insurance a patient has is basic and often determined when the appointment is scheduled. Providers must have at least a basic working knowledge of services and equipment covered by various insurance plans. At this time, Medicare offers no prescription medication benefit. However, a secondary or Medigap insurance program may cover prescription medications with only a minimal copayment by the patient. Many persons over 65 years of age choose to participate in a health maintenance organization (HMO) or health plan. These plans may dictate which medications, consultants, and even laboratory and radiology service the patient may use. A provider who is unaware of these requirements will do his or her patients a great disservice by inadvertently sending them to an unauthorized facility for laboratory work or x-ray examinations for which they will be forced to pay out of pocket. Services or equipment for which the patient has no cov-

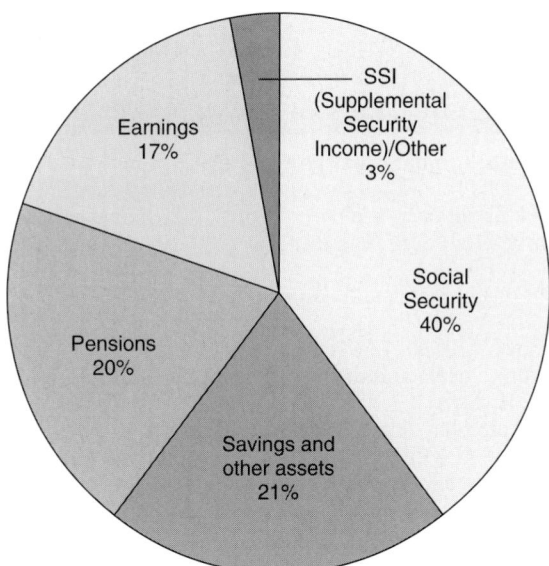

Figure 1-5 Sources of income for people 85 years of age and older. (From U.S. Department of Health and Human Services, Social Security Administration, and Office of Research and Statistics: *Income of the aged chartbook, 1992,* SSA Pub. No. 13-11727, Washington, DC, 1994, U.S. Government Printing Office.)

erage should be discussed in terms of its costs and benefits. For example, hearing aids, which are not covered by any insurance programs, including Medicare, may not be a priority for an individual with hearing loss and a limited income. However, some persons may consider them vital and be willing to adjust their budget for the anticipated benefits derived from obtaining these assistive devices. The practitioner should become familiar with free or low-cost alternatives to care recommendations that may be available through public or private agencies.

FUNCTIONAL ASSESSMENT
Activities of Daily Living

The practitioner may not know that a patient requires assistance with specific tasks without formal questioning. Family members often say that a parent never needed help with dressing until the death of the spouse, when in reality the parent did require assistance but the functional deficit (or cognitive impairment) was not realized until the caregiver was no longer available. Functional abilities involving self-care are discussed in terms of activities of daily living (ADLs), which are typically divided into the following categories (ABCDETT):

Ambulation: Mobility with or without an assistive device
Bathing: Sponge baths, traditional baths, or showers
Continence: Sphincter control (bowel and bladder; not the ability to get to a commode)
Dressing: Selecting and getting clothes as well as the act of dressing
Eating: The ability to feed oneself (not the ability to prepare meals)
Toileting: Getting to the commode, undressing and redressing, and cleaning oneself
Transferring: Getting in and out of a bed or chair

The Katz index of ADLs is a tool to assess a patient's ability to perform these functions (Box 1-5). Each function is rated on a three-point scale, with a maximum score of 18. The task classification is based on what the patient is *actually* doing, not what he or she is *capable* of doing. Another functional assessment tool that focuses on ADL performance is the Barthel Index (Table 1-2). A patient scoring 100 on this tool is continent; feeds, dresses, and bathes

Box 1-5

Katz Index of Activities of Daily Living*

1. **Bathing (either sponge bath, tub bath, or shower)**
   a. Receives no assistance (gets in and out of tub by self if tub is usual means of bathing)
   b. Receives assistance in bathing only one part of body such as the back or a leg
   c. Receives assistance in bathing more than one part of body or is not bathed
2. **Continence**
   a. Controls urination and bowel movement completely by self
   b. Has occasional "accidents"
   c. Needs supervision to keep urine or bowel control, uses catheter, or is incontinent
3. **Dressing (gets clothes from closets and drawers, including underclothes, outer garments; uses fasteners, including braces, if worn)**
   a. Gets clothes and gets completely dressed without assistance
   b. Gets clothes and gets dressed without assistance except in tying shoes
   c. Receives assistance in getting clothes or getting dressed or stays partly or completely undressed
4. **Eating**
   a. Feeds self without assistance
   b. Feeds self except for assistance in cutting meat or buttering bread
   c. Receives assistance in feeding or is fed partly or completely by using tubes or intravenous fluids
5. **Toileting (going to the "toilet room" for bowel and urine elimination; cleaning self after elimination and arranging clothes)**
   a. Goes to "toilet room," cleans self, and arranges clothes without assistance (may use object for support such as cane, walker, or wheelchair and may manage night bedpan or commode and emptying same in morning)
   b. Receives assistance in going to "toilet room," cleaning self, or arranging clothes after elimination or receives assistance in using night bedpan or commode
   c. Does not go to room termed "toilet" for the elimination process
6. **Transferring**
   a. Moves in and out of bed or chair without assistance (may use object for support such as cane or walker)
   b. Moves in and out of bed or chair with assistance
   c. Does not get out of bed

---

*Response a., 3 points; b., 2 points; c., 1 point; maximum score, 18 points.

himself or herself; gets up out of bed and chairs; walks at least a block; and can ascend and descend stairs.

The instrumental activities of daily living (IADLs) are higher-level abilities that allow a person to function independently in the home and community:

- Using the telephone
- Shopping
- Preparing meals
- Doing laundry
- Housekeeping
- Taking medications
- Managing money
- Traveling

Some clinicians also include reading, writing, climbing stairs, and paid employment. The five-item questionnaire for IADLs allows the practitioner to assess the patient's skills in these areas (Box 1-6).

TABLE 1-2	Barthel Index		

Action	With Help	Independently
1. Feeding (if food needs to be cut up = help)	5	10
2. Moving from wheelchair to bed and return (includes sitting up in bed)	5-10	15
3. Personal toilet (washing face, combing hair, shaving, cleaning teeth)	0	5
4. Getting on and off toilet (handling clothes, wiping, flushing)	5	10
5. Bathing self	0	5
6. Walking on level surface (or if unable to walk, propelling wheelchair)	0*	5*
7. Ascending and descending stairs	5	10
8. Dressing (includes tying shoes, fastening fasteners)	5	10
9. Controlling bowels	5	10
10. Controlling bladder	5	10

A patient scoring 100 BDI is continent, feeds himself, dresses himself, gets up out of bed and chairs, bathes himself, walks at least a block, and can ascend and descend stairs. This does not mean that he is able to live alone—he may not be able to cook, keep house, and meet the public—but he is able to get along without attendant care.

Definition and Discussion of Scoring

1. Feeding
   10 = Independent. The patient can feed himself a meal from a tray or table when someone puts the food within his reach. He must put on an assistive device if this is needed, cut up the food, use salt and pepper, spread butter, etc. He must accomplish this in a reasonable time.
   5 = Some help is necessary (e.g., with cutting up food, as listed previously).

2. Moving from wheelchair to bed and return
   15 = Independent in all phases of this activity. Patient can safely approach the bed in his wheelchair, lock brakes, lift footrests, move safely to bed, lie down, come to a sitting position on the side of the bed, and change the position of the wheelchair, if necessary, to transfer back into it safely and return to the wheelchair.
   10 = Either some minimal help is needed in some step of this activity or the patient needs to be reminded or supervised for safety of one or more parts of this activity.
   5 = Patient can come to a sitting position without the help of a second person but needs to be lifted out of bed, or he transfers with a great deal of help.

3. Doing personal toilet
   5 = Patient can wash hands and face, comb hair, clean teeth, and shave. He may use any kind of razor, but he must put in blade or plug in razor without help, as well as get it from the drawer or cabinet. Female patients must put on own makeup, if used, but need not braid or style hair.

4. Getting on and off toilet
   10 = Patient is able to get on and off toilet, fasten and unfasten clothes, prevent soiling of clothes, and use toilet paper without help. He may use a wall bar or other stable object for support if needed. If it is necessary to use a bed pan instead of toilet, he must be able to place it on a chair, empty it, and clean it.
   5 = Patient needs help because of imbalance or in handling clothes or in using toilet paper.

From Mahoney FI, Barthel DW: Functional evaluation: the Barthel Index, *Maryland State Med J* 14:62, 1965. Reprinted with permission.
*Score only if unable to walk.

Continued

TABLE 1-2	**Barthel Index—cont'd**

5. Bathing self
> 5 = Patient may use a bathtub, shower, or take a complete sponge bath. He must be able to do all the steps involved in whichever method is employed without another person being present.

6. Walking on a level surface
> 15 = Patient can walk at least 50 yards without help or supervision. He may wear braces or prostheses and use crutches, canes, or a walkerette, but not a rolling walker. He must be able to lock and unlock braces if used, assume the standing position and sit down, get the necessary mechanical aids into position for use, and dispose of them when he sits. (Putting on and taking off braces is scored under dressing.)

6a. Propelling a wheelchair
> 5 = Patient cannot ambulate but can propel a wheelchair independently. He must be able to go around corners, turn around, maneuver the chair to a table, toilet, etc. He must be able to push a chair at least 50 yards. Do not score this item if the patient gets a score for walking.

7. Ascending and descending stairs
> 10 = Patient is able to go up and down a flight of stairs safely without help or supervision. He may and should use handrails, canes, or crutches when needed. He must be able to carry canes or crutches as he ascends or descends stairs.
> 5 = Patient needs help with or supervision of any one of the above items.

8. Dressing and undressing
> 10 = Patient is able to put on and remove and fasten all clothing and tie shoelaces (unless it is necessary to use adaptations for this). This activity includes putting on and removing and fastening corset or braces when these are prescribed. Such special clothing as suspenders, loafer shoes, or dresses that open down the front may be used when necessary.
> 5 = Patient needs help in putting on and removing or fastening any clothing. He must do at least half the work himself. He must accomplish this in a reasonable time. Women need not be scored on use of a brassiere or girdle unless these are prescribed garments.

9. Continence of bowels
> 10 = Patient is able to control his bowels and have no accidents. He can use a suppository or take an enema when necessary (as for spinal cord injury patients who have had bowel training).
> 5 = Patient needs help in using a suppository or taking an enema or has occasional accidents.

10. Controlling bladder
> 10 = Patient is able to control his bladder day and night. Spinal cord injury patients who wear an external device and leg bag must put them on independently, clean and empty bag, and stay dry day and night.
> 5 = Patient has occasional accidents or cannot wait for the bed pan or get to the toilet in time or needs help with an external device.

The total score is not as significant or meaningful as the breakdown into individual items, since these indicate where the deficiencies are.

Any applicant to a chronic hospital who scores 100 BDI should be evaluated carefully before admission to see whether such hospitalization is indicated. Discharged patients with 100 BDI should not require further physical therapy but may benefit from a home visit to see whether any environmental adjustments are indicated.

Five-Item Instrumental Activities of Daily Living Screening

1. **Can you get to places out of walking distance?**
   a. Without help (can travel alone on bus, taxi, or drive own car)
   b. With some help (need someone to help or go with you when traveling)
   c. Unable to travel unless emergency arrangements are made for a specialized vehicle such as an ambulance
2. **Can you go shopping for groceries or clothes (assuming that you have transportation)?**
   a. Without help (can take care of all your shopping needs yourself)
   b. With some help (need someone to go with you on all shopping trips)
   c. Completely unable to do any shopping
3. **Can you prepare your own meals?**
   a. Without help (can plan and cook meals yourself)
   b. With some help (can prepare some things but unable to cook full meals yourself)
   c. Unable to do any meal preparation
4. **Can you do your housework?**
   a. Without help (can scrub floors, etc.)
   b. With some help (can do light housework but need help with heavy work)
   c. Unable to do any housework
5. **Can you handle your own money?**
   a. Without help (can write checks, pay bills, etc.)
   b. With some help (can manage day-to-day buying but need help with managing your checkbook and paying your bills)
   c. Completely unable to handle money

Loss of ability in any of these areas may signify the beginning of a more severe functional decline. When a patient states that he or she does not perform a particular task, the practitioner should determine whether this reflects a functional inability or a "social norm" (e.g., a husband may have never done the grocery shopping or prepared meals). These deficits may exist but do not become apparent until the patient is required to perform these tasks (e.g., after the death of the spouse).

Gait and Mobility

The formal assessment of gait and mobility does not take long and is important to assess the patient's ability to ambulate safely. The performance-oriented mobility assessment examines both the balance and gait components and is particularly useful in assessing the patient's risk of falling (Table 1-3). Another tool is the Tinetti Balance and Gait Evaluation instrument (Figure 1-6). The Rancho functional assessment screen (Table 1-4) focuses on the patient's upper extremity strength, range of motion, and ambulatory status. Each test correlates with a particular function and provides the practitioner with insight into the patient's ability to carry out routine daily activities and identifies areas in which therapies may be beneficial to enhance function.

Safety

In gathering information regarding safety, the practitioner must explore factors other than the patient's gait and balance. Many safety risks, especially in the home, can be corrected, which will enhance the patient's ability to safely remain in a more independent setting while avoiding injury. In an epidemiologic model, safety risks are considered as an interrelationship between three factors: the agent (e.g., electricity, chemicals, gravity), the person (e.g., health and cognitive status, knowledge, biologic defense mechanisms), and the environment (e.g., space, lighting, sanitation, furnishings, pets, other people). Each of these factors must be considered in the evaluation of safety risk. Cognitive impairment and memory deficit, poor vision, and impaired sensation may place a person at risk for burns in the kitchen or bath. Impaired hand strength and coordination may place a person at risk of injury when cutting food with a sharp knife. Falls are a particularly common risk that older adults face.

Summary

The comprehensive geriatric assessment is a multifaceted process that plays a critical role in the quality of life of older adults. The information obtained can be used in many ways to maintain or improve the person's health and function. Health promotion, disease prevention, and diagnosis are only the beginning. Referral to appropriate community resources such as case management; physical, occupational, and speech therapies; and assistance with facility placement, if necessary, can dramatically improve the quality of life of both the patient and the family who may be coping with a difficult situation. A practitioner who is knowledgeable of available resources and support agencies will always be able to offer assistance and guidance to patients and families, even if limited medical and nursing interventions are offered. Not all providers who care for older adult patients have

---

TABLE 1-3	Performance-oriented Mobility Assessment

Position Change or Balance Maneuver	Observations
Balance Component	
Getting up from chair*	Potential risk of fall if patient does not get up with single movement; pushes up with arms or moves forward in chair first; unsteady on first standing
Sitting down in chair	Plops in chair; does not land in center
Withstanding nudge on sternum	Moves feet; grabs object for support
Romberg test (eyes closed)	Same as above; tests patient's reliance on visual input for balance
Neck turning	Moves feet; grabs object for support; complains of vertigo, dizziness, or unsteadiness
Reaching up	Unable to reach up to full shoulder flexion standing on tiptoes; unsteady; grabs object for support
Bending over	Unable to bend over to pick up small object (e.g., pen) from floor; grabs object to pull up on; requires multiple attempts to rise
Gait Component	
Initiation	Hesitates; stumbles; grabs object for support
Step height	Does not clear floor consistently (scrapes or shuffles); raises foot too high (more than 2 inches)
Step continuity	After first few steps, does not consistently begin raising one foot as other foot touches floor
Step symmetry	Step length not equal; pathologic side usually has longer step length (problem may be in hip, knee, ankle, or surrounding muscles)
Path deviation	Does not walk in straight line; weaves side to side
Turning	Stops before initiating turn; staggers; sways; grabs object for support

*Use hard, armless chair.

Tinetti Balance and Gait Evaluation
BALANCE

Instructions: Subject is seated in hard armless chair.
The following maneuvers are tested.

1. **Sitting balance**

Leans or slides in chair	= 0
Steady, safe	= 1 ____

2. **Arises**

Unable without help	= 0
Able but uses arms to help	= 1
Able without use of arms	= 2 ____

3. **Attempts to arise**

Unable without help	= 0
Able but requires more than 1 attempt	= 1
Able to arise with 1 attempt	= 2 ____

4. **Immediate standing balance** (first 5 sec)

Unsteady (staggers, moves feet, marked trunk sway)	= 0
Steady but uses walker or cane or grabs other objects for support	= 1
Steady without walker, cane, or other support	= 2 ____

5. **Standing balance**

Unsteady	= 0
Steady but wide stance (medial heels more than 4 in. apart) or uses cane, walker, or other support	= 1
Narrow stance without support	= 2 ____

6. **Nudged** (subject at maximum position with feet as close together as possible, examiner pushes lightly on subject's sternum with palm of hand 3 times)

Begins to fall	= 0
Staggers, grabs, but catches self	= 1
Steady	= 2 ____

7. **Eyes closed** (at maximum position No. 6)

Unsteady	= 0
Steady	= 1 ____

8. **Turning 360 degrees**

Discontinuous steps	= 0
Continuous	= 1 ____
Unsteady (grabs, staggers)	= 0
Steady	= 1 ____

9. **Sitting down**

Unsafe (misjudged distance, falls into chair)	= 0
Uses arms or not a smooth motion	= 1
Safe, smooth motion	= 2 ____

Balance score: ____ /16

Figure 1-6 Tinetti Balance and Gait Evaluation. (From Tinetti M: Performance-oriented assessment of mobility problems in elderly patients, *J Am Geriatr Soc* 34:119-126, 1986.)

Tinetti Balance and Gait Evaluation
GAIT

Instructions: Subject stands with examiner; walks down hallway or across room, first at his "usual" pace, then back at "rapid, but safe" pace (using usual walking aid such as cane, walker).

10. **Initiation of gait** (immediately after told to "go")
Any hesitancy or multiple attempts to start   = 0
No hesitancy   = 1   ____

11. **Step length and height**
a. Right swing foot
Does not pass left stance foot with step   = 0
Passes left stance foot   = 1
Right foot does *not* clear floor completely with step   = 0
Right foot completely clears floor   = 1   ____
b. Left swing foot
Does not pass right stance foot with step   = 0
Passes right stance foot   = 1
Left foot does *not* clear floor completely with step   = 0
Left foot completely clears floor   = 1   ____

12. **Step symmetry**
Right and left step length not equal (estimate)   = 0
Right and left step appear equal   = 1   ____

13. **Step continuity**
Stopping or discontinuity between steps   = 0
Steps appear continuous   = 1   ____

14. **Path** (estimated in relation to floor tiles, 12-in. diameter; observe excursion of 1 foot over about 10 ft of the course)
Marked deviation   = 0
Mild/moderate deviation *or* uses walking aid   = 1
Straight without walking aid   = 2   ____

15. **Trunk**
Marked sway or uses walking aid   = 0
No sway but flexion of knees or back or spreads arms
out while walking   = 1
No sway, no flexion, no use of arms, and no use of
walking aid   = 2   ____

16. **Walking stance**
Heels apart   = 0
Heels almost touching while walking   = 1   ____

Gait score: ____ /12
Total score: ____ /28

Figure 1-6   cont'd

| TABLE 1-4 | **Rancho Functional Assessment Screen** | | | |

Test	Functions Tested	Normal	Limited	Unable
Put both hands together behind head	Combing hair; washing back, etc.			
Put both hands together in back of waist	Managing clothing; washing lower back			
Sitting, touch great toe with opposite hand	Lower extremity dressing; hygiene			
Squeeze examiner's two fingers with each hand	Grasp strength (approximately 20 lb of pressure needed for functional activities)			
Hold paper between thumb and lateral side of index finger while examiner tries to pull it out	Pinch strength (approximately 3 lb of pressure needed for functional activities)			
Stand from chair without using hand	Transfer ability; fall risk			
Walk 15-30 m	Velocity; household ambulatory status			

been trained in the skills and expertise of geriatric clinicians. The medical and nursing community as a whole benefits when those with these skills share them with others, providing assistance and insights that may make a difference in that provider's ability to best manage the older adult patient's complicated needs.

Resources

AGENET Eldercare Network
17 Applegate Court, Suite 200
Madison, WI 53713
(608) 256-3944
www.agenet.com

U.S. Department of Health and Human Services Healthfinder
www.healthfinder.org

References

Federal Interagency Forum on Aging-Related Statistics. Available at www.agingstats.gov. Accessed March, 2003.

Goldberg T, Chavin S: Preventive medicine and screening in older adults, *J Am Geriatr Soc* 45:345-354, 1997.

Gudmundsson A, Carnes M: Geriatric assessment: making it work in primary care practice, *Geriatrics* 51(3): 53-57, 1996.

Hayward RSA, Steinberg EP, Ford DE: Preventive care guidelines, *Ann Intern Med* 111(9):761-762, 1991.

Markides K, Rudkin L: Racial and ethnic diversity. In Birren J, editor: *Encyclopedia of gerontology: age, aging, and the aged,* Los Angeles, 1996, Academic Press.

Mayfield D, McLeod G, Hall P: The CAGE questionnaire: validation of a new alcoholism screening instrument, *Am J Psychiatry* 131:1121-1123, 1974.

Mezey M, Mitty E, Ramsey G: Assessment of decision-making capacity: nursing's role, *J Gerontol Nurs* 23(3):28-35, 1997.

Rubenstein L: Geriatric assessment: physical. In Birren J, editor: *Encyclopedia of gerontology: age, aging, and the aged,* Los Angeles, 1996, Academic Press.

Schiavenato M: The Hispanic elderly: implications for nursing care, *J Gerontol Nurs* 23(6):10-15, 1997.

Shua-Haim J et al: Depression in the elderly, *Hosp Med* 33(7):44-58, 1997.

U.S. Census Bureau: Population Projections of the United States by Age, Sex, Race, Hispanic Origin, and Nativity: 1999-2100, January 2000. Available at www.census.gov/population. Accessed March, 2003.

U.S. Department of Health and Human Services, Office of Public Health and Science, Office of Disease Prevention and Health Promotion: *U.S. Preventive Services Task force guide to clinical preventive services,* ed 2, Washington, DC, 1996, USDHHS.

Williams T: Comprehensive functional assessment: an overview, *J Am Geriatr Soc* 31:637-641, 1983.

Woolery WA: Occult HIV infection: diagnosis and treatment of older patients, *Geriatrics* 52(11):51-61, 1997.

Yoshikawa T, Cobbs E, Brummel-Smith K: *Ambulatory geriatric care,* St Louis, 1993, Mosby.

2

Exercise

The extent to which exercise can delay the physical decline associated with aging is a complicated subject that has received new attention in the last decade. In the year 2030, there will be more than 70 million Americans over 65 years of age, with the over-85 group the fastest growing segment of the population.

The MacArthur Studies of Successful Aging conclude that regular physical activity provides older adults a consistently protective effect with respect to adverse changes in physical functioning (Seeman and Chin, 2002). Recent studies have shown that older adults can adapt and respond to both endurance and strength training. Outcomes of regular moderate to intense exercise include improved cardiovascular health, lower fasting glucose levels, decreased age-related muscle loss, improved bone health, improved postural stability, increased flexibility and range of motion (ROM), and increased life expectancy (Mazzeo and Tanaka, 2001).

Regrettably, what is also known is that two thirds of all adults 65 years of age and older are either irregularly active or completely sedentary. By 75 years of age, one in three men and one in two women engage in no regular activity (U.S. Department of Health and Human Services, 2000). Certain characteristics are associated with low rates of physical activity. Women are generally less physically active than men; persons with low incomes and less education are less active than those with higher incomes and education (Boyette et al, 2002). With inactivity comes an increased risk of chronic disease, including coronary heart disease, hypertension, diabetes, obesity, back problems, constipation, osteoporosis, and depression. Findings in gerontology and sports science suggest that regular physical activity and exercise can help maintain and enhance the functioning, health, and psychologic well-being of older adults.

Even national public health directives support the routine prescription of physical activity for the older adult (Centers for Disease Control and Prevention, 1998). Experts recognize that physical activity can prevent or delay many of the physical and psychologic problems that commonly occur with aging (Fillit et al, 2002; Mather et al, 2002). The American Heart Association (AHA) Guidelines for Primary Prevention of Cardiovascular Disease and Stroke: 2002 Update lists physical activity as one of the nine risk interventions (Pearson et al, 2002) (Table 2-1). In addition, regular physical exercise may have broader significance for the control of hypertension, lower occurrence of depressive symptoms, and improved balance in diabetic patients with peripheral neuropathy (Brandao Rondon et al, 2002; Mather et al, 2002; Richardson, Sandman, and Vela, 2001).

TABLE 2-1	Risk Intervention: Physical Activity

Goal	Recommendation
At least 30 min of moderate-intensity physical activity on most (and preferably all) days of the week	If cardiovascular, respiratory, metabolic, orthopedic or neurologic disorders are suspected or if patient is middle-age or older and is sedentary, consult physician before initiating vigorous exercise program. Moderate-intensity activities (40% to 60% of maximum capacity) are equivalent to a brisk walk (15-20 min per mile). Additional benefits are gained from vigorous-intensity activity (>60% maximum capacity) for 20-40 min 3 to 5 days a week. Recommend resistance training with 8 to 10 different exercises 1-2 sets per exercise and 10-15 repetitions at moderate intensity (2 days or more a week). Flexibility training and an increase in daily lifestyle activities should complement this regimen.

Pearson TA et al: AHA guidelines for primary prevention of cardiovascular disease and stroke: 2002 update: consensus panel guide to comprehensive risk reduction for adult patients without coronary or other atherosclerotic vascular diseases, *Circulation* 106:388-391, 2002.

Experts suggest that loss of muscle mass and strength has less to do with aging than with chronic inactivity. Researchers have examined flexibility, strength, and cardiovascular fitness in older adults and found that, regardless of age, the musculoskeletal and cardiovascular systems respond to both resistance and aerobic training (Beere et al, 1999). Studies have shown that strength training can counteract muscle weakness in very elderly people and resistance exercises especially appeared to increase muscle strength significantly (Vincent et al, 2002). Moreover, many older participants involved in exercise studies significantly reduce their level of disability, improve their functional ambulatory level, and increase their general sense of well-being (Pennix et al, 2002).

The overwhelming evidence reported in most studies supports the premise that regular appropriate exercise in older adults is a potential means of reducing the burden of impairments and ultimately improving function and quality of life; however, not all older adults are candidates for regular physical activity. For example, persons with diagnosed contraindications to acute exercise, such as severe seizure disorders, severe cardiovascular disease, and severe obstructive pulmonary diseases, require close attention and physician-directed involvement. Patients with extreme motor, neurologic (e.g., spasticity, plegia), or musculoskeletal (e.g., joint inflammation, chronic subluxation) limitations also require a specialized approach to exercise and careful intervention by the practitioner. In general, regular physical activity and exercise are appropriate for healthy older adults with evidence of diminished flexibility, strength, and functional capacity because of chronic inactivity. This chapter focuses on exercise for the functionally independent, community-dwelling older well adult.

Perspectives on Exercise in Older Adults

A typical exercise program includes activities aimed at increasing musculoskeletal flexibility and strength and at improving cardiovascular fitness. All these components are important, and different types of activity are required for each.

Exercise objectives can be either therapeutic or preventive. Accomplishing these objectives can be related to specific types of exercise. Table 2-2 describes types of exercise and the associated physiologic effects.

TABLE 2-2	Physiologic Effects of Various Types of Exercise	

Type of Exercise	Description	Physiologic Effect(s)
Stretching	Stretching exercise routine moving joint beyond initial point of resistance	Reduction of contractures in periarticular tissues
Strengthening		
Isometric	Contraction of muscle *without* moving the joint (muscle length does not change)	Reduction of blood flow to contracting muscle, increase in BP
Isotonic	Contraction of muscle *with* ROM (muscle length changes)	Increase in blood flow to contracting muscles, decrease in BP
	Work is generated by resistance and repetitions	High resistance, low repetition for maximal strength and hypertrophy; low resistance, high repetitions for maximal endurance
Isokinetic	Machine controls speed of movement and offers accommodating resistance to movement	Increase in BP, increases blood flow to muscles
Endurance		
Aerobic	Sustained reciprocal motion of large muscle groups to induce metabolic and circulatory stress	Increases endurance capacity of skeletal and cardiac muscle for work

Modified from Ytterberg SR, Mahowald ML, Krug HE: Exercise for arthritis, *Bailliere's Clin Rheumatol* 8:1, 1994. *BP,* Blood pressure; *ROM,* range of motion.

STRETCHING

Clinical experience shows that stretching exercise is often overlooked. In sporting and recreational activities, many musculoskeletal injuries can be associated with an oversight in stretching. Stretching exercises are intended to maintain or improve ROM and flexibility and to prepare patients for activity and function. It can also be used during an exercise cool-down period.

In the older adult, lack of flexibility usually limits an activity rather than decreases strength. The lack of flexibility imposed by years of inactivity can yield an enormous degree of joint and motor limitation. This physiologic limitation can cause burdensome functional limitations and, in the extreme, serious subsequent dependency. Activities such as grooming, dressing, sitting at a standard-height toilet or in a straight-back chair, reaching, and even stair climbing can be impaired by the joint limitation caused by lack of flexibility.

Stretching exercises are the only exercises that will increase flexibility. Stretching exercises do not increase strength or cardiovascular fitness. Static stretching (a controlled, sustained stretch of the muscle tendon unit to the point of mild discomfort) is generally recommended as the best way to maintain muscle length and correct muscle imbalance. Stretching exercises should always be part of a strengthening or cardiovascular fitness program in the form of the warm-up and cool-down segments of an exercise program. Generally, stretches should be focused on the low back, hamstrings, quadriceps, pelvic, and shoulder girdle muscle groups. Figure 2-1 provides examples of stretching exercises that can be used by the older well adult. The correct position is important; however, each patient's position may vary a little according to his or her own available degree of flexibility. The patient should feel mild tension in the muscle tendon group targeted to be stretched. The stretching action should be performed slowly and carefully, maintaining tension on the muscle for 10 to 20 seconds and then slowly releasing the stretch. A stretch is never to the point of pain. A stretching session usually centers around 15 to 20 minutes of stretching exercises per day. When used as the warm-up and cool-down segments of an exercise program, the stretching session can be limited to 5 to 8 minutes. The optimal duration and intensity of stretching and the effects of temperature are still being questioned in the literature. Local or national professional associations can provide information on acquiring patient education material, such as simple pictorials and techniques. Supply and medical equipment vendors who support hospital and medical clinics are also an excellent resource.

STRENGTHENING

The musculoskeletal system protects vital organs and governs a person's mobility. Normal age-related changes in the musculoskeletal and neurologic systems result in a decline in function for the older patient. For example, signs and symptoms of osteoarthritis, especially in weight-bearing joints, limit joint motion, flexibility, and overall mobility. Coordination, dexterity, proprioception, and vestibular integrity also show signs of decline with aging. Certainly for older adults the risk of functional loss is heightened when disease or a sedentary lifestyle accompanies the normal age-related changes.

Strength is essential to maintaining mobility and functional independence. Strengthening exercises should focus on the shoulder girdle and upper extremities and on the pelvic girdle and lower extremities. Studies support strength, particularly lower-extremity strength, as a strong predictor of success for functionally impaired older adults (Schenkman et al, 1996). Strength can also contribute to the prevention of joint and muscle injury and to sustaining bone strength (Bellew, 2002).

A main ingredient in building strength is to force the muscle to work. As explained later in this chapter, requiring a muscle to work against a load (e.g., dumbbell weights), through an arc of motion, and for a number of repetitions builds strength. The amount of rest taken between exercise intervals also contributes to strengthening. Another important requirement is that, in the course of exercising, enough work must be accomplished to reach a point of fatigue. If the exercise does not achieve fatigue, the muscles are not working sufficiently to gain a training response. Fatigue can be generally described as a tired feeling, in the body part being exercised, that makes the last two to three repetitions difficult to perform. No pain should be experienced during the last couple of exercise repetitions.

As an individual gains strength, more work (e.g., increasing the resistance, the number of repetitions, or the number of exercise sessions per week) is progressively added to repeat the strengthening scenario. Vigorous strengthening sessions require "a day of rest" between sessions; therefore three sessions per week (at a minimum) would usually be viewed as a typical frequency for an exercise program. With less vigorous strengthening programs, however, four to five sessions per week are not discouraged. Combining vigorous strengthening exercises with cardiac conditioning activities can also progress an exercise program. In this situation, the scheduled "day of rest" can be substituted with such aerobic activities as brisk walking, stationary cycling, or swimming.

Types of Strengthening Exercise

Exercises can generally be divided into three types: isometric, isotonic, and isokinetic.

ISOMETRIC EXERCISES. In isometric exercises, muscles are contracted without changing their length or causing joint movement. The contraction is held for a specified time, relaxed, and repeated for a specified number of times (i.e., repetitions). Isometric exercises are useful when pain or deformity restricts joint movement or as warm-up exercises for more strenuous exercises. Figure 2-2 illustrates an isometric exercise used for a painful knee(s). A combination of hip adduction and quadriceps muscle contractions is being used to maintain strength. Isometric exercises do not build strength and only delay a muscle's decline in strength. If acute pain inhibits joint movement or an extremity is immobilized (e.g., casted), isometric exercises are usually the patient's only source of exercise.

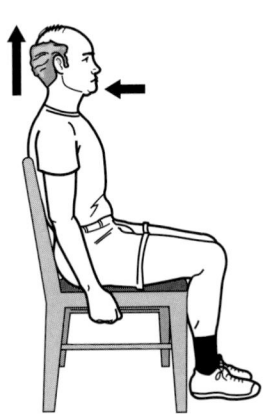

Gently pull chin in
while lengthening
back of neck.
Hold 10 seconds.

Repeat:_____Times
_____Times a day.

A

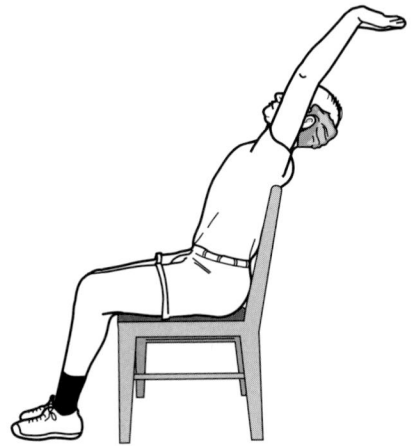

Bring arms straight up
over head and back
as far as possible,
causing back to arch
gently. Hold 10 seconds.

Repeat:_____Times
_____Times a day.

B

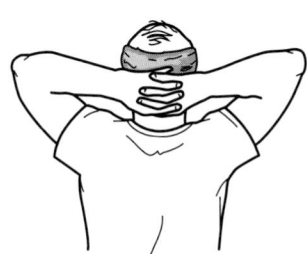

Place hands
behind your head
and pull elbows back
as far as possible.
Hold 10 seconds.

Repeat:_____Times
_____Times a day.

C

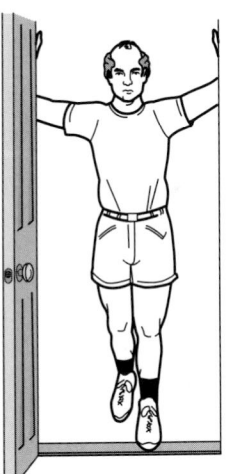

With arms
behind doorjamb,
gently lean forward.
Hold for ____ seconds.
Stretch is felt
across chest.

Repeat:_____Times
_____Times a day.

D

Figure 2-1 Examples of stretching exercises.

Sit or lie on a flat surface with your legs straight out. With a rolled towel between your knees, push knees together. Then, still keeping your knees together, tighten the muscles in the front of your thighs by forcing your knees backwards. Hold for 10 seconds.

Repeat:_____Times
           _____Times a day

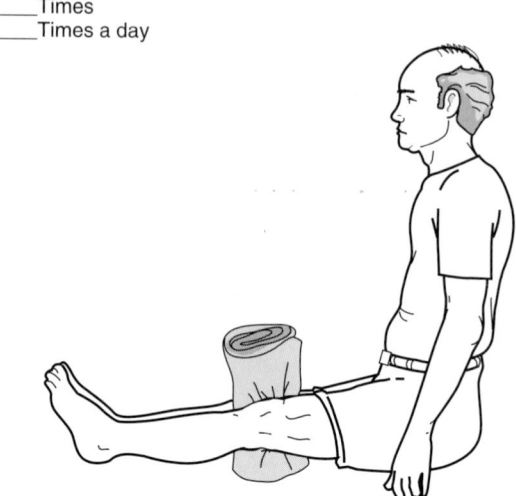

Figure 2-2   Example of an isometric exercise for the knees.

Isotonic Exercises. In isotonic exercises, muscle contraction with muscle shortening and lengthening occurs, causing the joint to move through an arc of motion. Resistance, caused by the weight of the body part and added resistance (e.g., cuff weight) that loads the muscle being exercised, makes the muscle work and builds strength. Guided resistance equipment (e.g., Cybex or Nautilus machine) or free weights are typically used to offer resistance during isotonic exercise. Figure 2-3 illustrates a set of dumbbells, an example of free weights. Free weights are inexpensive, versatile, and easy to organize for a home program. Figure 2-4 provides an example of guided resistance equipment. The gear uses gravity-loading systems (e.g., a stack of weighted plates) to offer resistance through particular movement patterns. The equipment is easy to use and generally is considered safer and more comfortable to use than free weights because there are no weights to drop, the exercise movements are guided, and solid support is provided during exercise. The equipment is popular and usually is found in private health clubs or community activity-oriented organizations (e.g., YMCA).

Isotonic exercise is usually the choice for physical activity prescribed to increase and maintain strength. The usual exercise format is a set number of repetitions with sufficient weight to cause the patient to sense fatigue in the exercised extremity toward the last few repetitions of the exercise routine. The program may progress by adding weight or by increasing the number of repetitions. Of extreme importance is the practitioner's responsibility for determining the most appropriate weight for the patient at the start of exercising. By keeping in the office a few cuff weights ranging between 1 and 5 pounds, the practitioner generally can find a weight that a patient can safely move throughout the arc of joint motion. Clinical experience recommends starting the older patient at half the weight found suitable during the patient's office visit. Attaching the selected weight to an extremity, instructing the patient to continue joint motion for 12 to 15 repetitions, listening to verbal feedback, and observing the quality of joint motion will assist the practitioner in determining a suitable work level for the patient's exercise program. If the practitioner needs further expertise (e.g., paresis, joint contracture), a referral to a physical therapist for an exercise program is certainly indicated.

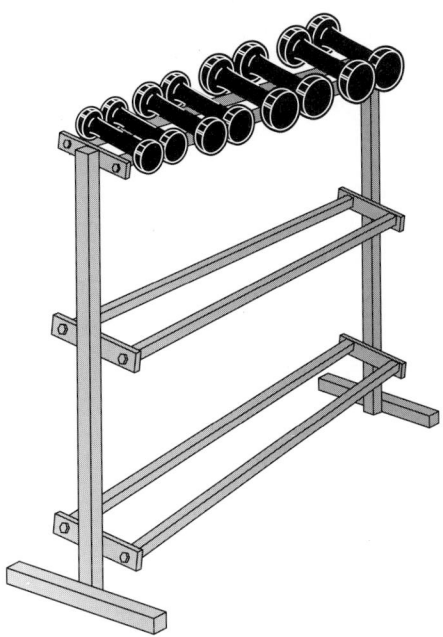

Figure 2-3 Graduated dumbbell weights. (Courtesy Sammons Preston, An AbilityOne Company, Bolingbrook, Ill.)

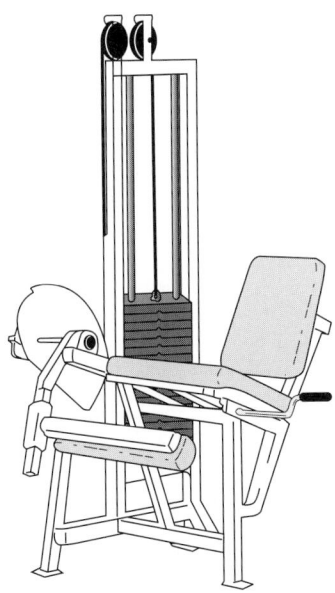

Figure 2-4 Weight-stacked, guided-resistance machine that can be used for knee extension exercises. (Redrawn from Cook BB, Stewart GW: *Strength basics: your guide to resistance training for health and optimal performance*, Champaign, Ill, 1996, Human Kinetics.)

Although numerous exercise progression techniques exist, one simple approach is to alter the following basic exercise variables: *resistance, repetitions, sets,* and the *rest interval. Resistance* is the weight or load against which a muscle works. A *repetition* (rep) is the single, complete action of an exercise from the start position to completion and back to the start position. A *set* is a given number of complete and continuous repetitions of an exercise. The *rest interval* is the amount of rest or recovery taken between sets of an exercise or between different exercises in a program. For example, 12 uninterrupted repetitions of an exercise equal one set of 12. The patient rests a minute, does 12 more repetitions performing two sets of 12, and so on. A written description of this format is as follows:

Shoulder shrugs	2	× 12	3 lb	2 min
(exercise)	(sets)	(reps)	(resistance)	(rest interval)

Manipulating any of these variables alters the intensity of an exercise. The patient can be instructed to increase the weight gradually by half a pound (i.e., resistance) over a period of 2 weeks (Figure 2-5). The workload can also be gradually increased by adding sets or repetitions or by shortening the rest intervals. If the patient encounters joint pain, any of these variables can be adjusted to accommodate the patient's level of work.

Strength gains can be further accelerated by practicing an exercise pattern of faster concentric (muscle-shortening) movements and slower eccentric (muscle-lengthening) movements. For example,

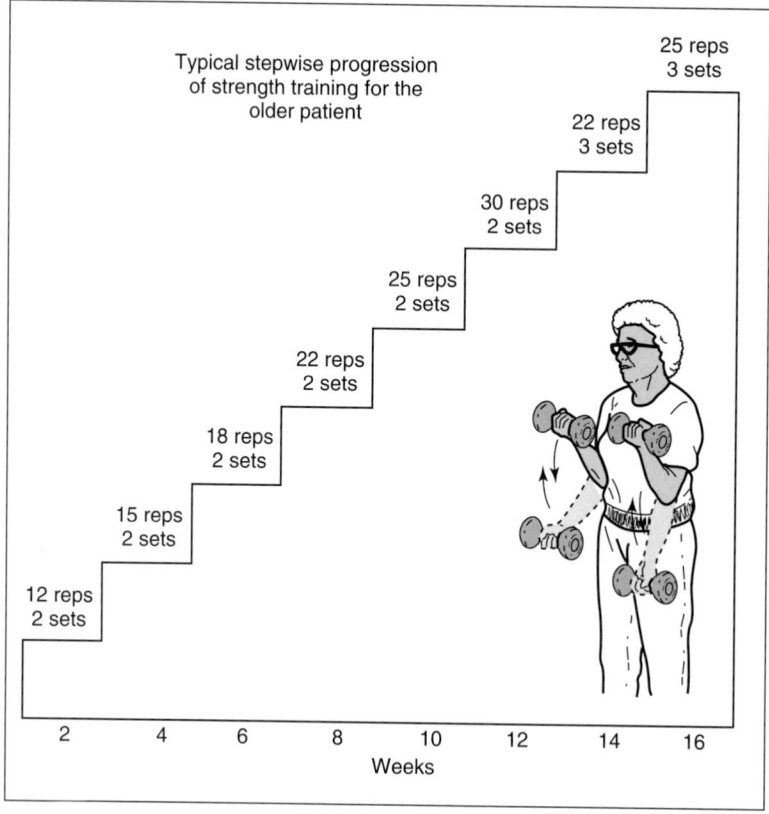

Typical stepwise progression of strength training for the older patient

25 reps 3 sets

22 reps 3 sets

30 reps 2 sets

25 reps 2 sets

22 reps 2 sets

18 reps 2 sets

15 reps 2 sets

12 reps 2 sets

Weeks

Figure 2-5 An approach used in progressing an older patient's dumbbell exercise program. The approach can be applied to other forms of strengthening programs. (Reproduced with permission from *Geriatrics* 47(8):34, 1992. Copyright by Advanstar Communications Inc. Advanstar Communications Inc. retains all rights to this article.)

while performing an exercise pattern, the patient should complete a concentric contraction (elbow bending) within 2 seconds and then take 4 seconds to complete the subsequent eccentric contraction (elbow straightening). The exercise session can occur once a day for three to four times per week.

Isokinetic Exercises. The third type of exercise is isokinetic, a form of isotonic exercise. Basically the difference between the two types is that isokinetic exercise is performed on specialized equipment designed to control the speed of movement and offer accommodating resistance to an isotonic exercise. Generally, isokinetic equipment is found in specialized orthopedic training clinics and is used in the rehabilitation of severe musculoskeletal injuries. Isokinetic exercise is not discussed in this chapter.

CARDIOVASCULAR TRAINING

Cardiovascular training should be considered the foundation of any fitness program. Flexibility and strength exercises support this critical component of a balanced fitness program because the patient must be able to perform cardiovascular training (Fatouros et al, 2002). The impact of cardiovascular training, however, is of even greater importance. Not only does the activity offer extremely beneficial cardiovascular health outcomes, such as significant reduction in the risk of coronary heart disease and hypertension and improvements in arterial compliance (Mazzeo and Tanaka, 2001), but it also increases the ability to deliver oxygen to working muscle and increases the capacity of muscle to extract oxygen and eliminate metabolic by-products. From a functional perspective, this statement means that for every given functional task, there should be less relative work. In other words, for the older adult, performing the usual activities of daily living should no longer be so great a challenge. Clinicians should follow the physical activity goal recommendations of the AHA (Pearson et al, 2002).

Warm-up and cool-down periods should also help reduce the incidence of cardiac rhythm disturbances during cardiovascular exercise.

New Perspective on Physical Fitness

Two major national organizations, the AHA (Pearson et al, 2002) and the American College of Sport Medicine (ACSM, 1998), have issued recommendations regarding appropriate exercise training.

In 2002 the AHA published their update on guidelines for primary prevention of cardiovascular disease and stroke. One of the main recommendations concerned physical activity. Moderate activities were set at 40% to 60% of maximum capacity, and these types of exercise were encouraged for at least 30 minutes on most days of the week. See Table 2-1 for a more detailed description.

In 1995, the ACSM and the Centers for Disease Control and Prevention (CDC) issued a joint statement that was published in the *Journal of the American Medical Association.* The February 1995 article, entitled "Physical Activity and Public Health," recommended an alternative plan for those who have not been successful with the 3- to 5-days-a-week, 20-minute regimen. The new recommendation is moderate-intensity exercise for 30 minutes most days of the week. Those 30 minutes can be broken into smaller segments; for instance, a 10-minute walk taken three times a day will produce the same basic health benefit as a 30-minute walk (Pate et al, 1995). For many years, exercise scientists have recognized that fitness is related to enhanced health. Certainly future studies are necessary to determine whether loosening the model to make it more achievable and practical will actually promote activity. This new alternative in cardiovascular training is an encouraging approach for sedentary older adults or those with a poor fitness level who want to engage in a healthier lifestyle.

Designing an Exercise Program

The design of an exercise program for the older well adult should focus on prevention, restoration, and maintenance with three primary objectives in mind: (1) determining an adequate, challenging, and safe activity; (2) sustaining an effective level of habitual physical activity; and (3) ensuring that the fitness activity selected remains safe and effective.

DETERMINING AN ADEQUATE, CHALLENGING, AND SAFE ACTIVITY
Preexercise Office Assessment

Before prescribing physical activity for an older adult, the practitioner should conduct a preexercise assessment. Typically, the well older adult will have some form of chronic disease with factors that limit the activity or narrow the range of possibilities for exercise (e.g., medications, severe osteoarthritis, coronary artery disease, diabetes, orthostatic hypotension, painful feet, neuropathies, obesity, osteoporosis, incontinence, or restrictive pulmonary conditions). These factors certainly challenge the practitioner in designing a safe and effective exercise program. Therefore an assessment is imperative for providing the practitioner with adequate information to avoid injury or a worsening of underlying chronic diseases and for determining an appropriate level of activity that will be enjoyable and practical for the older adult.

The assessment should include cardiac risk, potential physical limitations, painful conditions, contraindications, and other medical complications. The history should include experience with exercise, an assessment of lifestyle risk factors that are potentially modifiable through exercise, previous activity levels to help set realistic goals, and a medication review. Medications commonly used by older patients that have pharmacologic effects interfering with physical activity include antihistamines, anticholinergics, antipsychotics, beta-blockers, diuretics, insulin, and oral hypoglycemic agents. These medications may require a careful cardiovascular and neurologic evaluation and may necessitate modifications of the patient's exercise prescription.

The physical examination should include measurement of vital signs and evaluation of the patient's cardiac function. Recent debate concerns the appropriateness of a cardiovascular stress test before starting an exercise program for sedentary, asymptomatic men and women over 75 years of age (Gill, DiPietro, and Krumholz, 2000). In the past, before an exercise program was undertaken, a stress test was recommended for older adults with or without symptoms suggestive of or known cardiovascular, pulmonary, or metabolic disease (ACSM, 1990). For some clinicians, experience encourages the use of cardiovascular stress testing to assess cardiovascular fitness in the older population.

Gill and colleagues cite the low rate of participation of older adults in exercise programs despite the overwhelming evidence of the benefits. They contend that the risks, expense, and unproved benefit of cardiac stress testing deter many older adults from participating in an exercise program. They offer a set of assessment recommendations that can be performed during an office visit; these recommendations are applicable to asymptomatic, previously sedentary older adults (Table 2-3). Clinicians must strive to balance the dual and sometimes conflicting goals of maximizing the health of the patient while at the same time minimizing the risk. Respiratory function should also be assessed by simply checking (i.e., spirometry) the patient's forced vital capacity (FVC) and forced expiratory volume in 1 second (FEV_1) (American Thoracic Society, 1979).

Quick Assessment Tools for the Neuromusculoskeletal System

The assessment should also include a gross assessment of flexibility and joint motion, muscle strength, and balance. In the office, immediate observations of the patient's behavior should cue the practitioner about the areas on which the assessment should focus. For example, simple observations such as a slow nonantalgic gait, labored breathing, difficulty in turning, and problems in mounting the examination table should provide a sense that strength, balance, gait, and aerobic capability must be examined. Other information that may help the practitioner design a safe and effective exercise program include the patient's use of an assistive device, quality of vision or hearing, and ability to follow directions.

Flexibility. Flexibility in the older adult should be assessed functionally. Such an assessment can be accomplished by asking the patient to perform functional activities such as sitting and rising in a standard-height chair, reaching for an object overhead, clasping the hands behind the head and the small of the back, climbing on and off the examination table, and rising from lying on the floor. For example, the findings would be based on the patient's ability to reach fully behind the head or

TABLE 2-3	Office Preexercise Cardiovascular Risk Assessment of Sedentary Symptomatic 75-Year-Old Persons

Goal: To minimize the risk of adverse cardiac events.
1. Complete history and physical examination to identify potential cardiac contraindications to exercise, including the following:
   - Myocardial infarction within 6 mo
   - Angina
   - Congestive heart failure signs or symptoms (bilateral rales, shortness of breath)
   - Resting systolic blood pressure ≥200 mm Hg or diastolic blood pressure ≥110
   - Cardiovascular reserve testing: Climbing a flight of stairs without shortness of breath or developing any type of chest pain
   - Resting electrocardiogram (ECG) reviewed for new Q-waves, ST-segment depressions or T-wave inversion
2. Low-intensity exercise program selecting from one of the following modalities:
   - Gait training
   - Balance exercises
   - Tai chi
   - Self-paced walking
   - Lower-extremity resistance training with elastic tubing or ankle weights

All programs should have as a minimum one session of supervision and training. Intensity and amount of exercise should be gradually increase in accordance with the older person's capacity. Each session should have a warm-up and a cool-down period. If chest pain, shortness of breath, or dizziness occurs, the patient should receive oral and written instructions to rest and to see his or her physician if these symptoms persist or recur.

Adapted from Gill TM, DiPietro L, Krumholz HM: Role of exercise stress testing and safety monitoring for older persons starting an exercise program, *JAMA* 284(3):342-348, 2000.

the small of the back when clasping hands. An inability to reach behind either body area usually indicates a marked limitation in shoulder ROM. Another concern would be the patient's inability to bend forward when rising from a chair, which usually indicates a lack of adequate hip flexion. Certainly, if the need arises, goniometric measurements of joints identified as limited in motion can be recorded (American Academy of Orthopedic Surgeons, 1996).

Always important but often overlooked is testing the flexibility of the hip, hamstring, and lower back. Lack of flexibility in the hip, knee, and ankle can be an indicator for gait and balance problems. Also, physical activity in patients with moderate tightness in these areas, whether the patients are young or old, usually promotes complaints of low back pain. Interestingly, some investigators have recently noted a strong relationship between hip flexor tightness (i.e., greater than 10 degrees) and limited ankle dorsiflexion (i.e., at least zero degrees) causing hip and low back pain in more than 60% of their walking and jogging exercise participants (Brown, 1993). Therefore if an older adult is a candidate for walking or jogging, the practitioner should assess hip flexor tightness (Figure 2-6) and ankle dorsiflexion range. Accordingly, testing should also include the sit-and-reach test to grossly assess hamstring, hip, and lower back flexibility (Chandler, 2000). In this simple test the patient is asked to sit in a stable chair, reach forward, and then reach to each side, with the practitioner noting the patient's ability to perform the task. An object to be picked up can be placed at a reasonable distance from the patient to facilitate reach and gross trunk movements.

The sit and cross-uncross leg test is a quick test of hip flexibility. While sitting in a chair, the patient is asked to cross one thigh over the other. The patient is then asked to uncross his or her thigh and place the lateral side of his or her foot on the opposite knee. This simple test determines whether gross restriction is present.

Strength. Strength can be assessed with a number of sophisticated methods, such as manual muscle testing, dynamometer testing (e.g., strain gauges, hand-grip dynamometers), and progressive mobility testing (Chandler, 2000). These tests are appropriate for definitive testing, especially after a significant strength deficiency is identified. For the office, however, a gross strength assessment can be adequate for assessing the physical capability of the older adult and reliable enough to identify quickly and easily particular problems that the practitioner may wish to self-investigate more intently or refer to a specialist for a definitive assessment and prescribed treatment. The following are examples of gross strength tests that the practitioner can use in an office or clinic environment.

Rising-on-Toes Test. The rising-on-toes test can be used to determine the strength of the gastrocnemius-soleus muscle group. The quick test involves asking the patient to hold on to the back of a chair and rise up on the toes, one leg at a time, 10 times. The patient must be able to complete the 10 repetitions with full ankle excursions. Inability to complete the test indicates moderate weakness,

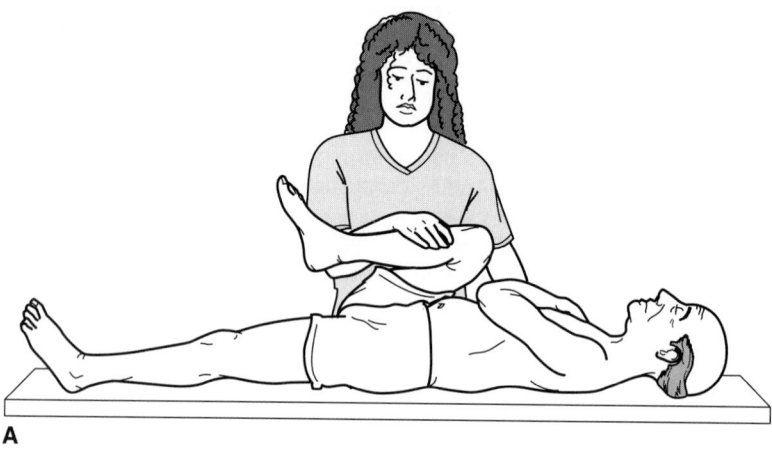

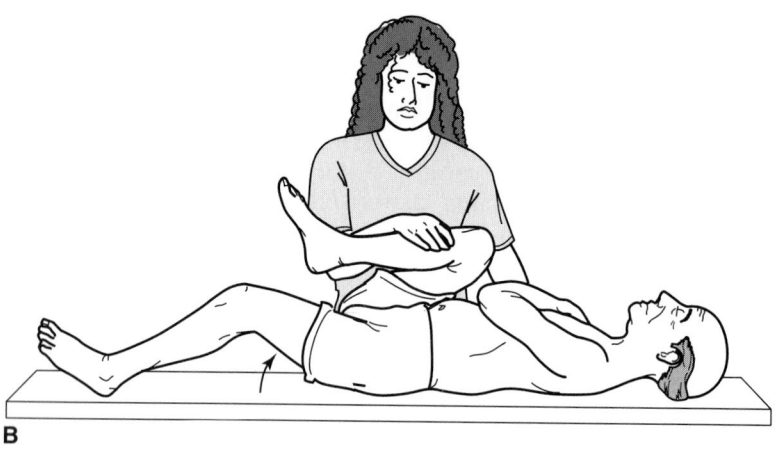

Figure 2-6   Thomas test for flexion contracture of the hip. **A,** Normal range of hip flexion. **B,** Hip flexion demonstrating flexion contracture.

and strengthening must be accomplished if the patient is considering a fitness program of walking, jogging, tai chi, or dance aerobics. For the agile older patient, this test can be enhanced by having the patient walk (supported by the practitioner's hand or unsupported) on his or her toes for a short distance (e.g., 8 to 10 feet).

Walking-on-Heels Test. The walking-on-heels test can be used to examine quickly the patient's ability to dorsiflex at the ankle. This test has the patient walk in place on his or her heels (10 steps for each leg). Again the patient must be able to complete the 10 repetitions with full ankle excursions. Like the rising-on-toes test, this test can be enhanced by having the patient walk (supported by the practitioner's hand or unsupported) on his or her heels for a short distance (e.g., 8 to 10 feet). Inability to complete the test indicates moderate weakness, and strengthening must be accomplished if the patient is considering a fitness program of walking, jogging, tai chi, or dance aerobics.

To a lesser extent, ankle inversion and eversion can be tested by having the patient walk on the lateral borders of his or her feet to test eversion and to test inversion by instructing the patient to walk on the medial borders of his or her feet. Besides strength, the test can determine whether the patient has any gross restriction in his or her ROM of the ankle and foot.

Hip-Drop Test. The hip-drop test, shown in Figure 2-7, can be used to assess grossly gluteus medius strength. The integrity of this hip stabilizer muscle is essential in weight-bearing activities because the pelvis drops every time the patient takes a step. In this test the practitioner stands behind the patient and uses as landmarks the skin dimples overlying the posterior superior iliac

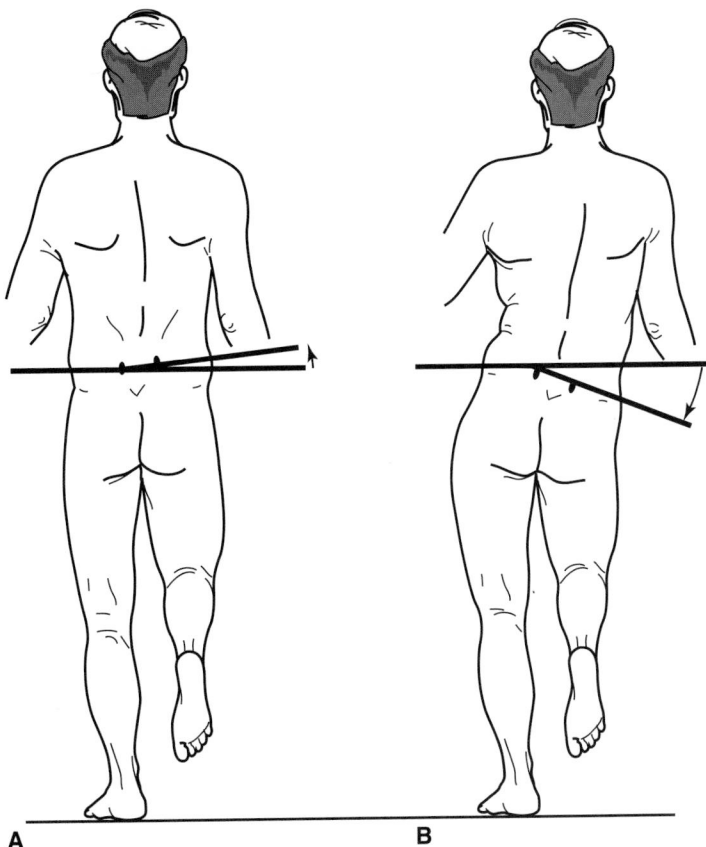

Figure 2-7 Hip-drop test. **A,** Normal. **B,** Abnormal.

spines. Normally the skin dimples should appear level when the patient bears weight equally on both legs. The patient is then asked to stand on one leg. The skin dimple and pelvis on the non–weight-bearing side should elevate, indicating that the gluteus medius muscle on the weight-bearing side is functioning properly (negative Trendelenburg sign). If the dimple and pelvis on the non–weight-bearing side remain in position or actually drop, the gluteus medius muscle on the weight-bearing side is weak (positive Trendelenburg sign). A strengthening program is indicated before a weight-bearing exercise program can begin.

Hip-Extension Test. The hip-extension test is used to determine hip extension strength. Figure 2-8 illustrates the test. The patient is asked to lie prone and raise the entire lower extremity, against gravity, through the full ROM (i.e., 0 to 30 degrees). If the patient is unable to raise even his or her leg though the arc of motion, a strengthening program is indicated. If the patient accomplishes the hip extension, the practitioner then offers manual resistance to determine whether the position can be maintained. Again, if weakness is detected, a strengthening program is necessary before a weight-bearing exercise program can begin. This test can also be performed by asking the patient to rise from a chair with arms folded across the chest and the back straight. Care must be taken to guard the patient from falling, which might happen to patients with weak hip extensors. Most patients with "weak hip extensors" tend to stand and walk with an exaggerated lurch. Some patients exhibit a forward trunk. In any case, the poor posture held during sustained physical activity will promote low back pain. The practitioner should be cautioned in strength testing the hip in older adults with a history of hip fracture. This caution can be extended to strength testing the trunk for older adults with strong history of vertebral fractures. Strength assessments under these conditions should be performed under the supervision of a rehabilitation physician or physical therapist.

Balance. Balance is a major determinant of functional independence. A patient's ability to balance can be compromised by disease or injury, medication, and the process of aging. Impaired balance poses a threat to physical safety and can lead to self-imposed restrictions on activities. Therefore an exercise program for the older adult should include activities that improve balance control.

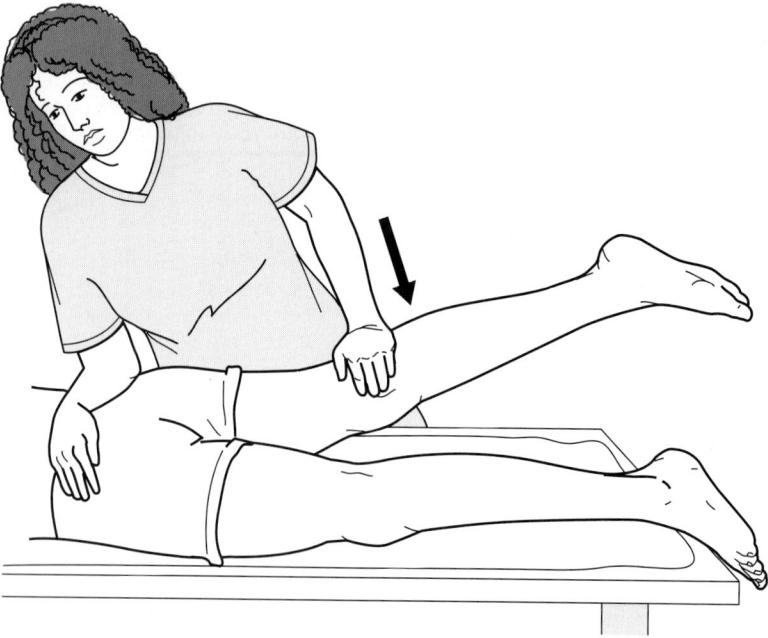

Figure 2-8   Hip-extension test. The normal limit for hip extension is approximately 30 degrees.

Balance can be considered to have three basic properties: maintenance of a stable position, stabilization during voluntary movements, and reaction to external disturbance. Basically, the body does its best to keep its center of gravity close to the center of the base of support. The body's ability to maintain this stable position is supported by postural reactions and subsequent adjustments that occur before, during, and after voluntary movement or external perturbations.

Balance is usually thought of as either static or dynamic. *Static balance* can be viewed as the patient's ability to maintain a stable upright position in unsupported sitting or standing and to withstand reasonable perturbations such as the external force of a sternal nudge. In *dynamic balance,* the same patient's ability is determined by adding the dimension of movement in space, such as walking, bending, or reaching.

Quantitative performance-oriented scales for assessing static and dynamic balance have been developed and tested. In addition, a posturography evaluation can be achieved by the use of sophisticated movable platforms, which are extremely expensive and somewhat large pieces of equipment that require extensive operating space not normally found in the usual office or clinic environment. In certain clinical situations, referring the patient to a local posturography testing center is appropriate. In an office setting, however, the practitioner may want to choose certain simple and relatively quick tests to assess balance. For example, static balance can be evaluated by the stand-on-one-leg test, the sharpened Romberg, and the reach test. For dynamic balance, tests can include the get-up-and-go test, imaginary-balance-beam test, and walking through a simple office setting obstacle course.

Static Balance. Standing on one leg (Chandler, 2000) with the eyes open for a period of time is an easy and simple test to assess quickly any significant deficits in static balance. Although no generally accepted standard for time values associated with the one-leg stand test have been established, the inability of a patient to stand on one leg for less than 5 seconds is certainly indicative of a significant deficit. The practitioner should conduct several patient trials to account for a patient's learning curve and to ensure reliable findings. The practitioner is cautioned from allowing the patient to place the non–weight-bearing leg on the stance leg, shifting the position of the stance leg, or hopping because these alterations are considered "cheating."

The sharpened Romberg can also be used to assess static balance quickly. Table 2-4 illustrates the test, which involves six segments with a simple grading of either "able or not able" to complete the requested task. Figure 2-9 should clarify the patient's foot placements for testing. This relatively comprehensive test is easy to administer and is a reliable assessment tool.

The reach test (Chandler, 2000) is a must add-on for assessing static balance (Figure 2-10). The test requires the practitioner to use a yardstick to measure the distance the patient is able to reach before losing his or her balance. To perform the test, the practitioner places the flat side of a yardstick on a wall. The patient is asked to stand comfortably with the reaching shoulder sideways next to the wall and yardstick. The patient is then asked to reach forward as far as possible along the yardstick until the practitioner notes the patient's loss of balance. The distance reached is recorded. The practitioner should ensure that he or she is in a position to catch the patient if balance is completely lost.

Dynamic Balance. The get-up-and-go test (Mathias, Nayak, and Isaacs, 1987) has the patient rise from a chair and proceed as quickly as possible toward a preplanned destination (e.g., use of a particular clinic hallway that has been measured for distance). The complexity of the test can be upgraded by incorporating turns, controlling the patient's base of support, and adding simple functionally driven tasks into the test protocol. For example, the patient can be asked to rise from a chair and walk down a 30-foot hallway. While walking, the patient is asked to walk for 15 feet with one foot immediately in front of the other, heel to toe (i.e., imaginary balance beam test). The patient is then asked to turn around, return to the chair, and sit. Stepping over obstacles such as a telephone book(s) can be added to the protocol (i.e., obstacle course test). The trial is timed, and any difficulties are recorded. Several trials are recommended to ensure testing reliability.

Obviously, depending on the patient's capabilities, the practitioner may want to take into account in the preexercise assessment other considerations, such as the patient's gait, speed of movement, and skills in the activities of daily living, that are not elaborated here. Nevertheless, this chapter has

TABLE 2-4	Sharpened Romberg for Testing Balance		
Task	**Activity**	**Performance**	
	Circle "able" or "not able" in completing the requested task.		
	Standing with feet together with the eyes open for 10 s	Able	Not able
	Standing with feet together with the eyes open for 10 s and with eyes closed	Able	Not able
	Standing with feet in a semitandem (1 foot ahead of the other by a half a foot length) position for 10 s, eyes open	Able	Not able
	Standing with feet in a semitandem (one foot ahead of the other by a half a foot length) position for 10 s, eyes closed	Able	Not able
	Standing in full tandem position (one foot immediately in front of the other, heel to toe), eyes open	Able	Not able
	Standing in full tandem position (one foot immediately in front of the other, heel to toe), eyes closed	Able	Not able

Adapted from Chandler JM: Balance and falls in the elderly. In Guccione AA: *Geriatric physical therapy*, ed 2, St Louis, 2000, Mosby.

presented a number of options to assist the practitioner in determining a safe activity and an appropriate fitness level for the well older adult. Once the information gathered during the assessment is integrated into the patient's overall medical and physical condition, a fitness plan will emerge that includes commonsense goals and addresses the patient's personal needs.

THE EXERCISE PRESCRIPTION

An exercise prescription should be designed to meet the exercise history, functional status, painful conditions, medical problems, and health needs of an individual patient. Clinical traits found during the office preexercise assessment can also assist the practitioner in determining the type of exercise and an appropriate activity level for a particular older patient. For example, patients who have

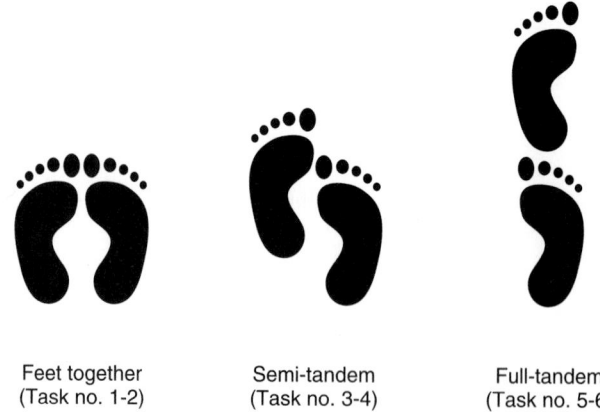

Feet together   Semi-tandem   Full-tandem
(Task no. 1-2)   (Task no. 3-4)   (Task no. 5-6)

Figure 2-9   Foot placements for sharpened Romberg test. (From Guccione AA: *Geriatric physical therapy*, ed 2, St Louis, 2000, Mosby.)

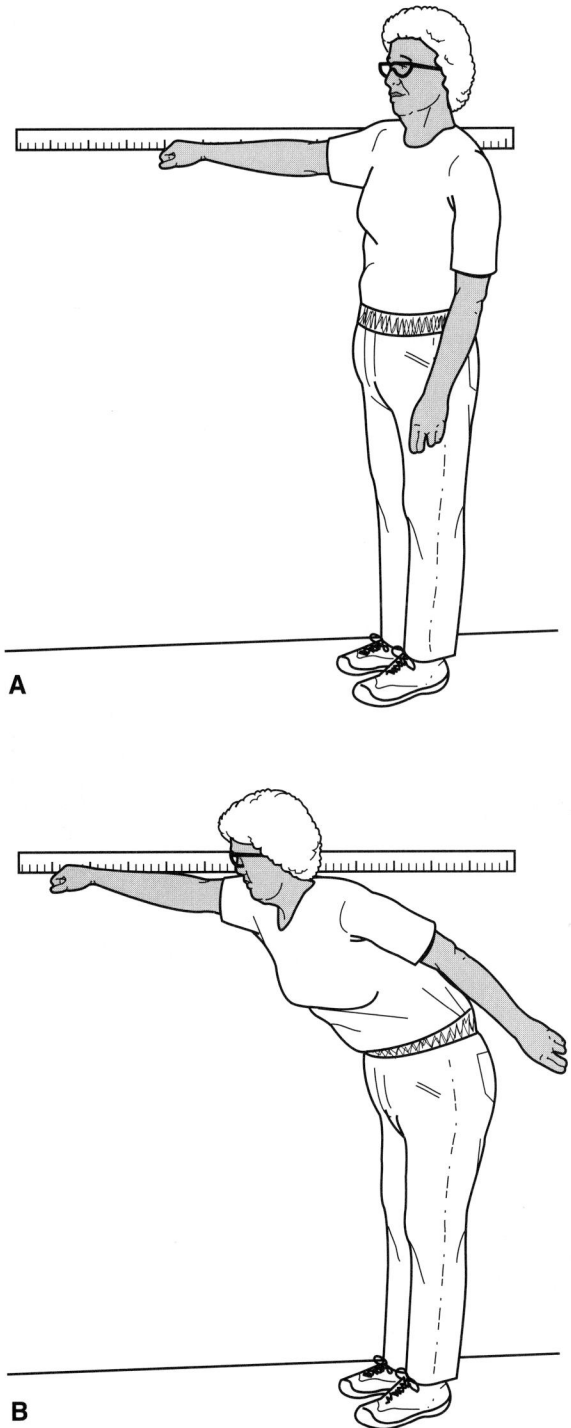

A

B

Figure 2-10   Functional reach. **A,** Starting position. **B,** Ending position. (Redrawn from Guccione AA: *Geriatric physical therapy*, ed 2, St Louis, 2000, Mosby.)

a lengthy history of being sedentary or frail may drive the prescription design toward a stretching, strengthening, and balance fitness program (e.g., versus aerobic training). Also, patients with such complications as orthostatic hypotension, impaired equilibrium, and gait disturbances may need to begin their exercise program in a supervised setting. For the apparently healthy and active older adult, however, the prescription may be immediately directed toward a moderate aerobic conditioning program. The individual's specific goals also help design the parameters of the exercise prescription (e.g., decrease cardiovascular risk, reduce weight, improve physical function or cardiovascular fitness). All patients should be counseled to be aware of the development of signs or symptoms of cardiac risk.

The prescription for any type of exercise activity should always include the *f*requency of the activity, the *i*ntensity, and the *t*ime (FIT model). As discussed earlier, when setting ranges for these parameters, the settings should be sufficient to generate a training response (e.g., for strengthening, the training response can be a sense of muscle fatigue encountered during the last few exercise repetitions). For aerobic activities the target heart rate within an established training zone is the training response benchmark. The maximum heart rate is the highest rate at which the heart can safely pump (beats per minute) during exercise.

As discussed earlier, aerobic exercise program progresses by slowly increasing the exercise frequency, intensity, and time. The practitioner should also keep in mind that although progression is important to maintain an adequate training response, progressive increases in vigorous exercise levels also increase the risk of physical and medical complications such as musculoskeletal sprains, painful joints, and tendinitis. Therefore the key in setting these exercise parameters is to establish an optimal range for each of these components without maximizing the high risk of complications.

In addition to prescribing a conditioning phase, the exercise prescription should also include activities for warm-up and cool-down phases. For example, the warm-up and cool-down phases can be stretching or slowed walking, and the conditioning phase necessitates a brisk walk (i.e., the actual vigorous activity). Both the warm-up and cool-down phases are essential components of an exercise program. Including such information on the prescription as aerobic exercise for 20 minutes with 5 minutes of warm-up and 5 minutes of cool-down, for a total of 30 minutes, is sufficient to remind the patient and (if applicable) the community program of the need for warm-up and cool-down periods. The frequency in this example can be three to five times a week with a duration of 20 minutes and intensity to target heart rate.

As discussed earlier, for strength training, the appropriate intensity is generally 50% to 80% of the patient's maximum repetitive lifting ability as estimated during the preexercise office assessment. Duration can start at two sets of 12 repetitions and gradually increase as the patient begins to feel no training response. The prescribed frequency should be no less often than three times a week. Elastic tubing can be substituted for a weight program. Weight or tubing tensile resistance can be gradually increased over a period of weeks. The practitioner must ensure that 5 minutes of warm-up and 5 minutes of cool-down are included in the strengthening program, just as they are in aerobic training. For the older adult, some form of aerobic activity should always be part of a strengthening program. Suggesting a simple 15- to 20-minute walk or even the use of a stationary cycle for most sedentary older adults would not be unreasonable.

Examples of Typical Exercise Activities

Clinical experience suggests that the older adult's exercise program should include multiple forms of activities aimed at increasing musculoskeletal flexibility, strength, and cardiovascular endurance. Stretching should be part of every exercise session as warm-up and cool-down from the conditioning period. The following are examples of typical exercise activities that may be modified for the older well adult.

Walking. Walking is a form of total-body exercise that can be considered the most prescribed exercise by practitioners. Walking is appropriate for 80% of healthy older adults and has the additional benefit of improving performance in important activities of daily living. The walk can be brisk walking, hill walking, or treadmill walking. Mall walking has become a popular type of exercise among well older adults. It must be stressed, however, that exercise walks must be performed at a higher intensity than a normal walking pace. Figure 2-11 illustrates a typical walking program. Intensity is increased by slowly adding time and the number of walking sessions while maintaining at least 40% to 60% of a patient's maximal heart rate. The activity can improve the efficiency of the heart and lungs, burn fat and calories, build musculoskeletal strength and endurance, and improve balance and coordination. Certainly aerobic dancing and running can also accomplish the same benefits; however, walking is easier on the joints and spine. For instance, running or aerobic dance movements exert a force equal to three to four times body weight during weight bearing. Walking transmits forces of only one to one and a half times the patient's weight on the joints and spine, which is about 60% to 75% less than the force transmitted in high-impact sports such as running and aerobics. Moreover, walking is accessible; that is, no special equipment except comfortable shoes and clothing is necessary. The activity is inexpensive and can be incorporated into a patient's daily routine. It also has variety; that is, it can be social (e.g., group walking) or individual. It is appropriate for all fitness levels and all ages, especially the older adult. Walking programs can be a fitness model for patients with obesity, arthritis, heart disease and hypertension, type 2 diabetes, osteoporosis, and certain pulmonary disorders.

Multiple Endurance Programs. Multiple endurance exercise programs are activity programs less likely to cause muscle and joint overuse and fatigue (Brown, 2000). Endurance exercises may include

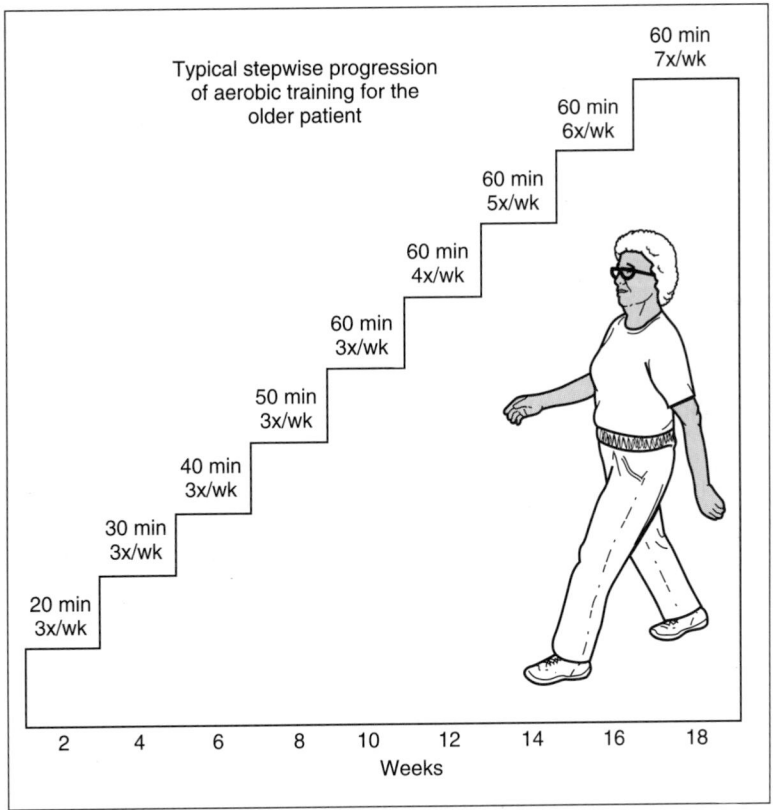

Figure 2-11 An approach used in progressing an older patient's walking program. The approach can be applied to other types of aerobic programs. (Reproduced with permission from *Geriatrics* 47(8):34, 1992. Copyright by Advanstar Communications Inc. Advanstar Communications Inc. retains all rights to this article.)

walking, brisk walking, treadmill walking, stationary cycling, indoor rowing and ski machines, swimming, and calisthenics. Running, bicycling, cross-country skiing, and ice-skating are also activities that build aerobic capacity but have a higher tendency for falls and should be considered carefully, especially for elderly women. One 60-minute exercise session may include a warm-up; brisk walking, riding a stationary bicycle, and rowing while maintaining a comparable heart rate for all three activities; and a cool-down. Substituting for the conditioning activity with an aerobic videotape, stair climbing, and a stationary bike can be adequate for an indoor exercise program.

Aquatic Programs. Aquatic programs are also popular with older adults. An aquatic program can be designed to help a broad range of people achieve fitness and function, especially patients with such limitations as joint pain from severe osteoarthritis, painful feet, coronary artery disease, obesity, lung disease, postural deformities, and severe deconditioning (Takeshima et al, 2002). Studies have validated the usefulness of aquatic programs meeting the metabolic and cardiovascular responses that fulfill the ACSM exercise prescription guidelines for realizing health benefits (D'Acquisto, D'Acquisto, and Renne, 2001).

Community-based aquatic fitness programs are popular, and access is relatively simple. These programs are especially helpful to older adults who migrate according to the change in seasons. Community aquatic programs are geographically widespread, which lessens the occurrence of "a break in training." Aquatic programs are usually group sessions, which can promote socialization and lead to a level of habitual physical activity.

Tai Chi. Tai chi has been used for centuries in Asian cultures as a form of Chinese exercise. Although health benefits have not been fully established in Western scientific literature, evidence suggests that it is a safe form of moderate exercise that can provide physiologic benefits and enhance balance and body awareness (Yalden and Chun, 2001). Studies conducted by S. Wolf and colleagues (1996, 1997) at the Atlanta Frailty and Injuries Cooperative Studies on Intervention Techniques found that tai chi delayed the onset of first or multiple falls 47.5% longer than computerized platform balance training or education. It also reduced the subjects' fear of falling. This finding is extremely relevant because falls in the older population constitute a major risk in physical safety and an obstacle to maintaining their independence. Although other studies have demonstrated that a combined strengthening and weight-training program and most exercise programs for older patients reduce the risk of falls (Gardner et al, 2002; Jensen et al, 2002; Wu, 2002), tai chi can serve as a favored alternative to the traditional exercise programs aimed at reducing falls in older adults. Like aquatic fitness programs, tai chi can be a group activity that promotes socialization, provides multiple benefits, and increases self-assessed health (Taggart, 2001). Unlike aquatic programs, however, this form of fitness requires no special equipment or space. Tai chi programs have become so popular that they can be accessed through local community organizations and senior citizen groups.

Elastic Therapy. Elastic therapy can also be used to strengthen muscle groups. Commonly referred to as elastic bands (e.g., Theraband) or tubes (e.g., surgical tubing), these popular and widely used elastic tools can add resistance (as does using weights) in an isotonic exercise program. The bands come in different widths that are color coded for specific resistance (i.e., elastic tensile resistance) levels. When using surgical tubing, practitioners can select different tube diameters to match the available strength and endurance of the muscle being exercised. Such accommodation reduces the risk of overloading the patient. The smaller the tube diameter, the lower the resistance for the patient. Selection of the tensile strength of the elastic tube actually is determined by what muscle is being addressed and how strong that muscle is at the present time. A good rule is to pick a tubing size that will continually resist the muscle yet allow full (or available) motion around the joint in a controlled manner. For example, in weak muscles, thin elastic tubing, which offers very little resistance, can be used. The patient who becomes stronger graduates to a thicker, more resistive type of tubing. A person should not be unstable or unable to complete the exercise.

Figure 2-12 illustrates exercise movements that use elastic material. A typical elastic exercise program consists of 12 to 15 repetitions with the appropriate size of tubing for three to five sets per exercise session. As the patient becomes stronger, tubing can be upgraded to provide more resistance. Although no aerobic capability benefit is obtained from tubing programs, the activity can be prescribed for the homebound older adult who may need strengthening of particularly large muscle groups. A general practitioner should contact a physical therapist to design an effective and safe tubing program for the older adult.

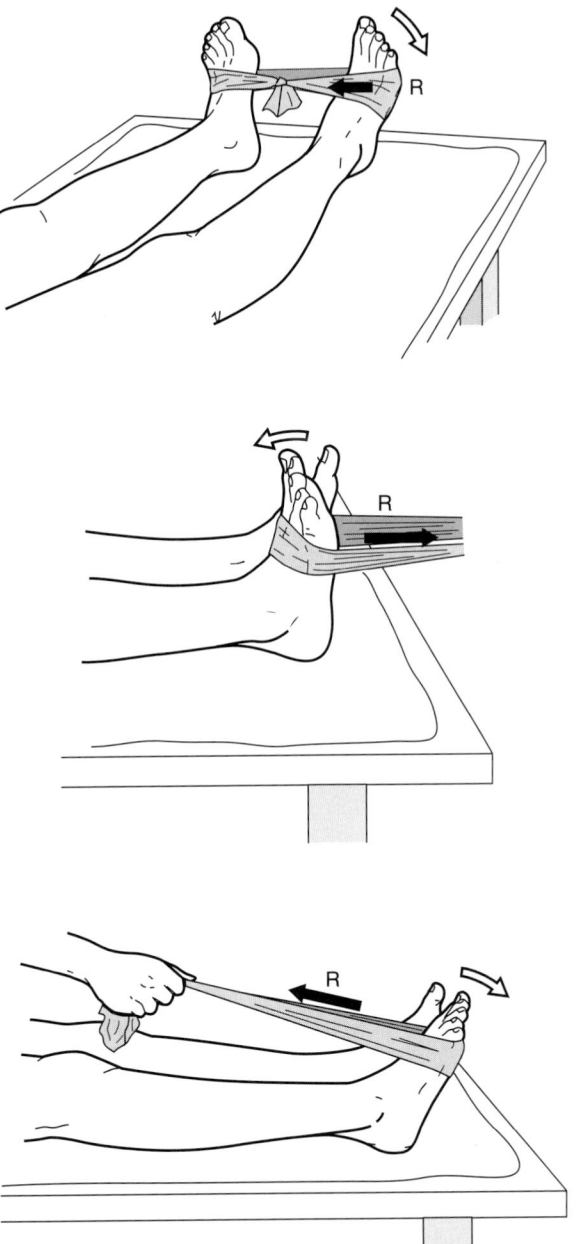

Figure 2-12 Examples of exercise using elastic bands. *R* and *dark arrow* indicate direction of resistance. *Light arrow* indicates direction of foot movement while exercising. (Redrawn from Kisner C, Lynn AC: *Therapeutic exercise: foundations and techniques*, ed 4, Philadelphia, 2002, FA Davis.)

    Functional Programs. Strengthening programs can also be functional. Activities usually focus on certain dynamic components of a particular functional activity. Figures 2-13 and 2-14 are examples of exercises used to encourage such functional components as reaching overhead and to the side, bending forward while sitting, and pushing. The exercise program can be performed solo or with a partner, such as a family caregiver. Exercises may also include upper-extremity lateral raises, shoulder shrugs, bicep curls, triceps presses, side bends, rising and sitting from a chair, wall slides, marching in place, stair climbing, and stool step-ups. A pair of cuff weights can be used to add more effort to the activity. Functional strengthening programs are usually moderate to low-level types of exercise. Nevertheless, modest physiologic benefits can occur at these lower-end exercises; even for many slightly impaired older adults, exercise may forestall further declines in physiologic reserves.

SUSTAINING AN EFFECTIVE LEVEL OF HABITUAL PHYSICAL ACTIVITY

Researchers have shown that the greatest improvements in flexibility, strength, and cardiovascular fitness occur within the first few months of an exercise program, with the performance plateau occurring shortly thereafter (Cunningham, Imgram, and Rechnitzer, 1979; Sidney and Shephard, 1978). Improvements in cardiovascular function and flexibility achieved in the early stages of an

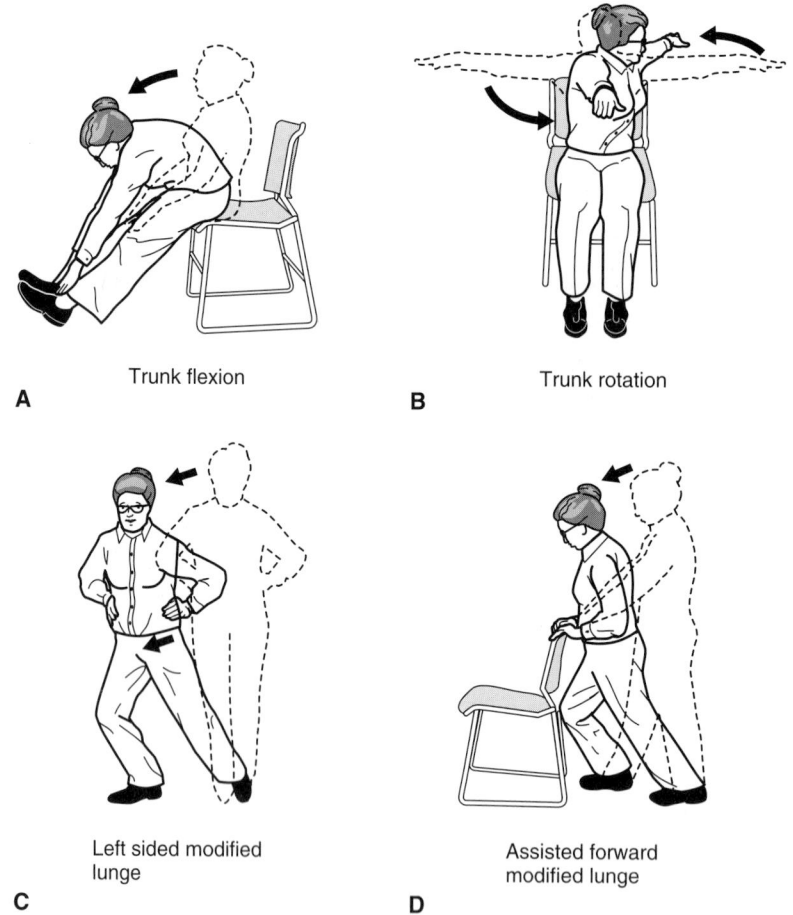

Trunk flexion

A

Trunk rotation

B

Left sided modified
lunge

C

Assisted forward
modified lunge

D

Figure 2-13   Functional solo exercise patterns. **A,** Trunk flexion. **B,** Trunk rotation. **C,** Left-sided modified lunge. **D,** Assisted forward modified lunge.

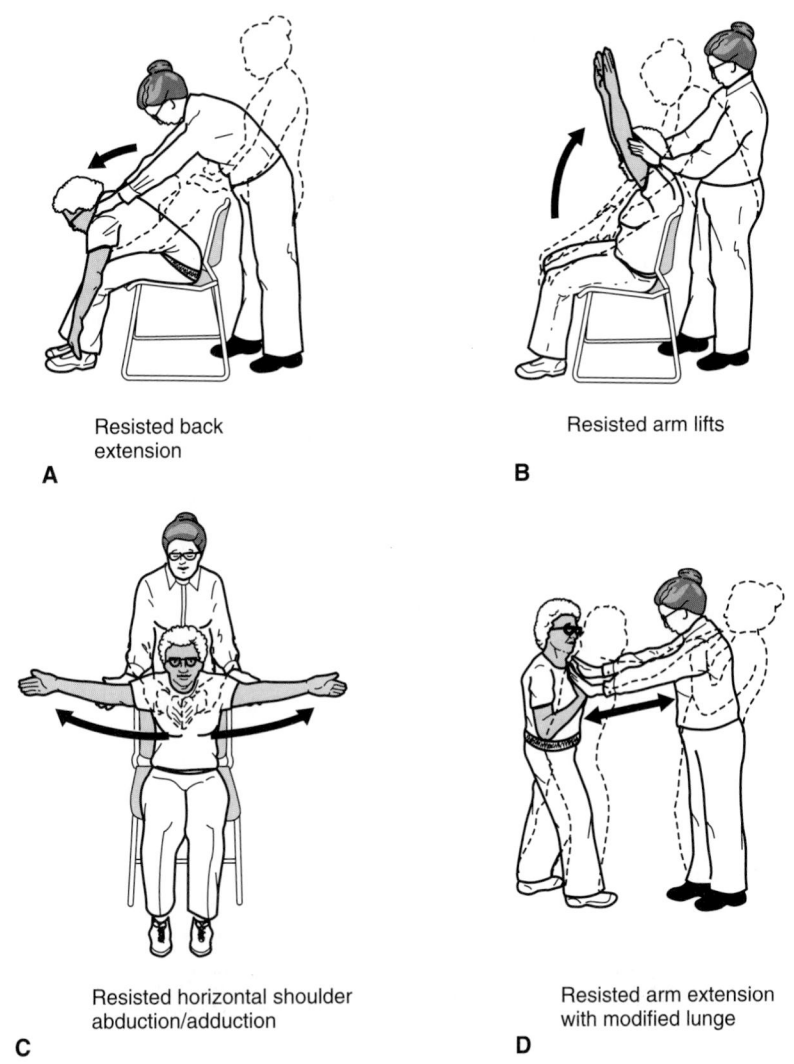

A, **Resisted back extension**

B, **Resisted arm lifts**

C, **Resisted horizontal shoulder abduction/adduction**

D, **Resisted arm extension with modified lunge**

Figure 2-14 Functional partnered exercise patterns. **A,** Resisted back extension. **B,** Resisted arm lifts. **C,** Resisted horizontal shoulder abduction/adduction. **D,** Resisted arm extension with modified lunge.

exercise program can be maintained for at least 2 years (Morey et al, 1996). Findings indicate that exercise, when performed in the course of everyday life situations, may have a significant role and meaning for older adults. Many factors, however, can affect the older adult's continued commitment to adopting and sustaining an effective level of habitual physical activity. A change in environment resulting from a geographic move, poor access to equipment or services, cost, and an exacerbation of a chronic ailment are only a few of the circumstances that may be faced in real life. Any of these interruptions may contribute to "a break in training"; however, emphasis must be placed on continuous training, which is necessary to maintain the health benefits from exercise.

Although self-paced exercise protocols have shown promise as safe, effective, and acceptable exercise models for primary and secondary prevention in the general population of community-dwelling older adults (Morey et al, 1996; Rooks et al, 1997), experts suggest that more than 50% of patients drop out of recommended exercise programs within the first 6 months (Kligman and Pepin,

1992). Experts note that exercise is unique among all health behaviors because it takes more time and effort than any other health behavior. For instance, a 30-minute exercise session is not really limited to half an hour. The individual may have to travel somewhere, change clothes, and shower afterwards, adding up to a large portion of time in a person's day. Exercise is a complex set of acts that includes planning for participation, initial adoption of physical activity, and continued participation or maintenance. Experts estimate that beginning exercisers probably spend 2 minutes of preparation to exercise 1 minute; thus the burden on a person's schedule is significant. With that in mind, if people are not enjoying themselves, the risk of discontinuing exercise is quite high.

Practitioners can enhance exercise compliance by clearly defining the expected health benefits of exercise for the individual patient and by selecting a type of activity the patient enjoys. The exercise, whether it is walking for 10 minutes three times a day, stepping up and down on benches or stools, or simply dancing to music in the living room, must not be simply repetitive, meaningless exercise but purposeful and engaging for the person on more than just a muscular level. Patients should be encouraged to exercise regularly, increase their pace gradually, and vary their activity to maximize both compliance and enjoyment. Recommending simple modifications of routine daily activities can be instrumental in reaching fitness goals. If the recommended activities fit into the patient's daily schedule and lifestyle, an exercise program is more likely to be followed.

ENSURING THAT FITNESS ACTIVITY REMAINS SAFE AND EFFECTIVE

Periodic assessment is critical given the normal age-related changes in the musculoskeletal, neurologic, and cardiopulmonary systems that, over time, result in patient-specific declines in function for the older patient. Physical fitness programs must accommodate these age-associated changes to remain safe and effective. Therefore the practitioner must periodically assess and, if applicable, modify the exercise program to fit normal age-related changes or the insult of a new disability.

Providing routine follow-up visits after the initial assessment is also important to encourage patients to continue with their fitness program. Without encouragement, many patients discontinue the exercise and lose the progress made in slowing the decline associated with the normal aging process. Suggested follow-up intervals include quarterly for the first year, every 6 months for the next 2 years, and annually in the fourth and fifth years. The follow-up, with measurements compared with the initial assessment, can provide a feeling of accomplishment and motivate patients.

Follow-up by the practitioner or office staff is recommended. Maintaining a simple list in an office personal computer of patients with care plans that include exercise can prompt occasional telephone calls to verify compliance. Telephone contact should be made 2 weeks and then 3 months after the evaluations to ensure patient compliance with the exercise program. Follow-up testing can be performed at 6 months or 1 year to assess improvement in physical fitness and provide further motivation to continue the exercise program. This visit is a good time to repeat an exercise stress test to assess the impact of the exercise program.

Special Considerations for the Older Adult

Pain and discomfort, such as angina pectoris, dyspnea, intermittent claudication, or joint pain, are likely to be observed in older patients and are reasons for decreasing or even stopping an exercise session. Skin color, changes in coordination, cognition, equilibrium, and blood pressure should be monitored, especially within the first 5 minutes of recovery after exercise; older adults may tend to have blood pooled in the lower extremities, which limits the adequacy of regional blood flow. The exercise intensity needs to be decreased if these complications occur.

Some clinicians who deal with exercise and injury in older adults have reported relatively no complaints of orthopedic discomfort in most of their deconditioned exercisers who completed 3 months of low-intensity flexibility and strengthening activities (Brown, 2000). On the other hand, these same clinicians did report pain complaints in a significant percentage of their patients who completed 6 months of high-intensity training. Most painful episodes were classified as nonspecific joint pain, probably of osteoarthritic origin and usually at the knee or ankle-foot. The point is that some form of orthopedic discomfort should be expected when older adults do endurance training. The clinicians recommend that patients should be told up front to expect the potential discomfort and pain and that the practitioner is there to provide needed care for such problems. Conservative measures such as icing, rest, elastic wrapping, nonsteroidal antiinflammatory drugs, and modification of the exercise program succeed in managing almost all pain.

At times, pain complaints may be attributed to musculotendinous injuries. Muscle injuries include strains, sprains, overuse, contusions, and compartment syndrome. The injured muscle or tendon is placed at significant risk for complete rupture of the muscle or tendon if subjected to high tensile force. Therefore premature return to activity may magnify the risk of rupture. If the injury is not addressed adequately and the patient continues to perform at a higher level of activity, a cycle of repetitive tissue failure develops.

Osteoporosis is common in older adults, especially in women. The risk of osteoporotic fractures in older adults, especially of the wrist, spine, or hip, is also prevalent. Exercise programs to help delay loss of bone mass should include flexibility and strength training in the major (large) muscle groups; weight-bearing activities; and certain aerobic activities that can increase flexibility, strength, and static and dynamic balance (e.g., tai chi, stair-climbing, or walking). Patients who have severe osteoporosis should exercise caution.

- Avoid high-impact activities such as jogging.
- Avoid activities in which participants tend to fall (e.g., ice-skating, bicycling).
- Gradually increase the intensity and complexity of activities, especially those that exert sudden ballistic movements of the extremities (e.g., tennis, golf).
- Adapt weight-bearing activities to patients' movement abilities.

Back pain is also prevalent, and for most patients a simple treatment approach of rest and reduction of the activities that cause the pain should be the first intervention. Heat or cold and nonsteroidal antiinflammatory medication can also reduce pain.

For patients experiencing cervical pain, home cervical traction (over the door) and an isometric program with gradual progression to isotonic cervical exercises may be useful. Swimming with a face mask and snorkel to limit cervical ROM and take advantage of the water buoyancy can be done to continue a moderate level of physical fitness.

For thoracolumbar pain, traditional back exercises such as Williams' flexion exercises and MacKenzie extension exercises may encourage thoracolumbar flexibility and strength. If the patient is overweight, weight reduction is mandatory to reduce loading of the spine. Fitness activities for patients who have a propensity for thoracolumbar pain include walking (level surfaces), swimming, and aquatic exercise. If sitting is tolerated, sessions of 15 minutes two to three times a day on a stationary bike can also be beneficial. Chronic thoracolumbar pain patients should avoid high-impact and vigorous anaerobic types of activities and focus on aerobic activities.

Wearing shoes for exercising is important. The selection of an appropriate shoe depends on the type of exercise and the patient's foot profile (e.g., rigid cavus foot, pes planus, hammer toes). The following characteristics should be considered:

- Cushioning is the resilient property of the midsole, shoe tongue, collar of the shoe, and heel. The purpose of cushioning is to protect the feet from pressure and friction.
- Firm heel counters that aid in rear foot stability are important during gait.
- Choose a wide and high toe box that is wide enough to allow the foot and toes to splay outward when the person is standing. The toe box should be high enough so that the toes are not touching the top of the box.
- Flexibility is important at the ball of the foot with the forefoot.
- Shock absorption is usually found at the heel and sometimes at the ball of the foot. Shoes with no shock absorption can promote muscle fatigue and pain in the feet and legs.
- Variable lacing systems allow fitting the shoe to the foot and accommodate structural irregularities, swelling or contracting from the weather or the time of day, and shoe wear.

Summary

Regular physical exercise for the older adult delays many physical and psychologic problems that commonly occur with aging. It can provide the foundation to support an older adult's ability to achieve activities of daily living and ultimately to improve overall function and quality of life. National recognition of a new training alternative in cardiorespiratory and muscular fitness should certainly encourage greater participation by older well adults and inspire engagement in a healthier lifestyle.

Designing an appropriate physical exercise program is a complex task. A preexercise assessment is a required step that the practitioner must take before prescribing a program for well older adults. By including a limited physical examination, cardiovascular testing, and assessments of flexibility, strength, and balance, the practitioner will be able to prescribe a safe, effective, and individualized program that will help ensure continued patient participation. Taking this opportunity to record baseline information and establishing an office habit of contacting patients at a later time (i.e., follow-up contacts) will not only encourage continued participation but also ensure that the patient's physical exercise program remains safe and effective in meeting the changing health needs that occur with aging. Routine physical exercise is an inexpensive approach toward maintaining a healthier lifestyle and overall well-being for the older well adult.

Resources

American Physical Therapy Association
www.geriatricspt.org

Senior Site Web Page
www.senior-infosite.com

References

American Academy of Orthopedic Surgeons: *Joint motion: method of measuring and recording,* Edinburgh, 1996, Churchill Livingstone.

American College of Sports Medicine: Position stand on the recommended quantity and quality of exercise for developing and maintaining cardiorespiratory and muscular fitness in adults, *Med Sci Sports Exerc* 22:265-274, 1990.

American College of Sports Medicine: The recommended quantity and quality of exercise for developing and maintaining cardiorespiratory and muscular fitness and flexibility in healthy adults, *Med Sci Sports Exerc* 30(6):975-991, 1998.

American Thoracic Society: ATS statement: snowbird workshop on standardization of spirometry, *Am Rev Respir Dis* 119:831, 1979.

Beere PA et al: Aerobic exercise training can reverse age-related peripheral circulatory changes in healthy older men, *Circulation* 100(10):1085-1094, 1999.

Bellew JW: The effect of strength training on control of force in older men and women, *Aging* 14(1):35-41, 2002.

Boyette LW et al: Personal characteristics that influence exercise behavior of older adults, *J Rehabil Res Dev* 39(1):95-103, 2002.

Brandao Rondon MU et al: Postexercise blood pressure reduction in elderly hypertensive patients, *J Am Coll Cardiol* 39(4):676-682, 2002.

Brown M: Muscle fatigue and impaired endurance in older adults. In Guccione AA, editor: *Geriatric physical therapy,* ed 2, St Louis, 2000, Mosby.

Centers for Disease Control and Prevention: Surgeon General's workshop on health promotion and aging: summary recommendations of the Physical Fitness and Exercise Working Group, *MMWR* 38(41):700-707, 1989.

Chandler JM: Balance and falls in the elderly. In Guccione AA, editor: *Geriatric physical therapy,* ed 2, St Louis, 2000, Mosby.

Cunningham DA, Imgram KJ, Rechnitzer PA: The effect of training: physiological responses, *Med Sci Sports Exerc* 11:379, 1979.

D'Acquisto LJ, D'Acquisto DM, Renne D: Metabolic and cardiovascular responses in older women during shallow-water exercise, *J Strength Cond Res* 15(1):12-19, 2001.

Fatouros IG et al: The effects of strength training, cardiovascular training and their combination on flexibility of inactive older adults, *Int J Sports Med* 23(2):112-119, 2002

Fillit HM et al: Achieving and maintaining cognitive vitality with aging, *Mayo Clin Proc* 77(7):681-696, 2002.

Gardner MM et al: Application of a falls prevention program for older people to primary care practice, *Prev Med* 34(5):546-553, 2002.

Gill TM, DiPietro L, Krumholz HM: Role of exercise stress testing and safety monitoring for older persons starting an exercise program, *JAMA* 284(3):342-348, 2002.

Jensen J, Lundin-Olsson L et al: Fall and injury prevention in older people living in residential care facilities. a cluster randomized trial, *Ann Intern Med* 136(100):733-741, 2002.

Kligman EW, Pepin E: Prescribing physical activity for older patients, *Geriatrics* 47(8):34, 1992.

Mather AS et al: Effects of exercise on depressive symptoms in older adults with poorly responsive depressive disorder: randomized controlled trial, *Br J Psychiatry* 180;411-415, 2002.

Mathias S, Nayak U, Isaacs B: Balance in elderly patients: the get-up and go test, *Arch Phys Med Rehabil* 68:305, 1987.

Mazzeo RS, Tanaka H: Exercise prescription for the elderly: current recommendations, *Sports Med* 31(11):809-818, 2001.

Morey MC et al: Five-year performance trends for older exercises: a hierarchical model of endurance, strength, and flexibility, *J Am Geriatr Soc* 44(10):1226-1231, 1996.

Pate RR et al: Physical activity and public health. A recommendation from the Centers for Disease Control and Prevention and the American College of Sports Medicine, *JAMA* 273(5):402-407, 1995.

Pearson TA et al: AHA guidelines for primary prevention of cardiovascular disease and stroke: 2002 update: consensus panel guide to comprehensive risk reduction for adult patients without coronary or other atherosclerotic vascular diseases, *Circulation* 106:388-391, 2002.

Penninx BW et al: Exercise and depressive symptoms: a comparison of aerobic and resistance exercise effects on emotional and physical function in older persons with high and low depressive symptomatology, *J Gerontol B Psychol Sci Soc Sci* 57(2):P124-P132, 2002.

Richardson JK, Sandman D, Vela S: A focused exercise regimen improves clinical measures of balance in patients with peripheral neuropathy, *Arch Phys Med Rehabil* 82(2):205-209, 2001.

Rooks DS et al: Self-paced resistance training and walking exercise in community-dwelling older adults: effects on neuromotor performance, *J Gerontol A Biol Sci Med Sci* 52(3):161-168, 1997.

Schenkman M et al: The relative importance of strength and balance in chair rise by functionally impaired older individuals, *J Am Geriatr Soc* 44:1441-1446, 1996.

Seeman T, Chen X: Risk and protective factors for physical functioning in older adults with and without chronic conditions: MacArthur Studies of Successful Aging, *J Gerontol B Psychol Sci Soc Sci* 57(3):S135-S144, 2002.

Sidney KH, Shephard RJ: Frequency and intensity of exercise training for elderly subjects, *Med Sci Sports Exerc* 10:125, 1978.

Taggart HM: Self-reported benefits of t'ai chi practice by older women, *J Holist Nurs* 19(3):223-32, 2001.

Takeshima N et al: Water-based exercise improves health-related aspects of fitness in older women, *Med Sci Sports Exerc* 34(3):544-551.2, 2002.

U.S. Department of Health and Human Services: *Healthy people 2010: understanding and improving health*, ed 2, Washington, DC, 2000, US Government Printing Office.

Vincent KR et al: Resistance exercise and physical performance in adults aged 60 to 83, *J Am Geriatr Soc* 50(6):1100-1107, 2002.

Wolf S et al: The effect of tai chi and computerized balance training on postural stability in older subjects, *Phys Ther* 77:371-381, 1997.

Wolf S et al: Reducing frailty and falls in older persons: an investigation of tai chi and computerized balance training, *J Am Geriatr Soc* 44:489-497, 1996.

Wu G: Evaluation of the effectiveness of Tai Chi for improving balance and prevention falls in the older population—a review, *J Am Geriatr Soc* 50(4):746-754, 2002.

Yalden J, Chung L: Tai Chi: towards an exercise program for the older person, *Aust J Holist Nurs* 8(1):4-13, 2001.

3

Nutrition

Health promotion is an integral aspect of primary care. Changes in diet and exercise patterns of older adults can be effective in the promotion of healthy lifestyles and in the prevention of certain nutrition-related conditions (Chernoff, 2001). Primary care practitioners need to assess their patients' health practices in relation to diet and exercise regularly. For older healthy adults assessment includes weight measurement and a review of normal dietary intake and normal physical activity. At each visit a review of medications with the intent to check for any interaction with food is a consideration that is frequently overlooked.

General Guidelines

The 2000 Dietary Guidelines for Americans cosponsored and issued by the U.S. Department of Health and Human Services and the U.S. Department of Agriculture (2001) offer practical advice and scientific information for the American consumer. The guidelines give 10 recommendations that are grouped in three areas: "Aim for Fitness," "Build a Healthy Base," and "Choose Sensibly" (Box 3-1). There is new emphasis on the relationship of maintaining a healthy weight and physical activity (Figure 3-1). See Chapter 2 for appropriate physical exercise recommendations.

The guidelines continue to stress balance and moderation in food choices with reliance on the 1992 Food Pyramid (Figure 3-2 and Box 3-2). Choosing the best foods that meet the dietary guidelines is not an intuitive process. Boxes 3-3 and 3-4 show how to assist patients in maximizing their food choices.

In response to the recent and continuing outbreaks of food-borne illnesses, the guidelines for the first time address the important issue of food safety in regard to storage and preparation of food in the home (Box 3-5). The guidelines can be downloaded from the Internet at www.health.gov/dietaryguidelines.

Supplements

Vitamins are a type of nutrient that is not produced by the body and must be obtained from food. They are classified as fat-soluble or water-soluble vitamins. Fat-soluble vitamins like vitamin A can accumulate in the body, whereas water-soluble vitamins such as vitamin C do not. A review of the

Aim for Fitness

1. Aim for a healthy weight.
2. Be physically active each day

Build a Healthy Base

3. Let the Pyramid guide your food choices.
4. Choose a variety of grains daily, especially whole grains.
5. Choose a variety of fruits and vegetables daily.
6. Keep food safe to eat.

Choose Sensibly

7. Choose a diet that is low in saturated fat and cholesterol and moderate in total fat.
8. Choose beverages and foods to moderate your intake of sugars.
9. Choose and prepare foods with less salt.
10. If you drink alcoholic beverages, do so in moderation.

From U.S. Department of Health and Human Services, U.S. Department of Agriculture: *Nutrition and your health: dietary guidelines for Americans*, ed 5, Washington, DC, 2001, US Government Printing Office.

research investigating the benefits and risks of antioxidant supplements is beyond the scope of this chapter. An excellent review from the Harvard Medical School Guide to Healthy Eating was written for the public (Willett, 2001), and Griffith wrote an excellent handbook for practitioners on vitamins (Griffith, 2000).

Vitamin and mineral supplements cannot replace food as the mainstay of a healthy diet. Some people need a supplement to meet a specific nutrient deficiency, but most do not. What is needed is a rational approach to supplements, not a response to whatever the newest fad or advertisement claims. Primary care practitioners need to stress the risks of toxicity if older adults are taking several multiple vitamins, herbal remedies, mineral supplements, and megadoses of certain vitamins such as vitamin A.

For older adults a recommended daily allowance (RDA)-level multivitamin, especially if the label indicates it meets the standards of the United States Pharmacopeia (USP), is the best insurance for a healthy diet. One recommendation that is being made more frequently is for older adults to consider taking an extra 400-mg vitamin E supplement on a daily basis, but not a megadose; more is not better (Willett, 2001).

Optimizing Intake for Debilitating Conditions/Malnutrition

For patients with debilitating conditions, the goal of the diet may be to maximize calorie and protein intake to promote healing. Emphasis should then be placed on substituting lower-calorie and lower-protein foods with those containing higher quantities. Examples of food choices include the following:

Dairy: Encourage whole milk, cheeses, cottage cheese, puddings, and custards made from whole milk; use cheese or cream sauces on entrees and vegetables. Fortified milk can be made by adding dry milk powder to milk for an increased nutrition content. Persons who are lactose intolerant can use Lactaid milk.

Meats and meat substitutes: Encourage meats (all varieties), fish, eggs, peanut butter, and beans.

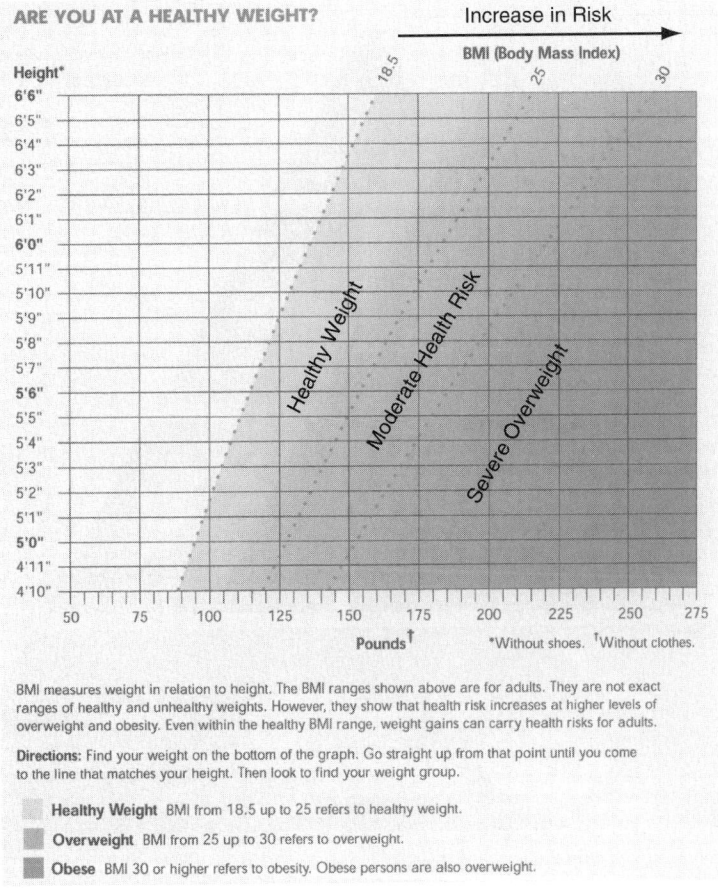

Figure 3-1   Body mass index (BMI) chart. (From U.S. Department of Health and Human Services, U.S. Department of Agriculture: *Nutrition and your health: dietary guidelines for Americans*, ed 5, Washington, DC, 2001, US Government Printing Office.)

Fats: Add margarine or butter on breads, hot cereals, and vegetables; use oils in cooking.

Soups: Substitute cream soups for broth-based varieties.

Supplements: Commercial nutritional supplements can be used but may be expensive for many; a lower-cost alternate is powdered breakfast mix (use with whole milk).

It may also be helpful to encourage multiple small meals and snacks throughout the day in place of three larger meals, especially if early satiety or poor appetite is a problem. Numerous studies of the prevalence of malnutrition in hospitals have been conducted in the past 25 years. They indicate that the incidence of malnutrition ranges from 30% to 50% (Coats et al, 1993). Nutrition screening programs of geriatric populations in both institutional and community settings report malnutrition risk rates ranging from 25% to 85% (Wellman et al, 1997). Typical causes of malnutrition in older persons are chewing or swallowing disorders, cardiac insufficiency, depression, social deprivation, and loneliness (Pirlich and Lochs, 2001), decreased food intake, sedentary lifestyle, reduced energy expenditure, and residing alone in a large urban area (Meydani, 2001; Millen and Silliman, 2001). Malnutrition may not be identified in older adults because the changes that occur with malnutrition may instead be attributed to those that occur with aging. Patients who are mildly or moderately

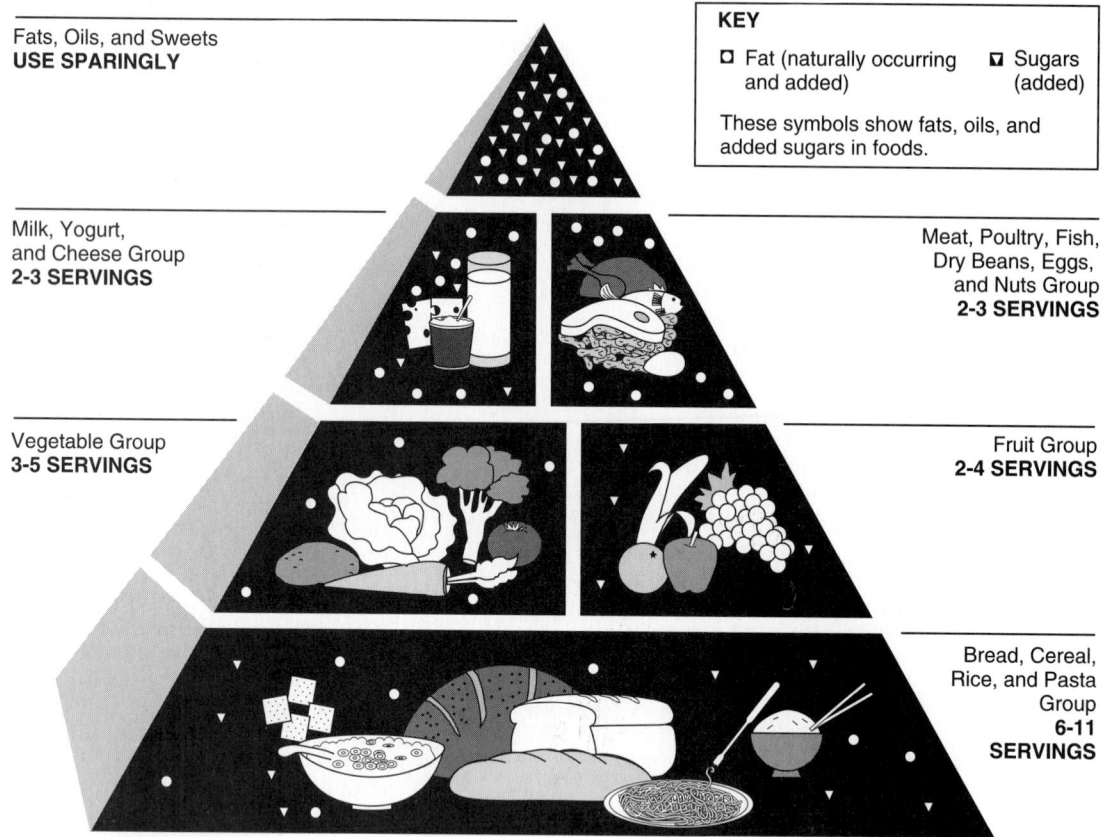

Fats, Oils, and Sweets
USE SPARINGLY

KEY
◻ Fat (naturally occurring   ▼ Sugars
   and added)   (added)
These symbols show fats, oils, and
added sugars in foods.

Milk, Yogurt,
and Cheese Group
2-3 SERVINGS

Meat, Poultry, Fish,
Dry Beans, Eggs,
and Nuts Group
2-3 SERVINGS

Vegetable Group
3-5 SERVINGS

Fruit Group
2-4 SERVINGS

Bread, Cereal,
Rice, and Pasta
Group
**6-11
SERVINGS**

What Counts as a Serving?

With the Food Guide Pyramid, what counts as a "serving"
may not always be a typical "helping" of what you eat.
Here are some examples of servings:

Bread, Cereal, Rice and Pasta - 6-11 servings recommended
Examples of one serving:
1 slice of bread
1 oz. of ready-to-eat cereal
1/2 cup of cooked cereal, rice, or pasta
3 or 4 small plain crackers

Vegetables - 3-5 servings recommended
Examples of one serving:
1 cup of raw leafy vegetables
1/2 cup of other vegetables, cooked or chopped raw
3/4 cup of vegetable juice

Fruits - 2-4 servings recommended
Examples of one serving:
1 medium apple, banana, or orange
1/2 cup of chopped, cooked, or canned fruit
3/4 cup of fruit juice

Milk, Yogurt, and Cheese - 2-3 servings
recommended
Examples of one serving:
1 cup of milk or yogurt
1 1/2 oz. of natural cheese
2 oz. of process cheese

Meat, Poultry, Fish, Dry Beans, Eggs, and Nuts -
2-3 servings recommended
Examples of one serving:
2-3 oz. of cooked lean meat, poultry, or fish
1/2 cup of cooked dry beans,
1 egg, or 2 tablespoons
of peanut butter = 1 oz. of lean meat

How Much Is an Ounce of Meat?

Here's a handy guide to determining how much
meat, chicken, fish, or cheese weigh:
1 ounce is the size of a **match box.**
3 ounces are the size of a **deck of cards.**
8 ounces are the size of a **paperback book.**

Figure 3-2 Food guide pyramid. (Source: U.S. Department of Agriculture.)

Box 3-2

The Food Guide Pyramid: Putting the Dietary Guidelines into Action

Learning to eat right is now made simpler with the new Food Guide Pyramid by the U.S. Department of Agriculture (USDA). The Pyramid is a graphic description of what registered dietitians and other nutrition experts have been advising for years: Build your diet on a base of grains, vegetables, and fruits. Add moderate quantities of lean meat (poultry, fish, eggs, legumes) and dairy products, and limit the intake of fats and sweets.

The Food Guide Pyramid illustrates how to turn the Dietary Guidelines for Americans (issued by USDHHS/USDA in 1990) into real food choices.

The Dietary Guidelines—and their relationship to the Food Guide Pyramid—are as follows:

- **Eat a variety of foods**. The body needs more than 40 different nutrients for good health, and because no single food can supply all these nutrients, variety is crucial. Variety can be ensured by choosing foods each day from the five major groups shown in the Pyramid: (1) Breads, Cereals, Rice & Pasta (6-11 servings); vegetables (3-5 servings); (3) fruits (2-4 servings), (4) milk, yogurt & cheese (2-3 servings); (5) meat, poultry, fish, dry beans, eggs and nuts (2-3 servings) and (6) fats, oils and sweets (use sparingly).
- **Maintain healthy weight**. Being overweight or underweight increases the risk of developing health problems, so it is important to consume the right amount of calories each day. The number of calories needed for ideal weight (which varies according to height, frame, age, and activity) will generally determine how many servings in the Pyramid are needed.
- **Choose a diet low in fat, saturated fat, and cholesterol**. As shown in the Pyramid, fats and oils should be used sparingly because diets high in fat are associated with obesity, certain types

of cancer, and heart disease. A diet low in fat also makes it easier to include a variety of foods because fat contains more than twice the calories of an equal amount of carbohydrates or protein.
- **Choose a diet with plenty of vegetables, fruits, and grain products**. Vegetables, fruits, and grains provide the complex carbohydrates, vitamins, minerals, and dietary fiber needed for good health. Also, they are generally low in fat. To obtain the different kinds of fiber contained in these foods, it is best to eat a variety.
- **Use sugars only in moderation**. Sugars, and many foods containing large amounts of sugars, supply calories but are limited in nutrients. Thus they should be used in moderation by most healthy people and sparingly by those with low calorie needs. Sugars, as well as foods that contain starch (which breaks down into sugars), can also contribute to tooth decay. The longer foods containing sugars or starches remain in the mouth before teeth are brushed, the greater the risk for tooth decay. Some examples of foods that contain starches are milk, fruits, some vegetables, breads, and cereals.
- **Use salt and sodium only in moderation**. Table salt contains sodium and chloride, which are essential to good health; however, most Americans eat more than they need. Much of the sodium in people's diets comes from salt they add while cooking and at the table. Sodium is also added during food processing and manufacturing.
- **If you drink alcoholic beverages, do so in moderation**. Alcoholic beverages contain calories but little or no nutrients. Consumption of alcohol is linked with many health problems, causes many accidents, and can lead to addiction. Therefore alcohol consumption is not recommended.

Adapted from *At the Center*, National Center for Nutrition and Dietetics, Chicago, Summer 1992.

malnourished may not be diagnosed as being malnourished. The consequences of malnutrition can be dramatic. Malnourished patients experience 2 to 20 times more complications and have up to 100% longer hospital stays, which can cost $2000 to $10,000 more per stay. Along with these longer and more expensive hospitalizations, malnourished patients have more frequent readmissions, riskier surgeries, delayed recovery times, and premature nursing home admissions. All these factors contribute to a decreased quality of life and significantly increased health care costs (Wellman et al, 1997).

Box 3-3

How to Increase Your Intake of Whole Grain Foods

Choose foods that name one of the following ingredients *first* on the label's ingredient list:
- Brown rice
- Oatmeal
- Whole oats
- Bulgur (cracked wheat)
- Popcorn
- Whole rye
- Graham flour
- Pearl barley
- Whole wheat
- Whole grain corn

Try some of these whole grain foods: whole wheat bread, whole grain ready-to-eat cereal, low-fat whole wheat crackers, oatmeal, whole wheat pasta, whole barley in soup, tabouli salad.

From U.S. Department of Health and Human Services, U.S. Department of Agriculture: *Nutrition and your health: dietary guidelines for Americans,* ed 5, Washington, DC, 2001, US Government Printing Office.
NOTE: Wheat flour, enriched flour, and degerminated corn meal are not whole grains.

Age-related Changes

Numerous body composition changes accompany aging. They include a decrease in lean body mass (which results in a decline in the basal metabolic rate), an increase in the relative amount of adipose tissue, a decline in total body water, and a decrease in bone density. Physiologic function of organs may change with age. Gastrointestinal motility and digestive or absorptive capacity may decrease. Maintenance of bowel function through exercise, adequate fluids, and fiber will be an important goal. Oral health may decline; typically dentition decreases, and cavities increase. Finally, there are declines in thirst, taste, and smell sensitivity.

Risk Factors and Indicators of Poor Nutritional Status

Nutritional risk factors are characteristics that increase the likelihood that a patient has or will have problems with nutritional status. They include an inappropriate food intake, poverty, social isolation, dependency or disability, acute or chronic diseases or conditions, chronic medication use, and advanced age.

Specific indicators of poor nutritional status provide evidence that poor nutritional status is present. They are broken down into major and minor indicators as follows.

MAJOR INDICATORS OF POOR NUTRITIONAL STATUS

- Weight loss of 10 or more pounds
- Underweight or overweight
- Serum albumin below 3.5 g/dl
- Nutrition-related disorders
- Inappropriate food intake
- Triceps skinfold < 10th percentile or > 95th percentile
- Change in functional status
- Midarm muscle circumference < 10th percentile

Which Fruits and Vegetables Provide the Most Nutrients?

The lists below show which fruits and vegetables are the best sources of vitamin A (carotenoids), vitamin C, folate, and potassium. Eat at least two servings of fruits and at least three servings of vegetables each day:

Sources of Vitamin A (Carotenoids)

- Orange vegetables such as carrots, sweet potatoes, pumpkin
- Dark-green leafy vegetables such as spinach, collard greens, turnip greens
- Orange fruits such as mango, cantaloupe, apricots
- Tomatoes

Sources of Vitamin C

- Citrus fruits and juices, kiwi fruit, strawberries, cantaloupe
- Broccoli, peppers, tomatoes, cabbage, potatoes
- Leafy greens such as romaine lettuce, turnip greens, spinach

Sources of Folate

- Cooked dry beans and peas, peanuts
- Oranges, orange juice
- Dark-green leafy vegetables such as spinach, mustard greens, romaine lettuce
- Green peas

Sources of Potassium

- Baked white or sweet potatoes, cooked greens such as spinach, winter (orange) squash
- Bananas, plantains, dried fruits such as apricots and prunes, orange juice
- Cooked dry beans such as baked beans, lentils

From U.S. Department of Health and Human Services, U.S. Department of Agriculture: *Nutrition and your health: dietary guidelines for Americans,* ed 5, Washington, DC, 2001, US Government Printing Office.

MINOR INDICATORS OF POOR NUTRITIONAL STATUS

- Alcoholism
- Cognitive impairment
- Chronic renal insufficiency
- Multiple concurrent medications
- Malabsorption syndromes
- Anorexia, nausea, dysphagia
- Change in bowel habit
- Fatigue, apathy, memory loss
- Poor oral or dental status
- Dehydration
- Poorly healing wounds
- Loss of subcutaneous fat or muscle mass
- Fluid retention
- Reduced iron, ascorbic acid, zinc

The presence of these risk factors or indicators should serve as a warning that the patient's nutritional status may be poor, and further assessment is warranted. The Determine Your Nutritional

Box 3-5
Food Safety

1. **Clean. Wash hands and surfaces often**
   Wash your hands with warm soapy water for 20 seconds (count to 30) before you handle food or food utensils. Wash your hands after handling or preparing food, especially after handling raw meat, poultry, fish, shellfish, or eggs. Right after you prepare these raw foods, clean the utensils and surfaces you used with hot soapy water. Replace cutting boards once they have become worn or develop hard-to-clean grooves. Wash raw fruit and vegetables under running water before eating. Use a vegetable brush to remove surface dirt if necessary. Always wash your hands after using the bathroom, changing diapers, or playing with pets. When eating out, if the tables, dinnerware, and restrooms look dirty, the kitchen may be, too—so you may want to eat somewhere else.

2. **Separate. Separate raw, cooked, and ready-to-eat foods while shopping, preparing, or storing**
   Keep raw meat, poultry, eggs, fish, and shellfish away from other foods, surfaces, utensils, or serving plates. This prevents cross-contamination from one food to another. Store raw meat, poultry, fish, and shellfish in containers in the refrigerator so that the juices don't drip onto other foods.

3. **Cook. Cook foods to a safe temperature**
   Uncooked and undercooked animal foods are potentially unsafe. Proper cooking makes most uncooked foods safe. The best way to tell if meat, poultry, or egg dishes are cooked to a safe temperature is to use a food thermometer. Several kinds of inexpensive food thermometers are available in many stores.

   Reheat sauces, soups, marinades, and gravies to a boil. Reheat leftovers thoroughly to at least 165°F. If using a microwave oven, cover the container and turn or stir the food to make sure it is heated evenly throughout. Cook eggs until whites and yolks are firm. Don't eat raw or partially cooked eggs, or foods containing raw eggs, raw (unpasteurized) milk, or cheeses made with raw milk. Choose pasteurized juices. The risk of contamination is high from undercooked hamburger, and from raw fish (including sushi), clams, and oysters. Cook fish and shellfish until it is opaque; fish should flake easily with a fork. When eating out, order foods thoroughly cooked and make sure they are served piping hot.

4. **Chill. Refrigerate perishable foods promptly**
   When shopping, buy perishable foods last, and take them straight home. At home, refrigerate or freeze meat, poultry, eggs, fish, shellfish, ready-to-eat foods, and leftovers promptly. Refrigerate within 2 hours of purchasing or preparation—and within 1 hour if the air temperature is above 90°F. Refrigerate at or below 40°F, or freeze at or below 0°F. Use refrigerated leftovers within 3 to 4 days. Freeze fresh meat, poultry, fish, and shellfish that cannot be used in a few days. Thaw frozen meat, poultry, fish, and shellfish in the refrigerator, microwave, or cold water changed every 30 minutes. (This keeps the surface chilled.) Cook foods immediately after thawing. Never thaw meat, poultry, fish, or shellfish at room temperature. When eating out, make sure that any foods you order that should be refrigerated are served chilled.

5. **Follow the label**
   Read the label and follow safety instructions on the package such as "KEEP REFRIGERATED" and the "SAFE HANDLING INSTRUCTIONS."

6. **Serve safely**
   Keep hot foods hot (140°F or above) and cold foods cold (40°F or below). Harmful bacteria can grow rapidly in the "danger zone" between these temperatures. Whether raw or cooked, never leave meat, poultry, eggs, fish, or shellfish out at room temperature for more than 2 h (1 h in hot weather 90°F or above). Be sure to chill leftovers as soon as you are finished eating. These guidelines also apply to carry-out meals, restaurant leftovers, and home-packed meals-to-go.

7. **When in doubt, throw it out**
   If you are unsure that food has been prepared, served, or stored safely, throw it out. You may not be able to make food safe if it has been handled in an unsafe manner. For example, a food that has been left at room temperature too long may contain a toxin produced by bacteria—one that can't be destroyed by cooking. So if meat, poultry, fish, shellfish, or eggs have been left out for more than 2 h, or if the food has been kept in the refrigerator too long, don't taste it. Just throw it out. Even if it looks and smells fine, it may not be safe to eat. If you have doubt when you're shopping or eating out, choose something else.

From U.S. Departments of Health and Human Services, U.S. Department of Agriculture: *Nutrition and your health: dietary guidelines for Americans*, ed 5, 2001, Washington, DC, U.S. Government Printing Office.

The Warning Signs of poor nutritional health are often overlooked. Use this checklist to find out if you or someone you know is at nutritional risk.

Read the statements below. Circle the number in the yes column for those that apply to you or someone you know. For each yes answer, score the number in the box. Total your nutritional score.

DETERMINE YOUR NUTRITIONAL HEALTH

	YES
I have an illness or condition that made me change the kind and/or amount of food I eat.	2
I eat fewer than 2 meals per day.	3
I eat few fruits or vegetables, or milk products.	2
I have 3 or more drinks of beer, liquor or wine almost every day.	2
I have tooth or mouth problems that make it hard for me to eat.	2
I don't always have enough money to buy the food I need.	4
I eat alone most of the time.	1
I take 3 or more different prescribed or over-the-counter drugs a day.	1
Without wanting to, I have lost or gained 10 pounds in the last 6 months.	2
I am not always physically able to shop, cook and/or feed myself.	2
TOTAL	

Total Your Nutritional Score. If it's —

0-2   **Good!** Recheck your nutritional score in 6 months.

3-5   **You are at moderate nutritional risk.** See what can be done to improve your eating habits and lifestyle. Your office on aging, senior nutrition program, senior citizens center or health department can help. Recheck your nutritional score in 3 months.

6 or more   **You are at high nutritional risk.** Bring this checklist the next time you see your doctor, dietitian or other qualified health or social service professional. Talk with them about any problems you may have. Ask for help to improve your nutritional health.

These materials developed and distributed by the Nutrition Screening Initiative, a project of:

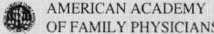 AMERICAN ACADEMY OF FAMILY PHYSICIANS

THE AMERICAN DIETETIC ASSOCIATION

NATIONAL COUNCIL ON THE AGING

Remember that warning signs suggest risk, but do not represent diagnosis of any condition. Turn the page to learn more about the Warning Signs of poor nutritional health.

The Nutrition Screening Initiative is funded in part by a grant from Ross Laboratories, a division of Abbott Laboratories.

Figure 3-3 Checklist to determine nutritional health. (Reprinted with permission of the Nutrition Screening Initiative, a project of the American Academy of Family Physicians, the American Dietetic Association, and the National Council on the Aging, Inc., and funded in part by a grant from Ross Products Division, Abbott Laboratories, Inc.)

Continued

DISEASE

Any disease, illness or chronic condition which causes you to change the way you eat, or makes it hard for you to eat, puts your nutritional health at risk. Four out of five adults have chronic diseases that are affected by diet. Confusion or memory loss that keeps getting worse is estimated to affect one out of five or more of older adults. This can make it hard to remember what, when or if you've eaten. Feeling sad or depressed, which happens to about one in eight older adults, can cause big changes in appetite, digestion, energy level, weight and well-being.

EATING POORLY

Eating too little and eating too much both lead to poor health. Eating the same foods day after day or not eating fruit, vegetables, and milk products daily will also cause poor nutritional health. One in five adults skip meals daily. Only 13% of adults eat the minimum amount of fruit and vegetables needed. One in four older adults drink too much alcohol. Many health problems become worse if you drink more than one or two alcoholic beverages per day.

TOOTH LOSS/ MOUTH PAIN

A healthy mouth, teeth and gums are needed to eat. Missing, loose or rotten teeth or dentures which don't fit well or cause mouth sores make it hard to eat.

ECONOMIC HARDSHIP

As many as 40% of older Americans have incomes of less than $6,000 per year. Having less--or choosing to spend less--than $25-30 per week for food makes it very hard to get the foods you need to stay healthy.

REDUCED SOCIAL CONTACT

One-third of all older people live alone. Being with people daily has a positive effect on morale, well-being and eating.

MULTIPLE MEDICINES

Many older Americans must take medicines for health problems. Almost half of older Americans take multiple medicines daily. Growing old may change the way we respond to drugs. The more medicines you take, the greater the chance for side effects such as increased or decreased appetite, change in taste, constipation, weakness, drowsiness, diarrhea, nausea, and others. Vitamins or minerals when taken in large doses act like drugs and can cause harm. Alert your doctor to everything you take.

INVOLUNTARY WEIGHT LOSS/GAIN

Losing or gaining a lot of weight when you are not trying to do so is an important warning sign that must not be ignored. Being overweight or underweight also increases your chance of poor health.

NEEDS ASSISTANCE IN SELF CARE

Although most older people are able to eat, one of every five have trouble walking, shopping, buying and cooking food, especially as they get older.

ELDER YEARS ABOVE AGE 80

Most older people lead full and productive lives. But as age increases, risk of frailty and health problems increase. Checking your nutritional health regularly makes good sense.

Figure 3-3,   cont'd.

Health checklist (Figure 3-3), developed by the Nutrition Screening Initiative (1992), is a good educational tool for increasing patients' and their families' awareness of nutritional risk factors. It enables early identification of potential nutrition-related problems and timely intervention to correct these problems (Sahyoun et al, 1997).

Assessment of Nutritional Status

Several parameters are used in assessing a patient's nutritional status.

WEIGHT

An ideal weight can be estimated by using the following formula:

For men 100 lb for the first 5 ft + 5 lb for each additional inch

Because older adults can vary greatly from such estimations of ideal body weight or from standard weights from the Metropolitan Life Insurance tables, a comparison of current to usual body weight is the most revealing on an individual basis (Posthauer and Russell, 1997). Significant involuntary weight loss is considered 5% in 1 month, 7.5% in 3 months, or 10% in 6 months. Weight loss is considered severe with losses greater than these percentages in the time frame specified (Posthauer and Russell, 1997). If actual weights are impossible to obtain, the next step is to determine whether clothes are now looser or observe for signs of weight loss such as loose, sagging skin or temporal wasting. In clinic or office settings, an actual weight should be obtained at each visit, with a note on whether clothes and shoes were worn when weight was taken.

The major causes of weight loss in older adults are social or psychiatric problems, medical conditions, and age-related changes. Older patients with unintentional weight loss are at higher risk for infection, depression, and death (Huffman, 2002). Often depression is a leading cause of unintentional weight loss, but other factors should be investigated, such as number and type of medications, cardiac disorders, malignancies, and gastrointestinal disorders. In at least 25% of cases no specific cause is identified. Each patient should receive a complete history and physical examination, fecal occult blood test, complete blood count, a chemistry panel, thyroid-stimulating hormone measurement, and a urinalysis. Management will focus on the underlying cause and nutritional support (Huffman, 2002). A period of watchful waiting with regular monitoring of the patient is appropriate before additional diagnostic testing is done (Moriguti and Moriguti, 2001).

BIOCHEMICAL ASSESSMENT

The biochemical assessment is another valuable element in a nutritional evaluation. Interpretation levels of the following laboratory values may vary slightly from institution to institution.

Albumin

Albumin is a carrier protein that is needed for the maintenance of oncotic pressure. Levels correlate well with the degree of malnutrition and the risk of mortality and morbidity (Fischbach, 1999). It is one of the most reliable biochemical indexes of malnutrition in older adults.
Interpretation:
2.8 to 3.5 g/dl: Mild depletion
2.1 to 2.7 g/dl: Moderate depletion
< 2.1 g/dl: Severe depletion

The limitations of using albumin (Covinsky and Covinsky, 2002) include its long half-life of 21 days, which makes it insensitive to acute changes in nutrition status. In addition, albumin values can be low because of nonnutritional factors such as liver disease, infection, fluid imbalances (edema, overhydration), nephrotic syndrome, postoperative states, and metabolic stress. It can be falsely elevated because of dehydration. If any of these factors are currently an issue for the patient, it may be helpful to recheck the value as the condition resolves. For instance, a severely dehydrated patient may present with a normal albumin, but once the patient is hydrated, obtaining an additional albumin will provide a more accurate interpretation of protein stores.

Prealbumin

Prealbumin is a more sensitive indicator of visceral protein status because of its short half-life of 2 to 3 days. An upward trend is a good indicator of appropriate intake and improving nutritional status.
Interpretation:
10 to 15 mg/dl: Mild depletion
5 to 10 mg/dl: Moderate depletion
< 5 mg/dl: Severe depletion

With adequate nutritional support, prealbumin levels increase by 4 to 5 mg/dl a week. An increase of less than 2 mg/dl a week reflects either an inadequate intake of protein or kilocalories or an inadequate protein response (Fischbach, 1999). As with albumin, prealbumin can be low because of nonnutritional factors, including acute metabolic states, postsurgery status, liver disease, infection, and dialysis. Prealbumin can be falsely elevated because of steroids, acute or chronic renal failure, and dehydration. In the case of steroids or renal failure, trends should be monitored rather than looking at a single value.

Nitrogen Balance

Nitrogen balance is one of the most widely used nutritional indicators for patients receiving enteral or parenteral nutrition support. The desired N_2 balance for anabolism is +2 to +6. For the N_2 balance to be accurate, the following is needed: an accurate 24-hour urine collection (e.g., 24-hour urine urea nitrogen [UUN]), a minimal creatinine clearance of 50 ml/minute, and adequate caloric intake. N_2 balance is not an optimal nutritional indicator immediately following surgery or injury, for patients with acute sepsis or severe stress or acute or chronic renal failure (because of decreased creatinine clearance), or following spinal cord injury.

PATIENT INTERVIEW

The patient interview is perhaps the most important component of assessing a patient's nutritional status and devising a plan of care. All possible barriers to a person's food intake must be identified. The following areas should be reviewed with the patient or caregiver:
Oral health examination: Does the patient have loose or lost teeth? Dentures? Mouth pain? Dry mouth? Is there any evidence of difficulty in swallowing (drooling, coughing after swallows, hoarseness, wet gargling voice, repeated cases of pneumonia)?
Presence of gastrointestinal complaints: Does the patient complain of anorexia? Nausea? Vomiting? Diarrhea? Constipation? Is the patient lactose intolerant?
Disabilities and function: Is there loss of vision or hearing or taste or smell changes? Is the patient able to feed herself or himself? Is assistance needed for tray setup versus total feed? Are modified utensils needed? Does cognitive impairment affect eating?
Dietary history: What is the patient's usual intake? Who cooks the meals and shops for food? Are there specific diet restrictions? Ethnic or religious considerations? How much alcohol is consumed?
Social history: Is the patient isolated or depressed? Are support systems adequate? Is a fixed or low income preventing the purchase of adequate, nutritious food?
The development of a care plan will directly result from what is obtained in the patient interview and assessed via the weight and biochemical data.

Nutritional Requirements of the Geriatric Patient

A variety of calculations are available to estimate calorie and protein requirements.

ENERGY

The *Harris-Benedict equation* is often used for calculating basal energy expenditure (BEE) because it takes into account the person's height, weight, age, and activity level (American Dietetic

Association, 1992). Individualization for the variable geriatric population is necessary in applying stress factors.

$$Male: 66 + (13.8 \times weight\ in\ kg) + (5 \times height\ in\ cm) - (6.8 \times age)$$
$$Female: 655 + (9.6 \times weight\ in\ kg) + (1.8 \times height\ in\ cm) - (4.7 \times age)$$
$$Total\ caloric\ needs = BEE \times activity\ factor \times injury\ factor$$
$$Activity\ factors\ include,\ in\ bed,\ 1.2;\ out\ of\ bed,\ 1.3.$$

Examples of injury factors include mild infection, 1 to 1.2; moderate infection, 1.2 to 1.4; severe infection, 1.4 to 1.8; minor surgery, 1 to 1.1; major surgery, 1.1 to 1.2 (American Dietetic Association, 1992).

If the patient's body weight is above 125% ideal body weight, use adjusted body weight for calculations:

$$Adjusted\ wt = [(Actual\ wt - Ideal\ wt) \times 0.25] + Ideal\ wt$$

The Harris-Benedict equation was developed with normal-weight, healthy adults; therefore it may not be as accurate for assessing critically ill or injured patients (Ireton-Jones et al, 1998).

PROTEIN

Evidence exists for slightly increased protein requirements in the elderly of 1 to 1.1 g/kg compared with the RDA of 0.8 g/kg. Needs are higher for conditions that cause an increased metabolic rate or increased protein losses such as wound healing or fighting infection. For example, a stage IV pressure ulcer may require 2 g of protein per kilogram of body weight.

Consider the preceding calculations as merely estimations of calorie and protein requirements. Continued observance of trends in weights, laboratory values, and food intake is essential in determining whether these estimations are adequate.

FLUID/TUBE FEEDING

Maintenance of water balance is essential to normal physiologic function; however, despite the imperative to maintain water balance, older adults frequently experience alterations in their fluid level and subsequently and at times rapidly become dehydrated (Sheehy et al, 1999). Conditions that increase the risk of dehydration include the following:

- Natural response to thirst decreased
- Mental or physical incapacitates that reduce the ability to recognize thirst, create an inability to express thirst, or decrease access to water
- Self-restriction for convenience
- Increased fluid output resulting from less efficient kidneys
- Some drugs, such as diuretics, that increase urine output (Kenney and Chiu, 2001)

Most people require 30 ml of fluid per kilogram of body weight unless a fluid restriction is indicated. In general, 1 kcal/cc formulas provide approximately 85% water, 1.2 to 1.5 kcal/cc formulas provide approximately 80% water, and 2 kcal/cc formulas provide about 70% water. Water not provided by the formula should be provided via water flushes. Additional water may be needed in cases of fever, elevated environmental temperature, low environmental humidity, dry oxygen, and air-fluidized bed therapy, all of which cause evaporative water loss. Losses from vomiting, diarrhea, excessive ostomy drainage, and other gastrointestinal fluid losses should be replaced with an oral or intravenous rehydration solution because of the loss of water and electrolytes.

Nutrition Support Issues
DO NOT RESUSCITATE STATUS AND PATIENT PROGNOSIS

If food intake is deemed inadequate, the ramifications of initiating nutrition support need to be considered. First and foremost, the health professional must determine whether an advance directive addresses the issue. Informed consent, which truly informs the patient or guardian of the risks and benefits, must be obtained if there is no advance directive dealing with nutritional support (Brett and Rosenberg, 2001). Invasive therapeutic intervention, such as percutaneous endoscopic gastrostomy placement (PEG), is common procedure in patients with limited life expectancy. Outcomes have been disappointing, with at least 20% of patients dying within 30 days of the procedure; many who survive have severely impaired functional status (Post, 2001; Skelly, 2002). When considering whether artificial feedings will help the frail older patient regain useful function, it is useful to determine whether the possible benefits from nutrition support may be outweighed by the burdens. Benefits may include increased ability to recover, the possibility of returning to useful functioning, improved physiologic state, increased resistance to infection, and improved healing of skin and wounds. Burdens may include physical pain, spiritual and emotional pain and suffering, denial of a peaceful death, invasive procedures, indignity, and emotional and financial burden on the family (Dorner et al, 1997). Furthermore, data concerning the effectiveness of tube feeding in terms of improvement of wound healing survival or even preventing aspiration do not support the widespread use in terminally ill older patients (Daly, 2000). On the other hand, 30% to 50% of family members and patients with dementia express a preference for artificial feeding if it becomes necessary (Daly, 2000). The use of PEG placement and feeding in vulnerable, frail older patients presents a difficult, complex situation with moral, cultural, social, and political influences that often conflict with one another (Mackie, 2001). There is no single, easy answer to this situation. Each case must be handled with the highest regard for the older patient; when possible the wishes of the patient are the deciding factor.

MONITORING

If nutritional support is initiated, monitoring of trends in weight and laboratory values (weekly UUN and prealbumin, if appropriate) is done to ensure that the nutritional support is appropriately meeting the patient's needs.

Strategies for Improving a Patient's Nutritional Status

- Assess all possible barriers to an adequate intake.
- Enlist family assistance. Use home health services. If they are available, experts in nutrition, physical therapy, occupational therapy, speech, or social work should be consulted as indicated to address barriers.
- Use snacks and supplements to boost intake. Encourage smaller, more frequent meals and high-calorie, high-protein foods wherever possible.
- Monitor weight on a regular basis.
- Supplement daily with a multivitamin and mineral supplement. It is often difficult for the older patients to consume adequate amounts of nutrients from food alone.

    When prescribing diet therapy, it is important to look at the overall medical picture of the individual patient. The optimal method for nutritionally supporting patients who are at risk for malnutrition is to feed them a nutritionally dense, well-balanced diet. Liberalizing diet restrictions may lead to a more palatable diet and more interest in food.

Summary

This chapter addresses a fundamental physiologic need that many times is ignored by primary care providers to the detriment of the older person's health and well-being. It is an astute practitioner who always assesses the nutritional status and everyday practices of the older patient. This chapter provides an important knowledge base and practical considerations for potential risk factors, normal nutritional requirements for a healthy life, and assessment and treatment of malnutrition.

Resources

Administration on Aging
Nutrition in the Elderly
oig.hhs.gov/oas/reports/region1/19302510.pdf
www.aoa.dhhs.gov/ELDFAM/nutrition/nutrition.asp

American Academy of Family Physicians
Nutrition Screening Initiative
www.aafp.org/nsi

References

American Dietetic Association: *Handbook of clinical dietetics,* ed 2, New Haven, Conn, 1992, Yale University Press.

Brett AS, Rosenberg JC: The adequacy of informed consent for placement of gastrostomy tubes, *Arch Intern Med* 161(5):745-748, 2001.

Chernoff R: Nutrition and health promotion in older adults, *J Gerontol A Biol Sci Med Sci* 56(2):47-53, 2001.

Coats KG et al: Hospital malnutrition: a reevaluation 12 years later, *J Am Diet Assoc* 93:27-33, 1993.

Covinsky KE et al: Serum albumin concentration and clinical assessments of nutritional status in hospitalized older people: different sides of different coins, *J Am Geriatr Soc* 50(4):631-637, 2002.

Daly BJ: Special challenges of withholding artificial nutrition and hydration, *J Gerontol Nurs* 6(9):21-31, 2000.

Dorner B et al: The "to feed or not to feed" dilemma, *J Am Diet Assoc* 97(10 Suppl 2):S172-S176, 1997.

Fischbach F: *A manual laboratory and diagnostic tests,* ed 5, Philadelphia, 1999, Lippincott.

Griffith HW: *Minerals supplements and vitamins: the essential guide,* Tucson, Ariz, 2000, Fisher Books.

Huffman GB: Evaluating and treating unintentional weight loss in the elderly, *Am Fam Physician* 65(4):640-650, 2002.

Ireton-Jones C et al: Should predictive equations or indirect calorimetry be used to design nutrition support regimens? Point-Counterpoint, *Nutr Clin Pract* 13:141-145, 1998.

Kenney WL, Chiu P: Influence of age on thirst and fluid intake, *Med Sci Sports Exerc* 33(9):1524-1532, 2001.

Mackie SB: PEGS and ethics, *Gastroenterol Nurs* 24(3):138-142, 2001.

Meydani M: Nutrition interventions in aging and age associated disease, *Ann N Y Acad Sci*, 928:226-235, 2001.

Millen BE et al: Nutritional risk in an urban homebound older population: the nutrition and healthy aging project, *J Nutr Health Aging* 5(4):269-277, 2001.

Moriguti JC et al: Involuntary weight loss in elderly individuals: assessment and treatment, *San Paulo Med J* 119(2):72-77, 2001.

Nutrition Screening Initiative: *Nutrition interventions manual for professionals caring for older Americans,* Washington, DC, 1992, Author.

Pirlich M, Lochs H: Nutrition in the elderly, *Best Pract Res Clin Gastroenterol* 15(6):869-884, 2001.

Post SG: Comments on research in the social sciences pertaining to Alzheimer's disease: a more humble approach, *Aging Ment Health* 5(Suppl 1):S17-S19, 2001.

Sahyoun NR et al: Nutritional screening initiative checklist may be a better awareness/educational tool than a screening one, *J Am Diet Assoc* 97:760-764, 1997.

Sheey CM, Perry PA, Cromwell SL: Dehydration: biological considerations, age-related changes and risk factors in older adults, *Biol Res Nurs* 1(1):30-37, 1999.

Skelly RH: Are we using percutaneous endoscopic gastrostomy appropriately in the elderly? *Curr Opin Clin Nutr Metab Care* 5(1):35-42, 2002.

U.S. Department of Health and Human Services, U.S. Department of Agriculture: *Nutrition and your health: dietary guidelines for Americans,* ed 5, Washington, DC, 2001, US Government Printing Office.

Wellman NS et al: Elder insecurities: poverty, hunger, and malnutrition, *J Am Diet Assoc* 97(suppl 2): S120-S122, 1997.

Willett W: *Eat, drink, and be healthy: the Harvard Medical School guide to healthy eating,* New York, 2001, Simon and Schuster.

4

Cancer: Risk Assessment and Screening

Because of the many benefits of early detection and early treatment of illness, a great deal of attention is paid to screening for acute and chronic disease in all populations. Cancer is one condition that is more easily treated when diagnosed early; however, several factors make the diagnosis and treatment of cancer more complicated in the older population. In general, older persons should be considered eligible for the same approach to screening, assessment, and treatment as younger patients. *Age alone is not a reason to forgo appropriate medical care.* Comorbid conditions, social and financial issues, and goals of care, however, significantly impact clinical decision making when a cancer is discovered in an older person.

These same factors must be taken into consideration in making decisions about screening for illness such as cancer. Questions to be asked include the following: What are the overall risks and benefits to screening, diagnosis, and treatment in this individual patient? Can the patient tolerate the screening procedure? Could the patient withstand aggressive treatment in the event a cancer is detected? Are there comorbid conditions that would preclude surgery or chemotherapy? How would treatment (or no treatment) affect the individual's quality of life? What are the goals of care for this individual?

Less is known about the risks and benefits of cancer screening and treatment in the older population as a result of their exclusion from clinical trials because of comorbid conditions and other factors. Whereas many groups have developed recommendations regarding whom and when to screen for specific cancers, little consensus has been established for the older population.

The decision to screen for cancer in older persons requires consideration of the risks and benefits for the individual and discussions with the patient (or caregiver) regarding the goals of care (survival versus quality of life). It is important to understand the risks associated with specific cancers as they apply to the individual patient (i.e., family history, occupational and environmental exposure, and other factors) as well as how various treatment options might be tolerated in light of comorbid conditions. An important role of the primary care provider is to provide information and support so that that patients and caregivers can make informed, appropriate decisions.

Prevalence of Cancer in the Older Population

Fifty percent of cancers occur in patients older than 65 years of age, and it is thought that by the year 2030, 65% of cancers will occur in older persons (Krasnow, 2002). Whereas heart disease is the most common cause of death in older persons, cancer is a close second. In fact, in persons 65 to 74 years of age, cancer is the most common cause of death in women and is roughly equal to heart disease as a cause of death in men (Hayman et al, 2001). In addition, the proportion of the population that is over 65 years of age is expected to grow significantly over the next three decades. Currently 34 million, or one in nine, persons are 65 years of age or older; by 2030 this number will have more than doubled to about 70 million, or one in five (Hayman et al, 2001).

It is not fully understood why the older adults are more likely to develop cancer. Several theories of cancer causation in older people exist, including decreased immune surveillance, prolonged duration of exposure to carcinogens, and increased susceptibility of aged cells to carcinogens; however, no single theory has been accepted universally (Sial and Catalano, 2001).

The two main approaches to cancer prevention are (1) primary prevention, which may be less applicable to older than to younger people, involves changes in lifestyle, exercise, and diet to prevent the development of cancer; and (2) secondary prevention, which involves screening tests and examinations to aid in the early detection of cancer, decreasing morbidity and mortality from cancer, and increasing the chance for cure (Sial and Catalano, 2001).

During the past few decades, medical advances have led to a decline in the age-specific mortality of most malignancies. Screening for occult disease has played an important role in this progress, allowing more effective treatment through early detection. Conditions such as chronic renal insufficiency, congestive heart failure, liver disease, dementia, prior malignancies, and poor performance status, however, are common exclusion criteria for cancer clinical trials. Older patients typically present with a high level of these comorbidities and as a result have traditionally been excluded from studies of both screening and treatment for cancers. Therefore, both the screening test and the available treatment often have not been tested in the older adults (Heflin and Cohen, 2001). As a result, providers must extrapolate data about the effectiveness of screening in younger patients and apply it to older patients, and the decision to offer cancer screening to the older person becomes quite complex.

Numerous medical organizations have developed guidelines for cancer screening. The range of recommendations is broad and sometimes conflicting, leaving primary care providers to determine the most reasonable method of screening for each individual patient. Several studies show that as a result of the lack of consistent recommendations primary care providers do not always comply with cancer screening guidelines (Zoorob et al, 2001). Like many medical decisions, cancer screening decisions require weighing quantitative information, such as risk of cancer death and likelihood of beneficial and adverse outcomes, as well as qualitative factors, such as the individual patient's values and preferences (Walter and Covinsky, 2001). Although most health care professionals would agree that clinical judgment should supercede age-cutoff guidelines when the potential harms or benefits from a screening test strongly weigh in a particular direction, there is little guidance about how to apply clinical judgment to screening decisions concerning older patients (Walter and Covinsky, 2001).

The availability of insurance coverage also influences whether patients receive screening for various health issues. The 1992 National Health Interview Survey revealed that persons 40 to 64 years of age with Medicaid coverage and those with private fee-for-service coverage were more likely to be screened (70% higher) than those who had no coverage. In contrast, persons 65 years of age and older who had supplemental private fee-for-service insurance in addition to Medicare were more likely to receive testing than those with Medicare and Medicaid or those with Medicare only. Managed care enrollees at all ages were about 10% more likely to be screened than those enrolled in private fee-for-service plans (Potosky et al, 1998).

Risk Assessment

Assessment of an older patient's ability to tolerate cancer treatments must take into account comorbid conditions. A variety of comorbidity indexes are available to assist with the determination of the mortality risk for individual patients. One example is the Charlson Comorbidity Index (Table 4-1) (Aapro, Extermann, and Repetto, 2000), which is a standardized instrument based on 1-year mortality risk. It considers 19 different diseases weighted from 1 to 6 points. Another is the Cumulative Illness Rating Scale Geriatrics (CIRS-G), which classifies comorbidities by organ systems and grades each condition from 0 (no problems) to 4 (several incapacitating or life-threatening conditions). See Table 4-2 (Aapro, Extermann, and Repetto, 2000).

The Comprehensive Geriatric Assessment is a valuable tool in determining the appropriateness of aggressive evaluation and treatment of cancer (or any illness) in the older patient. The approach investigates functional, nutritional, psychological, and cognitive status and socioeconomic factors that affect the older person's overall functional status. The assessment of the older person for oncology treatment should include past medical history, physical examination, psychiatric history, and formal evaluation of cognitive abilities as well as visual and auditory abilities. In addition, the social resources of the older person need to be determined because these may dictate care needs, the feasibility of the plan of care, and discharge planning. For example, a patient with no reliable transportation to daily radiation treatments may require a temporary stay in a palliative care unit or other inpatient setting while treatment is completed.

TABLE 4-1	Charlson Comorbidity Index

Comorbidity	*Points*
Myocardial infarct	1
Congestive heart failure	1
Peripheral vascular disease	1
Cerebrovascular disease (except hemiplegia)	1
Dementia	1
Chronic pulmonary disease	1
Connective tissue disease	1
Ulcer disease	1
Mild liver disease	1
Diabetes (without complications)	1
Diabetes with end-organ damage	2
Hemiplegia	2
Moderate or severe renal disease	2
Second solid tumor (nonmetastatic)	2
Leukemia	2
Lymphoma, multiple myeloma	2
Moderate or severe liver disease	3
Second metastatic solid tumour	6
Acquired immunodeficiency syndrome (AIDS)	6
Total points _____	

From Aapro M, Extermann M, Repetto L: Evaluation of the elderly with cancer, *Ann Oncol* 11(suppl 11):223-229, 2000.

TABLE 4-2	Cumulative Illness Rating Scale Geriatrics (CIRS-G)

	Score
Heart	.....
Vascular	.....
Hematopoietic	.....
Respiratory	.....
Eyes, ears, nose and throat, larynx	.....
Upper GI	.....
Lower GI	.....
Liver	.....
Renal	.....
Genitourinary	.....
Musculoskeletal/integument	.....
Neurologic	.....
Endocrine/metabolic and breast	.....
Psychiatric illness	.....
Total number of categories endorsed	.....
Total score	.....
Severity index:	
(total score/total number of categories)	.....
Number of categories at level 3 severity	.....
Number of categories at level 4 severity	.....
Rating strategy	
0 – No problem	
1 – Mild or past problem	
2 – Moderate problem requiring therapy	
3 – Severe or uncontrollable problem	
4 – Extremely severe problem or organ failure	
A manual is available to assist rating	

From Aapro M, Extermann M, Repetto L: Evaluation of the elderly with cancer, *Ann Oncol* 11(suppl 11):223-229, 2000.
GI, Gastrointestinal.

Walter and Covinsky (2001) developed a framework for individualized decision making for cancer screening in older patients. Their framework takes into consideration four issues: the risk of dying of a screen-detectable cancer; the benefits of screening for specific cancers; the harms of cancer screening (complications, potential treatment of clinically unimportant cancers, and psychological distress); and the patient's values and preferences. No universal agreement has been reached, however, on this multifaceted and complicated issue.

Environmental Issues

Decisions regarding whether to screen a particular patient for a specific type of cancer are influenced by several issues, such as medical and family history, social history, and habits. Also important is the history of occupational and environmental exposures to carcinogens, which requires obtaining information regarding each patient's exposures in their living environments (i.e., in what areas of the country they have lived, the presence of any known high-risk industrial exposures nearby) and workplaces over the patient's lifetime.

Associations have been made between cancer risk and extended exposure to fine particles of pollution from power plants and diesel engines. A study published by Pope and colleagues (2002) demonstrated that long-term exposure to combustion-related fine particulate air pollution is an important environmental risk factor for cardiopulmonary and lung cancer mortality. For example, persons who live within 25 to 30 miles of coal-burning power plants, generally the most polluting type of facility, appear to be at greatest risk for exposure to particulates.

Various occupational exposures are established carcinogens: asbestos (lung cancer, mesothelioma, some gastrointestinal cancers), benzene (leukemia), and cadmium (prostate cancer). Certain industrial processes are associated with elevated cancer risks, some without identified specific carcinogenic agents. An example is bladder and lung cancer in the rubber industry. In addition, exposure to ionizing and nonionizing radiation such as ultraviolet light exposure (skin cancers), radon (lung cancer), and gamma radiation and neutrons (leukemia, thyroid, and breast cancers, such as in atomic bomb survivors).

An example of an environmental risk concern is exposure to dioxins (e.g., chlorinated dibenzo-p-dioxins [CDDs], certain polychlorinated biphenyls [PCBs], chlorinated dibenzofurans [CDFs]), which are released into the air from combustion processes such as commercial or municipal waste incineration, from burning fuels (such as wood, coal, or oil), and from burning of household trash and during forest fires. Paper manufacturing and cigarettes are also sources of dioxins. Exposure to dioxins has been associated with severe skin ailments and possibly liver damage as well as cancer (Environmental Protection Agency, 2002).

The Integrated Risk Information System (IRIS), prepared and maintained by the U.S. Environmental Protection Agency (EPA), is an electronic data base containing information on human health effects that may result from exposure to various chemical in the environment (EPA, 2002).

Screening Issues

Cancer screening is the application of a test to detect the presence of a cancer in an asymptomatic person. The results of a screening test do not establish a diagnosis; they only identify persons with the highest likelihood of having cancer (Silverman et al, 2000).

The usefulness of a screening program can be evaluated by characteristics of both the disease and requirements of the screening test. The disease should meet the following criteria: high costs (morbidity, mortality, and economic), high incidence and prevalence, a known natural history and biology, a high prevalence in the preclinical phase, and effective treatments available. The screening test should be able to detect disease in the preclinical phase; have acceptable sensitivity and specificity; be acceptable to individual patients; and be simple, inexpensive, and safe (Silverman et al, 2000).

Screening tests are either positive or negative. The *sensitivity* of a screening test is the proportion of persons with a positive test result for the disease that the test is intended to reveal. The *specificity* of a test is the proportion of persons with negative test results for the disease that the test is intended to reveal. A *false-positive* test occurs when a disease-free person tests positive. A *false-negative* test occurs when a diseased person tests negative.

The *positive predictive value* of a screening test is the probability that a person has the disease given that the test is positive. The *negative predictive value* of a screening test is the probability that a person does not have the disease given that the test is negative. Predictive values depend of the sensitivity, specificity, and prevalence of the disease in the general population.

Major medical organizations have achieved some consensus on screening guidelines for breast, cervical, and colorectal cancer. In the absence of compelling evidence to indicate a high risk of endometrial cancer, lung cancer, oral cancer, and ovarian cancer, almost no medical organizations have developed screening guidelines for these types of cancer (Zoorob et al, 2001). Table 4-3 provides a summary of cancer screening recommendations for low-risk patients by medical organization. Table 4-4 provides information about Medicare coverage for cancer screening procedures.

TABLE 4-3	Summary of Cancer Screening Recommendations for Low-risk Patients

Medical Organization	Screening Recommendations
	Breast Cancer
	Mammography
AAFP	Every 1 to 2 yr, ages 50 to 69; counsel women ages 40 to 49 about potential risks and benefits of mammography and clinical breast examination.
ACOG	Every 1 to 2 yr starting at age 40, yearly after age 50
ACS	Annually after age 40 yr
AMA	Every 1 to 2 yr in women ages 40 to 49; annually beginning at age 50
CTFPHC	Every 1 to 2 yr, ages 50 to 59
NIH	Data currently available do not warrant a universal recommendation for mammography for women in their 40s; each woman should decide for herself whether to undergo mammography.
USPSTF	Every 1 to 2 yr, ages 50 to 69
	Clinical breast examination
AAFP	Every 1 to 2 yr, ages 50 to 69; counsel women ages 40 to 49 about potential risks and benefits of mammography and clinical breast examination.
ACOG	Yearly (or as appropriate) general health evaluation that includes examination to detect signs of premalignant or malignant conditions
ACS	Every 3 yr, ages 20 to 39; yearly after age 40; monthly breast self-examination beginning at age 20 yr
AMA	Continuation of clinical breast examinations in asymptomatic women older than age 40 yr
CTFPHC	Yearly, ages 50 to 69 yr
USPSTF	Insufficient evidence to recommend for or against using clinical breast examination alone; optional every 1 to 2 yr, ages 50 to 69 yr
	Cervical Cancer
AAFP	Pap test at least every 3 yr to women who have ever had sexual intercourse and who have a cervix
ACOG	Annual Pap test and pelvic examination beginning at age 18 or when sexually active; after three or more tests with normal results, Pap test may be performed less frequently on physician's advice.
ACS	Pap test annually starting at age 18 or when sexually active; after two to three normal (negative) tests, continue at discretion of physician.
AGS	Pap test every 3 yr until age 70; in women of any age who have never had a Pap test, **screening** with at least two negative smears 1 yr apart
AMA	Annual Pap test and pelvic examination starting at age 18 (or when sexually active); after three or more normal annual Pap tests, the Pap test may be performed less frequently at the physician's discretion.
CTFPHC	Pap test annually beginning at age 18 or following initiation of sexual activity; after two normal Pap results, perform Pap tests every 3 yr to age 69.

TABLE 4-3	Summary of Cancer Screening Recommendations for Low-risk Patients—cont'd

Medical Organization	*Screening Recommendations*
USPSTF	Pap test at least every 3 yr in women who have ever had sexual intercourse and who have a cervix; discontinue regular testing after 65 yr of age if Pap test results have been consistently normal.
	Colorectal Cancer
AAFP	No published standards or guidelines for low-risk patients
ACOG	After age 50, annual FOBT (DRE should accompany pelvic examination); sigmoidoscopy every 3 to 5 yr
ACS	After age 50, yearly FOBT plus flexible sigmoidoscopy and DRE every 5 yr or colonoscopy and DRE every 10 yr or double-contrast barium enema and DRE every 5 to 10 yr
AMA	Annual FOBT beginning at age 50, and flexible sigmoidoscopy every 3 to 5 yr beginning at age 50 yr
AGA	FOBT beginning at age 59 (frequency not specified); sigmoidoscopy every 5 yr, double-contrast barium enema every 5 to 10 yr or colonoscopy every 10 years.
CTFPHC	Insufficient evidence to recommend using FOBT **screening** in the periodic health examination of individuals older than age 40; insufficient evidence to recommend sigmoidoscopy in the periodic health examination; insufficient evidence to recommend **screening** with colonoscopy in the general population
USPSTF	After age 50, yearly FOBT and/or sigmoidoscopy (unspecified frequency for sigmoidoscopy)
	Prostate Cancer
AAFP	No published standards or guidelines for low-risk patients
ACP-ASIM	Physicians should describe potential benefits and known harms concerning diagnosis and treatment; listen to the patient's concerns, then indicate decision to **screen.**
ACS and AUA	Offer annual DRE and PSA **screening**, beginning at age 50, to men with at least a 10-yr life expectancy and to younger men at high risk.
AMA	Provide information regarding the risks and potential benefits of prostate **screening.**
CTFPHC AND USPSTF	DRE and PSA tests are not recommended for the general population.
	Skin Cancer
ACS	Cancer-related checkup, including skin examination every 3 yr between ages 20 and 40, and every year for anyone age 40 and older
AMA	Patients should talk to their physicians about the frequency of **screening** for skin cancer (those at modestly increased risk should see a primary care physician annually); skin self-examination should be performed monthly.
CTFPHC	Insufficient evidence to recommend for or against total-body skin examination or self-examination; counsel on avoiding sun exposure and wearing protective clothing.

Continued

TABLE 4-3	**Summary of Cancer Screening Recommendations for Low-risk Patients—cont'd**
Medical Organization	*Screening Recommendations*
USPSTF	Insufficient evidence to recommend for or against routine **screening** for skin cancer by primary care clinicians or counseling patients to perform periodic skin examination.
	Testicular Cancer
ACS	Examine testicles as part of a cancer-related checkup.
CTFPHC	Insufficient evidence to recommend routine examination of testes by physician or by patient self-examination
USPSTF	Insufficient evidence to recommend for or against routine **screening** of asymptomatic men in the general population by physician examination or patient self-examination

DRE, Digital rectal examination; *FOBT*, fecal occult blood testing; *Pap*, Papanicolaou; *PSA*, prostate-specific antigen. Abbreviations for medical organizations: *AAFP*, American Academy of Family Physicians; *ACOG*, American College of Obstetricians and Gynecologists; *ACP-ASIM*, American College of Physicians-American Society of Internal Medicine; *ACS*, American Cancer Society; *AGA*, American Gastroenterological Association; *ACS*, American Geriatrics Society; *AMA*, American Medical Association; *AUA*, American Urological Association; *CTFPHC*, Canadian Task Force on Preventive Health Care; *NIH*, National Institutes of Health; *USPSTF*, U.S. Preventive Services Task Force.
From Zoorob R et al: Cancer screening guidelines, *Am Fam Physician* 63(6):1101-1112, 2001.

TABLE 4-4	**Medicare Coverage for Cancer Screening Procedures**
Type of Cancer	*Description of Medicare Coverage*
Breast	Annual **screening** mammography for women older-than age 40 yr
Cervix	Pap testing and pelvic examination at three-year intervals. Yearly **screening** is allowed for women who are at a high risk of cervical or vaginal cancer or who have had an abnormal Pap smear in the preceding three years.
Colorectal	For individuals older than 50 yr, **screening** fecal occult blood testing is reimbursed by Medicare one time per year and flexible sigmoidoscopy is reimbursed once every four years or once every two years if the patient is at high risk. Colonoscopy is reimbursed every two years if the patient is at high risk for colon cancer (no age limit). Barium enema is reimbursed as a substitute for sigmoidoscopy or colonoscopy if the primary care physician deems it advisable.
Prostate	Annual digital rectal examination and prostate-specific antigen test in men older than 50 yr

From Zoorob R et al: Cancer screening guidelines, *Am Physician* 63(6):1101-1112, 2001. *Pap*, Papanicolaou.

LUNG CANCER

Lung cancer is the leading cause of death in men and women, accounting for an estimated 156,900 deaths in 2000, which equates to 28% of all cancer-related deaths. Cigarette smoking, which is well established as the major risk factor, has particular importance in older smokers because they have probably accumulated large exposures.

There is no evidence that screening for lung cancer in low-risk patients is effective. Neither cytologic screening of sputum nor chest radiographs have proved useful in this population. In general, medical organizations have not developed any official recommendations for lung cancer screening. Similarly, in high-risk patients, periodic screening with chest radiographs has not proved to reduce mortality from lung cancer. Instead, many organizations recommend that primary care providers counsel patients against tobacco use.

Two imaging techniques, fluorescence bronchoscopy and spiral computed tomography, have received recent attention for their potential benefit in lung cancer screening. Both techniques are currently being investigated in the United States.

Tobacco Cessation

Smoking is responsible for three million deaths per year worldwide (Bohadana et al, 2000) and is responsible for an estimated $100 billion annually in direct medical and indirect nonmedical costs (Okuyemi et al, 2001). Up to 60% of adult smokers began smoking by 13 years of age (American Heart Association, 2002), which means that many older smokers will not only have had several decades of exposure to carcinogens but also that they will have a decades-long habit to break. According to the Centers for Disease Control and Prevention (CDC), about 40% of America's 50 million smokers will try to stop smoking at least once this year, and on each attempt fewer than 1 in 10 will succeed. For each attempt, relapse rates approach 70% at 3 months and exceed 90% at 1 year (Lantz and Giambanco, 2001). The benefits of smoking cessation—reduction in smoking related-disability and increased life expectancy—still apply in the older smoker. Therefore practitioners need to be familiar with various smoking cessation programs and tools to be prepared to help the patient with this difficult task.

Two addictions are associated with smoking: the response behavior and the nicotine. A person who has smoked less than half a pack per day (10 cigarettes) may not require much more than moral support and assistance in substituting a different, healthier habit when the smoking "trigger" occurs. These triggers often include arising in the morning, commuting in a car, and after eating a meal. Substituting other behaviors, such as going for a walk, brushing the teeth, or chewing gum, may help to "break the habit" for lighter smokers. Heavier smokers will probably require a tapered nicotine replacement in addition to behavioral modifications.

Several nicotine-replacement systems are currently on the market. These include gum, titrated patches, nicotine nasal spray, and nicotine inhalers. When considering a nicotine-replacement patch, one must consider the number of cigarettes smoked in an average day. Two packs of cigarettes equal about 300 mg of nicotine. Patients who smoke two packs per day will require an appropriate dose (i.e., two nicotine patches) of replacement initially. The patient who smokes irregularly, or less than half a pack per day, may actually be increasing the nicotine dose by using a patch and may benefit from one of the other replacements. Table 4-5 reviews the pharmacologic interventions for smoking cessation.

In light of the recent significant advancements in the pharmacotherapies of smoking cessation, less attention has been paid to behavioral tobacco cessation treatments. The Clinical Practice Guidelines published by the United States Public Health Service (Fiore et al, 1996) recommend the "five A's" as an approach for clinicians to identify smokers and help them to quit:

1. Ask the patient whether he or she uses tobacco.
2. Advise the patient to quit tobacco use.
3. Assess the patient's willingness to quit tobacco use.

TABLE 4-5	Pharmacologic Interventions for Smoking Cessation			
Method	*Dose*	*Duration**	*Side effects*	*Precautions*
Nicotine replacement				
Nicotine gum (Nicorette, OTC)	2 or 4 mg/square max 24 mg/d	12 weeks, often used chronically	Mouth irritation, heartburn	Tachycardia if chewed rapidly
Nicotine patch† (Habitrol, Rx only; Nicoderm CQ, OTC in tapered doses)	21, 14, 7 mg/d	8 weeks, often used chronically	Skin irritation, insomnia	
(Nicotrol, OTC)	15 mg/d	16 hrs/d for 6 weeks; remove at night		For those using 10 cigarettes/day
(ProStep, OTC in tapered doses)	22, 11 mg/d	6 weeks, often used chronically	Skin irritation, insomnia	
Nicotine inhaler (Nicotrol Inhaler)	4 mg delivered, max 16 mg/d	Up to 6 months	Mouth and throat irritation	Tachycardia if used rapidly
Nicotine nasal spray (Nicotrol NS)	4 mg delivered, max 40 mg/d	Up to 6 months	Nose and throat irritation	Tachycardia if used in excess
Antidepressant				
Bupropion SR (Zyban)	150 mg/d for older adults	Initial 12 week course; can extend ≥6 months if history of depression	Insomnia, irritability	Contraindicated in patients with history of seizures

From Lantz MS, Giambanco V: Smoking cessation: The key to treating older smokers? Don't quit helping, *Geriatrics* 56(5):58-59, 2001.

OTC, Over-the-counter;

*The FDA has not approved these interventions for chronic use, but in many cases continuation beyond 6 months has resulted in safe and successful smoking cessation.

†The initial dose should be based on the number of cigarettes smoked per day. The highest dose for patients smoking ≥2 packs/day, the lowest dose for those smoking < 1 pack/day

4. Assist the patient in his or her attempt to quit.
5. Arrange follow-up contacts and relapse prevention.

Behavioral interventions include multicomponent coping skills training (also called coping response therapy, problem-focused treatment, relapse-prevention training, and cognitive-behavioral therapy). The common elements include social support; didactic information about nicotine dependence, withdrawal symptoms, and situations that are risks for relapse; and training in the use of cognitive and behavioral responses to cope with urges to smoke that reduce risk of relapse. Instruction on how to recover from an initial smoking lapse without progressing to full relapse also should be included.

Pharmacotherapy is often integrated into multicomponent programs (Brandon, 2001). Other approaches include rapid smoking (requiring deep inhalation of cigarette smoke every 6 seconds to induce an aversion response); scheduled reduced smoking (where gradually reduced smoking occurs on a predetermined schedule of when each cigarette is to be smoked that is not controlled by the patient); and depression-focused counseling (Brandon, 2001). It is also helpful to instruct patients to include the following strategies in their approach: involve family, friends, and co-workers for support; avoid alcohol; do not attempt to diet during this time; exercise regularly; and drink plenty of fluids.

Even if a patient has failed in the past, it is important to continue efforts at smoking cessation. The following contacts are useful resources in this effort:

American Cancer Society, 1599 Clifton Road NE Atlanta, GA (404) 320-3333
American Heart Association, 7272 Greenville Ave, Dallas, TX (800) AHA-USA1
American Lung Association, 1740 Broadway, 14th Floor, New York, NY (212) 315-8700
National Cancer Institute (NCI), 31 Center Drive, MSC 2580, Bethesda, MD (800) 4-CANCER

COLORECTAL CANCER

Colorectal cancer is the third most common cancer. About 130,200 new cases (93,800 of the colon and 36,400 of the rectum) were diagnosed in 2000, and this disease accounted for an estimated 56,300 deaths in 2000 (Zoorob et al, 2001). Colorectal cancer is a disease of late life with age-adjusted incidence and death rates increasing dramatically with age.

No specific causative agent for colorectal cancer has been identified. Risk factors include a personal and family history of colorectal, breast, or endometrial carcinoma; familial polyposis syndrome; inflammatory bowel disease; and the presence of adenomatous polyps. Other factors include age; obesity; and certain dietary factors, including a low-fiber, high-fat, and high-cholesterol diet, alcohol consumption, and a high phosphate and low calcium intake (Sial and Catalano, 2001).

Most colorectal cancers evolve from premalignant adenomas, and the estimated time of progression from polyp to cancer is 5 to 10 years. Removal of these slow-growing lesions prevents the development of cancer (Heflin and Cohen, 2001).

Commonly used screening tests include digital rectal examination (DRE), fecal occult blood testing (FOBT), flexible sigmoidoscopy, colonoscopy, and dual-contrast barium enema.

The FOBT is the least expensive and simplest screening test (e.g., Hemoccult). Colorectal cancers and adenomas larger than 2 cm in diameter bleed intermittently, and detection of fecal occult blood depends on the degree of blood loss. In general 2 ml of blood in the stool is necessary to produce a positive test (Sial and Catalano, 2001). Therefore the primary function of FOBT is to detect larger lesions, which are usually malignant.

Flexible sigmoidoscopy is performed using a 35- or 60-cm flexible scope. The primary advantage of sigmoidoscopy is that it permits direct visualization of the bowel, although only the distal portion of it. The 60-cm flexible scope can detect 40% to 60% of all adenomas and cancers (Anderson, 2000).

Dual-contrast barium enema alone has not been proven to reduce mortality; however, it is considered safer than sigmoidoscopy and colonoscopy. In addition, it can image the entire colon and can detect cancers and large polyps nearly as well as colonoscopy and better than FOBT or sigmoidoscopy. It does miss small polyps, however, and it does not permit removal or biopsy of polyps, often requiring subsequent examination with colonoscopy (Anderson, 2000).

Colonoscopy provides access to the rectum and colon, can detect polyps and cancers, permits biopsy or lesion removal during the procedure, and rarely produces false-positive results. The procedure can be painful, results vary according to the competence of the examiner, and accuracy of diagnosis can be affected by lesion size. The procedure also introduces the risk of significant complications, including intestinal perforation, hemorrhage, and respiratory sedation resulting from anemia and arrhythmia (Anderson, 2000).

Biopsy should be done of small polyps (<7 mm in diameter) found by screening flexible sigmoidoscopy. If the polyps are hyperplastic, no further action is required. If the polyps are adenomatous, colonoscopy is indicated. Larger polyps are usually adenomas requiring colonoscopy, and therefore biopsy is not necessary during flexible sigmoidoscopy (Silverman et al, 2000).

Colonoscopy is the procedure of choice for evaluating patients for symptoms or as a screening test for high-risk patients. Indications for colonoscopy include prior rectal cancer, prior colonic adenomas, ulcerative pancolitis of 8 years' duration, left-sided colitis of longer than 15 years' duration, familial adenomatous polyposis, hereditary nonpolyposis colorectal cancer, first-degree relatives with sporadic colorectal cancer or adenomas before 60 years of age, or several first-degree relatives with colorectal cancer or adenomas (Silverman et al, 2000).

The American Cancer Society and the Agency for Health Care Research and Quality issued a comprehensive set of recommendations in 1997. For adults over 50 years of age, one of the following is recommended: (1) FOBT every year, (2) flexible sigmoidoscopy every 5 years (first performed at age 50), (3) annual FOBT and flexible sigmoidoscopy every 5 years, (4) air-contrast barium enema every 5 to 10 years, or (5) colonoscopy every 10 years. They include no upper age limit at which screening should be suspended but state that "the age at which to stop screening depends on the judgment of individual patients and their clinicians" (Heflin and Cohen, 2001).

BLADDER CANCER

Bladder cancer is the sixth most commonly diagnosed cancer in the United States. About 54,300 new cases were expected to be diagnosed in 2001 (NCI, 2002). Bladder cancer is more than 2.5 times more common in men than in women and occurs almost twice as often in whites than in African Americans. The incidence of bladder cancer increases with age, with about 80% of newly diagnosed cases occurring in persons 60 years of age and older.

Risk factors for bladder cancer include cigarette smoking; prolonged exposures to urinary foreign bodies and infections; exposure to aminobiphenyl or other occupational or environmental exposures such as aromatic amines in dyes, combustion gases, and soot from coal; chlorination by-products in heated water; and certain aldehydes such as those used in the rubber and textile industries. Occupations reported to be associated with an increased risk of bladder cancer include those that involve organic chemicals, such as dry cleaners, paper manufacturers, rope and twine makers, and workers in apparel manufacturing (NCI, 2002).

The use of cystoscopies and bladder wash and cytologic examinations has proven quite successful in the surveillance of patients with previously treated bladder cancers. These means are not practical, however, because of expense, morbidity, and reluctance in persons without a history of bladder cancer. Single and repetitive hematuria testing also has not proved effective as a screening method.

PROSTATE CANCER

An estimated 180,400 cases of prostate cancer were diagnosed in 2000. Approximately 31,900 men died of the disease, making it the second leading cause of cancer-related death in men. The incidence of prostate cancer rises rapidly in each decade of life after 50 years of age; African American men and those with a family history of prostate cancer have an even higher incidence (Zoorob et al, 2001). Eighty-one percent of all cases of prostate cancer are diagnosed in men older than 65 years of age.

It has been difficult to demonstrate reductions in morbidity and mortality with prostate cancer screening because of two factors. First, most prostate cancers have a long detectable preclinical phase. As a result, men with an expected remaining life of less than 10 years derive little benefit from identification of a cancer that will not threaten the quantity or quality of their lives. Second, treatment of localized disease with prostatectomy or radiation can lead to incontinence and impotence, which reduce quality of life (Heflin and Cohen, 2001).

Available screening devices include DRE and prostate specific antigen (PSA) testing. The optimal sensitivity of DRE is thought to be 55% to 68% in asymptomatic men of any age. Serum PSA levels increase in men with prostate cancer; levels greater than 4 ng/dl are considered abnormal. The test has a sensitivity of 80% and a specificity of 91% (Heflin and Cohen, 2001). PSA misses 18% to 25% of prostate cancers and provides false-positive results about 60% of the time (Gambert, 2001).

Transrectal ultrasonography (TRUS) of the prostate gland may be used to provide additional information following an abnormal DRE or elevated PSA. It may also be used in the staging of a carcinoma and to guide a biopsy. TRUS is associated with a considerable number of false-positive results, however, and is therefore not a reliable screening modality (Gambert, 2001).

Screening for prostate cancer is a matter of debate, and recommendations differ widely. Most screening guidelines recommend using both DRE and PSA. Given the lower specificity rates of both tests among older men, however, an estimated 40% of men 70 to 79 years of age would undergo biopsies with this strategy, resulting in a biopsy yield of less than 10% (Heflin and Cohen, 2001). The American Cancer Society suggests annual DRE and PSA beginning at 50 years of age, but only after careful review of the risks and benefits. Screening should be continued for as long as the man has "at least a 10-year life expectancy." The U.S. Preventive Services Task Force states, however, that routine screening for prostate cancer is not recommended for men of any age. Many suggest, however, that high-risk patients, such as African American men and those with two first-degree relatives who have had the disease, should be considered for screening (Heflin and Cohen, 2001).

In an effort to improve the usefulness of the PSA, several modifications are being investigated, including age-adjusted values, PSA velocity, PSA density, and free circulating PSA. Measurements of free PSA concentrations are thought to allow better discrimination between cancer and benign prostatic hypertrophy.

BREAST CANCER

An estimated 182,800 new cases of breast cancer are diagnosed annually, accounting for about 48,000 deaths per year in the United States (Apantaku, 2000). Breast cancer ranks second as a cause of cancer-related deaths in women (Zoorob et al, 2001). The annual incidence among women older than 65 years of age is nearly six times that among women younger than 65, and more than 50% of breast cancer deaths occur among women older than 65 (Heflin and Cohen, 2001). Table 4-6 (Apantaku, 2000) provides data from the American Cancer Society regarding estimated numbers of new breast cancer cases by age.

Risk factors for breast cancer include being older than 50 years of age, prior history of breast cancer, positive family history, menarche before age 12, menopause after age 50, nulliparity, older than 30 years of age at first birth, obesity, high economic status, atypical hyperplasia on biopsy, and ionizing radiation exposure (Apantaku, 2000).

TABLE 4-6   **Estimated New Breast Cancer Cases in Women by Age**

Age (yr)	Estimate	Percentage of Total	Probability of Developing Invasive Cancer
< 30	600	0.3	1 in 235
30–39	8600	4.8	
40–49	32,600	18.1	1 in 25
50–59	33,000	18.3	
60–69	36,600	20.3	1 in 15
70–79	43,500	24.2	
80 and older	25,300	14.0	
Total	180,200	100.0	1 in 8

Reprinted with permission from the American Cancer Society, *Breast Cancer Facts and Figures.* Atlanta: American Cancer Society 1997:14.

Screening strategies include breast self-examination, clinical breast examination, and mammography. Breast self-examination has a low sensitivity (20%-30%). The sensitivity of clinical breast examination in older women is thought to be about 50%. The mammogram remains the cornerstone of breast cancer screening; its sensitivity is 75% to 90% (Heflin and Cohen, 2001); however, sensitivity varies with age, breast density, and screening interval. Of women 70 years of age and older, 8% will have an abnormal screening mammogram. Of these women 86% to 92% will be found on further testing not to have cancer (Silverman et al, 2000).

Most groups recommend performing clinical breast examination and mammography or mammography alone every 1 to 2 years beginning at 40 years of age. Regarding an upper age limit, the American Cancer Society recommends that screening be offered "as long as the woman is in good health." The U.S. Preventive Services Task Force recognizes that the most persuasive evidence supports breast cancer screening between ages 50 and 69. It acknowledges that women older than 70 with "reasonable life expectancy" may benefit from screening because of the significant impact that the disease has in older women (Heflin and Cohen, 2001). Indeed, data from studies such as McCarthy and colleagues (2000) support the use of regular mammography in women 85 years of age and older with a reduction in breast cancer mortality.

Older women with three or more major comorbidities (i.e., hypertension, diabetes, arthritis, myocardial infarction, stroke, respiratory disease, or other cancers) are 20 times more likely to die of a cause other than breast cancer within 3 years (Parnes et al, 2001). Some agreement exists that screening should not be performed in older women who have significant comorbidities, poor functional status, low bone mineral density, little interest in preventive care, or an unwillingness to accept the potential harm of screening (Parnes et al, 2001).

CERVICAL CANCER

An estimated 12,800 cases of invasive cervical cancer were diagnosed in 2000, and an estimated 4600 women died of the disease (Zoorob et al, 2001). As with breast cancer, the effect of invasive cervical cancer increases with age: 25% of new cases and 40% to 50% of cervical cancer deaths occur in women older than 65 years of age (Heflin and Cohen, 2001).

Risk factors include early sexual intercourse, multiple sexual partners, and a history of human papilloma virus (HPV) infection. For older patients, an additional risk is the lack of previous screening. If cervical dysplasia is detected and treated before the onset of invasive squamous cell cancer, the patient has a definite survival advantage. Successful early intervention also avoids the extensive surgery and radiation needed to treat invasive disease (Heflin and Cohen, 2001).

For the past 3 decades, the Papanicolaou (Pap) smear has been the standard screen for cervical cancer. For cervical cancer screening, most organizations recommend a Pap smear and pelvic examination at least every 3 years for patients between 20 and 65 years of age. Unfortunately, with age, the target region for cell collection, the squamocolumnar junction, recedes into the cervical canal, making sampling more difficult and less reliable in older women (Heflin and Cohen, 2001).

General agreement exists that Pap smears should be performed at least every 3 years in women who have a uterus and have had sexual intercourse. The American Cancer Society sets no specific upper age limit, whereas the U.S. Preventive Services Task Force recommends suspending screening at 65 years of age if the woman has had repeatedly normal smears. Others recommend offering continued screening beyond 65 years of age if the woman is sexually active and is expected to live for more than 5 to 7 years (Heflin and Cohen, 2001).

The American Geriatrics Society recommendations include the following: (1) regular Pap smear screening should be done at 1- to 3-year intervals until at least age 70; (2) an older woman of any age who has never had a Pap smear should be screened until two negative Pap smears 1 year apart have been taken; (3) individual circumstances, such as the patient's life expectancy, ability to undergo treatment if cancer is detected, and ability to cooperate with and tolerate the Pap smear procedure, may obviate the need for cervical cancer screening; (4) women who have had a hysterectomy may still have a cervix and, if one is present, these women may be screened under the same criteria as in the preceding; if no cervical tissue remains, no further Pap smear is needed provided the hysterectomy was performed for benign disease and risk factors for the development of cervical neoplasia are not present; (5) cervical sampling is carried out by means of gentle scraping of the ectocervix with a curved spatula, followed by insertion and rotation of an endocervical brush (American Geriatrics Society, 2001).

According to the U.S. Preventive Services Task Force, Pap smears are not necessary in women who have had a complete hysterectomy unless the surgery was performed because of cervical cancer or its precursors.

Interest in developing HPV DNA testing as an adjunct to screening in women is increasing because of the relationship between HPV types 16, 18, 33, and 35 and increased risk of cervical neoplasia (Silverman et al, 2000).

ENDOMETRIAL CANCER

An estimated 38,300 cases of cancer of the uterine corpus, usually of the endometrium, were expected to be diagnosed in 2001 (NCI, 2002). Endometrial cancer is the most common invasive gynecologic cancer in U.S. women. Incidence rates are higher among white women (22.4 per 100,000) than among African American women (15.3 per 100,000). About 6,500 deaths as a result of endometrial cancer were predicted in 2000. The incidence of endometrial cancer increases with age, peaking at 100.7 cases per 100,000 women between 70 and 75 years of age (Zoorob et al, 2001).

Risk factors for endometrial cancer include the use of estrogen replacement therapy unaccompanied by progesterone; obesity; high-fat diet; reproductive factors such as nulliparity, early menarche, and late menopause; and tamoxifen use. Hereditary nonpolyposis colorectal cancer syndrome is also associated with a markedly increased risk of endometrial cancer compared with women in the general population.

Routine screening of women for endometrial cancer is not of any proven benefit. No screening test has been evaluated for its impact on endometrial cancer mortality (NCI, 2002). Endometrial aspiration has been proposed as a potential screening technique with a sensitivity approaching 80%. Endometrial sampling and transvaginal ultrasound are more appropriate as diagnostic tools for symptomatic women than as a screening tools for the healthy population.

OVARIAN CANCER

Ovarian cancer is the second most common gynecologic cancer, with 23,100 new cases and 14,000 deaths estimated to have occurred in 2000. A woman has a 1-in-70 risk of ovarian cancer in her lifetime. The incidence of ovarian cancer increases with age, from 1.4 cases per 100,000 in women younger than 40 years of age to 45.0 cases per 100,000 in women 60 years of age and older. About 50% of all new cases of ovarian cancer and deaths occur in women over 65 years of age.

Ovarian cancer kills more women each year than cervical and endometrial cancers combined (Zoorob et al, 2001). Unfortunately, most women present with late-stage disease, mostly because of the lack of symptoms during the early stages.

Available screening techniques have been ineffective because of the low prevalence of ovarian cancer and the marginal specificity of available tools. The bimanual pelvic examination is neither sensitive enough nor specific enough to detect early stage cancer. The serologic marker CA-125 is shed by 80% to 85% of women with serous epithelial cancer (Heflin and Cohen, 2001). Unfortunately, increased serum levels of CA-125 are also found in patients with a number of nonmalignant conditions, including endometriosis, pelvic inflammatory disease, and leiomyomata.

Transvaginal ultrasound has a sensitivity of 91% to 97%; however, its specificity of only 52% to 70% leads to a large number of exploratory surgeries with identification of few malignancies (Heflin and Cohen, 2001).

SKIN CANCER

Skin cancer is the most frequently diagnosed cancer in the United States. About 1.3 million cases of highly curable basal or squamous cell cancer are diagnosed each year. In addition, about 47,700 cases of melanoma were diagnosed in 2000. An estimated 9600 persons died of skin cancer in 2000, with 7700 dying of melanoma and 1900 dying of other skin cancers (Zoorob et al, 2001). The incidence of melanoma rises rapidly in white persons after the age of 20 years. Fair-skinned persons exposed to the sun are at higher risk.

Unfortunately, routine skin screening has not proved to decrease mortality from skin cancer; however, regular skin self-assessments by patients (with assistance from family or friend to assess areas not easily viewed, such as the back), and annual skin examinations by a health care provider or dermatologist are generally recommended.

ORAL CANCER

An estimated 30,100 new cases of oral cancer were expected to be diagnosed in 2001 (NCI, 2002). Oral cancer accounts for 3% of cancers in men and 2% of cancers in women. More than 90% of oral cancers are diagnosed in persons over 45 years of age (Silverman et al, 2000), and oral cancer occurs more frequently in African Americans than in whites.

The primary risk factors in both men and women are the use of tobacco (including smokeless tobacco) and alcohol. Infection with HPV-16 virus has been associated with excess risk of developing squamous cell carcinoma of the oropharynx (NCI, 2002).

Most organizations recommend annual examination by a dentist or primary care provider for patients at high risk of oral cancer (i.e., those over 60 years of age who use tobacco or alcohol heavily). Screening examination should include inspection of the high-risk sites where 90% of all oral squamous cell cancers arise: the floor of the mouth, the ventrolateral aspect of the tongue, and the soft-palate complex. Screening in low-risk patients may aid in early detection of disease but unfortunately has not been shown to reduce mortality. It is important to counsel patients against the use of tobacco (especially chewing tobacco) as well as to use alcohol either moderately or not at all.

Care Issues for Older Patients Undergoing Cancer Treatment

When determining the appropriateness of oncologic treatments for older persons, several issues must be taken into consideration, depending on the proposed treatment course. Disease or stress can alter dramatically the delicate balance between existing functional reserves and normal physiologic functioning (Aapro et al, 2000). Not only cancer but also its treatment can significantly upset this balance, robbing older patients of their function as well as quality of life.

Several factors can affect older patients' ability to tolerate various cancer treatments. These include aforementioned comorbidities, decreased stem cell reserves, decreased DNA repair enzymes, and altered drug metabolism and clearance. Malignancies may develop and respond differently in older patients. For example, tumors of the breast, lung, and prostate tend to follow a more indolent course in the older adults. Acute myelogenous leukemia tends to be more resistant to treatment. Non-Hodgkin's lymphoma and ovarian cancers tend to have a shorter duration of remission, even if the initial response seems better than in younger patients. Cancers of the thyroid and central nervous system tend to follow a more aggressive course (Krasnow, 2002).

Operative risk assessment for older patients should include careful evaluation of kidney, liver, and cardiac function as well as cognitive status. A person's ability to tolerate radiation therapy may be limited by such factors as the need for supine positioning and immobilization during treatments. Chemotherapy agents cause stress on different organ systems, requiring a focused assessment of the systems that may be affected by the specific regimen to be used. Assessment may include renal and liver function as well as bone marrow reserves and the possible impact of drugs that are neurotoxic and ototoxic.

In addition to the medical evaluation, the availability of social resources is important in determining a plan of care for older persons. A patient undergoing cancer treatment must have reliable assistance at home when needed as well as transportation to appointments (which may include daily radiation treatments) and financial resources to obtain any needed medications, adaptive equipment, and other expenses.

Malnutrition is common in older patients and is even more common in cancer patients. This is often a subject of great concern for the patients and their caregivers. Because of a decreased thirst reflex, older patients are more likely to experience dehydration caused by nausea, vomiting, or diarrhea, especially if they have no close support. Nutritional status and dietary habits should be screened to prevent unwarranted complications of treatment and to ensure proper dietary advice and support (Extermann and Aapro, 2000).

Summary

Several issues must be considered in the determination of whether to screen the older patient for various types of cancer, including exposures, family history, social history, and comorbid conditions. The patient's remaining years of life and candidacy for further diagnostic testing and available therapies should be also assessed. Ultimately, the decision is a combination of information regarding expected outcome and the patient's individual preferences for care.

References

Aapro M, Extermann M, Repetto L: Evaluation of the elderly with cancer, *Ann Oncol* 11(Suppl 11):223-229, 2000.

American Geriatrics Society: Screening for cervical carcinoma in older women, position paper, Clinical Practice Committee, *J Am Geriatr Soc* 49(5):655-657, 2001.

Anderson J: Clinical practice guidelines: review of the recommendations for colorectal screening, *Geriatrics* 55(2):67-73, 2000.

Apantaku LM: Breast cancer diagnosis and screening, *Am Fam Physician* 62(3):596-602, 2000.

Bohadana A et al: Nicotine inhaler and nicotine patch as a combination therapy for smoking cessation, *Arch Intern Med* 160:3128-3134, 2000.

Brandon TH: Behavioral tobacco cessation treatments: yesterday's news or tomorrow's headlines? *J Clin Oncol* 19(18 suppl):64-68, 2001.

Environmental Protection Agency: *Questions and answers about dioxins.* Available at www.epa.gov. Accessed April 22, 2002.

Extermann M, Aapro M: Assessment of the older cancer patient, *Hematol Oncol Clin North Am* 14(1):63-77, 2000.

Fiore MC et al: *Smoking cessation: clinical practice guideline*, No. 18, Rockville, MD, 1996, US Department of Health and Human Services, Public Health Service, Agency for Health Care Policy and Research, AHCPR Publication No. 96-0692.

Gambert SR: Prostate cancer: when to offer screening in the primary care setting, *Geriatrics* 56(1):22-31, 2001.

Hayman JA et al: Estimating the cost of informal caregiving for elderly patients with cancer, *J Clin Oncol* 19(13):3219-3225, 2001.

Heflin MT, Cohen HJ: Cancer screening in the elderly, *Hosp Pract* 36(3):61-69, 2001.

Krasnow S: *Cancer in the elderly*, presentation at the Veterans' Affairs Medical Center, Washington, DC, 2002.

Lantz MS, Giambanco V: Smoking cessation: the key to treating older smokers? Don't quit helping, *Geriatrics* 56(5):58-59, 2001.

McCarthy EP et al: Mammography use, breast cancer stage at diagnosis, and survival among older women, *J Am Geriatr Soc* 48 (10), 2000.

Okuyemi K, Ahluwalia J, Wadland WC: The evaluation and treatment of tobacco use disorder, *J Fam Pract* 50(1):981-987, 2001.

Parnes BL et al: Question: when should we stop mammography screening for breast cancer in elderly women? *J Fam Pract* 50(2):110-111, 2001.

Pope CA et al: Lung cancer, cardiopulmonary mortality, and long-term exposure to fine particulate air pollution, *JAMA* 287(9):1132-1141, 2002.

Potosky AL et al: The association between health care coverage and the use of cancer screening tests: results from the 1992 National Health Interview Survey, *Med Care* 36(3):257-270, 1998.

Sial SH, Catalano MF: Gastrointestinal tract cancers in the elderly, *Gastroenterol Clin* 30(2):565-590, 2001.

Silverman MA et al: Cancer screening in the elderly population, *Hematol Oncol Clin North Am* 14(1):89-112, 2000.

Walter LC, Covinsky KE: Cancer screening in elderly patients: a framework for individualized decision making, *JAMA* 285(21):2750-2756, 2001.

Zoorob R et al: Cancer screening guidelines, *Am Fam Physician* 63(6):1101-1112, 2001.

5

Clinical Pharmacology

Prescribing drugs appropriately for older adults is an important component of both day-to-day primary care evaluation and comprehensive assessment of the older patient. The basic concepts of prescribing drugs appropriately differ significantly from those used for other age groups because the effects of a drug on the older patient can be magnified by certain changes that occur during the aging process. Changes may be secondary to an alteration of drug absorption, metabolism, or excretion of the drug; to structural and physiologic changes of aging organ systems; or to blunting of immune defenses.

Because of these changes and because older patients in general have significantly more illnesses, they take more prescription and over-the-counter drugs than other age groups. The average older American takes 4.5 prescriptions and 3.5 over-the-counter medications at any given time. That same person may refill about 15 prescriptions per year. As would be expected, the highest incidence of polypharmacy is in the nursing home population burdened with advanced age and chronic disease, averaging eight medications per patient.

Older patients are at greater risk for and experience greater severity of adverse drug reactions (ADRs) (Table 5-1). An ADR is the development of unwanted symptoms, signs, changes in laboratory values, or death directly related to the use of a medication (Cobbs et al, 2002-2004). It may occur secondary to alterations in drug absorption, metabolism, or elimination. It may also occur in the form of drug-drug or drug-disease interactions. This increased risk is not independently related to age, however. Two of the most common factors associated with ADRs involve a reduction in renal or hepatic function requiring dosage adjustment.

Older patients are also at greater risk for both polypharmacy and ADRs because they tend to be referred to or visit more specialist physicians. Further, they visit pharmacies more often and at more different sites. Their regular pharmacy may not have the drug in stock, and an apparent perceived urgent need to be taking the drug as soon as possible may encourage them to go elsewhere. Various family members serving as caregivers for an older loved one may use their own respective pharmacies when refilling the drug, which may also add to the confusion and the number of pill bottles. An older patient may not know that he or she is taking several different forms of aspirin or acetaminophen because he or she may not be aware of the basic ingredients of different brand names. The older patient may make the automatic but wrong assumption that it is appropriate to take all the various forms of a prescription or over-the-counter drugs such as aspirin prescribed by all the specialists (rheumatologist, cardiologist, primary care physician).

TABLE 5-1	Classes of Drugs Associated with Frequent Adverse Drug Reactions by Mechanism and Body System		
Body System	**Drug Class**	**Mechanism of ADR**	**Adverse Drug Reaction (ADR)**
Cardiovascular	Diuretics	Fluid contraction, hypokalemia, hyponatremia	Lethargy; inappropriate antidiuretic syndrome; postural hypotension, falls, hip and other fractures
	Alpha-blocker drugs	Arterial vasodilation	Presyncopal light-headedness and falls, especially in high doses
	Beta-blocker drugs	Nonselective blockade of beta receptors	Precipitation or exaggeration of congestive heart failure, masking of hypoglycemia, postural hypotension, masking of symptoms of endocrine disease, reduction in exercise capacity, exacerbation of chronic lung disease or bronchospasm, memory loss, depression, arthropathy
Central nervous system	Anticholinergic agents (antihistamines, antispasmodics, phenothiazine and tricyclic antidepressants)	Stimulation of parasympathetic nervous system, central anticholinergic disruption	Sedation, cognitive dysfunction, lethargy, acute confusion; postural hypotension, falls, hip fracture; constipation, fecal impaction, worsening of glaucoma, urinary retention, dry mouth
	Benzodiazepine tranquilizers, barbiturates, hypnotics	Depression of central nervous system	Sedation, cognitive dysfunction, lethargy, acute confusion; postural hypotension, falls, hip and other fractures
	Central-acting antihypertensive agents (methyldopa, reserpine, clonidine)	Depression of central nervous system	Sedation, cognitive dysfunction, lethargy, acute confusion; postural hypotension
	Nonsteroidal antiinflammatory drugs		Sedation, cognitive dysfunction, lethargy, acute confusion
	Fluoroquinolones		Seizures, blurred vision, diplopia, headache, drowsiness

TABLE 5-1	Classes of Drugs Associated with Frequent Adverse Drug Reactions by Mechanism and Body System—cont'd		
Body System	**Drug Class**	**Mechanism of ADR**	**Adverse Drug Reaction (ADR)**
Gastrointestinal system	H$_2$ blocking agents, sucralfate	Reduction in acid secretion leading to achlorhydria	Increased risk of aspiration pneumonia in the presence of swallowing dysfunction in bed-bound patients
	Nonsteroidal antiinflammatory drugs	Direct irritation of gastric and duodenal mucosa (inhibition of surface prostaglandin)	Diarrhea or constipation; malabsorption
	Antacids, iron preparations, tetracyclines	Binding between agents	
Liver	Anticoagulant (warfarin) Antiseizure medications (carbamazepine, phenytoin, barbiturates, meperidine)	Reduction in protein levels secondary to decreased intake, malabsorption decreased production, increased catabolism	Increased bleeding time (warfarin); sedation, lethargy, acute confusion, cognitive dysfunction (phenytoin, carbamazepine, barbiturates, meperidine); ataxia and incoordination (phenytoin)
	Barbiturates, meperidine, diphenhydramine, lidocaine, theophylline, ibuprofen, tolbutamide, salicylates, long-acting benzodiazepine tranquilizers (diazepam, chlordiazepoxide, flurazepam)	Reduction in phase 1 metabolism with normal aging	Increased risk of gastrointestinal or other bleeding (salicylates, ibuprofen); sedation, lethargy, acute confusion, cognitive dysfunction, postural hypotension, falls, hip fracture (barbiturates, meperidine, diphenhydramine, ibuprofen, diazepam, chlordiazepoxide, flurazepam); hypoglycemia (tolbutamide); postural hypotension, falls, anorexia, nausea, arrhythmias
Kidney	H$_2$ blocker drugs antibiotics (penicillins, aminoglycosides, fluoroquinolones)	Reduction in creatinine clearance	Confusion, irritability, drowsiness, lethargy, dizziness
	Digoxin	Reduction in creatinine clearance	Anorexia, decreased appetite, nausea; cardiac conduction problems; confusion, irritability, anxiety

Continued

TABLE 5-1	Classes of Drugs Associated with Frequent Adverse Drug Reactions by Mechanism and Body System—cont'd		
Body System	*Drug Class*	*Mechanism of ADR*	*Adverse Drug Reaction (ADR)*
	Nonsteroidal antiinflammatory drugs	Inhibition of prostaglandin-mediated renal vasodilation	Fluid retention, worsening hypertension, aggravation of congestive heart failure
	Fluoroquinolones		Hematuria
Skin	Tetracyclines	Photosensitivity	Dermatitis
	Fluoroquinolones	Photosensitivity	Pruritus, urticaria, rash

Older persons, especially the advanced age group (i.e., those at least 85 years old), have blunted immune defense systems to fight infection, leading to a greater risk of pneumonia and influenza and less chance of recovery. In many cases, this change is due to inadequate antibody production (Hazzard et al, 1999). Manifestations of this blunted response may be seen in the gastrointestinal (junction of the esophagus and the stomach-cardiac sphincter of the stomach) and genitourinary systems (junction of the urinary sphincter and urethra), where bacteria may tend to reflux beyond otherwise "sterile" areas proximal to these sphincters. Thus, older patients may have a greater risk of aspiration pneumonia or bladder infection in the presence of disease, as is explained later in this chapter. These patients lose the margin of reserve that allows the human body to fight off stresses, whether physiologic, psychologic, or physical. In the presence of various disease processes, this loss of reserve plays a significant role. An example is precipitation of congestive heart failure (CHF) in a patient with angina and cardiomegaly who is challenged with a "few" grams of extra dietary salt intake, failure to take a morning dose of fluid medication or digoxin after a mild upper respiratory tract infection, or slight excesses of physical exertion (Cobbs et al, 2002-2004).

Normal changes of aging include reduction in total body water, reduction in muscle mass, and an increase in total body fat. These changes may translate into a greater risk of ADRs. Water-soluble drugs such as digoxin, theophylline, and alcohol are distributed in a smaller compartment than at other age groups. These drugs may accumulate at toxic levels at the same dose. Fat-soluble, long-acting benzodiazepines accumulate in body fat to a greater extent, which may lead to greater sedation, lethargy, and risk of falls than in younger patients with less body fat. Reduction in muscle mass with "normal" aging translates into reductions in renal clearance, especially in the advanced age group. This difference holds true for drugs dependent on renal clearance, such as digoxin, H_2-blocking agents, fluoroquinolones, penicillins, and aminoglycosides.

The normal aging process is accompanied by the following reductions: total number of receptors (the nervous system) and number of functioning receptors (the pancreas), responsiveness of organ-specific receptors to a stimulus and the responsiveness of specific organ systems to stimuli, blood supply (liver), and mass of the organ (kidneys, liver, brain). An example of reduction of responsiveness of a specific organ (central nervous system, or CNS) to stimuli is increased refractory time between responses and difficulty learning new material with advancing age. An example of reduction of responsiveness of organ-specific receptors to a stimulus is reduction in maximum heart rate, or "blunted" heart rate increase, initiated by the carotid baroreceptors sensing an acute change in blood pressure. It is likely to occur when the patient stands or sits from a supine position. Normally the expected increase in heart rate would neutralize the negative effects of any transient reduction in blood pressure and prevent any symptoms of dizziness or light-headedness. The "blunted" process may precipitate postural hypotension in an otherwise "normal" older patient in 10% to 15%

of instances. *Postural hypotension* is defined as a reduction in systolic blood pressure of 15 mm Hg or more on standing or sitting from the supine. In addition, the presence of various disease processes and drugs may potentiate these responses. An example of drug-induced exaggeration of normal aging responses is the development of cognitive dysfunction secondary to alcohol and other drugs, including central-acting antihypertensive agents, psychotropics in high doses or with high anticholinergic activity, long-acting minor tranquilizers, anticholinergic agents, high doses of certain antibiotics (aminoglycosides, fluoroquinolones, penicillins), high doses of H_2-blocking agents, and nonsteroidal antiinflammatory drugs (NSAIDs). These agents might cause reduction in response time to stimuli, leading to confusion, sedation, or lethargy. An example of drug-induced exaggeration of reduced responsiveness of an organ-specific receptor to a stimulus is the use of cardiovascular agents that might cause heart block at high doses in older patients, including digoxin, antiarrhythmic drugs, and calcium channel blockers.

Drug Metabolism

Five body systems deserve mention in the absorption, metabolism, and excretion of drugs in older adults and in the development of ADRs. The least important system from this standpoint is the integumentary system. In the outer layers of the skin, 7-dehydrocholesterol is converted by ultraviolet light of the sun to vitamin D_3. Although sunlight is not the only source of vitamin D production, institutionalized older patients with chronic renal or liver failure who do not get regular exercise may develop vitamin D deficiency. This deficiency may lead to the development of osteomalacia because the metabolically active form of vitamin D requires metabolism in the liver and the kidney.

The CNS plays an important role in the development of ADRs in older patients, primarily because of normal structural and physiologic changes and changes secondary to Alzheimer's disease and related diseases. This process makes the patient more susceptible to acute confusion (delirium) and chronic confusion (cognitive dysfunction). Drugs with significant anticholinergic or muscarinic activity—such as antihistamines, antispasmodics, tricyclic antidepressants, phenothiazines, and narcotics—should be minimized or avoided in older patients. Common side effects of anticholinergic drugs include dry mouth, constipation, mental-status changes, dry eyes, difficulty with urination, blurred vision, drying of bronchial secretions, and prevention of sweating. Medical diseases such as glaucoma, benign prostatic hyperplasia, Sjögren syndrome (dry eyes and dry mouth), constipation, chronic bronchitis, and peripheral vascular disease may be aggravated by these drugs. They may further predispose the older patient to the development of fecal impaction, worsening glaucoma, urinary retention, hypothermia and hyperthermia, and exacerbations of chronic bronchitis secondary to mucus plugging (Cobbs et al, 2002-2004).

Another body system that deserves mention is the gastrointestinal tract. In the normal older adult, physiologic changes include a reduction in acid secretion, a reduction in motility, an increase in transit time, and a greater tendency toward constipation. These changes do not usually translate into clinically significant disease; however, certain drugs dependent on an acid medium in the stomach may be absorbed to a greater or lesser degree. Albumin decreases slightly with normal aging, which is of no clinical significance. In the presence of disease of the gastrointestinal tract (previous gastrectomy, Crohn's disease, ulcerative colitis, sprue), however, older patients may develop malabsorption syndromes leading to hypoproteinemia and hypoalbuminemia. Albumin and total protein levels may also decrease in older patients secondary to one or a combination of three other possible mechanisms: decreased metabolism secondary to liver diseases such as cirrhosis, increased catabolism secondary to malignancy, or decreased intake secondary to socioeconomic issues or the anorexia associated with dementia or depression. Certain drugs are highly bound to protein or albumin. A reduction in total protein or albumin level may lead to a greater fraction of free drug bioavailable, leading to toxicity. Examples include phenytoin, meperidine, digoxin, and warfarin. Reduction of the dose of these drugs may be necessary in the following instances: to prevent confusion and ataxia secondary to phenytoin; lethargy, drowsiness, falls, or cognitive dysfunction secondary to the meperidine; confusion, anorexia, and nausea secondary to digoxin use; or bleeding secondary to warfarin use. Specific formulas are available that allow dose-specific adjustments according to protein and albumin levels. Anticholinergic drugs or sucralfate may predispose the older patient to constipation or gastric reflux (by relaxation of the sphincter of the stomach) and subsequent aspiration risk. In addition, the use of H_2-blocking drugs to reduce acid secretion in the stomach of an older patient with peptic ulcer disease or hiatal hernia theoretically might seem to be a logical step in the treatment process. The use of such drugs, however, would lead to further reduction in acid secretion and a neutral or basic medium. This might be an appropriate environment for bacteria refluxing from the stomach cavity to the lower esophagus. The problem is compounded when the patient develops swallowing problems from a stroke, Parkinson's disease, or other esophageal disorder and becomes bed bound. The patient is then further predisposed to aspiration risk (Cobbs et al, 2002-2004).

An important system regarding the development of ADRs in the older patient is the liver, the most important organ for the two metabolism systems of various drugs. Phase 1 metabolism undergoes significant reduction in activity with age. Drugs metabolized in this phase are oxidized, reduced, or hydrolyzed. Their half-lives are prolonged because of this phase. These drugs include diazepam, chlordiazepoxide, flurazepam, barbiturates, meperidine, phenytoin, propranolol, quinidine, warfarin, theophylline, tolbutamide, salicylates, nortriptyline, diphenhydramine, lidocaine, and ibuprofen. Phase 2 metabolism, involving conjugation or deactivation, is not altered with age. Drugs metabolized in phase 2 include the short-acting benzodiazepines (lorazepam, oxazepam, temazepam, triazolam) with relatively short half-lives. This difference in metabolism and half-life is reflected clinically by studies indicating a difference in hip fracture risk between long-acting and short-acting benzodiazepines, with long-acting ones having a greater risk (Berggren et al, 1987).

Another important element involving metabolism is the cytochrome P450 system. It is further subclassified by specific components in which various drugs may act as inhibitors or substrates leading to inadequate or toxic levels of a specific agent. Components include 1A2, 3A4, and 2D6. In each component, specific drugs have been shown to function as either inhibitor or substrate.

The most important organ system involved in the elimination of drugs dependent on renal blood flow is the kidney and subsequent creatinine clearance. Creatinine clearance decreases with advancing age, even in the presence of normal blood urea nitrogen and serum creatinine levels. Examples of affected drugs are digoxin, penicillins, aminoglycosides, H_2-blocking agents, and fluoroquinolones. Significant reductions in the dosage of these drugs are necessary with reduced creatinine clearance to avoid ADRs (e.g., acute changes in mental status, cognitive dysfunction, dizziness, falls, or syncope). A formula useful for estimation of creatinine clearance is:

CrCl (creatinine clearance) = 140 - age of the patient × weight of patient in kilograms ÷ the serum creatinine (values < 1 rounded to 1) × 72

In the case of women, the creatinine clearance should be multiplied by 0.85. A useful rule of thumb is that if the serum blood urea nitrogen or serum creatinine is elevated above the normal range, the creatinine clearance will at least be below 50 ml/minute. In such instances, the dosage of these drugs could be reduced by one-half or more.

HIGH-RISK DRUGS

Certain categories of drugs that present a high risk of ADRs to the older patient warrant special consideration and discussion. Both new and older drugs can present a varying degree of risk for an older patient. The Food and Drug Administration (FDA) is tasked with approval and monitoring of pharmaceutical products used in the United States. Primary care providers have access to the FDA website, which maintains current information regarding ADRs (www.fda.gov/medwatch). This list includes NSAIDs, H_2-blocking drugs, beta-blocking drugs, diuretics, psychotropics, central-acting alpha-blocker drugs, ganglionic antihypertensive drugs, anticholinergic drugs, antibiotics, antiarrhythmic drugs, drugs for dementia, and a miscellaneous group (Table 5-2, p. 128).

H_2 Blockers

Studies show a correlation between advancing age, peptic ulcer disease, and the presence of *Helicobacter pylori*, gram-negative bacteria. These bacteria colonize the lining of the stomach, especially in the presence of chronic disease. H_2-blocking drugs have been shown to be inadequate for healing ulcers of the stomach and duodenum, with a greater chance of recurrence than those treated with a combination of 2 weeks of antibiotics, metronidazole, and milk of bismuth (Graham et al, 1992; Hentschel et al, 1993). Both H_2-blocking drugs and sucralfate have been used nonspecifically as prophylaxis to prevent ulceration of the stomach in older patients with or without a history of gastrointestinal disease who are placed on salicylates or NSAIDs. This practice has become widespread among physicians, although this regimen is not an accepted indication (*Physician's Desk Reference*, 2002). One study, however, indicates that high-dose famotidine (40 mg) decreases the incidence of gastric and duodenal ulceration in patients taking NSAIDs (Taha et al, 1996). A study of more than 700 nursing home patients revealed that 41% were taking H_2-blocking drugs for indications that had not been substantiated by clinical studies (Gurwitz, Noonan, and Soumerai, 1992). Another common protocol is for critically ill patients in the intensive care unit setting to receive one of these agents to prevent stress-related gastrointestinal bleeding. Another study indicated that only two conditions that warranted use of these agents in this setting to prevent this complication: respiratory failure or coagulopathy (Cook et al, 1994).

Omeprazole, lansoprazole, rabeprazole, pantoprazole, and esomeprazole are proton-pump inhibitors, a class of drugs used to treat duodenal ulcer and gastroesophageal reflux disease. These agents are indicated in the treatment of active duodenal ulcer, treatment of heartburn and other symptoms associated with gastroesophageal reflux disease, treatment of erosive esophagitis and maintaining healing of erosive esophagitis, and long-term treatment of Zollinger-Ellison syndrome and other rare conditions that cause pathologic hypersecretion. Atrophic gastritis has been occasionally noted in long-term use. The drug should be taken before meals (*Physician's Desk Reference*, 2002).

Nonsteroidal Antiinflammatory Drugs

The NSAIDs are a particularly hazardous category of drugs that should be avoided in older patients if at all possible. They can cause ADRs by three different mechanisms: precipitation of confusion, gastrointestinal bleeding, and renal insufficiency or failure. In one study, NSAID use caused or exacerbated medical conditions in 86% of the 500 emergency admissions to a general hospital ward (Jones, Berman, and Doherty, 1992). In high doses, all these drugs may cause acute or cognitive dysfunction. Indomethacin, because of its high affinity for penetrating the blood-brain barrier, brings the greatest risk of CNS side effects such as confusion, dizziness, lethargy, restlessness, and depression (*Physician's Desk Reference*, 2002). It is inappropriate for use by older patients. Studies, including the Baltimore Longitudinal Study of Aging, have shown an overall decreased relative risk of Alzheimer's disease in patients taking NSAIDs. Increased duration of use is associated with greater risk reduction. All data are suggestive of a protective function but are not confirmatory (Stewart et al, 1997; Zandi et al, 2002b).

The NSAIDs also cause direct irritation of the gastric and duodenal mucosa, leading to gastritis, peptic ulcer, and esophagitis after first-time or sustained use. Often a patient may develop bleeding from an undiagnosed asymptomatic hiatal hernia or reflux that was precipitated by the use of these drugs. Several studies indicate that in high enough dose all NSAIDs can cause gastrointestinal bleeding, with the least risk from low doses of ibuprofen (200 to 400 mg) (Langman et al, 1994). A meta-analysis of 12 studies compared the frequency of major gastrointestinal side effects of the various NSAIDs. The lowest risk again occurred with the use of ibuprofen. In the comparison of ibuprofen with the other NSAIDs, fenoprofen had a relative risk of 1.6, followed by aspirin (1.6), diclofenac (1.8), sulindac (2.1), diflunisal (2.2), naproxen (2.2), indomethacin (2.4), tolmetin (3.0), piroxicam (3.8), and ketoprofen (4.2) (Henry et al, 1991).

A third mechanism by which NSAIDs cause ADRs in older patients is by prostaglandin-mediated renal vasodilation, leading to fluid retention and subsequent renal injury via several mechanisms and resulting in renal failure and glomerulopathy. By causing fluid retention, NSAIDs may be responsible for worsening hypertension or an inability to control adequately any existing hypertension or precipitating or aggravating existing CHF. Discontinuation of NSAIDs in an older patient with hypertension may result in a statistically significant reduction in mean blood pressure (Gottlieb et al, 1992; Gurwitz et al, 1994). The use of NSAIDs is associated with acute liver injury and a hepatitis-like syndrome. A study comparing acetaminophen (4000 mg) with high (2400 mg) and low (1200 mg) daily doses of ibuprofen for osteoarthritis of the knee indicated no difference in relief of symptoms (Bradley et al, 1991). For acute flares of inflammation (swollen, warm, tender joints) for which an NSAID may be beneficial, however, some practical guidelines include (1) using the agent as needed, alternating it with acetaminophen; (2) using the agent in the lowest possible dose, and (3) using the agent for 5 to 7 days and then discontinuing it. Occasionally persistent patients will demand that they be prescribed an NSAID for continuous use. In such cases patients should be advised of the potential side effects. The patient should agree to routine (every 3 to 4 months) monitoring of the blood urea nitrogen for early signs of renal insufficiency. In addition, a hemogram should be routinely performed to monitor patients for early gastrointestinal bleeding. In these cases misoprostol, a cytoprotective agent given four times daily, may provide some protection of the mucosa from gastrointestinal problems. Disadvantages of the drug include its high cost, the necessity of administering it four times daily, and its common side effect of diarrhea. The NSAIDs should not be used concomitantly with aspirin or warfarin because of the higher risk of causing bleeding complications (*Physician's Desk Reference*, 2002). Two published studies indicate that the specific NSAID naproxen may confer protection against myocardial infarction by virtue of an antiplatelet effect (Solomon et al, 2002).

The newer cyclooxygenase-2 inhibitors (rofecoxib, celecoxib, valdecoxib) provide equal efficacy compared with the traditional NSAIDs for the relief of signs and symptoms of rheumatoid and osteoarthritis with a gastrointestinal risk profile similar to placebo and superior to traditional NSAIDs. Contraindications include patients with active gastrointestinal disease (Bombardier et al, 2002; *Physician's Desk Reference*, 2002; Silverstein et al, 2000). One study, however, indicated that rofecoxib compared with celecoxib caused significantly more hypertension and edema (Whelton et al, 2001). An advantage is once or twice daily dosing; the disadvantage is its higher cost.

Beta-blockers

Beta-blocker drugs should be used with caution in older patients, particularly propranolol, which is considered in most instances an inappropriate drug because of its side effects. These include precipitation of or exacerbation of CHF, masking of hypoglycemia, development of postural hypotension, masking of symptoms of endocrine disease such as hypothyroidism, reduction in exercise capacity, exacerbation of chronic lung disease or bronchospasm, depression, memory loss, and production of arthropathy (Cahill et al, 1994; Newbern, 1991). However, it may be beneficial for the treatment of anxiety in demented patients and tremor disorders in older patients. The drug was also used to prove the efficacy of treatment of systolic hypertension (systolic blood pressure greater than 160) for the prevention of stroke and mortality (SHEP Cooperative Research Group, 1991). Use of the drug should be based on a risk-benefit ratio for the particular patient, including an evaluation of the patient's medical conditions. Beta-blocker drugs may also produce adverse effects on lipid metabolism (*Physician's Desk Reference*, 2002). Pragmatically the use of beta-blocker drugs would seem illogical because of the low incidence of high-renin, high-aldosterone hypertension and because renin and aldosterone levels decrease with normal aging (Cobbs et al, 2002-2004). They may be used as first-line agents for the older hypertensive patient with a previous history of angina or myocardial infarction because they can reduce overall mortality by as much as 76% in this population (Park, Forman, and Wei, 1995). A review of 3737 Medicare patients in New Jersey who had survived a myocardial infarction at 30 days showed that only 21% treated up to 90 days after discharge from the hospital had received a beta-blocker (Soumerai et al, 1997). Beta-selective blocking drugs such as atenolol or metoprolol have fewer side effects and also have the advantage of once- or twice-daily dosing. Therefore compliance is also increased significantly. The use of atenolol compared with the use of placebo decreases mortality significantly at 2-year follow-up in older patients (average age, 68 years) who underwent cardiac surgery (Mangano et al, 1996). A North American observational analysis indicated that beta-blocker therapy before and after coronary artery bypass grafting (less than 30 days postoperative) was associated with a significant reduction in mortality with the exception of patients with an ejection fraction of less than 30% (Ferguson et al, 2002). They also may be particularly appropriate for older patients for dual indications of atrial arrhythmias and hypertension. Beta-blocker drugs used selectively in patients with good left ventricular function can decrease the risk of CHF and death over a 2-year period. A beta-blocker, carvedilol, with alpha-blocking and antioxidant properties, was approved by the FDA in mid-1997. Its approved use is for increasing left ventricular function in patients with mild to severe CHF. Its action is thought to occur by moderating the adverse effects of chronic activation of the sympathetic nervous system (Packer et al, 1996). In one study at 1-year follow-up, ejection fraction increased significantly in these patients, with a decrease in resting and maximum heart rates as well. At 19-months' follow-up, a 26% reduction in the risk of death or hospital admission was noted (Australia/New Zealand Heart Failure Research Collaborative Group, 1997). A published review of all English-language large, randomized controlled clinical trials assessing the mortality benefits of beta-blockers in patients with heart failure showed a 30% reduction in mortality and a 40% reduction in hospitalizations in patients with class II through IV heart failure compared with placebo. The two agents included in the analysis currently available in the United States were carvedilol and metoprolol (Foody et al, 2002).

   Conventional wisdom has been that beta-blocker use is associated with symptoms of depression, fatigue, and sexual dysfunction, particularly in older patients. A meta-analysis of English-language clinical trials involving the use of beta-blockers for hypertension, myocardial infarction, and CHF between 1996 and 2000 showed no significant risks for any of these symptoms (Ko et al, 2002).

Diuretics

Diuretics constitute another class of high-risk drugs that should be used with caution in older patients, in part because of the reduction in total body water with normal aging and other factors. Side effects include hypokalemia possibly linked to sudden death, worsening renal function, left ventricular hypertrophy, and increases in total cholesterol and triglycerides. These agents may cause a contraction alkalosis. In addition, they may precipitate an exaggerated postural hypotensive response, leading to light-headedness, falling, and further morbidity or mortality from a hip or other fracture (Cobbs et al, 2002-2004; *Physician's Desk Reference*, 2002). Extreme caution is advised in administering thiazides to older patients with dementia or depression because of their tendency to drink less or even forget to drink fluids because of the associated memory loss. Frail and advanced older patients over 85 years of age are also at high risk because of their greater tendency to develop postural hypotension. Older patients on diuretics should be advised to drink lots of isotonic fluids during the summer months, especially during times of exercise and sweating. Diuretics may actually be harmful in hypertensive patients with diabetes. Thiazides are generally not effective in the presence of renal insufficiency.

   Loop diuretics (metolazone, furosemide, bumetanide) are popular drugs used to treat dependent leg edema in older patients, but they also have the potential of exaggerating the postural hypotension caused by chronic venous insufficiency and stasis, further increasing the risk of inducing lightheadedness, dizziness, falls, and fracture or other morbidity (Cobbs et al, 2002-2004). These agents should be reserved for severe edema that is refractory to leg elevation, stockings, and exercise. Loop diuretics should be reserved for patients with renal insufficiency or CHF to mobilize fluid and promote brisk diuresis. By causing calciuria, they may serve a useful purpose in the initial treatment of hypercalcemia (Cobbs et al, 2002-2004). Both loop and thiazide diuretics may be a significant cause of urinary incontinence. Removal, minimizing the dose, or changing the time of day for administration from the afternoon to midmorning may alleviate the problem in many cases (Cobbs et al, 2002-2004). The advantages of using thiazide diuretics in older patients for the treatment of mild hypertension include low cost and once-per-day dosing. The SHEP (systolic hypertension in the elderly) trial used a first-line drug, chlorthalidone, a long-acting diuretic. This study showed that reduction in systolic blood pressure below 160 mm Hg significantly reduced the incidence of stroke and cardiovascular disease and, to a lesser extent, cardiovascular deaths and total mortality (SHEP Cooperative Research Group, 1991). This effect was even greater for non-insulin-dependent diabetic patients than for nondiabetic patients (Curb et al, 1996). Much has been written about the adverse effects of thiazide diuretics on the lipid profile. A retrospective study of 9274 Medicare and Medicaid patients in New Jersey, 65 to 95 years of age, showed no significant effect of the use of these agents with the initiation of lipid-lowering agents (Monane et al, 1997). Doses above 50 mg are generally not effective in achieving blood pressure control. African-American patients seem to benefit more from thiazides than do white patients. For stepwise treatment of hypertension, diuretics in combination with other agents may potentiate the effect of other drugs but also have the disadvantage of being more expensive, especially in combined pill formulation.

Central-acting and Alpha-blocker Antihypertensive Drugs

Central-acting drugs such as clonidine, reserpine, and methyldopa can cause significant CNS side effects in older patients. These include headache, irritability, sedation, cognitive dysfunction, and depressive symptoms (*Physician's Desk Reference*, 2002). Alpha methyldopa, an older drug because of its short half-life, is given four times per day. The drug has a number of side effects: sedation, liver involvement, and multiple drug-drug interactions (*Physician's Desk Reference*, 2002). Reserpine offers the advantage of once-per-day dosing and is inexpensive, but it may produce bothersome side effects, including postural hypotension, dry mouth, constipation, bradycardia, bronchospasm, and hypersecretion of the digestive tract. It causes a hypertensive crisis when used in conjunction with food and drugs that contain a monoamine oxidase (MAO) inhibitor. The use of methyldopa and reserpine is inappropriate in older patients. Alpha-blocker drugs such as prazosin, terazosin, and doxazosin reduce blood pressure by causing vasodilation (*Physician's Desk Reference*, 2002). They have become popular because of their promotion as first-line agents for hypertension in the older patient with benign prostatic hyperplasia with associated signs and symptoms of urgency, frequency, or hesitancy. They have the added advantage of once- or twice-daily dosing. To achieve the dual role of blood pressure control and the control of prostatic symptoms, however, doses of 7 to 10 mg are often necessary. There is a risk of postural hypotension that can be minimized by taking the drug before bedtime.

Apresoline is an older drug that has traditionally been used for the treatment of hypertension. Its mechanism of action involves vasodilation, especially of the renal arteries. Side effects of the drug include negative effects on the cardiac muscle and an increase in heart rate, thereby increasing the workload of the heart. In some cases this may contribute to the development of CHF, especially in patients with impaired left ventricular function (*Physician's Desk Reference*, 2002). Disadvantages of the drug include a short half-life and its need to be taken four times per day. The drug may also cause a lupus-like syndrome. The dual-acting alpha- and beta-blocking drugs are agents that combine the advantages of beta-blockers with the vasodilating effects of alpha-blockers. They also do not increase heart rate and may be useful antihypertensive agents in patients with a history of stable heart failure. These combination drugs, however, tend to be more expensive than other classes of drugs in general. Other classes of drugs appropriate for the treatment of hypertension in older persons include the angiotensin-converting enzyme (ACE) inhibitor and calcium channel blocker drugs.

Antihypertensive Drugs

The ACE inhibitor drugs are a popular group of drugs used to treat hypertension. They have been shown in numerous studies to improve cardiac function in acute CHF secondary to diastolic dysfunction and to increase survival of patients with chronic severe CHF. Captopril, the first of these agents, reverses the reduction in renal blood flow that occurs with normal aging in healthy normotensive older patients by causing significant renal vasodilation. It also limits myocardial infarction expansion if given within 24 hours and subsequently to reduce short-term mortality at 5 weeks (ISIS-4 Collaborative Group, 1995). Enalapril has also been shown to slow the progression of renal disease, proteinuria, and albuminuria when it is taken for hypertension (compared with metoprolol) when patients were followed up for 3 years (Bjorck et al, 1992). Other positive effects of ACE inhibitor drugs are a slower rate of decline of renal function and a significant reduction in albuminuria. This effect has been shown using lisinopril compared with furosemide and atenolol in hypertensive patients with moderate diabetic renal insufficiency when patients were followed up for 18 months (Slataper et al, 1993). Captopril slows the progression of renal disease, reduces mortality rates, and alleviates the need for transplantation or dialysis as opposed to placebo when patients were followed up for 3 years (Lewis et al, 1993). Enalapril, compared with beta-blocker drugs, showed a significant reduction in proteinuria at 6 months and significant reduction in end-stage renal failure in patients with nondiabetic renal insufficiency who were followed up for 3 years (Hannedouche et al, 1994). In most cases, they offer the added advantage of once- or twice-daily dosing. ACE inhibitor drugs are contraindicated in the presence of renal artery stenosis. Frequent side effects of these drugs include cough and angioedema (*Physician's Desk Reference*, 2002). Potassium levels should be monitored in patients prescribed ACE inhibitors because of the tendency for these patients to develop hyperkalemia. The Heart Outcomes Prevention Evaluation (HOPE) study, a large multicenter randomized, placebo controlled trial, evaluated 9541 patients 55 years of age or older and considered at high risk of developing a major cardiovascular event because of a history of coronary artery disease, stroke, peripheral vascular disease, or diabetes accompanied by at least one other cardiovascular risk factor (hypertension, elevated total cholesterol levels, low high-density lipoprotein (HDL) levels, cigarette smoking, or documented microalbuminuria). Patients treated with ramipril versus placebo had a significant reduction in the risk of myocardial infarction, stroke, or death from cardiovascular causes (*Physician's Desk Reference*, 2002; Warner and Perry, 2002).

A new class of antihypertensive agents, the angiotensin II receptor antagonists, provides another option for older patients. The first of these agents, losartan, is significantly more effective than atenolol for treatment of patients with isolated hypertension and electrocardiographic evidence of left ventricular hypertrophy. Patients receiving losartan also have a significantly reduced incidence of cardiovascular mortality, nonfatal and fatal stroke, new-onset diabetes, and total mortality compared with atenolol. No difference was found in the incidence of myocardial infarction (Kjeldsen et al, 2002) with its use. A disadvantage is higher cost. Another agent, valsartan, was approved in late 2002 for the treatment of CHF.

Calcium channel-blocker drugs (antagonists) are also a popular group of drugs used to treat older hypertensive patients by producing vasodilation and promoting loss of sodium and water. Side effects include flushing, headache, dependent edema, and constipation, depending on the specific drug. They also offer the advantage of once- or twice-daily dosing, even though they are more expensive than diuretics or beta-blocker drugs. A case-control study, however, suggests increased mortality rates in hypertensive patients treated with these agents, with risk increasing as dosage increases. This risk was also increased with the use of short-acting agents, particularly nifedipine. Because of the possible limitations and criticisms of the study, a clinical trial is ongoing to prove or disprove these findings. Until further findings, long-acting agents are the preferred agents for hypertension according to the recommendations of the National Heart, Lung, and Blood Institute (Buring, Glynn, and Hennekens, 1995; Furberg, Psaty, and Meyer, 1995; Pinkowish, 1995). An encouraging controlled, open study compared short-acting nifedipine with diltiazem. After 5 years of follow-up, the risk of myocardial infarction, death, CHF, premature ventricular contractions, or hospitalization for worsening angina was significantly lower in patients treated with placebo or diltiazem compared with short-acting nifedipine. This effect did not reach statistical significance (Ishikawa et al, 1997).

Calcium antagonists have also been implicated in gastrointestinal hemorrhage because they inhibit platelet aggregation. One prospective study compared calcium antagonists with beta-blockers and ACE inhibitors in 1636 patients who were at least 68 years of age. Compared with beta-blockers, calcium antagonists had a relative risk of bleeding of 1.86 and ACE inhibitors a risk of 1.23. After adjustment for covariables, this risk was even greater than aspirin, with a relative risk of 1.51, and NSAIDs other than ibuprofen, with a relative risk of 1.4. The risk was similar to sodium warfarin (2.2) and steroids (1.9) (Pahor et al, 1996). Another prospective study evaluated 161 older postoperative hip fracture patients, 70 of whom were taking calcium antagonists. Patients taking calcium antagonists showed a 74% incidence of transfusion compared with 33% for those not taking these agents (Zuccala et al, 1997).

Calcium antagonists can worsen heart failure or increase mortality rates for patients with left ventricular dysfunction. A randomized, double-blind, placebo-controlled multicenter trial evaluated 186 patients with dilated cardiomyopathy and ejection fractions below 50% with no evidence of coronary artery disease who were using the short-acting version of the drug. Survival was the same for both the intervention and placebo groups. At 24-months' follow-up, no increased complications were found with diltiazem for patients with ejection fractions below 35%. Patients taking diltiazem had increased stroke volume and better endurance on exercise testing compared with patients receiving placebo. Patients taking diltiazem stated that they felt significantly better (Figulla et al, 1996). Amlodipine versus placebo has been shown to decrease significantly the risk of death and other end points (pulmonary edema, hypoperfusion, myocardial infarction, and sustained ventricular arrhythmia) in 1153 patients with nonischemic severe chronic heart failure (New York class IIIB or IV) with ejection fractions below 30%. Outcomes were similar in patients with ischemic disease (Packer et al, 1996b).

Verapamil, compared with placebo, is effective in increasing pain-free walking distance in patients with symptomatic peripheral vascular disease (Bagger et al, 1997). A recent study indicates calcium antagonists are used significantly more often than are beta-blockers for conditions such as previous myocardial infarction, coronary artery disease, and hypertension in older outpatients in a hospital-based academic geriatric practice (Fishkind, Paris, and Aronow, 1997).

Psychotropic Drugs

Psychotropic drugs, including minor tranquilizers, major tranquilizers, antidepressants, barbiturates, and hypnotics, are also a high-risk group. Adverse effects of these drugs in general include cognitive dysfunction, sedation, drowsiness, lethargy, and functional decline. Inappropriately high doses for the older patient may produce or exaggerate postural hypotension, leading to lightheadedness on standing or sitting from a supine position, falls, fractures, and other morbidity (Cobbs et al, 2002-2004). Because of their side-effect profile and their traditional overuse in institutional settings for such nonspecific conditions as insomnia, general agitation, and anxiety or for dementia syndromes, a 1987 federal law, the Omnibus Budget Reconciliation Act (OBRA), limits their use in these settings for specific indications only and in a time-limited fashion. Proper documentation in the medical record is also required. A retrospective review of 856 older medical and surgical hospital patients showed that those receiving sedative hypnotic medications have higher hospitalization costs, longer lengths of stay, and greater severity of illness (Zisselman et al, 1996). Major and minor tranquilizers are indicated only for psychotic behavior, hallucinations, or delusions that are potentially harmful to patients or their surroundings or for the prevention of aggressive, hostile, or combative behavior. Antidepressants should be used only for depressive symptoms. Antianxiety drugs should be used only to alleviate these symptoms in a patient with anxiety that is potentially harmful to the patient's medical or social condition. Barbiturates should be used only for the prevention of specific seizures. Hypnotics should be used for only occasional sleep, not on a daily basis. The first component of the law involving the use of major tranquilizers was implemented in 1994. As a result, the use of these agents has decreased significantly.

The major tranquilizers, commonly known as the *phenothiazines*, can also cause a drug-induced parkinsonian syndrome consisting of bradykinesia, resting tremor, and cogwheel rigidity of the extremities (Cobbs et al, 2002-2004). It has been traditional to prescribe them prophylactically with an anticholinergic drug (diphenhydramine, benztropine, trihexyphenidyl) to prevent the nuisance side effect of tremor. The older patient presenting with this syndrome, however, may not have the associated tremor, therefore alleviating the need for these agents, especially considering their additional troublesome side effects previously mentioned. In many cases, older patients are inappropriately treated for presumed Parkinson disease instead of removing or lowering the dose of the phenothiazine. The phenothiazine drugs have a particularly disturbing and in many cases irreversible side effect of tardive dyskinesia, characterized by abnormal, involuntary, repetitious muscle movements. Increasing the dose of the drug may temporarily suppress the involuntary movements, but with subsequent breakthrough and worsening of the involuntary movements. Removal of the drug may help to alleviate the movement disorder, but there is no predictable pattern to the syndrome. Anticholinergic drugs used to treat the parkinsonian side effects of phenothiazine major tranquilizers usually are of no benefit for this condition. The risk of tardive dyskinesia for older patients may be as high as six times that of younger patients using the phenothiazine drugs.

The choice of major tranquilizer (phenothiazine) prescribed for the older patient depends on the side effects of the agent matched to the signs and symptoms of the patient. All the phenothiazine major tranquilizers cause tardive dyskinesia and varying degrees of postural hypotension, anticholinergic side effects, sedation, and potency. For instance, an older patient with sleep-wake cycle problems secondary to sundowning from Alzheimer disease may benefit from the sedative properties of chlorpromazine, 10 to 25 mg, or thioridazine, 25 mg at bedtime. In dosage range, they produce sleep without inducing postural hypotension or significant anticholinergic disruption. The latter may lead to the development of delirium, worsening cognitive dysfunction, or other anticholinergic or parkinsonian side effects. By contrast, haloperidol, in a dose of 0.5 to 1 mg, may be an appropriate drug to treat aggressive, hostile, combative, or psychotic behavior in an agitated patient with dementia during the day. It is the least sedating and least hypotensive, and it has the fewest anticholinergic side effects of these agents; yet it is the most potent. The use of haloperidol at night for sleep might be counterproductive, however. These agents, especially in high doses, may reduce the self-care of the older patient with dementia. Functional decline may develop, manifested by a reduction in independent mobility, bathing, feeding, dressing, eating, and toileting. It may further lead to fecal and urinary incontinence and subsequent hygiene problems (Cobbs et al, 2002-2004).

Risperidone is a newer agent classified as a dopaminergic/serotonergic antagonist. It has a lower risk of tardive dyskinesia (4% to 10%), but it may cause prolactin level elevations and associated galactorrhea or gynecomastia. Recent studies show its effectiveness in the management of agitation in older patients with dementia (Madhusoodanan and Brenner, 2001; *Physician's Desk Reference*, 2002).

The newer antipsychotic agents, olanzapine, clozapine, quetiapine, and ziprasidone, provide a safer option than the traditional phenothiazine tranquilizers because they have a significantly lower risk of tardive dyskinesia (1% to 4%), but they also have the disadvantage of being much more expensive (*Physician's Desk Reference*, 2002). Clozapine is highly anticholinergic and may precipitate seizures. Regular monitoring of the white blood count is required because of the side effect of agranulocytosis. Olanzapine is also highly anticholinergic and causes weight gain. It is useful in patients with Parkinson disease or levodopa-induced psychotic symptoms. Quetiapine causes sedation and somnolence but is useful for nighttime sedation (*Physician's Desk Reference*, 2002).

The tricyclic antidepressants should be used with caution because of their side-effect profile, which is similar to that of the phenothiazines. Side effects include postural hypotension, anticholinergic side effects (dry mouth, blurred vision, tachycardia, constipation, urinary retention), sedation, and cognitive dysfunction (*Physician's Desk Reference*, 2002). They nonselectively block the reuptake of various neurotransmitters, including norepinephrine, serotonin, and dopamine. In low doses these agents promote a "quieting" or quinidine-like effect on the myocardium and, in high doses, an arrhythmogenic effect. These drugs can cause significant risk to some older patients because of cardiac involvement.

Suicide as a risk is related to antidepressants in general, not to the specific class, but rather related by dose, with higher doses associated with increased risk. Higher doses may also be associated with postural hypotension and falls, especially for amitriptyline. Tricyclic drugs with the fewest anticholinergic properties should be chosen over those with high anticholinergic side effects to limit the risk of precipitating acute confusion or precipitating or worsening cognitive dysfunction, especially at high doses. Desipramine and nortriptyline should be given during the morning because of their nonsedating properties. They also offer the safest profile; imipramine and amitriptyline offer the worst. The last of these drugs is considered inappropriate for older patients in most cases. Amitriptyline should not be given during the day because of its high risk of sedation and postural hypotension, and it should be avoided in doses exceeding 25 mg. Few current indications exist for its use, except to treat chronic pain syndromes in association with depressed mood or depression associated with both insomnia and anorexia. A beneficial effect is its ability to stimulate appetite. It should not be prescribed for patients with Alzheimer's disease.

The most popular class of agents to treat depression in older patients is the selective serotonin reuptake inhibitors (SSRIs). They achieve the same efficacy as the tricyclic agents but often are better tolerated because of their selectivity. Studies indicate that depression may be mediated primarily by a deficiency of serotonin, among other chemical agents in the brain. These agents offer an advantage over traditional tricyclic antidepressants because of their lack of significant anticholinergic side effects and quicker onset of action (i.e., 2 to 4 weeks). Theoretically, their use in patients with Alzheimer disease would seem appropriate to avoid worsening the structural anticholinergic disruption that typically occurs in these patients as the disease process worsens (Hazzard et al, 1999; Mach et al, 1995). Side effects of these agents include insomnia, agitation, decreased appetite, and nausea. Fluoxetine, the first of these agents, and its metabolite have a combined half-life of 4 to 16 days. It is less selective in its side-effect profile. Newer agents such as sertraline, paroxetine, and citalopram (*Physician's Desk Reference*, 2002) have half-lives approximating 24 to 48 hours. Being more selective for serotonin receptors, they are more appropriate for the older patient. The SSRIs are strong inhibitors of the cytochrome P-450 system, which is involved in the metabolism of many medications. Because of their tendency to cause withdrawal side effects, the dosage should be tapered before discontinuance of the drug. Used with other agents, such as the tricyclic agents, antihistamines, theophylline, erythromycin, benzodiazepines, and steroids, they can double or triple the levels of these agents, leading to a greater risk of ADRs (Sheikh, 1995). Caution should be exercised when using these drugs to treat depressive symptoms with or without dementia and in the malnourished patient because these drugs may magnify the symptoms of weight loss, nausea, and anorexia related to the disease process itself. This class of drugs also has the advantage of once-daily dosing and rapid onset of action compared with the slower-onset tricyclic antidepressants. These drugs should be administered in the morning because of their side effect profile.

Because of its direct serotonergic effects, trazodone, in an initial dose of 25 to 50 mg at bedtime, provides an excellent option for the dual purpose of treating the patients with dementia or depression exhibiting insomnia or sundowning. Side effects include postural hypotension and rarely priapism, usually in much higher doses than normally used in older patients, 150 to 300 mg (Cobbs et al, 2002-2004; *Physician's Desk Reference*, 2002). The SSRIs are also used in combination with trazodone for the treatment of depression; this is referred to as *augmentation therapy*. Patients receiving this combination should be monitored for signs and symptoms of the so-called serotonin syndrome, which is associated with restlessness and increased anxiety (Hazzard et al, 1999); this is due to the fact that both classes of drugs cause the accumulation of serotonin, even though by different mechanisms.

Atypical antidepressants include venlafaxine and bupropion. Venlafaxine has a chemical structure unrelated to tricyclic, tetracyclic, or other agents. Its side-effect profile is similar to that of the SSRIs, with the additional possibility of increasing diastolic blood pressure with increasing dose. It has a broader spectrum of reuptake of neurotransmitters than serotonin, but it does not inhibit the cytochrome P-450 system. Therefore the risk of ADRs in combination with other drugs may be lower. All the SSRIs listed herein have recently been used to treat chronic anxiety states and for the prevention of comorbidities of chronic anxiety, such as depression and alcohol and drug abuse. Various agents have received FDA indications recently for panic disorder, generalized or socialized anxiety disorder, posttraumatic stress disorder, or obsessive-compulsive disorder (*Physician's Desk Reference*, 2002).

Bupropion is a relatively safe drug with low anticholinergic and antiadrenergic side effects that is useful for the treatment of depression. It should be used with caution in patients with a history of seizure disorder, however, because it lowers the seizure threshold (Cobbs et al, 2002-2004). Mirtazapine is a combined agent different in structure from the SSRIs in that it is thought to enhance central serotonergic and noradrenergic activity. Increasing dosage is associated with increasing sedation. Another side effect that may be beneficial is increased appetite and weight gain (Cobbs et al, 2002-2004; *Physician's Desk Reference*, 2002).

Methylphenidate is an older drug that is regaining popularity for the treatment of retarded depression associated with psychomotor slowing, excessive sleepiness, and increased appetite. It should be administered in the morning because of its side effect of insomnia (Cobbs et al, 2002-2004). Because of its short half-life and quick onset of action, the drug can serve an equally useful purpose in hospitalized older patients with recent unexplained confusion. In such cases a major question is whether the patient's mental status is secondary to dementia or depression. The protocol involves an initial dose of 5 to 10 mg (the Ritalin challenge) and doubling the dose every day for up to 5 days. The mental status of the patient in whom confusion is mostly secondary to depression will improve in mood and orientation, and the patient primarily affected with dementia will become more confused. Results can be seen as early as the second or third day of administration. Because of its side effect of anorexia, patients taking this drug should be monitored for appetite problems. It should be used with caution for patients with a history of malnutrition or dementia. It should be used with caution for patients with significant cardiovascular disease because of its basic properties as an alpha stimulant and its tendency to worsen hypertension and anxiety and to cause arrhythmias.

Lithium is used to treat bipolar (manic-depressive) disorder. Regular monitoring of serum levels is recommended because of the frequency of adverse side effects with this drug, especially when used with other agents. Because the drug is distributed in the total body water content, excretion depends on adequate renal function. Dosages should be reduced for renal insufficiency. Levels of the drug may be increased for patients taking an ACE inhibitor and NSAIDs. Other agents, such as acetazolamide, urea, xanthine preparations (theophylline), and alkalinizing agents, may decrease serum levels. Lithium may interfere with blood monitoring for thyroid disease. Use with calcium channel blocker drugs can increase the risk of nervous system toxicity. Use of lithium with diuretics or in patients with restricted sodium diets for treatment of CHF or hypertension decreases sodium resorption by the renal tubules, which may lead to an increased risk of hyponatremia and lithium toxicity (*Physician's Desk Reference*, 2002). Other agents that may interfere with lithium metabolism include antipsychotics, calcium-channel blockers, and medications containing iodine. Early symptoms of toxicity include diarrhea, drowsiness, loss of appetite, muscle weakness, nausea or vomiting, slurred speech, or trembling. Late symptoms include confusion, unsteadiness, blurred vision, convulsions, dizziness, and increased urination. Less common side effects include postural hypotension, weight gain, bradycardia, cardiac arrhythmias, and heart block.

The benzodiazepine minor tranquilizers are useful agents for the treatment of agitation, anxiety, and insomnia in older patients. In this category, short-acting ones such as lorazepam (0.5 to 1 mg) and oxazepam (15 mg) are the recommended drugs of choice to prevent the worrisome side effects encountered with the long-acting agents, as previously mentioned (Cobbs et al, 2002-2004; Ensrud et al, 2002; *Physician's Desk Reference*, 2002). For this reason, flurazepam, chlordiazepoxide, and diazepam are inappropriate for older patients. Alprazolam is a short-acting benzodiazepine that requires metabolism by the liver. It should be used in a low dose (0.25 mg) twice or three times daily. It has minor antidepressant effects in addition to its antianxiety effect (*Physician's Desk Reference*, 2002). Other relatively short-acting benzodiazepines (triazolam and temazepam) serve a useful purpose for the occasional treatment of insomnia. Triazolam has a half-life of 4 to 6 hours. Temazepam has a half-life of 6 to 8 hours. Triazolam is useful to induce sleep, and temazepam will maintain sleep. Triazolam, in doses higher than 0.125 mg and used on a regular basis, has been implicated as a cause of delayed recall of tasks in older patients. For this reason, it should be used only occasionally in a dose of 0.125 mg. The benzodiazepines in general are known to cause short-term impairment in memory, even though their long-term effect is unknown.

Chloral hydrate is an old agent used for the treatment of insomnia in older patients. Because of its anticholinergic activity, other agents have a better side-effect profile (Sherrill and Reifler, 1999). Meprobamate is an older drug used to treat anxiety; however, its use in older patients is inappropriate because of the risk of causing sedation, confusion, and lethargy. Buspirone is a useful agent to treat chronic anxiety but must be given on a regular basis to be effective. Because onset of action requires 7 to 10 days, use of a short-acting benzodiazepine for this period may be necessary to relieve anxiety.

Zolpidem tartrate is a short-acting nonbenzodiazepine hypnotic with a chemical structure unrelated to the benzodiazepines, barbiturates, or other hypnotic drugs. It interacts with GABA-receptor sites. Therefore, it shares some of the properties of the benzodiazepines, including the potential to depress the CNS and impair motor and cognitive performance in older patients but less so and with an incidence of next-day drowsiness and rebound insomnia secondary to discontinuation. Unlike the benzodiazepines, physical dependence does not occur with regular use. It is indicated for the occasional use of insomnia. Although experience in older persons is limited, a 5-mg dose is recommended for this group of patients (*Physician's Desk Reference*, 2002). Zaleplon, recently approved by the FDA, is also a nonbenzodiazepine hypnotic similar to zolpidem, but it is ultra-short acting in the range of 1.5 to 3 hours. It is indicated for occasional use by patients who have difficulty falling asleep or wake up in the middle of the night (*Physician's Desk Reference*, 2002). Like zolpidem, it is indicated only for occasional use with the same potential for side-effect profile. A dose of 5 mg rather than 10 mg is initially indicated in the older patients.

Agents useful for the treatment of agitation and anxiety associated with dementia syndromes include trazodone and buspirone. Carbamazepine and valproic acid in lower doses traditionally used to treat seizure disorder (i.e., 100 to 200 mg twice daily) have also recently become popular agents for the treatment of agitation and aggressive, hostile, and combative behavior in these patients. These agents offer a safer side-effect profile than the traditional psychotropic agents and cause little toxicity. Regular laboratory monitoring (every 4 to 6 months) of the liver and bone marrow (hemogram) are advisable when using carbamazepine because the drug can cause liver and bone marrow depression (Tariot et al, 1994, 1995). Carbamazepine is indicated, however, for the management of seizures and trigeminal neuralgia (*Physician's Desk Reference*, 2002).

These psychotropic agents (major and minor tranquilizers, antidepressants, and hypnotics) should be withdrawn slowly because abrupt withdrawal can cause side effects. Common effects include agitation, anxiety, confusion, tachycardia, hypertension, and diaphoresis, depending on the specific category. A rare side effect is seizure. A good rule of thumb for tapering the benzodiazepines is to taper with a long-acting agent. In addition, for every year the patient has been using the drug, the dosage should be tapered over a month's time frame.

Levodopa is a dopaminergic agent that is useful for treating the symptoms of Parkinson's disease. Large doses of this drug are necessary, causing nausea as a major side effect. It is rapidly metabolized in the peripheral tissues to dopamine, and only a small amount gets to the CNS unchanged and metabolically active. In addition, the ingestion of protein can inhibit its absorption. Therefore carbidopa is administered with levodopa. The former inhibits the degradation of peripheral levodopa and does not cross the blood-brain barrier. The preparation is available in a convenient single oral dose form. Other side effects of carbidopa-levodopa include involuntary (choreiform, dystonic) movements, depression, paranoid or psychotic behavior, cognitive dysfunction, and suicidal ideation. Less common side effects include cardiac irregularities, postural hypotension, urinary retention, and bradykinetic episodes ("wearing off" effect indicating a more frequent dosing regimen is necessary) (*Physician's Desk Reference*, 2002).

Selegiline is a selective MAO inhibitor that has been used to treat early symptoms of Parkinson's disease to delay the need to start levodopa. Dopamine agonists (bromocriptine, pergolide, pramipexole, and ropinirole) can be used as first-line agents for older patients with Parkinson's disease and in patients with normal physical and cognitive function. Patients with dementia are at greater risk of side effects, including confusion, hallucinations, hypotension, nausea and vomiting, and daytime sedation (Dubois and Pillon, 1990; *Physician's Desk Reference*, 2002). The catechol-0-methyltransferase inhibitors (COMT), entacapone, and tolcapone may be used as adjuncts to levodopa therapy with concomitant slow reduction of the dosage of levodopa during initial administration to prevent dopaminergic side effects (*Physician's Desk Reference*, 2002). Benztropine and trihexyphenidyl are anticholinergic agents used to treat the tremor associated with Parkinson's disease or drug-induced Parkinson syndrome secondary to phenothiazine use (*Physician's Desk Reference*, 2002). Amantadine and rimantadine, antiviral agents, have also been used as adjuncts to anticholinergic therapy to treat Parkinson's disease. Doses higher than 100 mg in frail older patients or with renal impairment may be associated with an increased risk of side effects, including nausea, dizziness, light-headedness, insomnia, depression, anxiety, hallucinations, confusion, anorexia, dry mouth, constipation, orthostatic hypotension, and leg edema (*Physician's Desk Reference*, 2002).

The barbiturate class of drugs must be metabolized in the liver. As phase I metabolism slows with normal aging, caution is advised in the use and dosing of these agents in older patients. For this reason and because of their properties of physical dependence with continued use and tolerance, barbiturates should not be used in older patients for the management of general anxiety or for insomnia. Their use, as mentioned previously, should be restricted to treatment for seizure disorder in older patients. Most common side effects include sedation, somnolence, confusion, drowsiness, depression, and incoordination (*Physician's Desk Reference*, 2002).

Phenytoin is an agent with multiple uses in older persons. It has traditionally been used to treat seizure disorder. It has also become popular to treat the chronic pain of neuropathy, particularly in diabetic patients. It must be metabolized by the liver and it is highly protein bound. Only the free (unbound) portion of the drug is active in the serum, and the drug has unique pharmacokinetic properties. Therefore, regular serum monitoring is recommended. Caution is also advised in patients with chronic liver disease or malnutrition, in which side effects are likely to be magnified. These effects most commonly include CNS (nystagmus, ataxia, slurred speech, decreased coordination, mental confusion), nausea, vomiting, constipation, dermatitis, leukopenia, agranulocytosis, thrombocytopenia, and pancytopenia (*Physician's Desk Reference*, 2002).

Gabapentin is a newer agent used for the same purposes. Most common side effects include dizziness, somnolence, peripheral edema, asthenia, and diarrhea (*Physician's Desk Reference*, 2002). In late 2002 it also received an FDA indication for the treatment of postherpetic neuralgia.

Topiramate and zonisamide are new agents recently approved for partial seizures and partial or generalized seizures respectively. Dosage reduction is necessary in patients with renal insufficiency (*Physician's Desk Reference*, 2002). Zonisamide is contraindicated in patients with a history of sulfur allergy.

Drugs for Dementia

Various agents have been recommended for the treatment of Alzheimer's disease since the recognition that lecithin and acetylcholine deficiencies may play a role in its development. These agents include lecithin-containing health foods and megadoses of other vitamins. Even though these agents are popularly used, clinical trials have not proved their efficacy. Ergoloid mesylates, an older drug, has been used for the treatment of dementia but has shown no clinically significant effects (Cobbs et al., 2002-2004). Cerebral vasodilators were a popular group of drugs for the treatment of organic brain syndrome, Alzheimer's disease, or vascular dementia in the past. The theory behind the use of these agents was to increase vascular and oxygen supply to the brain. These drugs are contraindicated because of their risk of causing postural hypotension or "steal syndrome" (diverting blood from the brain to other tissues), which can lead to dizziness causing falls, fractures, and other morbidity. Pentoxifylline, a drug approved for use in treating peripheral vascular insufficiency, has been shown to slow the cognitive deterioration in patients with multiinfarct dementia, but it has little effect on memory.

Tacrine, an acetylcholinesterase inhibitor, is the first of a class of drugs approved for Alzheimer's disease. Studies prove its effectiveness for mild cases of the disease and only for short-term benefit (up to 30 weeks). Long-term studies are not available. In addition to cost, its disadvantages include the need for regular blood monitoring because the drug causes asymptomatic elevation of the liver function tests. This toxicity is usually associated with higher doses of the drug. Removal of the drug usually resolves the problem. Another disadvantage is a high frequency of other side effects, including diarrhea and nausea, occurring in up to 74% of patients, with 59% of patients stopping the drug (Knapp et al, 1994; Maltby et al, 1994). Newer agents introduced since tacrine indicated for the management of mild to moderate Alzheimer's disease include donepezil, rivastigmine, and galanthamine. These agents are considered safer and more practical because they do not require monitoring of liver function studies and can be given once or twice daily (Rogers and Friedhoff, 1996).

Donepezil is a reverse inhibitor of the enzyme acetylcholinesterase that slows the degradation of acetylcholine. Its advantage is that its dosing is once daily. It should be used in a patient with a Mini-Mental status of between 10 and 26 (Feldman et al, 2001). Rivastigmine is a dual-acting agent that inhibits both acetylcholinesterase and butyrylcholinesterase, a second enzyme identified in excess levels in the brains of patients with Alzheimer's disease. A study found that elevated butyrylcholinesterase levels were associated with amyloid plaque formation, also a finding in the pathology of Alzheimer's disease (Greig et al, 2001). Rivastigmine is available in four strengths: 1.5 mg, 3 mg, 4.5 mg, and 6 mg and is administered twice daily. It is recommended that the dose be slowly titrated to 6 to 12 mg for maximum effectiveness. A fourth agent, galanthamine, has gained popularity in having a "dual" action of inhibition of acetylcholinesterase as well as being an allosteric modulator of the nicotinic acetylcholine receptors. It is likely, however, that this action is not unique to galanthamine only. It is given in a dose of 16 and 24 mg twice daily (Tariot et al., 2000). Donepezil, rivastigmine, and galanthamine are indicated for mild to moderate cases of Alzheimer's disease and should be initiated as early as possible to prevent and slow cognitive decline. Studies lasting from 6 months to 2 years for the various agents indicate their effectiveness in slowing cognitive decline. It has been shown to slow the progression of the disease. Although not indicated, these agents have been shown to be effective for patients with vascular dementia and for patients with moderate to severe Alzheimer's disease. Major side effects include nausea, vomiting, diarrhea, decreased appetite, and agitation (*Physician's Desk Reference*, 2002). A major disadvantage is their cost.

Antibiotics

Classes of antibiotics for which the dosage should be reduced in older persons consistent with creatinine clearance, as mentioned earlier, include oral and parenterally administered penicillins and fluoroquinolones because of their risk of causing confusion, sedation, and lethargy (Cobbs et al, 2002-2004). Aminoglycosides, used in high doses and on a regular basis, may cause hearing loss, vestibular damage, and acute and chronic renal failure. In addition, the appropriate use of antibiotics in older patients is important to prevent the development of resistant strains of bacteria, an increasingly alarming concern among health care and public health officials. This includes penicillin-resistant pneumococci *(Streptococcus pneumoniae)* secondary to inappropriate use of penicillin for treatment of viral upper respiratory infection and allergic or chronic sinusitis. In addition, vancomycin-resistant *Enterococcus* species and methicillin-resistant *Staphylococcus aureus* have emerged in increasing numbers secondary to inappropriate use of vancomycin as a first-line agent for broad coverage of suspected sepsis and for general surgical prophylaxis. Fluoroquinolones have been inappropriately used as first-line agents for the treatment of community-acquired pneumonia in the healthy older adult, with resultant overwhelming sepsis and death in occasional cases. Appropriate general indications for the use of antibiotics include a productive colored sputum, evidence of bacteria, and leukocytes in the urine if symptomatic, evidence of cellulitis or suspected osteomyelitis or bacterial meningitis, or abscess formation.

A newer quinolone group of antibiotics provides an option for treatment of penicillin-resistant pneumococcus, including sparfloxacin, grepafloxacin, levofloxacin, gatifloxacin, and moxifloxacin. Rare side effects include nausea, vomiting, and diarrhea. Other rare side effects at high dosages include dizziness, insomnia, prolonged Q-T interval (determined by electrocardiographic monitoring), rash, photosensitivity, confusion, depression, psychosis, seizure, paresthesia, irritability, lethargy, cardiovascular collapse, arrhythmia, and, rarely, cardiorespiratory arrest (*Physician's Desk Reference*, 2002).

A new class of antibiotics, the ketolides, provides the promise of broad-spectrum activity similar to the macrolide antibiotics with particular activity against gram-positive, gram-negative, and atypical organisms. The first drug of this class is to be released in 2003 (Douthwaite, 2001). Rare side effects include prolonged Q-T interval (determined by electrocardiographic monitoring), elevated liver function enzymes, and diarrhea. The indiscriminate use of these agents can lead to diarrhea secondary to *Clostridium difficile* and related morbidity and mortality from pseudomembranous colitis (Cobbs et al, 2002-2004). Mild cases should be treated with oral metronidazole 250 mg three times daily for 10 days. Moderate to severe cases with systemic symptoms of fever and leukocytosis should be treated with intravenous vancomycin (Cobbs et al, 2002-2004; *Physician's Desk Reference*, 2002). The fluoroquinolone group of antibiotics should be given 4 hours before or 2 hours after administration of antacids or sucralfate because these agents may interfere with the effectiveness of fluoroquinolone. Side effects include photosensitivity, rash, urticaria, seizures, monoclonus, or renal failure. Reduced levels may occur in patients taking nitrofurantoin, zinc, multiple vitamins, antacids, and sucralfate. Elevated levels may occur in patients taking cyclosporine, theophylline, or caffeine.

A frequent misperception among health care professionals is that the presence of bacteria or leukocytes in the urine of a patient with a chronic indwelling urinary catheter or foul-smelling or pustular drainage from a pressure ulcer requires antibiotic administration. Patients with either chronic condition commonly develop colonization of the urinary tract or ulcer site, respectively. The use of oral antibiotics in such cases is both ineffective and apt to promote resistance. Indications for the administration of parental antibiotics in such cases are the presence of fever greater than 102° F rectally; elevation of the serum leukocyte count above 15,000 with a shift to granulocytosis; and other signs of systemic sepsis, including hypotension, a change in mental status, central pallor, peripheral cyanosis, diaphoresis, and tachycardia (Cobbs et al, 2002-2004). Surrounding cellulitis and suspicion of osteomyelitis are additional indications for parental antibiotics for patients with necrotic pressure ulcers.

Acyclovir is an antiviral agent used to treat herpes zoster (shingles). Initially approved for the treatment of herpes type 2 infections, the dosage for zoster is at a much higher dose of 800 mg every 4 hours five times daily for 7 to 10 days. If given within 48 hours of the infection, it has been shown to reduce the duration and severity of symptoms. The dosage of the drug, the frequency of administration, or both should be lowered in patients with creatinine clearance below 25 ml per minute to prevent neurologic side effects such as confusion, dizziness, hallucinations, paresthesia, and lethargy (*Physician's Desk Reference*, 2002). Side effects include skin rash, itching, myalgia, diarrhea, nausea, fever, headache, peripheral edema, lymphadenopathy, and leukopenia. The drug can be administered intravenously in severe cases associated with systemic involvement (ocular) or when associated with immune-deficiency states (*Physician's Desk Reference*, 2002). It also significantly decreased the incidence of postherpetic neuralgia at 6 months' follow-up in a meta-analysis of five randomized placebo-controlled trials. The patients' average age was 60 years. They were treated with 800 mg five times daily within 72 hours of onset of rash (Jackson et al, 1997).

Famciclovir, an antiviral agent for acute zoster infection, has the advantage of less frequent dosing (three times per day) and a better side effect profile. Dosage should also be reduced for renal insufficiency (*Physician's Desk Reference*, 2002).

Agents for Dizziness

It is common practice to prescribe meclizine for a patient who complains of "dizziness," especially in a hurried office visit. Older patients may be exhibiting one or a combination of three different syndromes in such cases, including "true" dizziness, presyncopal light-headedness, or disequilibrium. True dizziness implies a vertical or horizontal spinning of the surroundings that may or may not be associated with sensory or neurologic signs or symptoms. It can be secondary to a multitude of causes related to the inner ear or the CNS. Disequilibrium usually implies unsteadiness on the feet and usually on walking or turning. Disequilibrium may be secondary to a host of other disease processes as well. Presyncopal light-headedness implies a "feeling of being faint," usually on standing or sitting from the supine position and lasting 1 to 2 minutes in most cases. Various disease states and drugs previously mentioned in other sections may cause this syndrome. Appropriate evaluation of the type of dizziness as well as the associated signs and symptoms, time frame, and circumstance is necessary before prescribing meclizine for true dizziness because the treatment of the three syndromes is different. In addition, meclizine is an anticholinergic drug that should be used in the lowest dose possible, preferably 12.5 mg, to prevent side effects.

Cardiac Drugs

The few current indications for the use of digoxin include systolic dysfunction of the myocardium and treatment of atrial arrhythmias. The drug is useful in such patients to improve cardiac function, but it does not increase survival. This drug should be avoided if possible in older patients because it is excreted 90% unchanged in the urine and is highly dependent on creatinine clearance. Inappropriately high doses of digoxin may cause confusion, agitation, anxiety, nausea, vomiting, heart block, arrhythmias, and the visual perception of yellow or green colors. An early sign of digitalis toxicity is usually anorexia. In a study of 19 patients with moderate failure and left ventricular ejection fractions below 45%, the dose of digoxin was increased within the therapeutic range from 0.125 to 0.25 mg (low to moderate dose: mean levels of 0.8 to 1.5 ng/L) in patients with New York Heart Association class II or III heart failure. This dose adjustment did not significantly improve function (Slatton et al, 1997). When used concomitantly with other cardiac drugs such as quinidine, verapamil, or amiodarone, the dosage should be monitored closely and reduced accordingly because of the potentiating effects of these drugs. Digoxin is contraindicated in certain cardiac disease states such as incomplete heart block, pericarditis, aortic stenosis, and hypertrophic cardiomyopathy. The drug may also worsen myocardial ischemia with acute pulmonary edema. A retrospective study of 416 women and 112 men in an academic hospital-based geriatric practice showed that 17% of patients were taking digoxin. In addition to the indications for heart failure and atrial fibrillation, 9% of patients were on the drug for the inappropriate indication of coronary artery disease (Fishkind, Paris, and Aronow, 1997).

Quinidine is an older drug traditionally used to treat ventricular and atrial arrhythmias, including atrial fibrillation. A meta-analysis of controlled trials using quinidine to control normal heart rhythm after conversion indicated that its use increased mortality rate (Coplen et al, 1990). Common side effects of quinidine include ringing in the ears, diarrhea, flushing of the skin, bitter taste, nausea, stomach pain or cramping, headache, dizziness, light-headedness, blurred vision, skin rash, and wheezing. Rare side effects include confusion, fatigue, increased bleeding, and hemolytic anemia. Compared with sotalol, quinidine was significantly more effective (60% versus 20%) in attempting to convert 50 patients with persistent atrial fibrillation to normal sinus rhythm. These patients were randomized to one of these two drug regimens over a 7-day period. At 6 months' follow-up, quinidine was still more effective (86% versus 77%); however, patients on quinidine reported more proarrhythmic side effects (Hohnloser, van de Loo, and Baedeker, 1995). Another meta-analysis comparing amiodarone to flecainide involving 315 patients showed that 73% of patients on amiodarone, compared with 48% on flecainide, converted to normal sinus rhythm at 3 months, with 60% and 40%, respectively, still converted at 12 months (Zarembski et al, 1995).

Although flecainide and encainide are more recent and more potent antiarrhythmic agents, they have also been shown to increase mortality in patients with ventricular arrhythmias after acute myocardial infarction, with age being an independent risk factor (Akiyama et al, 1992). Procainamide has been shown to decrease short-term survival after cardiac arrest and resuscitation outside the hospital (Hallstrom et al, 1991). The side effects include nausea, vomiting, diarrhea, light-headedness, hypotension, edema, dizziness, and depression (*Physician's Desk Reference*, 2002). Procainamide can also cause a lupus syndrome. Because of the limited benefit-risk ratio for these drugs, they should be prescribed only under the close supervision and monitoring of a cardiologist.

Nitroglycerin preparations (nitrates), both orally and applied to the skin for treatment of ischemic heart disease and angina, may predispose the older patient to the development of light-headedness, postural hypotension, syncope, and falls, especially when used in an increasing dosage. Other common side effects include headache, faint or rapid heartbeat, nausea, and vomiting. Rare side effects include blurred vision, dry mouth, and skin rash occurring at the site of administration for topical preparations. Seizures may also occur in very high doses. Patients who use the patch preparations should remove the patch for 4 to 6 hours daily to prevent the development of tolerance from the drug.

HYPOLIPIDEMIC AGENTS

Hypocholesterolemic agents should be used with discretion in older patients. A recent meta-analysis of 35 randomized trials of cholesterol-lowering treatments questions the value of intensive treatment of hypercholesterolemia. These agents are likely to benefit only people with significant risk factors for coronary heart disease, including smoking, hypertension, sedentary activity, previous stroke or myocardial infarction, and family history of risk factors. Two studies indicate that serum lipid levels (elevated cholesterol and low HDL cholesterol) by themselves are poor predictors of coronary risk, coronary heart disease mortality, hospitalization for myocardial infarction, or unstable angina (Grover, Palmer, and Coupal, 1994; Krumholz et al, 1994). A meta-analysis of clinical trials involving cholesterol reduction has also failed to show any correlation with stroke risk (Hebert, Gaziano, and Hennekens, 1995). Serum cholesterol screening in healthy postmenopausal women has shown that serum cholesterol levels do not significantly change over the long term (7 to 10 years). Therefore a serum cholesterol performed every 5 to 10 years in older women without cardiovascular risk factors is sufficient (Hetland, Haarbo, and Christiansen, 1992). In addition, cholesterol-lowering agents used for patients with levels above 309 mg in the general population have not been shown to be cost effective. In general, these agents cost $190,000 per extra year of life saved as opposed to population-based promotion of better eating habits at a cost of $20 per extra year of life saved (Kristiansen, Eggen, and Thelle, 1991). A recent study involving a population-based study of Canadians using lipid-lowering agents indicated a lower risk of dementia and specifically Alzheimer's disease in patients less than 80 years of age (Rockwood et al, 2002).

Normal aging is accompanied by the dulling of taste and smell sensations (Cobbs et al, 2002-2004). Certain conditions—anorexia secondary to dementia, depression, or malignancy; visual or oral sensory deficits; living alone, with low income, lack of transportation; or living in an institutional setting (Cobbs et al, 2002-2004)—predispose older patients to the development of malnutritional states. Inappropriate dietary cholesterol restriction in these patients is unnecessary because it may worsen the process, leading to further anorexia, weight loss, and death. Liberalization of salt, carbohydrate, protein, and cholesterol restrictions for these patients may be one of the few quality-of-life measures that may make life worth living. Hypocholesterolemia (4 mmol/L) has been linked to increased mortality in older patients. It is probably secondary to chronic inflammatory processes producing a catabolic state. Restricted diets found in most malnourished nursing home patients can contribute to the situation (Buckler, Kelber, and Goodwin, 1994).

For patients with cardiovascular risk factors and a higher than normal low-density lipoprotein (LDL) cholesterol level, the statin (HMG-CoA reductase inhibitors) drugs are effective in lowering the LDL and total cholesterol. They also have the disadvantages of higher cost and the need for regular monitoring of liver function tests because of the development of rare hepatitis (Mach et al, 1995). These agents should not be used in combination with cyclosporine, gemfibrozil, or niacin because the combination may cause rhabdomyolysis and renal failure (*Physician's Desk Reference*, 2002).

Nicotinic acid lowers total cholesterol to some extent but significantly elevates the HDL cholesterol (Vega and Grundy, 1994). Gemfibrozil reduces total cholesterol and elevates HDL cholesterol to a lesser extent than nicotinic acid and the statin drugs (Vega and Grundy, 1994). Niacin and gemfibrozil also reduce serum triglyceride levels. They should be used after an adequate trial of diet has failed, for patients who have a history of pancreatitis or recurrent abdominal pain resembling pancreatitis, and for patients with triglyceride levels greater than 2000 mg/dl (*Physician's Desk Reference*, 2002). Frequent bothersome side effects of niacin include pruritus, flushing, tingling, headache, and diarrhea, especially in high doses of several grams per day. Concomitant administration with aspirin can prevent cutaneous side effects (Whelan et al, 1992). Common side effects of gemfibrozil include dyspepsia, abdominal pain, and acute appendicitis. Less frequent side effects include diarrhea, nausea or vomiting, and fatigue. This agent should not be used concomitantly with anticoagulants because it may increase the risk of bleeding. Use of the drug may increase the severity of gallstones and can necessitate gallbladder surgery. Use of the drug in the presence of liver disease may increase levels of the drug and subsequently the chances of side effects (*Physician's Desk Reference*, 2002).

Clofibrate is a drug that causes modest reduction in cholesterol with a somewhat greater reduction in triglyceride levels. It is associated with potentially bothersome gastrointestinal side effects, including diarrhea and nausea. It is a relatively weak agent. It may potentiate the effect of anticoagulants when used concomitantly. Clofibrate also has been shown to increase the incidence of cholelithiasis and subsequent morbidity and mortality from surgery (*Physician's Desk Reference*, 2002).

Regular isotonic (walking, running, swimming, bicycling) exercise for 20 to 30 minutes three times per week is an effective way of raising HDL cholesterol and can be effective in causing slow, progressive weight loss. It also has been shown to reduce mortality significantly in postmenopausal women. The reduction was smallest in those performing moderate exercise (gardening, golfing, taking long walks) once per week (24%) and greatest in those performing it more than four times per week (38%) (Kushi et al, 1997). Moderate alcohol intake (one or more drinks per day) has been shown to be effective in elevating HDL cholesterol and reducing the subsequent risk of stroke, myocardial infarction, and total and cardiovascular mortality. The studies relative to alcohol consumption and risk of dementia point to moderation as the key to prevention. One study involved a sample of the national cohort of the Canadian Study of Health and Aging and comprised 2873 patients followed up for 18 months. This study showed that the occurrence of all types of dementia, except Alzheimer's disease, and overall mortality were higher in those with questionable or definite alcohol abuse (Thomas and Rockwood, 2001). A prospective population-based study of 7983 persons 55 years of age and older with follow-up for an average of 6 years showed that light to moderate drinking was significantly associated with lower risk of any dementia and vascular dementia (Ruitenberg et al, 2002). Alcohol has been shown to increase threefold the levels of estradiol according to a study of 12 postmenopausal women on hormone replacement therapy (Ginsburg et al, 1996). The latter agent is thought to be one of the most potent lipid-lowering agents because it increases HDL, reduces LDL, and lowers total cholesterol.

Conventional wisdom and past studies have touted estrogen as being effective in retarding osteoporosis and reducing fracture risk at all bone sites (Daly et al, 1993; Robinson et al, 1994). Other positive effects of estrogen shown in studies have included vasomotor symptom and improvement of mood and cognition (Miller et al, 2002) and a lower incidence of osteoarthritis of the hip in white women (Nevitt et al, 1996). Numerous studies have also touted estrogen for the prevention of cardiovascular disease and mortality: less intimal thickening of the carotid arteries and less risk of stroke in postmenopausal women (Finucane et al, 1993; Manolio et al, 1993; Psaty et al, 1994); and decreased incidence of myocardial infarction or death after angioplasty at 5.5 years' follow-up (O'Keefe et al, 1997). Previous studies regarding the effect of estrogen and the risk of breast cancer are conflicting. One study showed a slight increased risk of breast cancer with consecutive use (Daly et al, 1993); however, another study contradicted this association (Evans, Fleming, and Evans, 1995). The risk of epithelial ovarian cancer is not increased by the use of hormone replacement therapy according to one study (Hempling et al, 1997). A recent study also showed that prior hormone replacement therapy but not current use (unless exceeded by 10 years) was associated with a decreased risk of Alzheimer's disease (Zandi et al, 2002a). Another recent study involving the Nurses' Health Study, an ongoing prospective cohort study, showed only improvement in verbal fluency but not for overall cognitive function (Grodstein et al, 2000). The effect on Alzheimer's disease is thought to be secondary to promoting the growth of cholinergic neurons and decreasing deposition of cerebral amyloid (Tang et al, 1996).

In older women with a history of hysterectomy and in the presence of cardiovascular risk factors and an elevated total cholesterol, low HDL, and high LDL component, it was thought that estrogen might offer a substantial advantage to the conventional cholesterol-lowering agents. In women without hysterectomies, estrogen has been used sequentially or in combination with progesterone to reduce the slight risk of endometrial cancer in patients taking unopposed estrogen. Formulations also include transdermal progesterone and or estrogen.

The Women's Health Initiative, a study involving 16,608 postmenopausal women, supported by the National Institute of Health was terminated prematurely in 2002 after the disturbing results showed that hormone replacement therapy as opposed to placebo was associated with an increase in the relative risk of cardiovascular disease (relative risk, or RR, = 1.29), breast cancer (RR = 1.26), stroke (RR = 1.41), and pulmonary embolus (RR = 2.13). The risk of colorectal cancer (RR = 0.63) and endometrial cancer (RR = 0.83) was reduced. The relative risk for death was 0.92 for patients using hormone replacement therapy. The study did show that hormone replacement therapy was significantly effective in increasing bone mineral density and reducing hip fracture incidence (RR = 0.66). As a result of these findings, health care professionals are rethinking the issue of use of hormone replacement therapy for the prevention and treatment of postmenopausal osteoporosis and prevention of cardiovascular disease. At best, expert consensus includes use of estrogen for perimenopausal symptom relief only and to taper use of estrogen as soon as possible when using it for prevention of osteoporosis during this period (1 to 2 years). The results of this study are not applicable to the estrogen-only arm, which is still ongoing (Rossouw et al, 2002).

Relative contraindications to estrogen use include fibrocystic disease and a history of migraine headaches. Absolute contraindications include a previous history or family history of breast cancer, previous pelvic cancer, and abnormal blood clotting (*Physician's Desk Reference*, 2002). The effect of estrogen for osteoporosis can be enhanced by the concomitant use of calcium in a dose of at least 1000 mg daily and vitamin D, 400 IU. The best absorption occurs with calcium carbonate and citrate (Hazzard et al, 1999). Risk of gallbladder disease in postmenopausal women and inflammation of the pancreas in women with high triglycerides is substantial (*Physician's Desk Reference*, 2002).

Tamoxifen is a nonsteroidal antiestrogen useful for the treatment of node-negative breast cancer in women after total mastectomy, segmental mastectomy, axillary node dissection, or breast irradiation. It also may be used for male and female patients with metastatic breast cancer (*Physician's Desk Reference*, 2002). It reduces significantly the risk of myocardial infarction and also to increase the risk of thromboembolic events in one study. Its positive effect on the heart is probably mediated by its effect on the lipid profile (McDonald et al, 1995).

DRUGS FOR THE PREVENTION OF OSTEOPOROSIS

Drugs beneficial in the treatment of osteoporosis for the patient who has relative or absolute contraindications to estrogen include calcitonin-salmon, sodium fluoride, and the bisphosphonates.

Until recently, calcitonin-salmon had to be given subcutaneously; a nasal spray is now available, although one disadvantage of the drug is its high cost. Another disadvantage is that the drug is indicated for the treatment, but not prevention of, postmenopausal osteoporosis and only in women who are 5 years postmenopausal and with low bone mass because it did not significantly reduce the incidence of hip fractures in clinical trials (*Physician's Desk Reference*, 2002). Calcitonin-salmon has also been shown to be clinically useful and effective in reducing the acute pain of a vertebral compression fracture for up to 12 weeks, alleviating the need for narcotics in some cases and the associated side effect profile (Pun et al, 1989).

Sodium fluoride has been shown to increase bone formation, but it also increases risk of fracture because the bone that is formed is more brittle (Hazzard et al, 1999). It is still considered experimental. Etidronate, a bisphosphonate, has been shown to be effective for the prevention of recurrent vertebral compression fractures in older women with osteoporosis when it is used cyclically in combination with calcium. Its disadvantages are cost and side effects, including, most commonly, diarrhea.

Sodium alendronate, the first bisphosponhate, is approved for primary prevention of postmenopausal osteoporosis. It significantly decreases the risk of vertebral and other fractures when used over a 3-year period. Follow-up studies also show its effectiveness for up to 7 years in increasing bone mineral density. Common side effects include abdominal pain, musculoskeletal pain, acid reflux, dyspepsia, esophageal ulcer, vomiting, abdominal distention, and gastritis in 1% to 3% of patients (Liberman et al, 1995). Because of its gastrointestinal side effect profile, the drug should be taken in the morning with at least 8 ounces of water and at least 1 hour before other liquids or food. A second bisphosphonate, risedronate, was approved recently and has a similar efficacy profile to that of alendronate (Harris et al, 1999; *Physician's Desk Reference*, 2002). It has a similar mode of administration as alendronate. One study showed that risedronate had a lower risk of gastrointestinal ulceration than did alendronate (Lanza et al, 2002). Both alendronate and risedronate are indicated in a once weekly dosage form in an attempt to increase compliance rates for therapy (Brown et al, 2002; *Physician's Desk Reference*, 2002). This dosage regimen has increased only bone mineral density significantly without evidence of a reduction in fracture risk. Both bisphosphonates share the disadvantage of being expensive.

Another option for management of postmenopausal osteoporosis is raloxifene. The second selective estrogen receptor modulator (SERM) approved for use in the United States, raloxifene is indicated for the prevention and treatment of postmenopausal osteoporosis. In the Multiple Outcomes of Raloxifene Evaluation study (MORE) at 3 years' follow-up, raloxifene was shown to increase significantly bone mineral density and to reduce the risk of first time and recurrent vertebral compression fractures versus placebo at 4 years' follow-up. It did not decrease, however, significantly the risk of hip fractures. Although not indicated, several caveats for this therapeutic option increase its utility in the clinical setting. Raloxifene did not significantly increase the risk of uterine bleeding or carcinoma compared with placebo. It has a similar effect on the lipid profile in significantly lowering cholesterol and in lowering LDL, but it has little to no effect in increasing HDL cholesterol. It does not increase triglyceride levels, as does estrogen. Raloxifene also significantly reduced the risk of breast cancer in the MORE trial by 76% compared with placebo but had the same incidence of thromboembolic disease. As with other newer therapies, raloxifene is expensive (Cummings et al, 1999; *Physician's Desk Reference*, 2002).

In late 2002 parathyroid hormone (PTH 1-34) was approved by the FDA. It is indicated for the treatment of postmenopausal women who are at high risk of fracture. In clinical trials, PTH at 19 months' follow-up, significantly and markedly increased bone mineral density in the spine and to a lesser extent in the femoral neck compared with placebo. It also significantly reduced the risk of new vertebral fractures and new nonvertebral fractures. Administration route is subcutaneous and daily. Side effects included headache, nausea, vomiting, and transient elevations of serum calcium. There was no evidence of significant hypertension (Neer et al, 2001).

DRUGS THAT CAUSE ANOREXIA

In the evaluation of causes of anorexia in older persons, a review of the patient's drug list with prompt removal of the suspected offending agent is a simple but expedient method of resolving the problem. It is preferable to instituting a potentially unnecessary extensive workup to rule out organic causes such as malignancy, dementia, and depression. Drugs known to cause anorexia include digoxin, procainamide, thyroxine, theophylline, nitrofurantoin, and the SSRIs (Thompson and Morris, 1991).

Inappropriately high doses of thyroxine may also cause agitation, insomnia, unexpected weight loss, tachycardia, arrhythmias, and premature osteoporosis (*Physician's Desk Reference*, 2002). Dietary fiber or psyllium may interact with oral thyroxine and reduce the subsequent absorption and efficacy of the drug. In such cases hypothyroid patients may require unusually higher doses of thyroid to normalize the thyroid-stimulating hormone level (Liel, Harmon-Boehm, and Shany, 1996). Theophylline may also precipitate anxiety, arrhythmias, postural hypotension, nausea, insomnia, and even seizures (Hazzard et al, 1999). Because of these side effects, a higher incidence of comorbid disease, and the concomitant use of other drugs, theophylline is more difficult to use for older patients. The concomitant use of theophylline and fluoroquinolones can cause a severe ADR secondary to doubling of the concentration of theophylline. This reaction may include seizures, agitation, confusion, nausea, and vomiting. For these reasons, if theophylline is to be used at all, a dose in the lower therapeutic range is appropriate (Hazzard et al, 1999). It is also prudent to use theophylline only for selected instances such as wheezing and asthma. The beta-agonist drugs, oral or inhaled, are the first line of treatment for chronic lung disease (Hazzard et al, 1999). Theophylline may be beneficial in the future for sleep-disordered breathing in patients with CHF and reduced left ventricular ejection fraction; a crossover study of 15 patients showed a significant reduction in the number of central apneas per hour compared with placebo (Javaheri et al, 1996).

Drugs such as cotrimoxazole, tetracycline, and nitrofurantoin should be avoided in older patients and patients with renal dysfunction. They should be used with caution in older patients in general because of their dependence on renal excretion. Chronic administration of tetracycline may cause staining of the teeth and skin, photosensitivity of the skin, diarrhea, or stomach cramping. They also chelate with other drugs taken orally, including antacids, iron preparations, laxatives, and calcium supplements, and prevent absorption.

DRUGS FOR HEALTH MAINTENANCE, GENERAL PROPHYLAXIS, MINERALS, VITAMINS, AND ANTIOXIDANTS

Because of the greater risk of malnutrition secondary to multiple diseases, limited income, social isolation, or dental problems, patients who are 62 years of age or older should be prescribed a general multiple vitamin. Recent advertisements on television and radio and in newspapers and periodicals encourage megadoses of specific vitamins, particularly A, C, and E. These vitamins are used primarily to prevent premature aging, especially with case-control studies, indicating that vitamins A and C may reduce the incidence of heart disease and stroke (Gale et al, 1995; Riemersma et al, 1991). A popular theory of aging involves the production of free ionizing and chemical radical formation causing damage to deoxyribonucleic acid and ribonucleic acid responsible for the production of proteins and enzymes and for cell function (Kristal and Yu, 1992). These vitamins may function as scavengers against free radicals or as antioxidants, preventing the aging process. Other studies of these vitamins, however, have shown unimpressive results. A trial compared 50 mg per day of vitamin E, 20 mg per day of β-carotene, a combination, and placebo in 22,269 male Finnish smokers without known coronary disease. Patients taking vitamin E showed no evidence of protection from the development of angina (Rapola et al, 1996). Another trial evaluated 1188 men and 532 women enrolled in a skin cancer prevention program using 50 mg per day of β-carotene or placebo for 4 years. At 8.2 years' follow-up, there was no difference in all causes of mortality, including cardiovascular death (Greenberg et al, 1996). The effect of vitamin E alone on coronary atherosclerosis also 's had mixed results. In a randomized controlled trial in 2002, patients with angiography-proven ꞓase using doses of 400 to 800 IU showed a dose-response effect, with a significant reduction in cardiovascular deaths and nonfatal myocardial infarction but not overall mortality at 1.4 years' follow-up (Stephens et al, 1996).

Low folate level has also been implicated as a cause of coronary artery disease according to a retrospective study of 5056 Canadian men and women (35 to 79 years of age) enrolled in a nutritional survey. The lowest serum quartile folate level was associated with a 69% increase in coronary artery disease (Morrison et al, 1996). A more recent randomized double-blind study showed that supplementation with folic acid, vitamin B_{12} and Vitamin B_6 versus placebo after percutaneous coronary intervention decreased the incidence of major adverse events (target lesion revascularization) and a nonsignificant trend toward decreased death and nonfatal myocardial infarction (Schnyder et al, 2002).

More disconcerting than these results is the association of β-carotene with cancer mortality. A trial of 18,000 current or former smokers and workers exposed to asbestos used a combination of 30 mg of β-carotene plus 25,000 IU of vitamin A compared with placebo. At 4 years' follow-up, the intervention group had a significantly increased risk of lung cancer (Omenn et al, 1996). Another prospective study of 72,337 registered nurses (postmenopausal) within 11 states with 18 years of follow-up showed an increased incidence of hip fractures in those women taking supplemental Vitamin A and using multivitamins versus those who did not (Feskanich et al, 2002).

Vitamins A, C, and E have been shown to increase cell-mediated immunity in older patients (Penn et al, 1991). In addition, higher β-carotene and vitamin C levels have been correlated with better memory performance according to a longitudinal study of 442 patients ages 65 to 94 (Perrig, Perrig, and Stahelin, 1997). Relative to the incidence or severity of upper respiratory tract infections in a population of individuals 60 years of age or older, a randomized, double-blind placebo-controlled trial showed no effect in patients receiving physiologic doses of multivitamin minerals and 200 IU of vitamin E. Instead, there was an increased incidence of adverse effects on illness severity (Graat, Schouten, and Kok, 2002).

Although popular among older persons, the use of specific vitamin and health food supplements should be discouraged until the results of numerous clinical trials definitely prove or disprove their effectiveness. Rather than a deficiency of vitamins, a more common problem among community-dwelling older adults is hypervitaminosis (Cobbs et al, 2002-2004). The fat-soluble vitamins A, D, E, and K accumulate in fat tissue with continued use, leading to vague and nonspecific but toxic symptoms that may be difficult to recognize. Specifically, megadoses of vitamin C can cause gastrointestinal irritability, a false-negative result on fecal occult testing, renal stones, and rebound scurvy. Megadoses of vitamin A can cause malaise, liver dysfunction, headache, hypercalcemia, and leukopenia (Cobbs et al, 2002-2004). Indications for specific vitamins include vitamin B_{12} for dementia, pernicious anemia, or malabsorption syndromes; vitamin C for pressure ulcers and for skin healing from incisions; vitamin D and calcium for osteomalacia and osteoporosis; vitamin K for bleeding problems; thiamine for chronic alcohol abuse; and folic acid supplementation for patients on phenytoin (phenytoin inhibits the production of folic acid) (Hazzard et al, 1999).

The need for supplemental iron therapy in older patients for nonspecific chronic anemia should be thoroughly investigated before prescription. Older patients in general tend to have a greater frequency of normal or increased tissue iron stores because of the high frequency of chronic diseases that cause iron-deficient erythropoiesis (Cobbs et al., 2002-2004). Side effects of oral iron therapy include constipation, black stools, hemosiderosis, and browning of the skin and teeth. The diagnosis of a microcytic hypochromic anemia related to iron deficiency in older adults should always be distinguished from other common causes, such as malignancies and acute or chronic inflammatory diseases. Blood studies such as serum iron, ferritin level, transferrin level, and total iron-binding capacity can easily distinguish between that secondary to iron and other disease states.

Trace metals have shown interesting results. Zinc lozenges have been shown to resolve upper respiratory symptoms sooner than placebo in a randomized trial of 100 employees of the Cleveland

Clinic (Mossad et al, 1996). A dose of 200 μg of selenium supplementation has been shown to reduce the total cancer incidence by 37% when comparing it with placebo in a multicenter, randomized trial of 1312 patients followed up for an average of 4.5 years (Clark et al, 1996). A case-control study recently indicated that high doses of alpha-tocopherol, gamma-tocopherol (isomers of Vitamin E), and selenium was shown in one study to prevent prostate cancer. Ongoing clinical trials are in process to answer this question definitively (Helzlsouer et al, 2000). An observational study showed that 3640 patients between 55 and 90 years of age with ophthalmologic evidence of macular degeneration who were followed up for an average of 6.3 years had less progression of the disease and better visual acuity in those taking high-dose vitamins C, E, β-carotene, and zinc supplements (Jampol et al, 2001).

A study involving dietary consumption and follow-up data from the 84,688 nurses enrolled in the Nurses' Health Study, 34 to 59 years of age and free of cardiovascular disease and cancer at baseline, showed that in the women with higher consumption of fish and omega-3 fatty acids, the risk of coronary artery disease and associated deaths was lower (Hu et al, 2002). Several recent cross-sectional and observational studies of older patients agree that dietary intake of various antioxidants (vitamins E, C, and β-carotene) are associated with a decreased risk of Alzheimer's disease and cognitive impairment (Engelhart et al, 2002; Morris et al, 2002; Perrig, Perrig, and Stahelin, 1997; Schmidt et al, 1998;).

Erythropoietin is one of the first of the new biotechnology drugs used to treat anemias of chronic disease. It is indicated for the treatment of anemia of chronic renal insufficiency, for anemia in zidovudine-treated human immunodeficiency virus (HIV) patients, for anemia in cancer patients on chemotherapy, and for the reduction of allogeneic blood transfusions in surgery patients (*Physician's Desk Reference*, 2002). Stimulating the production of erythropoietin increases mean hemoglobin levels and improve quality-of-life symptoms. It is a relatively safe drug with little risk of anaphylactic reactions. No contraindications for use by older adults have been noted. Because of its tendency to cause volume expansion, which could worsen blood control, its use should be monitored in patients with high blood pressure or chronic renal insufficiency. When using the drug, the patient should take an adequate substrate of iron supplementation for the production of red blood cells.

Aspirin in a dose of 81 mg is significantly more effective than placebo in reducing the incidence of cerebral infarction, fatal myocardial infarction, subsequent risk of stroke, subsequent transient ischemic attack, and death in older patients with a history of previous transient ischemic attack. An associated but insignificant increase in hemorrhagic stroke was found, however (the Swedish Aspirin Low-Dose Trial [SALT] Collaborative Group, 1991). It significantly reduces the risk of severe angina, myocardial infarction, and death at 6 and 12 months in older patients (under 70 years of age) with non-Q-wave myocardial infarction or unstable angina (Wallentin, 1991). It also has been effective in significantly reducing cardiovascular and all-cause mortality according to a survey of 2418 women with coronary artery disease at 3 years' follow-up. This risk reduction occurred in women over 60 years of age as well as in those with hypertension, diabetes, and previous myocardial infarction (Harpaz et al, 1996). Because of its relative safety, a baby aspirin should be a part of every older patient's medication regimen unless contraindicated by active gastrointestinal bleeding, a history of bleeding diathesis, other blood disorder, or a history of allergy to aspirin. A dose of 75 mg is as effective as 325 mg, with significantly less chance of gastrointestinal bleeding. This dose may be used safely as prophylaxis in asymptomatic patients with a history of peptic ulcer disease as well. It is equally as effective as warfarin in patients younger than 75 years of age with a history of nonrheumatic atrial fibrillation in preventing stroke. Exceptions include patients with risk factors such as a history of hypertension, previous thromboembolism, or heart failure (Stroke Prevention in Atrial Fibrillation Investigators, 1994). The 325-mg dose is also indicated in patients for the prevention of a recurrent thrombotic stroke instead of the 75-mg prophylactic dose. Aspirin has also been shown to reduce the risk of colon cancer.

Low-dose heparin in a dose of 5000 IU twice daily may be more effective than aspirin in preventing deep venous thrombosis (DVT) and subsequent fatal or nonfatal pulmonary embolus and death in older patients who are temporarily immobile secondary to an acute illness or in patients with a history of previous DVT or pulmonary embolus, obesity, a history of CHF, or chronic venous insufficiency (Cobbs et al, 2002-2004). This regimen is also recommended for general postoperative prophylaxis except for patients undergoing surgery for malignancies, repair of femoral or hip fracture, or lower-extremity joint replacement. In these instances, subcutaneous heparin used three times daily or preferably low-dose Coumadin (warfarin) starting on the day of surgery and for up to 10 weeks after surgery is recommended because these patients are at greater risk for DVT and embolization. To prevent significant bleeding, however, the international normalized ratio should be maintained at the lowest therapeutic level to prevent complications.

Enoxaparin, a low-molecular-weight heparin, alleviates the need for blood monitoring of prothrombin time and is equally as effective for the prevention of DVT after hip replacement. Periodic complete blood counts, including platelet count, are recommended during the course of treatment (*Physician's Desk Reference*, 2002). Although it is traditionally used up to 10 days after surgery, another study showed that 40 mg daily for up to 30 days can significantly prevent asymptomatic and symptomatic overall thromboembolism and proximal DVT compared with placebo (39% versus 18%) (Bergqvist et al, 1996). A multicenter, randomized, double-blind trial compared adjusted-dose warfarin with enoxaparin. After 14 days' follow-up, 30 mg of enoxaparin given every 12 hours subcutaneously was significantly better than warfarin in preventing DVT (37% versus 52%), with no difference between the two drugs in proximal venous thrombosis or bleeding (Leclerc et al, 1996). It is also as effective in the home setting as intravenous heparin at 90 days' follow-up in treating patients with DVT, with the additional advantage of fewer hospital days (1.1 versus 6.5) (Levine et al, 1996).

Whether to use warfarin or aspirin in an older patient is often a difficult question. A medical indication for the use of warfarin is a patient with a history of chronic atrial fibrillation secondary to rheumatic valvular heart disease to prevent embolic stroke (Hazzard et al, 1999). In addition, issues that should be factored into a decision include associated medical conditions, a history of gastrointestinal disease, compliance, economic or psychosocial issues, cognitive dysfunction, or risk of falling. In each case, the practitioner should weigh overall risk to expected benefit.

A recent study showed that anticoagulation does not prolong quality-adjusted life expectancy in the oldest old with nonrheumatic atrial fibrillation and those likely to benefit are those who have a high risk of stroke secondary to risk factors other than age alone (Desbiens, 2002).

Associated medical conditions such as liver disease, malabsorption syndromes, and malignancy may predispose the patient to a greater risk of ADRs (disease-drug) when using warfarin because of its protein-binding properties. In such instances, a reduction in the serum albumin may occur, which means less protein binding of the drug. Then a greater "free" portion of the drug is metabolically active, with a resultant increased chance of bleeding at the same dose. A patient with significant cognitive dysfunction may not be an ideal candidate because the patient may ultimately take too much in a single dose, which might predispose the patient to either increased risk of bleeding or insufficient amount to achieve the desired effect. The presence of other chronic medical conditions necessitating the use of other medications may increase the risk of drug-drug reactions as well.

The availability of a willing and able caregiver or interested party to administer the medication on a regular basis can resolve this issue. Pill-administration vehicles may also be of benefit. In addition, communication and understanding of the need for regular monitoring of the bleeding time, the physician and laboratory costs involved, the availability of transportation, and the distance from the medical facility for the patient are essential components. The absence of any of these factors makes the use of warfarin impractical.

A patient at increased risk of falls secondary to mobility problems, arthritis, neurologic disease, or specific drug therapy may be a less than optimal candidate for warfarin because of the increased risk of bleeding secondary to trauma. Patients taking warfarin after 80 years of age are at significantly increased risk of life-threatening and fatal bleeds (RR = 4.5) compared with those under 50 years of age (Fihn et al, 1996).

Patterned after the philosophy of the standard treatment of acute evolving transmural myocardial infarction, thrombolytic agents (streptokinase and recombinant tissue plasminogen activator) have also been used in the last several years in various clinical trials in an attempt to prove their efficacy for early treatment of ischemic cerebrovascular accident. Because of the conflicting data on outcomes such as short-term complications (bleeding and death) and short- and long-term neurologic outcomes, their use is not recommended at this time (Miyawaki,1997). Other indications include pulmonary embolus, DVT, arterial thrombosis or embolism, or occlusion of arteriovenous cannulas (*Physician's Desk Reference*, 2002).

Ticlopidine hydrochloride is a platelet aggregation inhibitor. It is indicated for the prevention of thrombotic stroke for patients with a history of previous transient ischemic attacks who have not responded to aspirin therapy or are intolerant to aspirin (allergy or previous bleeding). In patients with reductions in creatinine clearance (50 to 80 ml/minute), no significant difference has been found in the clinical effects of the drug. The drug has the potential to cause neutropenia in less than 2% of patients. This problem is usually reversible but can be life threatening in severe cases. Because of this problem, patients should have a neutrophil count initially before starting treatment and every 2 weeks for the first 3 months of therapy. Ticlopidine becomes 50% effective within 4 days of treatment and 60% to 70% effective in 10 to 11 days. It is contraindicated for patients who are hypersensitive to it and for patients with a history of hematopoietic disorders, severe liver impairment, or active peptic ulcer (*Physician's Desk Reference*, 2002). Clopidogrel is a newer agent that is similar to ticlopidine. It is indicated for the reduction of atherosclerotic events (myocardial infarction, stroke, and vascular death in patients with atherosclerosis documented by recent myocardial infarction, stroke, or established peripheral vascular disease. It is contraindicated for patients with sensitivity to it, or in patients with active bleeding. Rare side effects include the development of thrombotic thrombocytopenia purpura (TTP). An advantage over ticlopidine is that routine monitoring of blood components is not necessary (*Physician's Desk Reference*, 2002). A recent clinical trial showed that after percutaneous coronary intervention, patients receiving clopidogrel at 1-year follow-up had a 26.9% decrease in the combined risk of death, myocardial infarction, or stroke compared with placebo (Steinhubl et al, 2002).

Pentoxifylline is useful in treating intermittent claudication in patients with peripheral vascular disease by improving red blood cell flexibility, making it easier for these cells to pass through the microcirculation. This change translates clinically to greater pain-free walking distances (Cantwell-Gab, 1996). Cilostazol is a newer agent indicated for the reduction of symptoms of intermittent claudication. This agent is a potent inhibitor of the enzyme phosphodiesterase III and is therefore contraindicated for patients with CHF of any severity. No studies have evaluated its use concomitantly with platelet-aggregation inhibiting drugs. Most common side effects include headache, diarrhea, and palpitations (*Physician's Desk Reference*, 2002).

Influenza vaccine should be given yearly to all older adults, except those with a history of egg allergy; 90% of deaths caused by influenza epidemics are people older than 64 years of age. The vaccine is usually given between October and December. If influenza develops in a long-term-care institution, patients who have not been vaccinated or those allergic to the vaccine may be treated prophylactically with amantadine or rimantadine in a dose of 100 mg per day until the infection resolves. In high doses, common side effects of the drug include confusion, irritability, headache, rash, lethargy, nausea, and fluid retention. The drug can also shorten the duration and severity of influenza A if it is started within 24 to 48 hours of onset of symptoms, but it is not effective against influenza type B (Cobbs et al, 2002-2004; *Physician's Desk Reference*, 2002).

Pneumonia vaccine should be administered to all older patients at least once. Some geriatricians advocate a repeat vaccination 6 years from the date of the last one for those at high risk of pneumococcal pneumonia, such as asplenic and chronic obstructive pulmonary disease patients (Cobbs et al, 2002-2004). Patients who have received the older 18-polyvalent strain do not need a repeat injection. Even though older patients have the greatest need for these vaccinations, studies indicate that they often develop an inadequate antibody response to them because of their blunted immune responses. Because the rate of pneumococcal vaccination is much lower than that of influenza vaccination in older adults, administration of both simultaneously can improve the rate of vaccination of the latter. There is little difference in side effects when they are given together rather than separately (Honkanen, Keistinen, and Knela, 1996; *Physician's Desk Reference*, 2002).

Diphtheria tetanus prophylaxis is often ignored in older patients, but recent studies indicate that only about 20% to 60% of older adults have adequate antibody levels. Those especially at risk include diabetic patients with chronic foot ulcers and nursing home or homebound older patients with chronic pressure ulcers. Historically, many older adults were not exposed to childhood vaccinations, many of which were initiated after their youth. Any older patient who has not had vaccinations should receive three separate injections of diphtheria tetanus vaccination: initially, at 6 weeks, and at 1 year from the initial vaccine (Cobbs et al, 2002-2004; Gergen et al, 1995).

Older patients with a recent conversion (within 2 years) to positive tuberculin skin testing should be treated with isoniazid (300 mg per day for 6 months) because studies indicate a high degree of protection (69%) against conversion from tuberculous infection to disease. Patients with a history of positive skin testing of unknown duration should not be treated with this drug because of the risk of morbidity and subsequent mortality for patients who develop isoniazid-induced hepatitis. Exceptions to this rule include patients with diabetes mellitus, HIV disease, hematologic or reticuloendothelial malignancy, silicosis, previous gastrectomy, malnutrition, or scars of postprimary tuberculosis. Other exceptions include patients on 15 mg of steroids for more than 2 weeks, patients who have had close or household contact with an infected person, and those with scars of postprimary tuberculosis evidenced by chest radiograph (Hazzard et al, 1999). Patients taking the drug should have liver function tests performed every 6 weeks initially to monitor for the development of liver-function abnormalities. The drug should be administered with B_6 (pyridoxine) because the drug interferes with the metabolism of this vitamin.

STEROIDS

Oral corticosteroid use in the older patient population should be a last resort after conventional therapy has failed and for specific indications because of the side effects that occur after prolonged use. These side effects include dependence, weight gain, masking of infection, fluid retention, worsening or precipitation of hypertension, diabetes, cataracts, and osteoporosis. Steroids serve no purpose for the uncomplicated treatment of osteoarthritis and should be reserved for severe cases of active rheumatoid arthritis.

Steroids may be very beneficial for the treatment of asthma resistant to conventional therapy, initial treatment of certain dermatoses, polymyalgia rheumatica (15 to 20 mg daily), and temporal arteritis (40 to 60 mg daily) (Cobbs et al, 2002-2004). Inhaled steroids are as effective as oral steroids for the treatment of chronic lung conditions without producing the systemic side effects of the oral route (Cobbs et al, 2002-2004). The use of these agents in patients with asthma is associated with a 50% reduction in hospitalization as opposed to beta agonists (Donahue et al, 1997). Oral prednisolone has also been shown to improve survival for up to 1 year for patients with severe alcoholic hepatitis compared with placebo (Mathurin et al, 1996). Fludrocortisone acetate is an oral steroid specifically indicated for primary and secondary adrenocortical insufficiency of Addison disease or for salt-losing adrenogenital syndrome. Although not specifically indicated, it is also used to treat refractory postural hypotension. It works by causing fluid retention, leading to an increase in intravascular volume (*Physician's Desk Reference*, 2002).

LAXATIVES

The chronic use of stimulant (cascara, bisacodyl, senna) laxatives should be discouraged in older patients because of their tendency to produce a chemical denervation of the autonomic nerves as they detach from the mucosa of the large colon after many years of chronic use (Cefalu and Pike, 1981). This subsequently can lead to the development of a chronic nondilating megacolon syndrome, resulting in worsening constipation and even fecal impaction when the patient becomes immobile. Nonsystemic and bulk laxative agents (stool softener, psyllium) are the preferred agents of choice for the treatment of constipation. Prune juice serves an excellent purpose as a natural mild cathartic without long-term sequelae. Additional measures that should be used in conjunction with these agents include regular exercise; added fiber in the diet in the form of bran, fruits, and vegetables; and extra fluid intake (Cobbs et al, 2002-2004). An excellent laxative for the patient with gastrointestinal symptoms of hyperacidity is an inexpensive liquid magnesium containing antacid because these agents tend to cause diarrhea. Patients should also be advised that the frequency of regular bowel movements depends on a variety of factors, including associated medical conditions. What is "abnormal" for one patient may be "normal" for another. In addition to discouraging chronic laxative use, drugs known to cause constipation should be identified and removed, if possible. These drugs are most notably narcotics, anticholinergic agents, antispasmodics, antihistamines, major tranquilizers, tricyclic antidepressants, calcium-channel blocking agents, iron salts, and diuretics (Cefalu and Pike, 1981).

DIABETIC AGENTS

Chlorpropamide, a long-acting agent used for type 2 diabetes, is very potent and has been popular in the past; however, this agent has a half-life of 48 to 72 hours and an associated high risk of causing prolonged hypoglycemia, especially in patients with reduced appetite drive or cognitive dysfunction. It is generally considered an inappropriate drug for use in older patients. It should be reserved for cases of diabetes complicated with diabetes insipidus. The newer hypoglycemic (sulfonylurea) agents glipizide and glyburide are shorter acting and considered more appropriate for older patients; however, glyburide has the same risk of serious hypoglycemia as chlorpropamide according to a Tennessee case-control study of Medicaid enrollees. Serious hypoglycemia was defined as a blood sugar of below 50 mg per dilution or a level that resulted in hospitalization, emergency room admission, or even death associated with neuroglycopenia or autonomic symptoms, myocardial infarction, or stroke. Patients taking tolbutamide, tolazamide, and glipizide had lower risks of hypoglycemia than patients who took chlorpropamide and glyburide (Shorr et al, 1996). The main effect of glyburide and glipizide is to stimulate beta cells to release more insulin; they also have a peripheral effect. As a result, a major side effect is the development of insulin resistance, hyperinsulinemia, and subsequent weight gain. These agents should be used with caution in older patients with reduced thirst and appetite drives secondary to dementia, depression, liver disease, or malnutrition because of the risk of serious hypoglycemia.

Newer agents such as metformin and acarbose work by different mechanisms. They may be used in combination with the sulfonylureas to potentiate their effect or alone in patients who have not responded to them or have only a minor response (*Physician's Desk Reference*, 2002). The principal action of metformin is on the liver to reduce glucose production. Major advantages include weight loss and lowering insulin and lipid levels. It also does not cause hypoglycemia by itself. It should not be used for patients with liver or renal disease or for patients with heart failure because it may cause lactic acidosis. Disadvantages are gastrointestinal side effects of nausea, flatulence, diarrhea, and nausea. Acarbose functions to delay carbohydrate absorption in the gut by interfering with disaccharide (complex sugar) metabolism. As a result, it causes a blunting of postprandial hyperglycemia and subsequent lowering of elevated glycosylated hemoglobin. It causes a major side effect of flatulence. To be effective, the drug should be given with food and the dosage titrated up slowly.

The newest oral agents are the thiazolidinediones, including rosiglitazone and pioglitazone. These agents are indicated for non-insulin (type 2) diabetes and act primarily by reducing insulin resistance by improving insulin sensitivity in muscle and adipose tissue and inhibiting hepatic glucogenesis. In doing so, glucose levels are improved while reducing circulating insulin levels. These agents can be used alone or in combination with sulfonylurea, metformin, or insulin when diet and exercise plus the single agent fail to provide adequate glycemic control. Because these agents can cause elevations of the liver enzymes leading to rare liver failure, they should not be used in patients with active liver disease or in patients with liver alanine aminotransferase (ALT) levels 2.5 times or higher. In addition, initial and routine monitoring of liver function studies is recommended while the patient is receiving therapy. Other side effects include hypoglycemia, ovulation in pre-menopausal women, reduction in hemoglobin and hematocrit levels, edema, volume expansion and preload-induced cardiac hypertrophy (*Physician's Desk Reference*, 2002).

Insulin glargine is the first of the basal insulins approved by the FDA and is indicated for type 1 diabetes or adult patients with type 2 diabetes who require basal (long-acting) insulin for the control of hyperglycemia. It is given in a single subcutaneous nighttime injection. Dosage may need to be reduced in patients with liver or renal impairment. The most common side effect is hypoglycemia (*Physician's Desk Reference*, 2002).

MISCELLANEOUS DRUGS

Certain groups of drugs deserve special mention as being inappropriate and in some instances having no specific indications. Dipyridamole is an older drug that has been popular for the treatment of vascular problems by decreasing platelet "stickiness" and preventing stroke or myocardial infarction. It has not been shown to be superior to aspirin alone for the treatment of cerebral or coronary artery disease or in maintaining the patency of autologous grafts (Green and Miller, 1993).

Muscle relaxants can cause sedation, lethargy, confusion, and cognitive dysfunction. They should be avoided in older patients if possible (*Physician's Desk Reference*, 2002). The need for a "short-acting" muscle relaxer can best be served with a short-acting benzodiazepine such as lorazepam, 0.5 to 1 mg every 8 hours, used in a time-limited fashion.

Oxybutynin, an older drug with smooth muscle and anticholinergic/anti-muscarinic properties, has traditionally been used to treat detrusor hyperreflexia associated with temporary or chronic urge incontinence in older patients. It is an inappropriate agent for use in older patients (Willcox, Himmelstein, and Woolhandler, 1994). Another study indicated that oxybutynin caused cognitive impairment in older patients (Katz et al, 1998). A newer agent, tolterodine, may possess more antimuscarinic and site-specific muscarinic activity than oxybutynin with less cognitive side-effect profile in the older population (Malone et al, 2001; *Physician's Drug Reference*, 2002; Zinner et al, 2002). Phenazopyridine is an older drug that may be useful to treat the uncomfortable symptoms of urinary tract infection initially (48 to 72 hours) until the antibiotic can become effective. It stains the urine a dark orange color (*Physician's Drug Reference*, 2002).

Quinine is another older drug that has been used traditionally for the treatment of nonspecific nocturnal leg cramps. A meta-analysis of five clinical trials using doses from 200 to 500 mg indicated that it reduces the frequency but not the severity or duration of leg cramps (Man-Sons-Hing and Wells, 1995). Hydroquinine hydrobromide in a dose of 300 mg daily was significantly more effective than placebo for treatment of muscle cramps for 6 weeks in a clinical trial of 101 Danish patients (Jansen et al, 1997).

Ophthalmologic agents containing beta-blockers (timolol, levobetaxolol, and betaxolol) used to treat glaucoma in older patients may be associated with systemic side effects, especially in frail older patients. Most importantly, those references to the lung, heart or CNS include rare cases of CHF, hypotension, bronchospasm, bradycardia, arrhythmia, hypertension, heart block, claudication, confusion, depression, and hallucinations (Novack et al, 2002; *Physician's Desk Reference*, 2002).

Older patients may develop intractable anorexia and weight loss, especially when associated with a worsening dementia process or cancer. Cyproheptadine is a serotonin and histamine-blocking agent that may be effective for these patients by stimulating central appetite centers (Cobbs et al, 2002-2004). Some patients, especially those with Alzheimer's disease, should be monitored closely for the development of anticholinergic side effects, including constipation, dry mouth, agitation, confusion, sedation, dizziness, restlessness, tremor, irritability, hypotension, difficulty with urination, and urinary retention. Megestrol acetate is a synthetic derivative of the naturally occurring steroid progesterone. It is indicated for the treatment of anorexia, cachexia, or unexplained weight loss in patients with acquired immunodeficiency syndrome (AIDS). It has also been used to treat the cachexia and anorexia of dementia in older patients. Side effects include edema, hypertension, abdominal pain, chest pain, infection, moniliasis, sarcoma, cardiomyopathy, palpitations, constipation, dry mouth, hepatomegaly, leukopenia, depression, confusion, seizures, paresthesia, neuropathy, cough, shortness of breath, urinary incontinence, and alopecia (*Physician's Desk Reference*, 2002).

Midodrine, an alpha agonist, increases total peripheral vascular resistance. It has been proposed as a treatment for refractory (neurogenic) orthostatic hypotension. The drug is significantly more effective than placebo in increasing standing and supine systolic blood pressure and in decreasing the symptoms of light headedness but with more side effects at 2 weeks' follow-up (Low et al, 1997).

D-penicillamine, calcium disodium edetate (EDTA), and dimercaprol (BAL) have received notoriety in the past as possible useful agents for the treatment of atherosclerotic disease. The results of a recent randomized, controlled trial showed no evidence to support a beneficial effect of chelation therapy in patients with ischemic heart disease, stable angina, or a positive treadmill for ischemia (Knudtson et al, 2002).

Recreational cannabis has the potential for abuse even in the older population. A recent multisite retrospective cross-sectional study, however, confirms that long-term heavy cannabis users showed more impairments in memory and attention that endure beyond the stage of intoxication and worsen with increasing years of regular use (Solowij et al, 2002).

Ginkgo, another agent available as an over-the-counter item or in health food stores, has become popular, especially among the older adults, to improve memory. A recent 6-week randomized, placebo-controlled trial showed no improvement in performance on standard neuropsychological tests of learning, memory, attention, and concentration or naming and verbal fluency in older adults without cognitive impairment (Solomon et al, 2002).

Alosetron is a recently approved agent indicated for the treatment of severe diarrhea or predominant irritable bowel syndrome patients who have not responded to conventional therapy and whose symptoms are chronic (for 6 months or longer). Its use is not indicated in patients who are constipated or in patients with a history of sequelae for constipation such as intestinal obstruction, stricture, adhesions, history of ischemic colitis, impaired circulation, thrombophlebitis, hypercoagulable state, diverticulitis, Crohn disease, or ulcerative colitis (*Physician's Desk Reference*, 2002).

Drugs for Sexual Potency

Alprostadil (prostaglandin E$_1$) has been approved for use in the United States for the treatment of erectile dysfunction. The drug is administered by intracavernous injection and causes erections by relaxing arteriolar and cavernous smooth muscle. The response is dose related. The drug also has been shown to improve sexual satisfaction as reported by either partner in up to 86% of injections. Side effects include penis pain in 11% of injections, priapism (erection for more than 6 hours), and prolonged erections (lasting 4 to 6 hours). The latter two side effects occurred in 5% and 1% of men, respectively, at 16 months' follow-up. Study participants included those with vascular, neurogenic, and psychogenic causes of erectile dysfunction (Linet and Ogrinc, 1996).

The FDA approved sildenafil citrate (Viagra) in 1998 for the treatment of erectile dysfunction. It has since revolutionized the treatment of male impotence and therefore led to a sexual revolution. Sildenafil works by enhancing the effect of nitrous oxide, which is released in the corpus cavernosum during sexual stimulation, leading to an erection. Sildenafil is metabolized by the liver, and the dosage should be reduced in patients with hepatic cirrhosis. No dosage reduction is necessary for mild to moderate renal insufficiency (> 50 ml/minute creatinine clearance), but the dosage should be reduced for patients with severe renal insufficiency. Smaller starting dosages should also be used in healthy patients older than 65 years of age. Sildenafil is absolutely contraindicated for patients concurrently using nitroglycerin preparations; the combination can result in severe hypotension and cardiovascular death (*Physician's Desk Reference*, 1999). In more than 3000 patients 19 to 87 years of age with impotence for a mean duration of 5 years, it was significantly more effective than placebo for organic, psychogenic, and mixed types of impotence. A study of men with diabetes indicated that sildenafil was significantly more effective than placebo (54% versus 10%) in treating erectile dysfunction (Rendell et al, 1999).

The American College of Cardiology published an expert consensus document that lists patient categories for whom sildenafil is "potentially hazardous": (1) patients with stable coronary artery disease who are not using nitroglycerin preparations; (2) patients with CHF and borderline hypotension; (3) patients with hypertension using multiple antihypertensive regimens simultaneously; and (4) patients taking a long list of drugs that might prolong sildenafil's half-life (listed in publication). Dosage forms include 25-, 50-, and 100-mg tablets (*Physician's Desk Reference*, 2002).

Finasteride has been used in recent years for the treatment of initial symptomatic benign prostatic hyperplasia as a medical alternative to surgical treatment (transurethral resection of the prostate) or for the treatment of male-pattern baldness. It works by blocking the enzyme that converts testosterone to 5-alpha dihydrotestosterone. It has been effective in producing rapid regression of the size of the prostate, with 60% of treated patients experiencing a more than 10% improvement in urinary flow rate. Symptoms also improve in this group of patients by 30% or more. The drug should be used for at least 6 months. It should be used with caution because it can suppress serum prostatic antigen (PSA) levels in patients with prostate cancer. For this reason, a digital rectal examination should be performed initially and regularly while the patient is on the drug. Although not indicated for this purpose, PSA levels are used by clinicians to screen for the development of prostatic cancer while the patient is receiving the drug. A patient with a PSA level above 10 ng/ml and taking this drug should be referred to a urologist for workup of prostate cancer, and a level between 4 and 10 is advisable for the same (*Physician's Desk Reference*, 2002).

Terazosin, an alpha-blocker discussed previously, was compared with finasteride and placebo for the treatment of symptoms of benign prostatic hyperplasia in a 52-week multicenter trial of 1229 U.S. veterans. Symptom scores and urinary flow rates were significantly better with terazosin compared with placebo and finasteride alone, but no difference was found compared with using the combination together (Lepor, Williford, and Barry, 1996). Tamsulosin is an antagonist of alpha (la) adrenoreceptors in the prostate. It is indicated for the treatment of the signs and symptoms of benign prostatic hyperplasia. Its side-effect profile is similar to the alpha-blocker agents discussed previously (*Physician's Desk Reference*, 2002).

COLD AND OVER-THE-COUNTER PAIN MEDICATIONS

Older patients frequently seek advice about prescription and over-the-counter cold and cough medications. These agents usually have an antihistamine or decongestant component. In general, they should be avoided, especially in the presence of any medical illness that might contraindicate their use. Decongestants relieve nasal stuffiness, and antihistamines "dry up" bothersome watery secretions. Decongestants should be avoided for conditions such as anxiety and panic disorder, arrhythmias, and CHF. In addition, although studies in older patients are lacking, over-the-counter decongestant-antihistamine preparations have not been shown to improve symptoms in children (Hutton, Wilson, and Mellits, 1991). Patients with chronic nasal or allergic rhinitis or stuffiness should be instructed to use simple normal saline nasal spray three to four times daily to loosen secretions. If this remedy is insufficient and infection has been treated, topical steroid sprays combined with normal saltwater sprays are available by prescription to relieve symptoms as a safer alternative. Newer nonsedating antihistamines such as cetirizine, loratadine, and fexofenadine may offer a safer side-effect profile, especially as it relates to cognition (*Physician's Desk Reference*, 2002). Capsaicin is a topical agent that is useful for the symptoms associated with osteoarthritis. It must be applied three or four times daily with avoidance of the mucous membranes or eyes. Side effects include burning of the skin or rash, which may necessitate discontinuance (Hazzard et al, 1999).

Many older patients take over-the-counter analgesics for the relief of pain. These drugs often contain caffeine, which may be responsible for chronic symptoms of insomnia, especially if taken before bedtime (Brown et al, 1995). The most common categories of over-the-counter medications consumed by 1059 rural southwestern Pennsylvania older persons were analgesics (66.3%), followed by vitamin and mineral supplements (38.1%), antacids (27.9%), and laxatives (9.7%). The use of laxatives increased as that of analgesics decreased with increasing age (Stoehr et al, 1997).

STIMULANTS

Many dietary "natural" or "herbal" supplements used for weight loss, energy boosting, body building, or enhancement of performance contain ephedrine or related products. Frequent side effects of these agents include tachycardia, hypertension, coronary spasm, psychosis, seizures, and respiratory depression. Less frequent side effects include myocardial infarction, stroke, and death according to a 1995 Texas Department of Health report of 500 toxic reactions (Centers for Disease Control and Prevention, 1996). These effects can be magnified in older persons, many of whom have preexisting hypertension or atherosclerotic cerebral or coronary disease.

Dexfenfluramine and fenfluramine were initially approved for appetite suppression and only for patients with moderate to severe obesity (at least 30% heavier than ideal body weight). Their use is associated with a significantly greater risk for pulmonary hypertension (odds ratio 6:3) according to a case-control study (Abenhaim et al, 1996). These drugs were withdrawn from the U.S. market in 1997 because of reports of serious heart valvular defects detected among users.

CHRONIC PAIN CONTROL

Chronic pain is often the rule rather than the exception in older patients burdened by multiple chronic diseases, especially secondary to arthritis and malignancy. For these patients, the intensity and chronicity of perceived pain may produce or aggravate depressive symptoms. The latter can be a common symptom complex in older patients because of the loss of independence that occurs secondary to a myriad of problems: mobility problems; multiple sensory deficits in hearing, vision, taste, and smell; social isolation; institutionalization; and other losses, including financial, family, friends, and personal possessions.

Relieving chronic pain in an older patient in a pharmacologically safe and effective manner requires that certain principles be followed: (1) avoid high-risk drug administration that may increase the risk of ADRs and side effects; (2) avoid parenterally administered medications for the relief of pain; (3) preferably use oral route of administration and reserve parenteral treatment for alimentary dysfunction; (4) dependence should not be a concern, whereas tolerance is a minimal problem; (5) start with the simplest and safest drug available and switch to other categories as necessary; (6) always provide support for the patient in the form of counseling both informally from family, friends, and clergy and formally from social workers and psychologists as necessary; (7) never abandon the patient so that he or she feels alone or isolated; and (8) provide pharmacologic support for symptoms of depression (Patt, 1992; Rhymes, 1991).

Regarding specific drug therapy, acetaminophen given around the clock starting in a dose of 5 to 10 grains every 4 to 6 hours is often effective initially in providing pain relief secondary to arthritis. Caution is advised in using high doses of acetaminophen greater than 2 g per 24 hours. Use of acetaminophen in patients with liver disease or with regular use of alcohol is associated with an increased risk of liver pathology (Hazzard et al, 1999). In addition, a recent population-based cohort of 958,397 persons in the United Kingdom in a nested case-control analysis showed that acetaminophen at doses greater than 2 g was associated with a relative risk of upper gastrointestinal bleeding of 3.6, with corresponding relative risks for low to medium and high doses of NSAIDs of 2.4 and 4.9 (Garcia Rodriguez and Hernandez-Diaz, 2001). Tramadol is a centrally acting analgesic indicated for the treatment of moderate to moderately severe pain. It is not a narcotic and may offer an alternative to acetaminophen. It has no antiinflammatory activity. Side effects include seizures, especially for patients taking monamine oxidase inhibitors, SSRIs, tricyclic antidepressants, or neuroleptics. It may also cause sedation in patients using CNS-depressing agents such as alcohol, opioids, anesthetic agents, phenothiazine, tranquilizers, or sedative hypnotics (*Physician's Desk Reference*, 2002).

Patients with chronic pain and associated depressive symptoms often have associated insomnia and anorexia. In these cases, 25 to 50 mg of amitriptyline may be effective because of its sedating side effects and because it stimulates appetite. Trazodone is an alternative antidepressant for the patient with Alzheimer's dementia that lacks the significant anticholinergic side effects of amitriptyline. The starting dose is 25 to 50 mg at bedtime. If acetaminophen alone is not effective, propoxyphene and acetaminophen, a narcotic antagonist, may be more effective without the side-effect profile of NSAIDs or narcotics.

For patients with the chronic pain of bone metastasis from a terminal malignancy, NSAIDs are particularly useful, but increasing the dose provides a ceiling effect at which the patient gets no further relief of pain (Rhymes, 1991). Steroids may also be effective for the relief of this type of pain (Rhymes, 1991). A narcotic such as codeine used around the clock, with judicious use of laxatives, stool softeners, and a phenothiazine, may be the next step to relieving this type of pain. The phenothiazine may alleviate the side effect of the initial associated nausea and potentiate the effect of the narcotic. If this regimen is not effective, fentanyl patches with half-lives of 72 hours or morphine infusion pumps delivering a constant infusion with steady serum levels provide better relief (Psaty et al, 1994; Stampfer et al, 1991). Short-acting meperidine and meperidine-like preparations given orally or parenterally have the disadvantage, with their short half-lives, of allowing breakthrough pain and provide no added benefit over the use of morphine derivatives (Ishikawa et al, 1997). If used for acute pain, a dose of no more than 25 mg, in combination with an equal dose of a phenothiazine antiemetic (Promethazine), may be effective. Higher doses may induce anticholinergic delirium. Revised chronic pain guidelines developed by the American Geriatrics Society (AGS) in 2002 are an excellent practical source for the management of chronic pain in older patients (AGS Panel on Persistent Pain in Older Persons, 2002). The Cox-2 agents, celecoxib and rofecoxib, have been included in the treatment pyramid for treatment of chronic pain (AGS Panel on Persistent Pain in Older Persons, 2002).

ONCOLOGIC DRUGS

Ondansetron and granisetron are agents useful for the treatment of nausea and vomiting secondary to cancer chemotherapeutic treatment. They function by selectively blocking the 5-hydroxytryptamine serotonin receptors. Dosage forms are available for both parenteral and oral use. As more potent agents, they are significantly more effective than traditional antiemetic agents. Principal side effects include headache, constipation, weakness, fatigue, abdominal pain, diarrhea, and dizziness (*Physician's Desk Reference,* 2002). According to one study, ondansetron was significantly more effective than placebo for treatment of postoperative nausea (Tramer et al, 1997).

Pamidronate is a bisphosphonate that inhibits the bone resorption that occurs as a result of some metastatic cancers. When used intravenously, it is significantly more effective than placebo in reducing the frequency of nonvertebral fractures, hypercalcemia, bone surgery, and radiation therapy to bone. These results are from a randomized trial of 382 women with metastatic breast cancer and at least one lytic bone lesion (Hortobagyi et al, 1996).

BIOTECH DRUGS

Interferon-alfa shows promise as an adjuvant therapy for malignant melanoma according to a study of 280 patients followed up after surgical removal of the primary lesion, with and without regional lymph node involvement. Patients treated for 48 weeks of high-dose interferon alpha-2b had higher 5-year relapse-free and overall survival than those not treated (37% versus 26% and 36% versus 37%, respectively) (Balch and Buzaid, 1996). It also has been shown to be significantly more effective than no treatment in eliminating serum markers and improving histology in patients with chronic hepatitis after 50 months' of follow-up (Niederau et al, 1996). Interferon beta-1b has been shown to be significantly more effective than placebo in the treatment of patients with multiple sclerosis. Patients in the treatment group had fewer exacerbations of disease and less progression of disability than the placebo group at 2 years' follow-up (Jacobs et al, 1996).

Drug Compliance

Compliance with drug regimens is a significant problem in older adults more than in other age groups because of a host of factors: (1) multiplicity of diseases requiring multiple medications often obtained through multiple pharmacies, all of which may cause confusion for the patient; (2) cognitive dysfunction associated with memory loss and subsequent failure to take medication appropriately, leading to exacerbation of disease or toxicity states; (3) restricted income and inability to pay for medication, leading to exacerbation of disease; (4) difficulty in complying with office or hospital visits because of mobility problems for the patient or transportation problems in obtaining medication from the pharmacist promptly or, in some cases, at all; (5) visual problems that may increase the frequency of inappropriate medication or dose, leading to ADRs; and (6) medical diseases that may interfere with fine and gross coordination of the upper extremities for medication administration, such as stroke, Parkinson disease, cervical stenosis, dementia, and arthritis.

Drug compliance for the older patient can be enhanced in the following general ways: (1) educating the patient or family about the purpose of the medication and potential side effects; (2) educating the patient or family about the disease process and signs or symptoms of worsening disease; (3) asking the patient or family to bring all prescription and over-the-counter medications to each clinic or hospital visit for reevaluation; (4) assigning key family members or friends who may be of assistance in helping the patient secure needed medication from the pharmacy or clinic in a timely fashion; (5) asking family, friends, or nursing personnel when available to assist in or monitor medication administration for the older patient with visual, coordination, or cognitive problems; (6) using pill administration boxes that can be refilled weekly by the patient, family, friends, or nursing personnel; and (7) referring the patient to social service agencies, home health agencies, senior citizen centers, and volunteer agencies in order to assist in securing financial and transportation assistance as applicable.

Specific drug compliance can be increased for the older patient by encouraging the prescriber to (1) prescribe medication administered no more than once or twice daily, (2) administer one drug to treat two conditions when possible, (3) start with one-third to one-half the normal starting dose to decrease the risk of ADRs, (4) maximize the dose of one drug to treat a specific condition before adding a second agent to reduce the risk of ADRs, and (5) use the cheapest drug possible (Cobbs et al, 2002-2004).

Summary

Basic principles of drug therapy for older patients include an understanding of normal changes that occur during the aging process: reduced immune defenses, blunting and reduction of receptor sites, loss of physiologic reserve, and physiologic and structural changes in organ systems. These systems include the skin, gastrointestinal tract, liver, kidney, and brain. Advancing age is associated with the development of chronic disease, multiple diseases, and the need to take more over-the-counter and prescription medications. All these factors increase the risk of ADRs. The high incidence of sensory deficits, cognitive dysfunction, mobility problems, transportation difficulty, socioeconomic concerns, and arthritis necessitate extreme caution and attention to compliance issues as well. All these points make the topic of drug therapy in older patients much different from drug therapy in the general adult population.

| TABLE 5-2 | Appropriate and Inappropriate Drug Therapy in Older Adults |

Drug	Appropriate	Inappropriate	Special Considerations
Antiarrhythmic Agents			
Quinidine, procainamide, flecainide	Treatment of complicated arrhythmias	Treatment of routine arrhythmias	Use recommended for complicated cases under cardiologist supervision only
Antibiotics			
	Systemic symptoms of infected pressure ulcer or indwelling urinary catheter: fever, leucocytosis, hypotension, cellulitis, osteomyelitis, colored sputum	Surface exudate of pressure ulcers, bacteriuria and pyuria associated with indwelling urinary catheter; uncomplicated upper respiratory infection (viral)	May cause pseudomembranous colitis or promote resistance to antibiotics; adjust dose of penicillins, aminoglycosides, and fluoroquinolones consistent with creatinine clearance
Quinolones	Gram-negative infections	Community-acquired pneumonia	High doses associated with CNS toxicity-seizures, hallucinations, confusion, psychosis; rare side effects: photosensitivity; reduce dose with renal insufficiency; newer quinolones, sparfloxacin, grepafloxacin, levofloxacin indicated for penicillin-resistant pneumococcus
Ketolides	Gram-positive and some gram-negative-organisms and atypicals; potential for less resistance		
Anticholinergic Agents			
Antihistamines, tricyclic antidepressants, phenothiazine			Minimize or avoid use in patients with benign prostatic hyperplasia, glaucoma, chronic

TABLE 5-2	Appropriate and Inappropriate Drug Therapy in Older Adults—cont'd		
Drug	**Appropriate**	**Inappropriate**	**Special Considerations**
Anticholinergic Agents—cont'd			
tranquilizers, narcotics			constipation, peripheral vascular disease, chronic bronchitis, Alzheimer's disease
Antidizziness Agents			
Meclizine	"True" dizziness	Disequilibrium or presyncopal light-headedness	Use in low doses; anticholinergic affects may cause or worsen condition
Antihypertensive Agents			
Alpha-blocker drugs	Hypertension	High doses may cause postural hypotension or syncope	Dual indication for hypertension and benign prostatic hyperplasia
Beta-blocker drugs	Shorter-acting selective agents; atenolol or metoprolol	Propranolol	For dual indications: angina and high blood pressure or atrial arrhythmias, after myocardial infarction or angina to reduce cardiovascular mortality
Carvedilol and metoprolol	Management of congestive heart failure stages II-IV associated with improvement in ejection fracture, reduced resting and maximal heart rate, decreased mortality and hospitalization		
ACE inhibitors	Hypertension, chronic congestive heart failure, after acute myocardial infarction, slow renal function decline and reduced proteinuria in diabetics	Severe renal in-sufficiency	Monitor renal function periodically, rare angioedema, side effects of cough, contraindicated with renal artery stenosis, more expensive, hyperkalemia, once or twice daily dosing

Continued

| TABLE 5-2 | Appropriate and Inappropriate Drug Therapy in Older Adults—cont'd |

Drug	Appropriate	Inappropriate	Special Considerations
Antihypertensive Agents—cont'd			
Angiotensin II receptor antagonists	Hypertension		Expensive; safer option than ace inhibitors, no cough
Calcium antagonists	Hypertension, anginas, arrhythmias	Short-acting agents for hypertension, especially nifedipine	Cause vasodilation; side effects of flushing, pedal edema, constipation; verapamil useful in increasing pain-free walking distance in patients with intermittent claudication; increased mortality in patients taking short-acting agents for hypertension; increased risk of congestive heart failure or mortality in patients with left ventricular dysfunction; inhibit platelet function; increased risk for gastrointestinal hemorrhage; increased risk for transfusion postoperatively
Central-Acting Drugs			
Cold and OTC analgesic agents	See antihistamines and decongestants	See antihistamines and decongestants	Antihistamine-decongestant combination agents not found to be clinically effective in children
Antihistamines	For drying of excessive secretions	Alzheimer's patients	See anticholinergic drugs
Newer nonsedating agents (cetirizine, loratadine, fexofenadine)			More expensive
Decongestants	For relief of nasal stuffiness	For patients with congestive heart failure, arrhythmias, anxiety disorders	

TABLE 5-2	Appropriate and Inappropriate Drug Therapy in Older Adults—cont'd		
Drug	**Appropriate**	**Inappropriate**	**Special Considerations**
Analgesic agents	Pain relief	Patients with anxiety disorders or insomnia	Caffeine a frequent ingredient
Tramadol	Moderate to severe pain	Pain associated with bone metastasis, no antiinflammatory effect	Nonnarcotic
Acetaminophen	Mild to moderate pain	Moderate to severe pain; no antiinflammatory effect	Doses higher than 2 g daily associated with increased risk of gastrointestinal bleeding; use with alcohol or in presence of liver disease associated with increased liver toxicity
Dementia Drugs			
Hydergine			Not significantly effective
Tacrine	For mild impairment (Alzheimer's type) for up to 30 weeks	Moderate to severe Alzheimer's disease	Monitor liver function tests monthly while on drug because of potential liver toxicity; side effects of nausea, diarrhea, and vomiting
Donepezil	For mild impairment (Alzheimer's type) for up to 30 weeks	Mild to moderate Alzheimer's disease	No need to monitor liver function tests; side effects of nausea, diarrhea, and vomiting
Pentoxifylline	Multiinfarct dementia		Slows cognitive deterioration but not memory loss
Rivastigmine and galantamine	Mild to moderate dementia	Severe dementia	Long-term studies of cholinesterase inhibitors show retardation of cognitive decline and improvement in moderate to severe disease as well as with vascular dementia; expensive; side effects of nausea, vomiting, and diarrhea; slow

Continued

TABLE 5-2	Appropriate and Inappropriate Drug Therapy in Older Adults—cont'd		
Drug	**Appropriate**	**Inappropriate**	**Special Considerations**
Dementia Drugs—cont'd			titration to prevent side effects (at 2- to 4-wk intervals)
Vasodilators		Not effective	May cause postural hypotension
Digoxin	Congestive heart failure secondary to systolic dysfunction, atrial arrhythmias	Nonspecifically for other cardiac conditions	May cause anorexia, nausea, agitation, confusion; reduce dose according to creatinine clearance
Diuretics			
Loop	Treatment of fluid retention secondary to congestive heart failure or renal insufficiency; refractory and severe leg edema secondary to venous stasis or chronic venous insufficiency	Routine treatment of dependent edema or venous stasis secondary to chronic venous insufficiency, treatment of hypercalcemia; caution in using in advanced older adults or older adults with dementia or depression; treatment of uncomplicated hypertension	May cause contraction alkalosis, postural hypotension, hypokalemia, arrhythmias, and increased mortality; causes of hypercalciuria
Thiazide	Treatment of mild hypertension alone or in combination with other agents	Routine treatment of dependent edema or venous stasis secondary to chronic venous insufficiency; caution in using in advanced older adults or older adults with dementia or depression; doses	May cause contraction alkalosis, postural hypotension, hypokalemia, arrhythmias, and increased mortality; prevents loss of calcium in urine; may have secondary benefit in retarding osteoporosis; may adversely affect lipid

TABLE 5-2	Appropriate and Inappropriate Drug Therapy in Older Adults—cont'd		

Drug	Appropriate	Inappropriate	Special Considerations
		greater than 50 mg ineffective for hypertension	profile
Drugs for Diabetes			
Chlorpropamide		Long-acting (half-life of 48-72 hr), potent	Use only in patients with diabetes mellitus and diabetes insipidus
Acarbose	Type 2 diabetes in combination with sulfonylureas or alone in patients who have not responded to them		Major side effects of flatulence, causes blunting or postprandial hyperglycemia and lowering of elevated glycosylated hemoglobin; give with food
Glipizide and glyburide	Type 2 diabetes	Cautious use in patients with reduced appetite drive; dementia; malnutrition; depression	Side effects of weight gain, hyperinsulinemia, and hypoglycemia
Metformin	Type 2 diabetes in combination with sulfonylureas or alone in patients who have not responded to them	Patients with liver or renal disease or congestive heart failure	Side effects of diarrhea, nausea, vomiting, and flatulence; causes weight loss, lowering of insulin and lipid levels; serum creatinine monitoring
Thiazolidinediones (rosiglitazone and pioglitazone)	Monotherapy or in conjunction with sulfonylurea, metformin, or insulin when diet and exercise fails	Type 1 diabetes, liver disease, or ALT levels 2.5 times normal or greater	Regular monitoring of liver function studies necessary; expensive; reduces insulin resistance by improving insulin sensitivity in muscle and adipose tissue and inhibiting hepatic glucogenesis
Insulin glargine	Type 1 or type 2 diabetes		Given subcutaneously in a daily injection at bedtime; expensive; side effect of hypoglycemia

Continued

TABLE 5-2	Appropriate and Inappropriate Drug Therapy in Older Adults—cont'd

Drug	Appropriate	Inappropriate	Special Considerations
Gastrointestinal Agents			
H$_2$ blocker drugs	Treatment or prevention of peptic ulcer disease or gastroesophageal reflux	Used prophylactically to prevent NSAID-induced gastric or duodenal bleeding; prophylaxis to prevent bleeding secondary to stress-induced gastritis in intensive care unit patients	Increased risk of aspiration patients with swallowing abnormalities; indicated for prophylaxis against stress-induced gastritis in intensive care unit patients with a history of respiratory failure or bleeding disorders
Proton pump inhibitors (omeprazole, lansoprazole, rabeprazole, pantoprazole, and esomeprazole)	Severe or intractable gastrointestinal reflux disease	Treatment of uncomplicated peptic ulcer disease	Expensive
Sucralfate	Treatment of prevention of peptic ulcer disease	Used prophylactically to prevent NSAID-induced gastric or duodenal bleeding; prophylaxis to prevent bleeding secondary to stress-induced gastritis in intensive care unit patients	Increased risk of aspiration pneumonia in bed-bound patients with swallowing abnormalities; indicated for prophylaxis against stress-induced gastritis in intensive care unit patients with a history of respiratory failure or bleeding disorders
Hypolipidemic Agents			
Hypercholesterolemic drugs	For patients who have significant cardiovascular risk	Population-based treatment of hypercholesterolemia to prevent cardiovascular mortality	HMG-CoA reductase agents used with niacin, gemfibrozil, or cyclosporine may cause rhabdomyolysis and renal failure; need to monitor liver function tests when using HMG-CoA reductase (statin) agents; HMG-CoA agents more expensive; probucol can worsen cardiac conduction

TABLE 5-2	Appropriate and Inappropriate Drug Therapy in Older Adults		
Drug	**Appropriate**	**Inappropriate**	**Special Considerations**
Hypolipidemic Agents—cont'd			
			abnormalities; clofibrate may increase the incidence of cholelithiasis, subsequent morbidity and mortality from surgery; gemfibrozil and clofibrate may increase risk of bleeding when used with anticoagulants
Hypotriglyceridemic drugs	For patients in whom diet has failed, for triglyceride levels between 1000 and 2000 mg/dl, pancreatitis, recurrent abdominal pain resembling pancreatitis		See hypocholesterolemic drugs
Meperidine	Acute pain in low doses (25 mg)	Chronic pain	Short half-life
Miscellaneous Drugs			
Tolterodine	Treatment of overactive bladder	Not for patients with urinary retention, gastric retention, or narrow-angle glaucoma	Can cause blurred vision, dizziness
Dipyridamole			Not shown to be superior to aspirin for vascular disease or for autologous grafts
Muscle relaxers		May cause sedation, lethargy, cognitive dysfunction, postural hypotension, falls	

Continued

TABLE 5-2	Appropriate and Inappropriate Drug Therapy in Older Adults—cont'd		
Drug	**Appropriate**	**Inappropriate**	**Special Considerations**
Miscellaneous Drugs—cont'd			
Oxybutynin			Associated with cognitive impairment in the elderly in one study; considered inappropriate in older adults
Quinine	Metaanalysis indicates that it reduces the frequency but not the duration or severity of leg cramps		
Ophthalmologic agents (beta-blockers, timolol, levobetaxolol, betaxolol)			Rare systemic side effects in frail older patients (congestive heart failure, hypotension, bronchospasm, bradycardia, arrhythmia, hypertension, heart block, claudication, confusion, depression, and hallucinations)
Megestrol acetate	Refractory treatment of anorexia, cachexia, or unexplained weight loss in patients with AIDS		To treat refractory cachexia and anorexia of dementia in older patients; side effects (edema, hypertension, abdominal pain, chest pain, infection, moniliasis, sarcoma, cardiomyopathy, palpitations, constipation, dry mouth, hepatomegaly, leukopenia, depression, confusion, seizures, paresthesia, neuropathy, cough, shortness of breath, urinary incon-tinence, and alopecia)
D-penicillamine, calcium disodium edetate (EDTA), dimercaprol (BAL)		Treatment of atherosclerotic disease	

| TABLE 5-2 | Appropriate and Inappropriate Drug Therapy in Older Adults—cont'd |

Drug	Appropriate	Inappropriate	Special Considerations
Cannabis			Long-term heavy use associated with memory loss
Ginkgo		Recent controlled trial shows no effectiveness in improving memory; before surgery, concomitant use with warfarin, NSAIDs	Large amounts over time may be toxic; may cause bleeding
NSAIDs	PRN use, lowest possible dose, for acute flares of arthritis for 5-7 days	Indomethacin, chronic use of NSAIDs, active bleeding	Increased risk for gastrointestinal bleeding; may cause or worsen hypertension, congestive heart failure, renal insufficiency, or hepatitis; high doses associated with acute confusion and cognitive dysfunction, especially indomethacin; monitor hemogram and renal function with chronic use; acetaminophen as effective for osteoarthritis
Cyclooxygenase inhibitors (celecoxib, rofecoxib, valdecoxib)	Arthritis (osteoarthritis and rheumatoid arthritis)	Active gastrointestinal ulceration; patients with history of ischemic heart disease	Expensive, once or twice daily dosing; edema and hypertension with rofecoxib; increased risk for gastrointestinal bleeding
Osteoporosis Therapies			
Etidronate	Prevention of recurrent spinal compression fracture		
Alendronate	Prevention and treatment of postmenopausal osteoporosis		Increases bone mineral density; reduces spinal compression and hip fractures; once-weekly dosing; must be given with 8 oz of water and sitting up for 30 min

Continued

TABLE 5-2	Appropriate and Inappropriate Drug Therapy in Older Adults—cont'd

Drug	Appropriate	Inappropriate	Special Considerations
Osteoporosis Therapies—cont'd			
			before and after dose in-between meals; increased risk of GI disease
Risedronate	Prevention and treatment of postmenopausal osteoporosis		Increases bone mineral density; reduces spinal compression and hip fractures; once weekly dosing; must be given with 8 oz water and sitting up for 30 min before and after dose in between meals; increased risk of GI disease; one study showed better GI profile than alendronate
Tamoxifen	Osteoporosis, hormone replacement therapy		Ongoing clinical trials evaluating risk of breast cancer; increased risk of uterine bleeding and cancer; increases bone mineral density
Raloxifene	Prevention and treatment of postmenopausal osteoporosis		Increased bone mineral density; reduces risk of spinal compression fractures; no effect on hip fractures; positive effect on lipid profile, no elevation of triglycerides
Calcitonin salmon	Treatment of osteoporosis 5 yr postmenopausal		Increases bone mineral density; reduced risk of recurrent spinal compression fractures; no effect in reducing hip fractures; useful for acute management of spinal compression fractures (anesthetic effect)

TABLE 5-2	Appropriate and Inappropriate Drug Therapy in Older Adults—cont'd		
Drug	**Appropriate**	**Inappropriate**	**Special Considerations**
Calcium and vitamin D	Substrate to osteoporosis therapies	Used alone for osteoporosis	Increases bone mineral density; best form of calcium (gluconate or citrate)
Parathyroid hormone (1-34)	Postmenopausal women at risk of fracture	Prevention of osteoporosis	Increases bone mineral density; reduces risk of spinal compression fractures; no effect on the hip
Sodium fluoride		Osteoporosis	Increased bone formation associated with increased risk of fractures
Psychotropic Drugs			
Buspirone	Chronic anxiety	Depression	Delay in onset of action for 7-10 days
Tricyclic antidepressants	Depressive symptoms	Nonspecific treatment of insomnia or agitation	High doses of tricyclic agents can cause or worsen cognitive dysfunction, precipitate postural hypotension, and falls; suicide risk associated with death due to cardiotoxicity
Amitriptyline	Chronic pain, dose 10-25 mg, monitoring closely for side-effects	Nonspecific treatment of insomnia or agitation	Generally considered to be inappropriate for use to treat depression in older adults
Selective serotonin reuptake inhibitors (fluoxetine, paroxetine, citalopram, sertraline, venlafaxine)	Depressive symptoms; chronic anxiety		Can worsen appetite, insomnia, anxiety and weight loss in frail older adults or patients with dementia or depression
Venlafaxine			Dual-acting serotonergic and noradrenergic agent; higher dose may be associated with increase in blood pressure
Bupropion			Does not cause weight gain; contraindicated with a history of seizures

Continued

TABLE 5-2	Appropriate and Inappropriate Drug Therapy in Older Adults—cont'd		
Drug	**Appropriate**	**Inappropriate**	**Special Considerations**
Psychotropic Drugs—cont'd			
Mirtazapine			Side effect of increased appetite and weight gain; sedating; dual acting serotonergic and noradrenergic agent
Methylphenidate			Onset of action in 24 to 48 hr; higher dose may be associated with increase in blood pressure, arrhythmias, anxiety, weight loss and anorexia
Hypnotics	Occasional use for sleep	Regular use for sleep	Can cause sedation, cognitive dysfunction, falls; possible association with increased length of stay, hospital costs, and severity of illness
Zolpidem	Occasional insomnia	Daily use	Short-acting non-benzodiazepine, more specific action on the gaba receptors; no physical dependence or tolerance noted; minimal rebound insomnia or next-day drowsiness
Zaleplon	Occasional insomnia to maintain sleep	Daily use	Short-acting non-benzodiazepine, duration 6-8 hr, more specific action on the gaba receptors; no physical dependence or tolerance noted; minimal rebound insomnia or next-day drowsiness; indicated to initiate sleep or for awakening during the night; 5-mg dose recommended for the elderly
Meprobamate		For use in older adults	Causes sedation, confusion and lethargy
Chloral hydrate		Alzheimer's disease for insomnia, may cause hallucinations and delusions	

TABLE 5-2	Appropriate and Inappropriate Drug Therapy in Older Adults—cont'd		
Drug	*Appropriate*	*Inappropriate*	*Special Considerations*
Newer antipsychotic agents			
Risperidone	Psychosis, schizophrenia, disruptive hallucinations and delusions; studies show effectiveness to treat abnormal problem behaviors in dementia patients	Nonspecific agitation of dementia	Increased risk for cerebrovascular events, including stroke in older adult patients with dementia
Olanzapine, clozapine, ziprasidone, quetiapine	Psychosis, schizophrenia, disruptive hallucinations and delusions	Nonspecific agitation of dementia	Lower risk of tardive dyskinesia (1% to 4%); more expensive; clozapine, highly anticholinergic and may precipitate seizures, regular monitoring of the white blood count required, side effect of agranulocytosis; olanzapine, highly anti-cholinergic, causes weight gain, useful in patients with Parkinson's disease or patients with levodopa-induced psychotic symptoms; quetiapine, sedation
Trazodone			Sedating, useful for agitation of dementia
Buspirone			Delay of a week to 10 days for onset of action
Carbamazepine and valproic acid			Both agents used in doses lower than that for seizure disorder for troublesome abnormal behaviors of dementia; safer profile than psychotropics; routine monitoring of liver function studies and hemogram required when using carbamazepine (liver toxicity and bone marrow

Continued

TABLE 5-2	Appropriate and Inappropriate Drug Therapy in Older Adults—cont'd		
Drug	**Appropriate**	**Inappropriate**	**Special Considerations**
Psychotropic Drugs—cont'd			
			depression, toxicity); agents useful for the treatment of agitation and anxiety associated with dementia syndromes include trazodone and buspirone (Colenda, 1991)
Dopamine			Bradykinetic episodes "wearing off" effect requires more frequent dosing for Parkinson's disease; side effects of depression, paranoid or psychotic behavior, cognitive dysfunction, postural hypotension, urinary retention, cardiac irregularities; major side effect of nausea
Bromocriptine, pergolide, pramipexole, ropinirole	First-line agents for Parkinson's disease patients with normal physical and cognitive function	Parkinson's disease patients with dementia	Side effects of confusion, hallucinations, hypotension, nausea, vomiting, and daytime sedation
Cathechol-0-methylotransferase inhibitors (entacapone, tolcapone)			Used as adjuncts to levodopa therapy with concomitant slow reduction of the dosage of levodopa during initial administration to prevent dopaminergic side effects
Benztropine, trihexyphenidyl	To treat the tremor of Parkinson's disease or drug-induced Parkinson's syndrome secondary to phenothiazine use		Anticholinergic side effects
Amantadine, ramantidine	Used as an adjunct to anticholinergic therapy to treat Parkinson's disease		Doses higher than 100 mg in frail older patients or those with renal impairment may be associated with an increased risk of side-effects including nausea,

| TABLE 5-2 | Appropriate and Inappropriate Drug Therapy in Older Adults—cont'd | | |

Drug	Appropriate	Inappropriate	Special Considerations
			dizziness, light-headedness, insomnia, depression, anxiety, hallucinations, confusion, anorexia, dry mouth, constipation, orthostatic hypotension, and leg edema; useful as prophylaxis of or to shorten duration of influenza
Phenytoin	Seizure disorder; trigeminal neuralgia		Popular agent to treat the chronic pain of neuropathy, particularly diabetic; metabolized by the liver; highly protein bound; serum monitoring recommended; side effects of nystagmus, ataxia, slurred speech, decreased coordination, mental confusion), nausea, vomiting and constipation, dermatitis, leukopenia, agranulocytosis, thrombocytopenia, and pancytopenia
Gabapentin	Seizure disorder		Used for management of pain of neuropathy; new indication for postherpetic neuralgia
Major (phenothiazine) tranquilizers	Psychotic behavior, hallucinations or delusions that are troublesome for patient; aggressive, hostile, combative behavior in dementia patients	Nonspecific diagnosis of dementia	May cause or worsen cognitive dysfunction, functional decline, postural hypotension, and falls; parkinsonian side effects and risk of tardive dyskinesia; reduce dose and discontinue drug when possible; properly document need for drug
Minor (benzodiazepine)	Anxiety that is troublesome for	Nonspecific use for sleep	Reduce dose and discontinue drug when possible; avoid

Continued

TABLE 5-2	Appropriate and Inappropriate Drug Therapy in Older Adults—cont'd		
Drug	**Appropriate**	**Inappropriate**	**Special Considerations**
Psychotropic Drugs—cont'd			
tranquilizers	patients		PRN use; properly document need for drug
Barbiturates	Seizure disorder	Nonspecific treatment of insomnia or anxiety	Monitor drug levels, properly document need for drug; may cause or worsen cognitive dysfunction, postural hypotension, and falls
Miscellaneous Drugs			
Finasteride	Initial symptomatic benign prostatic hyperplasia	Patients with diagnosed or suspected prostate cancer	Should be used for at least 6 months; use with caution because it can suppress prostate-specific antigen levels in patients with prostate cancer
Steroids	Polymyalgia rheumatica (15-20 mg/day); temporal arteritis (40-60 mg/day); acute flares of rheumatoid arthritis, acute attacks of asthma resistant to conventional therapy; moderate to severe chronic lung disease; allergic rhinitis; initial treatment of certain dermatoses	Initial treatment of asthma; osteoarthritis	Side effects of weight gain; fluid retention; dependence; worsening or precipitation of hypertension or diabetes, cataracts, or osteoporosis
Fludrocortisone acetate	Replacement therapy for Addison's disease or adrenogenital syndrome	Not officially indicated for treatment of refractory postural hypotension	
Prostaglandin	Erectile dysfunction secondary to vascular, neurogenic, or psychogenic causes	General use to increase sexual potency	Side effects of penis pain, priapism, and prolonged erections
Tamsulosin	Signs and symptoms of benign prostatic hyperplasia		

| TABLE 5-2 | Appropriate and Inappropriate Drug Therapy in Older Adults—cont'd | | |

Drug	Appropriate	Inappropriate	Special Considerations
Stimulants			
Dexfenfluramine and fenfluramine		Cause pulmonary fibrosis and valvular heart defects	Withdrawn for use because of serious side effects
Theophylline	Acute wheezing or a diagnosis of asthma	Routine treatment of chronic obstructive lung disease	Can cause postural hypotension, nausea, anorexia, weight loss, arrhythmias, anxiety, insomnia insomnia
Vitamins and Prophylaxis			
Aspirin (81 mg)	Daily for all patients	Active gastrointestinal bleeding or history of bleeding diathesis or other blood disorders; allergy to aspirin	
Aspirin (325 mg)	For patients with a history of previous stroke	Active gastrointestinal bleeding or history of bleeding diathesis or other blood disorders; allergy to aspirin	
Heparin	Prophylaxis for transiently immobile patients with a history of deep vein thrombosis or pulmonary embolus; obesity, history of congestive heart failure, or chronic venous insufficiency		
Enoxaparin	Prevention of deep vein thrombosis and pulmonary embolism in patients after surgery for hip or knee replacement; home follow-up treatment for deep vein thrombosis	General postsurgical prophylaxis	Shown to be as effective as warfarin in preventing deep vein thrombosis; when used for home treatment of deep vein thrombosis, associated with decreased hospital stay

Continued

TABLE 5-2	Appropriate and Inappropriate Drug Therapy in Older Adults—cont'd

Drug	Appropriate	Inappropriate	Special Considerations
Vitamins and Prophylaxis—cont'd			
Warfarin	Prevention of deep vein thrombosis and pulmonary embolism in patients after surgery for cancer, hip fracture, or knee or hip replacement; prophylaxis for patients with chronic atrial fibrillation and rheumatic heart disease	General postsurgical prophylaxis; patients at risk for falls, with cognitive dysfunction or dementia, liver disease, or malnutrition	Maintain INR 2.0 to 3.0 normal to prevent excess bleeding tendency; increased bleeding in patients over 80 yr of age; use with caution in patients with liver disease and malnutrition; avoid use of NSAIDs and aspirin concomitantly because of increased risk of bleeding; weigh risk versus benefit; not associated with prolonged quality-adjusted life expectancy in the oldest old with nonrheumatic atrial fibrillation
Iron supplement	Proven iron deficiency	Nonspecific treatment of microcytic hypochromic anemia	
Zinc	Lozenges shown to be effective for reduction in severity and duration of upper respiratory symptoms; wound healing in event of pressure ulcers		Not yet approved by the FDA; associated with slowing of macular degeneration
Selenium	Shown to be effective in reduction in incidence of cancer		
Vitamins (antioxidants) A, C, E	For deficiency states only	For prophylazis against premature aging	Effective in increasing cell-mediated immunity; controversial regarding benefits for cancer and heart disease prevention; increased number of adverse effects in patients taking megadoses of vitamin E for upper

TABLE 5-2	Appropriate and Inappropriate Drug Therapy in Older Adults		

Drug	Appropriate	Inappropriate	Special Considerations
			respiratory tract infections; vitamin A associated with increased risk of hip fractures in postmenopausal women
Vitamins (multiple)	For all patients		
Estrogen	Symptom control of perimenopausal symptoms in women with a hysterectomy only		
Hormone replacement therapy	Symptom control of perimenopausal symptoms in women with a uterus	Postmenopausal osteoporosis; associated with increased cardiovascular morbidity (stroke, myocardial infarction, thromboembolic disease); increased incidence of breast cancer	
Alcohol			Higher risk of dementia and overall mortality with questionable or definite alcohol abuse; light to moderate drinking associated with lower risk of any dementia/vascular dementia; increases HDL, reduces LDL, and lowers total; moderate intake associated with reduced risk of stroke, myocardial infarction, and total and cardiovascular mortality
Erythropoietin	Anemia of chronic disease in zidovudine-treated immunodeficiency disease, anemia of chronic renal failure, and for reduction of		Associated with edema, hypertension, supplemental iron necessary as a substrate

| TABLE 5-2 | Appropriate and Inappropriate Drug Therapy in Older Adults—cont'd |

Drug	*Appropriate*	*Inappropriate*	*Special Considerations*
Vitamins and Prophylaxis—cont'd			
	allogeneic blood transfusions in surgery patients		
Clopidogrel	For reduction of atherosclerotic events (myocardial infarction, stroke and vascular death in patients with atherosclerosis documented by recent myocardial infarction, stroke, or established peripheral vascular disease		Contraindicated in states of active bleeding; rare side-effects, development of thrombotic thrombocytopenia purpura; advantage over ticlopidine, routine monitoring of blood components not necessary

CNS, Central nervous system; *FDA*, Food and Drug Administration; *ACE*, angiotensin-converting enzyme; *AIDS*, acquired immunodeficiency syndrome; *HDL*, high-density lipoprotein; *LDL*, low-density lipoprotein.

Resources

Center Watch, Inc.
Clinical Trials Listing Service
581 Boylston Street, Suite 200
Boston, MA 02116
www.centerwatch.com

Rx List Internet Drug Index
www.rxlist.com

References

Abenhaim L et al: Appetite-suppressant drugs and the risk of primary pulmonary hypertension, *N Engl J Med* 335:609-616, 1996.
Akiyama T et al: Effects of advancing age on the efficacy and side effects of antiarrhythmic drugs in post-myocardial infarction patients with ventricular arrhythmias, *J Am Geriatr Soc* 40:666-672, 1992.
American Geriatric Society Panel on Persistent Pain in Older Persons: The management of persistent pain in older persons, *J Am Geriatr Soc* 50:S205-S224, 2002.
Australia/New Zealand Heart Failure Research Collaborative Group. Randomised, placebo-controlled trial of carvedilol in patients with congestive heart failure due to ischemic heart disease, *Lancet* 349:375-380, 1997.
Bagger JP et al: Effect of verapamil in intermittent claudication: a randomized, double-blind, placebo-controlled, cross-over study after individual dose-response assessment, *Circulation* 95:411-414, 1997.

Balch CM, Buzaid AC: Finally, a successful adjuvant therapy for high-risk melanoma, *J Clin Oncol* 14:1-3, 1996.

Berggren D et al: Postoperative confusion after anesthesia in elderly patients with femoral neck fractures, *Anesth Analg* 66:497-504, 1987.

Bergqvist D et al: Low-molecular-weight heparin (Enoxaparin) as prophylaxis against venous thromboembolism after total hip replacement, *N Engl J Med* 335:696-700, 1996.

Bjorck S et al: Renal protective effect of enalapril in diabetic nephropathy, *BMJ* 304:339-343, 1992.

Bombardier C et al: Comparison of upper gastrointestinal toxicity of rofecoxib and naproxen in patients with rheumatoid arthritis. VIGOR Study Group, *N Engl J Med* 343:1520-1528, 2000

Bradley JD et al: Comparison of an antiinflammatory dose of ibuprofen, an analgesic dose of ibuprofen, and acetaminophen in the treatment of patients with osteoarthritis of the knee, *N Engl J Med* 325:87-91, 1991.

Brown JP et al: The efficacy and tolerability of risedronate once a week for the treatment of postmenopausal osteoporosis, *Calcified Tissue International* 71:103-112, 2002.

Brown SL et al: Occult caffeine as a source of sleep problems in an older population, *J Am Geriatr Soc* 43: 860-864, 1995.

Buckler DA, Kelber ST, Goodwin JS: The use of dietary restrictions in malnourished nursing home patients, *J Am Geriatr Soc* 42:1100-1102, 1994.

Buring JE, Glynn RJ, Hennekens CH: Calcium channel blockers and myocardial infarction: a hypothesis formulated but not yet tested, *JAMA* 274:654-655, 1995.

Cahill L et al: Beta-adrenergic activation and memory for emotional events, *Nature* 371:702-704, 1994.

Cantwell-Gab K: Identifying chronic peripheral arterial disease, *Am J Nurs* 96:44, 1996.

Cefalu CA, Pike J: Fecal impaction: a practical approach to the problem, *Geriatrics* 36:143-145, 1981.

Centers for Disease Control and Prevention: Adverse events associated with ephedrine-containing products: Texas, December 1993-September 1995, *MMWR Morb Mortal Wkly Rep* 45:689-693, 1996.

Clark LC et al: Effects of selenium supplementation for cancer prevention in patients with carcinoma of the skin: a randomized controlled trial, *JAMA* 276:1957-1963, 1996.

Cobbs E et al: GERIATRIC REVIEW SYLLABUS—A Core Curriculum in Geriatric Medicine. American Geriatrics Society, New York, NY, 2002-2004.

Cook DJ et al: Risk factors for gastrointestinal bleeding in critically ill patients, *N Engl J Med* 10:377-381, 1994.

Coplen SE et al: Efficacy and safety of quinidine therapy for maintenance of sinus rhythm after cardioversion, *Circulation* 82:1106-1116, 1990.

Cummings SR et al: The effect of raloxifene on risk of breast cancer in postmenopausal women: results from the MORE randomized trial, *JAMA* 281:2189-2196, 1999.

Curb JD et al: Effect of diuretic-based antihypertensive treatment on cardiovascular disease risk in older diabetic patients with isolated systolic hypertension, *JAMA* 276:1886-1892, 1996.

Daly E et al: Measuring the impact of menopausal symptoms on quality of life, *BMJ* 307:836-840, 1993.

Desbiens NA: Deciding on anticoagulating the oldest old with atrial fibrillation: Insights from cost-effectiveness analysis, *J Am Geriatr Soc* 50:863-869, 2002.

Donahue JG et al: Inhaled steroids and the risk of hospitalization for asthma, *JAMA* 277:887-891, 1997.

Douthwaite S: Structure-activity relationships of ketolides vs. macrolides, *Clin Microbiol Infect* 7 (suppl):11-17, 2001.

Dubois B, Pillon B: Cholinergic deficiency and frontal dysfunction in Parkinson's disease, *Ann Neurol* 28:117-121, 1990.

Engelhart MJ et al: Dietary intake of antioxidants and risk of Alzheimer's disease, *JAMA* 287:3223-3229, 2002.

Ensrud KE et al: Central nervous system-active medications and risk for falls in older women, *J Am Geriatr Soc* 50:1629-1637, 2002.

Evans MP, Fleming KC, Evans FM: Hormone replacement therapy: management of common problems, *Mayo Clin Proc* 70:800-805, 1995.

Feldman H et al: A 24 week, randomized, double-blind study of donepezil in moderate to severe Alzheimer's disease, *Neurology* 57:613-620, 2001.

Ferguson TB, Coombs LP, Peterson ED: Preoperative beta-blocker use and mortality and morbidity following CABG surgery in North America, *JAMA* 287:2221-2227, 2002.

Feskanich D et al: Vitamin A intake and hip fractures among postmenopausal women, *JAMA* 287:47-54, 2002.

Figulla HR et al: Diltiazem improves cardiac function and exercise capacity in patients with idiopathic dilated cardiomyopathy: results of the diltiazem in dilated cardiomyopathy trial, *Circulation* 94:346-352, 1996.

Fihn SD et al: The risk for and severity of bleeding complications in elderly patients treated with warfarin, *Ann Intern Med* 124:970-979, 1996.

Finucane FF et al: Decreased risk of stroke among postmenopausal hormone users: results from a national cohort, *Arch Intern Med* 153:73-79, 1993.

Fishkind D, Paris BE, Aronow WS: Use of digoxin, diuretics, beta blockers, angiotensin-converting enzyme inhibitors, and calcium channel blockers in older patients in an academic hospital-based geriatrics practice, *J Am Geriatr Soc* 45:809-812, 1997.

Foody MJ, Farrell MH, Krumholz HM: Beta blocker therapy in heart failure, *JAMA* 287:883-889, 2002.

Furberg CD, Psaty BM, Meyer JV: Nifedipine: dose-related increase in mortality in patients with coronary heart disease, *Circulation* 92:1326-1331, 1995.

Gale CR et al: Vitamin C and risk of death from stroke and coronary heart disease in cohort of elderly people, *BMJ* 310:1563-1566, 1995.

Garcia Rodriguez LA, Hernandez-Diaz S: Relative risk of upper gastrointestinal complications among users of acetaminophen and nonsteroidal anti-inflammatory drugs, *Epidemiology* 12:570-576, 2001.

Gergen PJ et al: A population-based serologic survey of immunity to tetanus in the United States, *N Engl J Med* 332:761-766, 1995.

Ginsburg ES et al: Effects of alcohol ingestion on estrogens in postmenopausal women, *JAMA* 276:1747-1751, 1996.

Gottlieb SS et al: Renal response to Indomethacin in congestive heart failure secondary to ischemic or idiopathic dilated cardiomyopathy, *Am J Cardiol* 70:890-893, 1992.

Graat JM, Schouten EG, Kok FJ: Effect of daily vitamin E and multivitamin-mineral supplementation on acute respiratory infections in elderly persons: a randomized controlled trial, *JAMA* 288:715-721, 2002.

Grady D et al: Hormone therapy to prevent disease and prolong life in postmenopausal women, *Ann Intern Med* 117:1016-1032, 1992.

Graham DY et al: Effect of treatment of *Helicobacter pylori* infection on the long-term recurrence rate of gastric or duodenal ulcer, *Ann Intern Med* 116:705-708, 1992.

Green D, Miller V: The role of dipyridamole in the therapy of vascular disease, *Geriatrics* 48:51-53, 57-58, 1993.

Greenberg ER et al: Mortality associated with low plasma concentration of beta carotene and the effect of oral supplementation, *JAMA* 275:699-703, 1996.

Greig NH et al: A new therapeutic target in Alzheimer's disease treatment: attention to butyrylcholinesterase, *Curr Med Res Opin* 17:158-165, 2001.

Grover SA, Palmer CS, Coupal L: Serum lipid screening to identify high-risk individuals for coronary death, *Arch Intern Med* 154:679-684, 1994.

Grodstein F et al: Postmenopausal hormone therapy and cognitive function in healthy older women, *J Am Geriatr Soc* 48:746-752, 2000.

Gurwitz JH et al: Initiation of antihypertensive treatment during nonsteroidal antiinflammatory drug therapy, *JAMA* 272:781-786, 1994.

Gurwitz JH, Noonan JD, Soumerai SB: Reducing the use of H_2-receptor antagonists in the long-term care setting, *J Am Geriatr Soc* 40:359-364, 1992.

Hallstrom AP et al: An antiarrhythmic drug experience in 941 patients resuscitated from an initial cardiac arrest between 1970 and 1985, *Am J Cardiol* 68:1025-1031, 1991.

Hannedouche T et al: Randomized controlled trial of enalapril and B blockers in nondiabetic chronic renal failure, *BMJ* 309:833-837, 1994.

Harpaz D et al: Effect of aspirin on mortality in women with symptomatic or silent myocardial ischemia, *Am J Cardiol* 78:1215-1219, 1996.

Harris ST et al: Effects of risedronate treatment on vertebral and nonvertebral fractures in women with postmenopausal osteoporosis, *JAMA* 282:1344-1352, 1999.

Hazzard WR et al: *Principles of geriatric medicine and gerontology,* ed 4, New York, 1999, McGraw-Hill.

Hebert PR, Gaziano JM, Hennekens CH: An overview of trials of cholesterol lowering and risk of stroke, *Arch Intern Med* 155:50-55, 1995.

Helzlsouer KJ et al: Association between alpha-tocopherol, gamma-tocopherol, selenium, and subsequent prostate cancer, *J Natl Cancer Inst* 92:2018-2023, 2000.

Hempling RE et al: Hormone replacement therapy as a risk factor for epithelial ovarian cancer: results of a case-control study, *Obstet Gynecol* 89:1012-1016, 1997.

Henry D et al: Meta-analysis workshop in upper gastrointestinal hemorrhage, *Gastroenterology* 100:1481-1482, 1991.

Hentschel E et al: Effect of ranitidine and amoxicillin plus metronidazole on the eradication of *Helicobacter pylori* and the recurrence of duodenal ulcer, *N Engl J Med* 328:308-312, 1993.

Hetland ML, Haarbo J, Christiansen C: One measurement of serum total cholesterol is enough to predict future levels in healthy postmenopausal women, *Am J Med* 92:25-28, 1992.

Hohnloser S, van de Loo A, Baedeker F: Efficacy and proarrhythmic hazards of pharmacologic cardioversion of atrial fibrillation: prospective comparison of sotalol versus quinidine, *J Am Coll Cardiol* 26:852-858, 1995.

Honkanen PO, Keistinen T, Knela SL: Reactions following administration of influenza vaccine alone or with pneumococcal vaccine to the elderly, *Arch Intern Med* 156:205-208, 1996.

Hortobagyi GN et al: Efficacy of pamidronate in reducing skeletal complications in patients with breast cancer and lytic bone metastases, *N Engl J Med* 335:1785-1791, 1996.

Hu FB et al: Fish and omega-3 fatty acid intake and risk of coronary heart disease in women, *JAMA* 287: 1815-1821, 2002.

Hutton N, Wilson MH, Mellits ED: Effectiveness of an antihistamine-decongestant combination for young children with the common cold: a randomized, controlled clinical trial, *J Pediatr* 118:125-130, 1991.

ISIS-4 Collaborative Group: ISIS-4: a randomized factorial trial assessing early oral captopril, oral mononitrate, and intravenous magnesium sulphate in 58,050 patients with suspected acute myocardial infarction, *Lancet* 345:669-685, 1995.

Jackson JL et al: The effect of treating herpes zoster with oral acyclovir in preventing postherpetic neuralgia: a meta-analysis, *Arch Intern Med* 157:909-912, 1997.

Jacobs LD et al: Intramuscular interferon beta-Ia for disease progression in relapsing multiple sclerosis, *Ann Neurol* 39:285-294, 1996.

Jampol LM: Antioxidants and zinc to prevent progression of age-related macular degeneration, *Arch Ophthalmol* 119:1417-1436, 2001.

Jansen PH et al: Randomised controlled trial of hydroquinine in muscle cramps, *Lancet* 349:528-532, 1997.

Javaheri S et al: Effect of theophylline on sleep-disordered breathing in heart failure, *N Engl J Med* 335: 562-567, 1996.

Jones AC, Berman P, Doherty M: Nonsteroidal antiinflammatory drug usage and requirement in elderly acute hospital admissions, *Br J Rheumatol* 31:45-48, 1992.

Katz IR et al: Identification of medications that cause cognitive impairment in older people: the case of oxybutynin chloride, *J Am Geriatr Soc*, 46:8-13, 1998.

Kjeldsen SE et al: Effects of losartan on cardiovascular morbidity and mortality in patients with isolated systolic hypertension and left ventricular hypertrophy: a Losartan Intervention for Endpoint Reduction (LIFE) substudy, *JAMA* 288:1491-1498, 2002.

Knapp MJ et al: A 30-week randomized controlled trial of high-dose tacrine in patients with Alzheimer's disease, *JAMA* 271:992-998, 1994.

Ko DT et al: Beta-blocker therapy and symptoms of depression, fatigue, and sexual dysfunction, *JAMA* 288: 351-357, 2002.

Kristal BS, Yu BP: An emerging hypothesis: synergistic induction of aging by free radical and Maillard reactions, *J Gerontol Biol Sci Med Sci* 47:B107-B114, 1992.

Kristiansen IS, Eggen AE, Thelle DS: Cost-effectiveness of incremental programmes for lowering serum cholesterol concentration: is individual intervention worthwhile? *BMJ* 302:1119-1122, 1991.

Knudtson ML et al: Chelation therapy for ischemic heart disease, *JAMA* 287:481-486, 2002.

Krumholz HM et al: Lack of association between cholesterol and coronary heart disease: mortality and morbidity and all-cause mortality in persons older than 70 years, *JAMA* 272:1335-1340, 1994.

Kushi LH et al: Physical activity and mortality in postmenopausal women, *JAMA* 277:1287-1292, 1997.

Langman MJ et al: Risks of bleeding peptic ulcer associated with individual nonsteroidal antiinflammatory drugs, *Lancet* 343:1075-1078, 1994.

Lanza Fl et al: Endoscopic comparison of esophageal and gastroduodenal effects of risedronate and alendronate in postmenopausal women, *Gastroenterology* 119:631-638, 2000.

Leclerc JR et al: Prevention of venous thromboembolism after knee arthroplasty, *Ann Intern Med* 124: 619-626, 1996.

Lepor H, Williford WO, Barry MJ: The efficacy of terazosin, finasteride, or both in benign prostatic hyperplasia, *N Engl J Med* 335:533-539, 1996.

Levine M et al: A comparison of low-molecular-weight heparin administered primarily at home with unfractionated heparin administered in the hospital for proximal deep-vein thrombosis, *N Engl J Med* 334:677-681, 1996.

Lewis EJ et al: The effect of angiotensin-converting-enzyme inhibition on diabetic nephropathy, *N Engl J Med* 329:1456-1462, 1993.

Liberman UA et al: Effect of oral alendronate on bone mineral density and the incidence of fractures in postmenopausal osteoporosis, *N Engl J Med* 333:1437-1443, 1995.

Liel Y, Harmon-Boehm I, Shany S: Evidence for a clinically important adverse effect of fiber-enriched diet on the bioavailability of levothyroxine in adult hypothyroid patients, *J Clin Endocrinol Metab* 81:857-859, 1996.

Linet OI, Ogrinc FC: Efficacy and safety of intracavernosal alprostadil in men with erectile dysfunction, *N Engl J Med* 334:873-877, 1996.

Low PA et al: Efficacy of midodrine versus placebo in neurogenic orthostatic hypotension: a randomized, double-blind multicenter study, *JAMA* 277:1046-1051, 1997.

Mach JR et al: Serum anticholinergic activity in hospitalized older persons with delirium: a preliminary study, *J Am Geriatr Soc* 43:491-495, 1995.

Madhusoodanan S, Brenner R: Update on risperidone use in elderly patients, *Clinical Geriatrics* 9:11; 32-40, 2001.

Malone JG et al: Tolterodine versus Oxybutynin-A geriatric perspective, *J Am Ger Soc*, 49:700-705, 2001.

Maltby N et al: Efficacy of tacrine and lecithin in mild to moderate Alzheimer's disease: double blind trial, *BMJ* 308:879-883, 1994.

Mangano DT et al: Effect of atenolol on mortality and cardiovascular morbidity after noncardiac surgery, *N Engl J Med* 335:1713-1720, 1996.

Manolio TA et al: Associations of postmenopausal estrogen use with cardiovascular disease and stroke risk factors in older women, *Circulation* 88:2163-2171, 1993.

Man-Sons-Hing M, Wells G: Meta-analysis of efficacy of quinine for treatment of nocturnal leg cramps in elderly people, *BMJ* 310:13-17, 1995.

Mathurin P et al: Survival and prognostic factors in patients with severe alcoholic hepatitis treated with prednisolone, *Gastroenterology* 110:1847-1853, 1996.

McDonald CC et al: Cardiac and vascular morbidity in women receiving adjuvant tamoxifen for breast cancer in a randomised trial, *BMJ* 311:977-980, 1995.

Miller KJ et al: Mood symptoms and cognitive performance in women estrogen users and nonusers and men, *J Am Geriatr Soc* 50:1826-1830, 2002.

Miyawaki E: Thrombolysis for stroke: some concern, some hope–an editorial, *Journal Watch* 16:51-52, 1997.

Monane M et al: The impact of thiazide diuretics on the initiation of lipid-reducing agents in older people: a population-based analysis, *J Am Geriatr Soc* 45:71-75, 1997.

Morris MC et al: Dietary intake of antioxidant nutrients and the risk of incidence Alzheimer disease in a biracial community study, *JAMA* 287:3230-3237, 2002.

Morrison HI et al: Serum folate and risk of fatal coronary heart disease, *JAMA* 275:1893-1896, 1996.

Mossad SB et al: Zinc gluconate lozenges for treating the common cold: a randomized, placebo-controlled study, *Ann Intern Med* 125:81-88, 1996.

Neer RM et al: Effect of parathyroid hormone (1-34) on fractures and bone mineral density in postmenopausal women with osteoporosis, *N Engl J Med* 344:19, 1434-1441, 2001.

Nevitt MC et al: Association of estrogen replacement therapy with the risk of osteoarthritis of the hip in elderly white women, *Arch Intern Med* 156:2073-2080, 1996.

Newbern VB: Cautionary tales on using beta blockers, *Geriatr Nurs* 12:119-122, 1991.

Niederau C et al: Long-term follow-up of HbeAG-positive patients treated with interferon alfa for chronic hepatitis B, *N Engl J Med* 334:1422-1427, 1996.

Novack GD et al: New glaucoma medications in the geriatric population: efficacy and safety, *J Am Geriatr Soc* 50:956-962, 2002.

O'Keefe JH Jr et al: Estrogen replacement therapy after coronary angioplasty in women, *J Am Coll Cardiol* 29:1-5, 1997.

Omenn GS et al: Effects of a combination of beta carotene and vitamin A on lung cancer and cardiovascular disease, *N Engl J Med* 334:1150-1155, 1996.

Packer M et al: Double-blind, placebo-controlled study of the effects of carvedilol in patients with moderate to severe heart failure: the precise trial, *Circulation* 94:2793-2799, 1996a.

Packer M et al: Effect of amlodipine on morbidity and mortality in severe chronic heart failure, *N Engl J Med* 335:1107-1114, 1996b.

Pahor M et al: Risk of gastrointestinal hemorrhage with calcium antagonists in hypertensive persons over 67 years old, *Lancet* 347:1061-1065, 1996.

Park KC, Forman DE, Wei JY: Utility of beta-blockade treatment for older postinfarction patients, *J Am Geriatr Soc* 43:751-755, 1995.

Patt RB: PCA: prescribing analgesia for home management of severe pain, *Geriatrics* 47:69-84, 1992.

Penn ND et al: The effects of dietary supplementation with vitamins A, C, and E on cell-mediated immune functions in elderly, long-stay patients, *Age Ageing* 20:169-174, 1991.

Perrig WJ, Perrig P, Stahelin HB: The relation between antioxidants and memory performance in the old and very old, *J Am Geriatr Soc* 45:718-724, 1997.

Physician's Desk Reference. Montvale, NJ, 2002, Medical Economics.

Pinkowish MD: Practical briefings: clinical news you can put into practice now, *Patient Care* 6-21, 1995.

Psaty BM et al: The risk of myocardial infarction associated with the combined use of estrogens and progestins in postmenopausal women, *Arch Intern Med* 154:1333-1339, 1994.

Punn KK et al: Calcitonin-salmon nasal spray: Analgesic effects on new vertebral fractures, *Clin Ther* 11:205-209, 1989.

Rapola JM et al: Effect of vitamin E and beta-carotene on the incidence of angina pectoris: a randomized, double-blind, controlled trial, *JAMA* 275:693-698, 1996.

Rendell MS et al: Sildenafil for treatment of erectile dysfunction in men with diabetes, *JAMA* 281:421-426, 1999.

Rhymes JA: Clinical management of the terminally ill, *Geriatrics* 46:57-67, 1991.

Riemersma RA et al: Risk of angina pectoris and plasma concentrations of vitamins A, C, and E and carotene, *Lancet* 337:1-5, 1991.

Rockwood K et al: Use of lipid-lowering agents, indication bias, and the risk of dementia in community-dwelling elderly people, *Arch Neurol* 59:223-227, 2000.

Rogers SL, Friedhoff LT: The efficacy and safety of donepezil in patients with Alzheimer's disease: results of a U.S. multicenter, randomized, double-blind, placebo-controlled trial: the Donepezil Study Group, *Dementia* 7:293-303, 1996.

Rossouw JE et al: Risks and benefits of estrogen plus progestin in healthy postmenopausal women: principle results from the women's health initiative randomized controlled trial, *JAMA* 288:321-331, 2002.

Ruitenberg A, et al: Alcohol consumption and risk of dementia: the Rotterdam study, *Lancet*, 359: 281-286, 2002.

The SALT Collaborative Group: Swedish aspirin low-dose trial (SALT) of 75 mg aspirin as secondary prophylaxis after cerebrovascular ischemic events, *Lancet* 338:1345-1349, 1991.

Schmidt R et al: Plasma antioxidants and cognitive performance in middle-aged and older adults: results of the stroke prevention study, *J Am Ger Soc* 46:1407-1410, 1998.

Schnyder G et al: Effect of homocysteine-lowering therapy with folic acid, vitamin B_{12} and vitamin B_6 on clinical outcome after percutaneous coronary intervention. The Swiss heart study: a randomized controlled trial, *JAMA* 288:973-979, 2002.

SHEP Cooperative Research Group: Prevention of stroke by antihypertensive drug treatment in older persons with isolated systolic hypertension: final results of the systolic hypertension in the elderly program (SHEP), *JAMA* 265:3255-3264, 1991.

Sherrill KA, Reifler BV: Psychotherapy and psychopharmacology. In Hazard et al: *Geriatric medicine and gerontology,* ed 4, New York, 1999, McGraw Hill.

Shorr RI et al: Individual sulfonylureas and serious hypoglycemia in older people, *J Am Geriatr Soc* 44: 751-755, 1996.

Silverstein et al: Gastrointestinal toxicity with celecoxib vs nonsteroidal anti-inflammatory drugs for osteoarthritis and rheumatoid arthritis: the CLASS study: a randomized controlled trial. Celecoxib Long-term Arthritis Safety Study, *JAMA* 284:1247-1245, 2000.

Slataper R et al: Comparative effects of different antihypertensive treatments on progression of diabetic renal disease, *Arch Intern Med* 153:973-980, 1993.

Slatton ML et al: Does digoxin provide additional hemodynamic and autonomic benefit at higher doses in patients with mild to moderate heart failure and normal sinus rhythm? *J Am Coll Cardiol* 29:1206-1213, 1997.

Solowij N et al: Cognitive functioning of long-term heavy cannabis users seeking treatment, *JAMA* 287:1123-1131, 2002.

Solomon DH et al: Nonsteroidal anti-inflammatory drug use and acute myocardial infarction, *Arch Intern Med* 162:1099-1104, 2002.

Soumerai SB et al: Adverse outcomes of underuse of beta-blockers in elderly survivors of acute myocardial infarction, *JAMA* 277:115-121, 1997.

Steinhubl SR et al: Early and sustained dual oral antiplatelet therapy following percutaneous coronary intervention, *JAMA* 288:2411-2420, 2002.

Stephens NG et al: Randomised controlled trial of vitamin E in patients with coronary disease: Cambridge Heart Antioxidant Study (CHAOS), *Lancet* 347:781-786, 1996.

Stewart WF et al: Risk of Alzheimer's disease and duration of NSAID use, *Neurology* 48: 626-632, 1997.

Stoehr GP et al: Over-the-counter medication use in an older rural community: the MoVIES Project, *J Am Geriatr Soc* 45:158-165, 1997.

Stroke Prevention in Atrial Fibrillation Investigators: Warfarin versus aspirin for prevention of thromboembolism in atrial fibrillation: stroke prevention in atrial fibrillation II study, *Lancet* 343:687-691, 1994.

Taha AS et al: Famotidine for the prevention of gastric and duodenal ulcers caused by nonsteroidal anti-inflammatory drugs, *N Engl J Med* 334:1435-1439, 1996.

Tang M et al: Effect of oestrogen during menopause on risk and age at onset of Alzheimer's disease, *Lancet* 348:429-432, 1996.

Tariot PN et al: Lack of carbamazepine toxicity in frail nursing home patients: a controlled study, *J Am Geriatr Soc* 43:1026-1029, 1995.

Tariot PN et al: Carbamazepine treatment of agitation in nursing home patients with dementia: a preliminary study, *J Am Geriatr Soc* 42:1160-1166, 1994.

Tariot PN et al: A 5-month, randomized, placebo-controlled trial of galantamine in AD, *Neurology* 54:12; 2269-2276, 2000.

Thomas VS, Rockwood KJ: Alcohol abuse, cognitive impairment, and mortality among older people, *J Am Geriatr Soc* 49:4; 415-420, 2001.

Thompson MP, Morris LK: Unexplained weight loss in the ambulatory elderly, *J Am Geriatr Soc* 39:497-500, 1991.

Tramer MR et al: A quantitative systematic review of ondansetron in treatment of established postoperative nausea and vomiting, *BMJ* 314:1088-1093, 1997.

Vega GL, Grundy SM: Lipoprotein responses to treatment with lovastatin, gemfibrozil, and nicotinic acid in normolipidemic patients with hypoalphalipoproteinemia, *Arch Intern Med* 154:73-82, 1994.

Wallentin LC: Aspirin (75 mg/day) after an episode of unstable coronary artery disease: long-term effects on the risk for myocardial infarction, occurrence of severe angina and the need for revascularization, *J Am Coll Cardiol* 18:1587-1593, 1991.

Warner GT, Perry CM: Ramipril: a review of its use in the prevention of cardiovascular outcomes, *Drugs* 62:1381-405, 2002.

Whelan AM et al: The effect of aspirin on niacin-induced cutaneous reactions, *J Fam Pract* 34:165-168, 1992.

Whelton A et al: Cyclooxygenase-2 inhibitors and cardiorenal function: a randomized, controlled trial of celecoxib and rofecoxib in older hypertensive osteoarthritis patients, *Am J Ther* 8: 85-95, 2001.

Zandi PP et al: Hormone replacement therapy and incidence of Alzheimer disease in older women: the Cache County Study, *JAMA* 288:2123-2129, 2002a.

Zandi PP et al: Reduced incidence of AD with NSAID but not H_2 receptor antagonists: the Cache County Study, *Neurology* 59(6):880-886, 2002b.

Zarembski DG et al: Treatment of resistant atrial fibrillation, *Arch Intern Med* 155:1885-1891, 1995.

Zinner NR, Mattiasson A, Stanton SL: Efficacy, safety, and tolerability of extended-release once-daily tolterodine treatment for overactive bladder in older versus younger patients, *J Am Geriatr Soc* 50:799-807, 2002.

Zisselman MH et al: Sedative-hypnotic use and increased hospital stay and costs in older people, *J Am Geriatr Soc* 44:1371-1374, 1996.

Zuccala G et al: Use of calcium antagonists and need for perioperative transfusion in older patients with hip fracture: observational study, *BMJ* 314:643-644, 1997.

6

Aging Skin

The skin of an older person serves as a window through which the body reveals much of its internal pathology. As part of comprehensive health care, providers should be encouraged to be attentive to the skin of their older patients.

People age at different rates, depending on a host of factors. Many older adults view skin problems as a normal consequence of the aging process and thus hesitate to mention them to their provider, even when they cause considerable discomfort or anxiety. This reticence must be considered and addressed by providers, who need to ask the older person about skin problems and changes in pigmentation, particularly in areas covered by clothing. This point cannot be overemphasized. Asking these questions may assist in a diagnosis and or prevent exacerbation of another disease.

Normal Skin and Age-related Changes

The human skin is composed of three layers: epidermis, dermis, and subcutaneous. These layers are a protective barrier between the body and the environment. The epidermis is the outer visible covering that reveals the physical changes of aging. The dermis and subcutaneous layer contain blood vessels and glands that provide pigmentation, insulation, and protection of the underlying organs. Table 6-1 outlines the multiple functions of the skin.

Changes in appearance and function over time are termed *intrinsic aging*. In most people, most unwanted changes are due not to aging alone but to a combination of aging and chronic environmental damage, largely sun exposure. The epidermis, dermis, subcutaneous fat, and appendages all change during the life of a person. Table 6-2 shows the age-related changes that occur with intrinsic aging.

EPIDERMIS

The epidermis of the skin is highly specialized stratified epithelia that functions to protect the body from physical and chemical damage, infection, dehydration, and heat loss. To maintain this critical barrier, epithelial tissues undergo constant renewal and repair (characteristically every 28 days). This turnover time is reduced by 50% between the third and eighth decades of life. This change can affect wound healing and causes drying of the epidermis. Vitamin D synthesis is a major function of the epidermis and keratinocytes, and it is significantly decreased in aged skin. Epithelial cells

| TABLE 6-1 | Functions of the Skin |

Skin Function	Mechanism
Protection	Intact skin covering creates a physical barrier against bacteria, minor physical trauma, and foreign substances
Synthesis of keratin	Keratinocytes are produced in the basal layer, develop, and then move to the surface of the skin
Excretion of wastes	Sweat, sodium chloride, urea, and lactic acid are excreted through the skin
Blood pressure regulation	Skin blood vessels can constrict, which promotes venous return and increases the cardiac output and blood pressure
Fluid regulation	Skin keeps fluids contained in the body
Temperature regulation	Skin blood vessels can (1) dilate to promote heat loss or to prevent tissue freezing (radiation), (2) constrict to conserve heat, or (3) regulate temperature by conduction, convection, and evaporation
Tissue repair	Skin replaces damaged skin cells and forms scar tissue
Production of vitamin D	In the presence of ultraviolet light, a precursor of vitamin D is converted to vitamin D in the skin
Sensory perception	Special sensors in the skin respond to touch, pain, heat, cold, pressure, vibration, tickling, itching, wetness, oiliness, and stickiness
Expression of emotional feelings	Surface of the skin can respond to emotions through sweating, pallor, or flushing

From Burke MM, Walsh MB: *Gerontologic nursing: wholistic care of the older adult*, ed 2, St Louis, 1997, Mosby.

(keratinocytes), which are the major barrier cells to chemical and microbial insults, undergo a program of terminal differentiation, expressing a set of structural proteins, keratins, which assemble into filaments and function to maintain cell and tissue integrity. Two types of cell adhesion structures, desmosomes and hemidesmosomes, function to glue keratinocytes to one another and to the basement membrane and connect the keratin cytoskeleton to the cell surface. Keratinizing epithelia, such as the epidermis and oral gingiva, which have to withstand severe physical and chemical forces, produce a toughened structure, the cornified cell envelope. This envelope is a major component of the epithelial barrier at the tissue surface (Presland and Jurevic, 2002).

Melanocytes and Langerhans' cells constitute the other epidermal cell types. Melanin determines skin color and tanning capacity and is the skin's major protection against damaging solar radiation. The number of enzymatically active melanocytes decreases by 10% to 20% each decade in both sun-protected and sun-exposed skin. Photosensitivity increases as the number of melanocytes declines. Loss of melanocytes results in graying hair and, coupled with a reduced capillary blood supply, fading normal skin color.

Langerhans' cells are derived from the bone marrow and are distributed diffusely throughout the epidermis. Their dendritic and immunocompetent capacities contribute to antigen recognition and presentation. In the aged skin Langerhans' cells are reduced by about 40%. This loss is believed to account for the observed age-associated decrease in delayed hypersensitivity. In sun-exposed skin, the loss of Langerhans' cells is greater. Organisms have a greater chance of invading the body through the skin.

DERMIS

Age-related changes in the dermis are numerous. The dermis, largely connective tissue, is inhabited by blood vessels, lymphatics, and multiple cellular components. It is involved in thermoregulation and

TABLE 6-2	Skin Changes Associated with Intrinsic Aging		
Compartment	**Component**	**Change**	**Biologic Consequence**
Epidermis	Keratinocytes	Decreased proliferative potential	↓ Wound healing, ↓ vitamin D production
	Melanocytes	Decreased 10%-20% per decade	↓ Photoprotection, white hairs
	Langerhans' cells	Decreased as much as 40%	↓ Delayed hypersensitivity reactions
	Basement membrane	Decreased surface area	↓ Epidermal-dermal adhesion, ↑ blistering
Dermis	Fibroblasts	Decreased collagen/elastin	↓ Tensile strength, ↓ elasticity
	Blood vessels	Decreased	↓ Thermoregulation, ↓ response to injury
	Mast cells	Decreased	↓ Immediate hypersensitivity reactions
	Neural elements	Decreased by one third	↓ Sensation, ↑ pain threshold
Subcutis	Fat	Decreased	↓ Mechanical protection and insulation
Appendages	Eccrine glands	Decreased number and output	↓ Thermoregulation
	Apocrine glands	Decreased number and output	Unknown
	Sebaceous glands	Increased size, decreased output	Unknown
	Hair	Decreased number and growth rate	Cosmetic

From Hazzard WR et al: *Principles of geriatric medicine and gerontology*, ed 3, New York, 1994, McGraw-Hill.

the inflammatory response as well as delivery of nutrients and oxygen to the skin. A 20% loss in dermal thickness occurs with aging, which often leads to the paper-thin or transparent skin appearance in older adults. In addition, the remaining dermis is relatively acellular and avascular, which interferes with its temperature-regulating capacity. This change predisposes older people to hypothermia and heat stroke during temperature extremes. With the decreased vascular supply (50% decrease in mast cells), there is a diminished response to cutaneous hypersensitivity reactions. These muted inflammatory reactions often fail to alert the physician or the patient to the need for intervention and therapy. These changes delay wound healing, which may be further compromised many times by the multiple chronic illnesses of an older adult.

SUBCUTANEOUS LAYER

The subcutaneous layer is composed of loose connective tissue, fat cells, and glands. Its main functions are to provide heat, insulation, and caloric reserves and to act as a shock absorber. Atrophy in this layer results in a reduction of many of these functions and primarily affects the face, extremities, hands, and soles of the feet. Because of the loss of the shock-absorber quality of the subcutaneous tissue, skin becomes more susceptible to trauma, particularly the soles of the feet. This change increases the trauma of walking and magnifies the many foot problems experienced by older people.

The cutaneous appendages are composed of eccrine, apocrine, and pilosebaceous units, which are hair follicles and sebaceous glands. The eccrine, or sweat, glands decrease with age, and apocrine glands in humans cause the characteristic odor associated with sweating. Sebaceous glands are found everywhere on the body with the exception of the palms, soles, and proximal nail folds. They secret sebum, a lipid-rich substance that decreases by 40% to 60% in the older adult.

Aging is associated with a gradual decrease in the number of hair follicles as well as a decrease in their growth rate. The hair of older people is sparse and thin, and it fails to grow with the same rapidity of a younger person. Loss of hair color and graying are also common because of the decrease in melanocytes. The nails thicken, develop longitudinal lines, and also have a decreased growth rate.

Environmental Effects on Skin

Environmental damage to the skin is due largely to sun exposure. Photoaging is a term that describes many of these preventable changes. Each person is affected differently by the sun, and varied chemical changes within the skin take place.

PHOTOAGING

Photoaging consists of changes in the cutaneous appearance and function that are a direct result of repeated sun exposure superimposed on intrinsic aging. Aged epidermis develops an abnormality in permeability barrier homeostasis, which is accentuated further in photoaged skin (Elias and Ghadially, 2002). Although many providers and patients perceive no difference between them, photoaging and chronologic aging are two distinct entities. This point must be made clear because it is estimated that more than 90% of cosmetically undesirable skin changes in older people are due to photoaging, and more than 90% of skin cancer arises in chronically sun-exposed (photoaged) compared with sun-protected skin. All changes caused by sun exposure can be grouped under the term *dermatoheliosis;* five parts of the skin are involved: epidermis (actinic keratosis), dermis (solar elastosis), blood vessels (telangiectasia), sebaceous glands (solar comedones), and melanocytes (diffuse or mottled brown patches) (Jackson, 2001). Table 6-3 lists changes associated with photoaging (Palmissano and Norman, 2000).

The skin of older patients must be carefully assessed and its protective aspects guarded. Although many of the intrinsic changes associated with aging cannot be diminished, many of their negative implications can be prevented if they are properly assessed by the provider. The changes associated with photoaging, particularly the high incidence of basal and squamous cell carcinomas, can be prevented. Many older people do not refer to their skin as problematic because they have come to accept their age and never critically see change. The provider needs to be conscious of this first organ that is seen.

More than 60% of older people are estimated to have a skin problem. The common manifestations of skin disorders in older persons follow.

Common Skin Disorders

As a person ages, neoplasms and infections are more prevalent. The disorders reviewed here address those found most commonly in older persons, but they are not exclusive to them.

BENIGN NEOPLASMS

Seborrheic keratoses are commonly found on sun-exposed skin. They appear as waxy, warty, greasy papules that have a "stuck-on" appearance. The color can vary from a flesh color to a darker brown. These lesions are most commonly found on the trunk, scalp, neck, extremities, and face. Size varies

TABLE 6-3	Photoaging

Clinical

- Actinic keratoses
- Fine and coarse wrinkling
- Telangiectasia
- Blotchiness and pigmentary changes
- Elastotic skin with giant comedones

Cellular Changes

- Irregular distribution of melanocytes
- Marked decrease in Langerhans' cells
- Dermal elastosis
- Decreased collagen
- Tortuosity of dermal blood vessels
- Epidermal atrophy and hyperplasia
- Increased photocarcinogenesis

From Palmissano C, Norman R Geriatric dermatology in chronic care and rehabilitation, *Dermatol Nurs* 12 (2):116-123, 2000.

from a few millimeters up to 5 cm. The etiology is not well known; however, a hereditary component is common in up to 50% of cases. Dermatosis papulosa nigra is a subtype of seborrhea found most commonly in older adults of African heritage. They appear on the face as dark papules that are sometimes pedunculated.

Treatment is usually light cautery or curettage. Another option is liquid nitrogen. Appearing most often in the older adult, usually beginning in the early fifties, seborrheic keratoses are benign and are removed for cosmetic purposes.

Acrochordons, or skin tags, are papillomas that are benign. They appear most often in middle-aged and older persons and are commonly found on the neck, axillae, and trunk. Treatment is usually scalpel removal or electrocautery.

Keratoacanthomas appear as nodules that enlarge rapidly. They have a keratin center, and the outline is smooth. Treatment is sometimes not necessary because keratoacanthomas may resolve on their own. They are often confused with squamous cell carcinoma. Although benign, treatment is based on diagnosis of a well-differentiated squamous cell carcinoma. Removal is performed by scalpel, curettage, or cautery.

PREMALIGNANT CONDITIONS

Actinickeratoses appear as raised, rough lesions that range in color from light tan to dark brown, well-defined patches. Mild to moderate erythema may also be present. If the practitioner is doubtful of the assessment, a skin biopsy is appropriate because the lesions may develop into squamous cell carcinoma. The location is the sun-exposed areas of the skin. Thus, treatment and prevention involve avoidance of sun and use of sunscreen with a high sun protection factor (SPF).

Treatment is cryotherapy with liquid nitrogen or curettage; 5-fluorouracil (5-FU) is also used in varying percentages, 1% to 2% for facial lesions and up to 5% for truncal lesions. Initially, erythema and burning occur, leading to ulceration in 2 to 4 weeks. Finally, vesiculation leads to ulceration and reepithelialization. This process takes up to 2 months, and the use of cream is stopped on ulceration.

If no results are seen with 5-FU alone, combination therapy with tretinoin cream is used on more resistant cases.

Bowen's disease is a chronic, scaly, erythematous plaque with well-defined margins. These plaques can occur in mucous membranes or anywhere else on the body. Often the patient's history includes arsenic exposure as a youth. Close monitoring is mandated because multiple lesions are associated with an increased incidence of internal malignancies. Treatment is with liquid nitrogen or curettage and cautery. Radiotherapy has been used; however, full-tumor doses are required.

Malignant Skin Conditions

Malignant skin conditions, for example, basal and squamous cell carcinomas, are common to the geriatric population. Factors such as sunlight, ultraviolet exposure, radiation, and carcinogenic chemicals predispose persons to such conditions (Box 6-1).

BASAL CELL CARCINOMA

Basal cell carcinoma (BCC) develops from the basal layer of the epidermis. It usually has a pearly appearance and is characterized as a firm nodule with rolled edges and an umbilicated center.

It occurs most often in those with freckled, fair, or ruddy skin and is the most common of all cancers, including skin cancer. Occasionally, BCC is confused with malignant melanoma. The warning signs for BCC are as follows:

- A sore that lasts for 3 weeks or more
- An irritated, reddened area that may be itchy or painful
- A smooth growth with an elevated, shiny border
- A pearly or translucent nodule resembling a mole
- A white or yellow lesion that resembles scar tissue

Before treatment for BCC, histologic confirmation is done. The biopsy techniques can be shave, punch, or excisional, depending on tumor size, tissue involvement, and location. Treatment of BCC is dependent on the carcinoma's size, level of invasion, and patient history. Curettage and cauterization are used to treat small tumors. The procedure is usually repeated to ensure complete removal. Cryotherapy is also used as an effective treatment for small tumors. Other treatment methods include

---

| **Box 6-1** |
| *Risk Factors for Skin Cancer* |

Overexposure to frost, wind, and UV radiation from the sun
Occupational exposure to radiation
Chemical carcinogen exposure
Genetic predisposition
Thermal burn scars
Chronic trauma and irritation to an area
X-ray therapy
Skin that is fair, ruddy, freckled, light hair or eyes; skin that burns easily
Precancerous skin lesions
Age over 50 yr
Indoor occupation with blasts of outdoor recreation
History of severe sunburn before age 18 yr

From Mayfield P: Skin. In Hogstel MO, editor: *Clinical manual of gerontological nursing*, St Louis, 1992, Mosby. *UV*, Ultraviolet.

complete excision and Mohs' cryosurgery for recurrent and high-risk BCC. If surgery is not an option, a common circumstance for older patients, radiotherapy is an option. Another alternative is topical 5-FU, which is used only on superficial lesions, especially when they present as numerous tumors. Unfortunately, there is a high recurrence, warranting close follow-up. All BCC patients should be monitored for recurrence or new lesions for 5 years.

SQUAMOUS CELL CARCINOMA

Like BCC, squamous cell carcinoma (SCC) usually develops on sun-damaged skin. It is the second most common skin cancer in white adults. It develops from the squamous epithelium and affects areas of chronic inflammation or chronic ulceration, such as the lower extremities. Venous stasis ulcers, systemic lupus erythematosus, and lupus vulgaris are often associated with SCC lesions. Initially the area affected becomes erythematous and indurated, causing the overlying layer to become hyperkeratotic or scaly, leading to ulceration. Unlike the translucent BCC nodule, SCC lesions present as opaque nodules. The carcinoma may appear as a red nodule with a rough, scaly nodule. Sometimes an ulcerated nodular mass occurs. Risk factors for SCC are a high occurrence of actinic keratoses, which are considered to be a premalignant form of SCC; and exposure to chemicals such as coal, pitch, asphalt, tar, soot, and creosote, all carcinogenic. There is a risk of metastases, depending on the tumor etiology. Lesions found on mucocutaneous junctions are most likely to metastasize.

Like BCC, SCC is treated initially by punch or incisional biopsy methods to confirm the diagnosis. Once it is confirmed, surgical excision involving at least 5 mm beyond the tumor's edges is used. Other methods include cryotherapy for small tumors and radiotherapy for poorly defined tumors.

MELANOMA

Malignant melanoma is a malignant neoplasm of pigmented cells called *melanocytes*. Different types of melanoma nodules exist. The etiology is unclear; however, sun exposure is thought to be a major contributing factor, especially a blistering sunburn before age 18. This trauma is believed to damage Langerhans' cells, affecting the cells' immune response. Malignant melanomas often occur in preexisting moles; a smaller portion of melanomas is seen in new moles. Thus any change in existing moles or the appearance of a new mole, especially after 40 years of age, warrants careful examination (Box 6-2).

Lentigo maligna (Hutchinson's freckle) presents as a pigmented macular lesion, usually less than 1 cm in diameter. It has an irregular border and is found on sun-exposed areas of the skin (face, neck, hands). One lesion may have areas that vary in color: brown, black, red, and white. Over time lentigo maligna enlarges, and pigmentation becomes irregular. About 5% to 7% of melanomas are lentigo maligna. It is referred to as a *freckle* because it occurs in persons over 60 years of age as a tan, flat lesion that gradually changes in size and color.

Box 6-2

Assessment Tool to Identify Moles at Risk of Developing into Malignant Conditions

The ABCD Rule
  A. Asymmetry: One half does not match the other half
  B. Border irregularity: Ragged, notched, or blurred edges
  C. Color: Not uniform in color, with differing shades of color such as brown, black, or a mottling of red, white or blue
  D. Diameter: A diameter greater than 6 mm or an increase in size

Data from McGovern M, Kwaiser-Kuhn J: Skin assessment of the elderly client, *J Gerontol Nurs* 1(4):39-43, 1992.

Treatment of lentigo maligna often involves a wide local incision, including a skin flap or skin graft. As with all melanoma patients, careful and routine follow-up is essential to detect any other areas of suspicion (bleeding moles, pigmentation changes).

Superficial spreading melanoma is the most common type of melanoma, accounting for about 65% to 75% of all melanomas. This melanoma spreads horizontally and peaks in middle age. It occurs on any area of the body and usually presents as a pigmented plaque with varying pigmentation and an irregular border. This type of melanoma is common to other melanomas because it is usually asymptomatic. If bleeding or pruritus is seen, the lesion is likely to be in an advanced stage. Treatment is discussed under nodular melanoma.

Nodular melanoma accounts for 20% of all melanomas. It occurs in a multitude of patients and is found on any body site. Initial manifestation is usually a vertically growing lesion with dark pigmentation. It can be seen as amelanotic (pink), although this is rare.

Treatment for superficial spreading and nodular melanoma involves an excisional or incisional biopsy for histologic interpretation. On diagnosis, referral to an experienced physician is needed for proper management. Further treatment involves excision with 1- to 3-cm margins, depending on the histologic diagnosis. Lymphadenectomy for prophylactic purposes has shown little, if any, benefit. Other treatment options include an isolated limb perfusion with chemotherapy or immunotherapy (interleukins, interferons). Table 6-4 describes the prognosis for melanomas of various depths.

Kaposi's sarcoma occurs as an indolent tumor in older persons of European origin, most often those of Jewish or Italian ancestry. It is also common in patients with acquired immunodeficiency syndrome (AIDS); however, the AIDS-related tumor is the lymphadenopathic form and is associated with a poor prognosis. Appearance is usually a dark blue or purple macula that gradually becomes a nodule or ulcer. On histologic examination, these cells are of endothelial origin, proliferating vessels, and connective tissue. Treatment is usually either simple excision or radiotherapy, if symptomatic. In older patients, this tumor often grows slowly and is benign.

Benign Skin Conditions
PRURITUS

Itching is a common complaint among older persons. A thorough examination for skin lesions should be performed. In addition, systemic disorders involving the liver or kidneys and diagnoses such as leukemia, iron-deficiency anemia, lymphoma, and polycythemia rubra vera may cause severe itching. A review of the drugs the patient takes may reveal side effects of itching. Although underlying conditions are often not the cause of the pruritus, it is important to investigate so that any reversible conditions may be detected and treated appropriately. Another fact to consider is that the dry, scaly skin common to older persons is extremely itchy.

Treatment for the patient who does not have an obvious skin lesion involves screening, such as a complete blood count, erythrocyte sedimentation rate, electrolyte and urea levels, and liver function

TABLE 6-4	Prognosis for Patients with Melanoma

Melanoma Depth	Prognosis
<0.85 mm	Highly curable; 99% of patients disease free at 8 yr
0.85-1.69 mm	Low metastatic risk; 93% of patients disease free at 8 yr
1.7-3.64 mm	Moderate metastatic risk; 67% of patients disease free at 8 yr
>3.65 mm	High metastatic risk; 35% of patients disease free at 8 yr

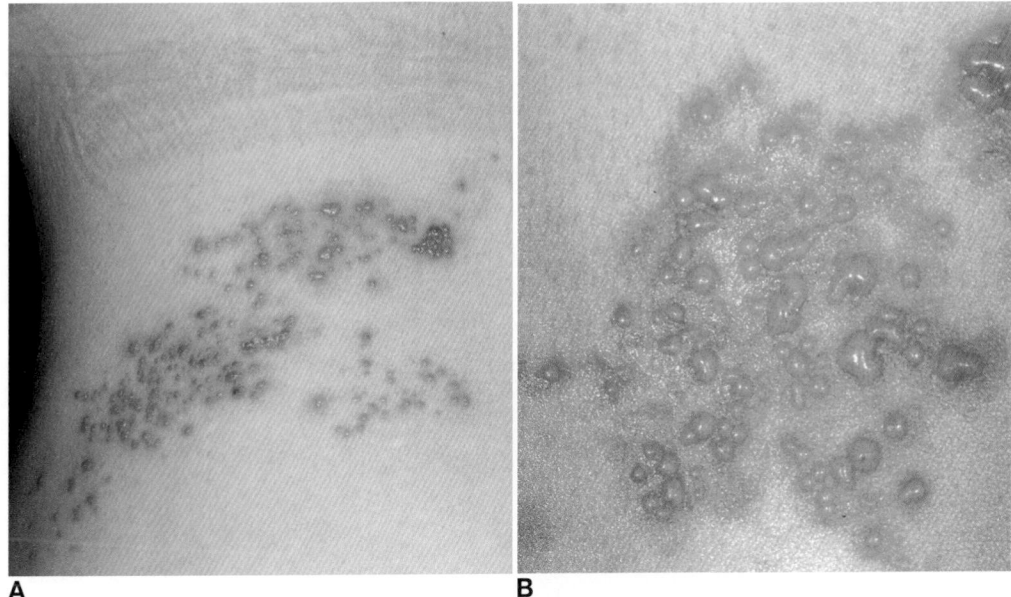

A **B**

Figure 6-1   Herpes zoster. **A,** A common presentation with involvement of a single thoracic dermatome. **B,** A group of vesicles that may vary in size. Vesicles of herpes simplex are a uniform size. (From Habif TP: *Clinical dermatology: a color guide to diagnosis and therapy,* ed 3, St Louis, 1996, Mosby.)

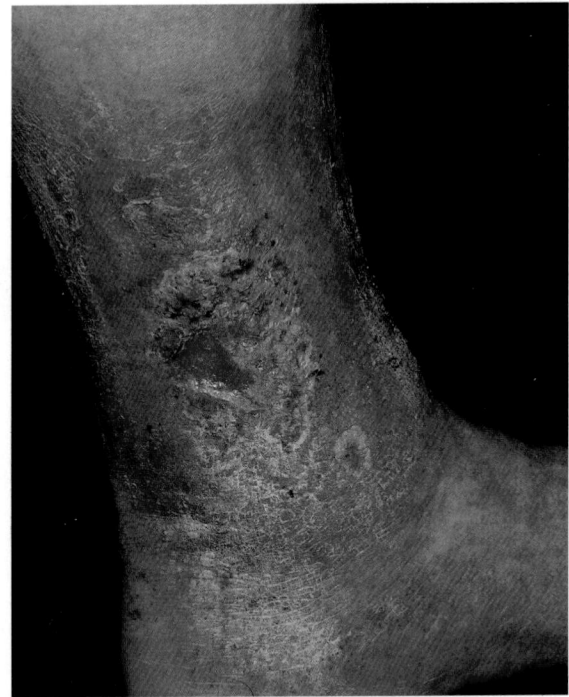

Figure 6-2   Venous stasis ulcer. (From Habif TP: *Clinical dermatology: a color guide to diagnosis and therapy,* ed 3, St Louis, 1996, Mosby.)

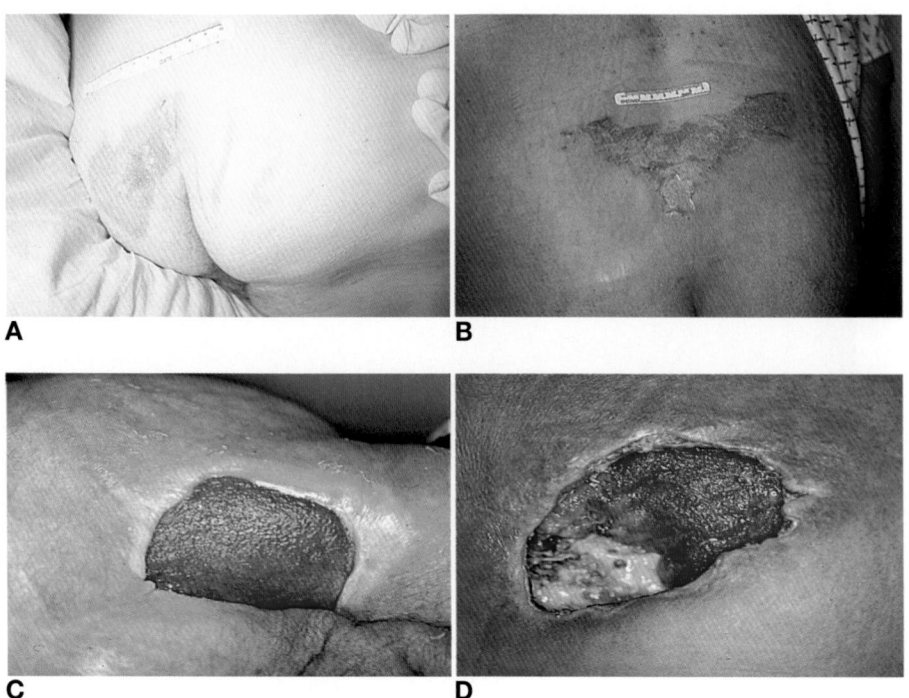

Figure 6-3 **A,** Stage I pressure ulcer. **B,** Stage II pressure ulcer. **C,** Stage III pressure ulcer. **D,** Stage IV pressure ulcer. (Courtesy Laurel Wiersema-Bryant, RN, MSN, Clinical Nurse Specialist, Barnes Hospital, St Louis. In Potter PA, Perry AG: *Basic nursing: a critical thinking approach,* ed 4, St Louis, 1999, Mosby.)

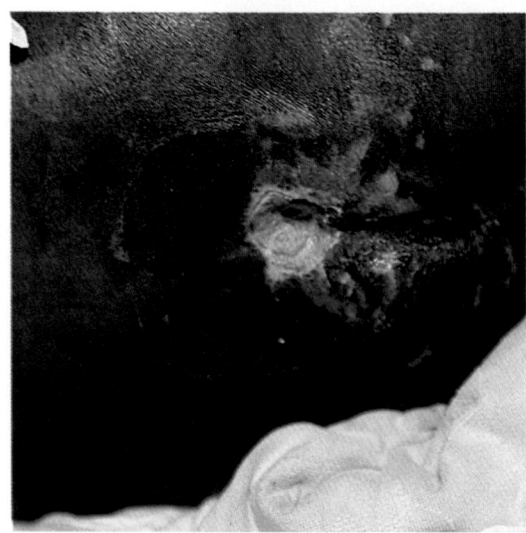

Figure 6-4 Pressure ulcer with tissue necrosis. (From Potter PA, Perry AG: *Basic nursing: a critical thinking approach,* ed 4, St Louis, 1999, Mosby.)

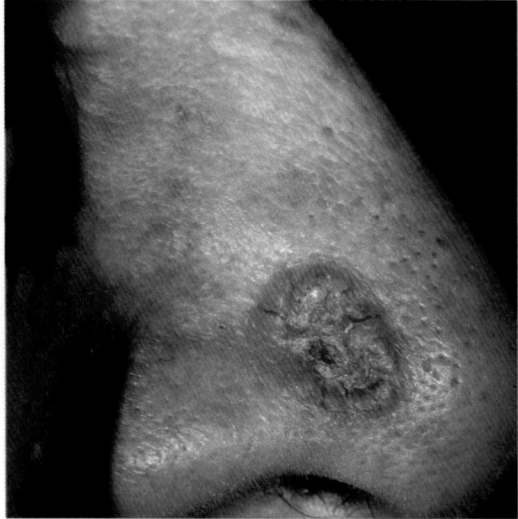

Figure 6-5 Basal cell carcinoma. (From Habif TP: *Clinical dermatology: a color guide to diagnosis and therapy,* ed 3, St Louis, 1996, Mosby.)

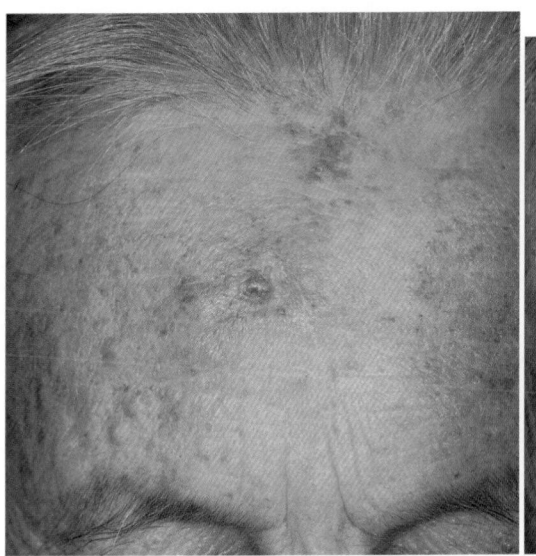

A

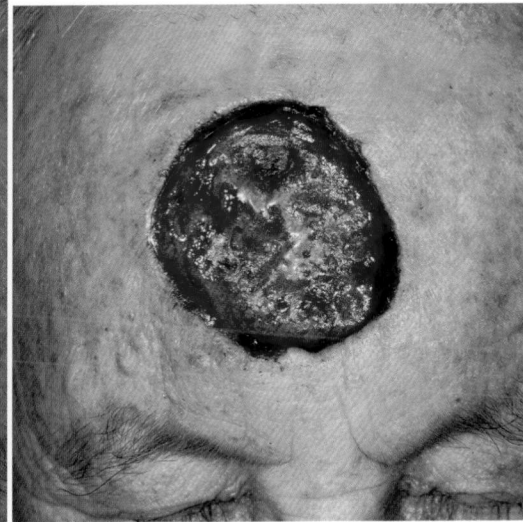

B

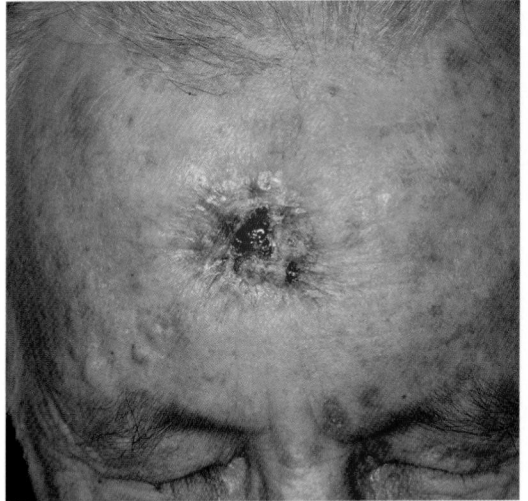

C

Figure 6-6 Basal cell carcinoma before **(A)** immediately after surgery **(B)**, and 6 weeks after surgery using Mohs' micrographic surgical technique **(C)**. (From Habif TP: *Clinical dermatology: a color guide to diagnosis and therapy,* ed 3, St Louis, 1996, Mosby.)

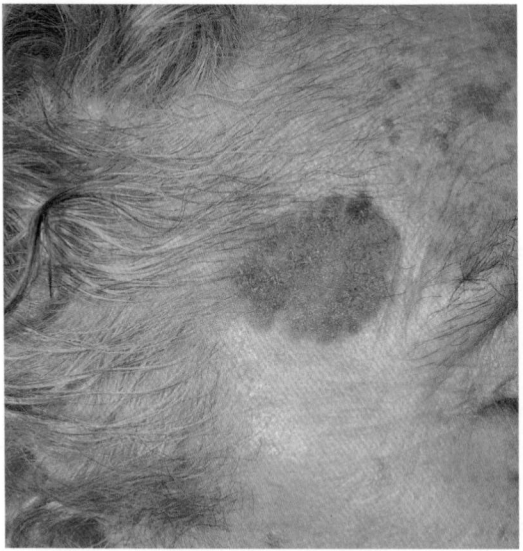

Figure 6-7 Seborrheic keratosis. (From Habif TP: *Clinical dermatology: a color* guide *to diagnosis and therapy,* ed 3, St Louis, 1996, Mosby.)

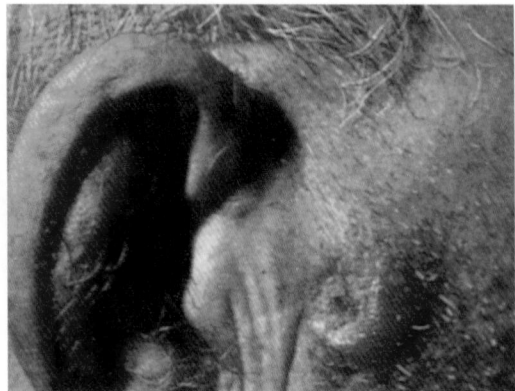

Figure 6-8 Squamous cell carcinoma. (Courtesy Gary Monheit, MD, University of Alabama at Birmingham School of Medicine.)

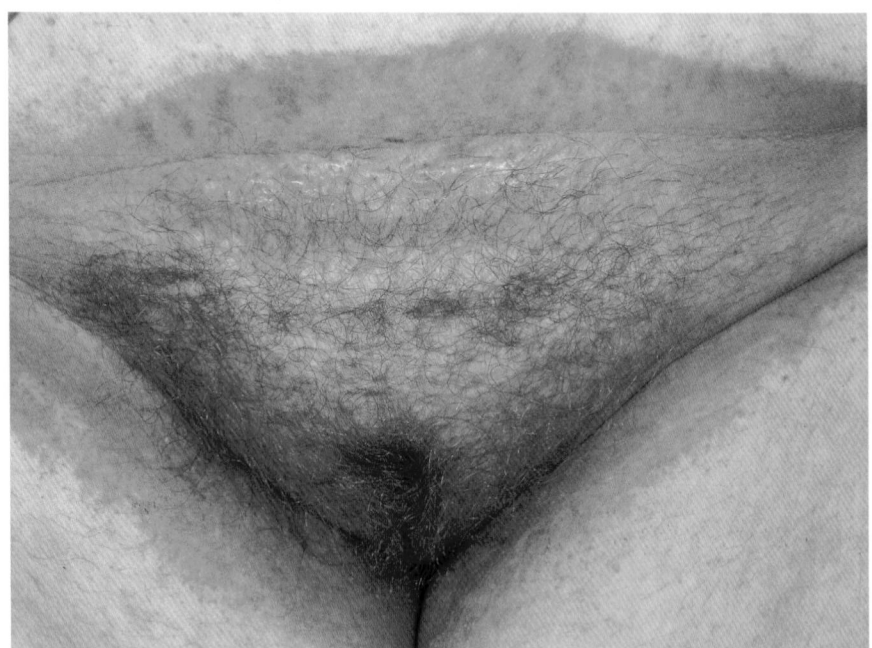

Figure 6-9 Candida intertrigo. (From Habif TP: *Clinical dermatology: a color guide to diagnosis and therapy,* ed 3, St. Louis, 1996, Mosby.)

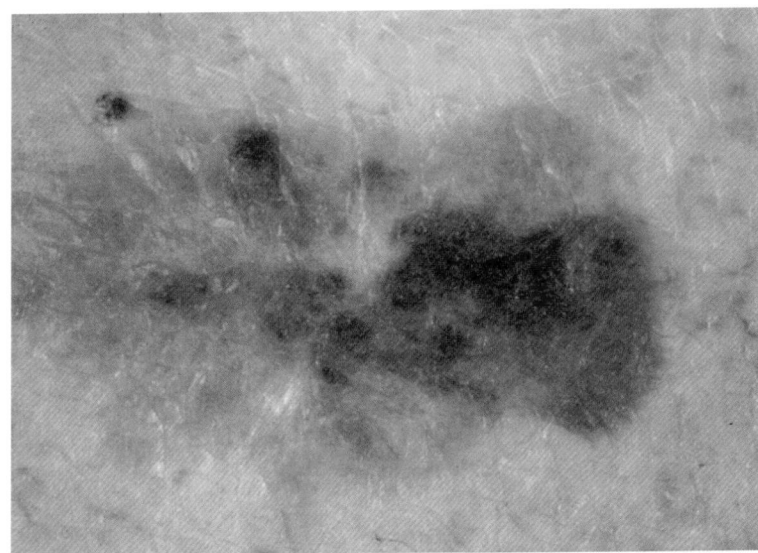

Figure 6-10 Lentigo malignant melanoma. (From Habif TP: *Clinical dermatology: a color guide to diagnosis and therapy,* ed 3, St Louis, 1996, Mosby.)

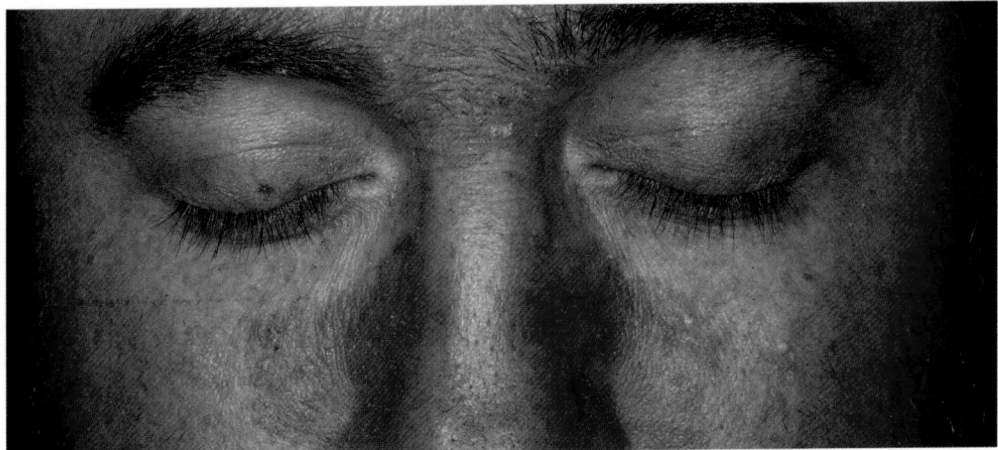

Figure 6-11 Seborrrheic dermatitis. (From Habif TP: *Clinical dermatology: a color guide to diagnosis and therapy,* ed 3, St Louis, 1996, Mosby.)

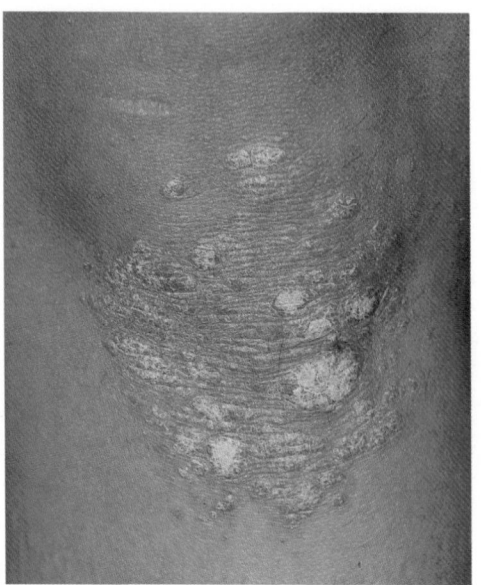

Figure 6-12 Psoriasis. (From Habif TP: *Clinical dermatology: a color guide to diagnosis and therapy,* ed 3, St Louis, 1996, Mosby.)

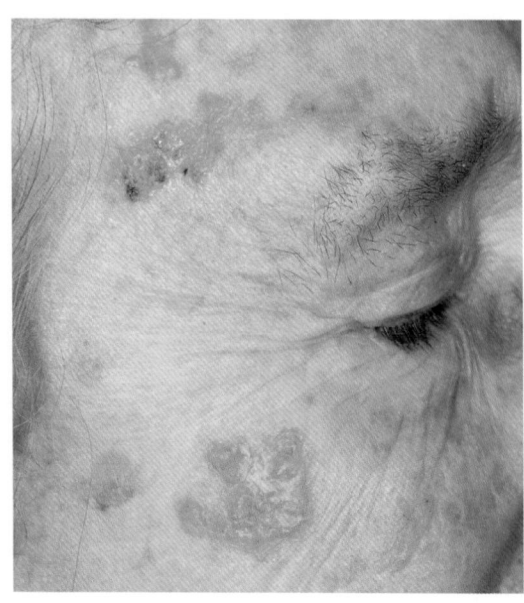

Figure 6-13 Actinic keratosis. (From Habif TP: *Clinical dermatology: a color guide to diagnosis and therapy,* ed 3, St Louis, 1996, Mosby.)

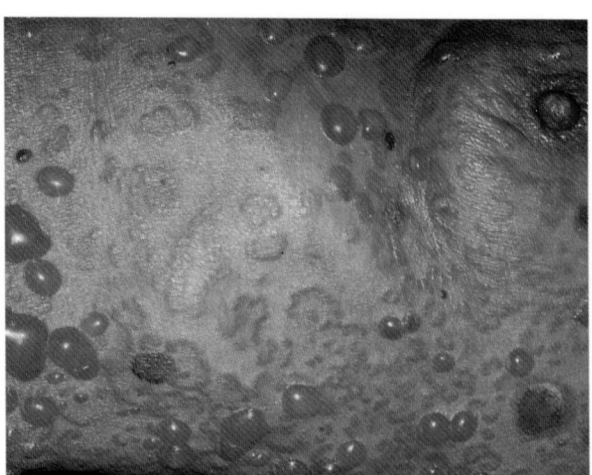

Figure 6-14 Bullous pemphigoid. Generalized eruption with tense blisters arising from an edematous, erythematous annular base. (From Habif TP: *Clinical dermatology: a color guide to diagnosis and therapy,* ed 3, St. Louis, 1996, Mosby.)

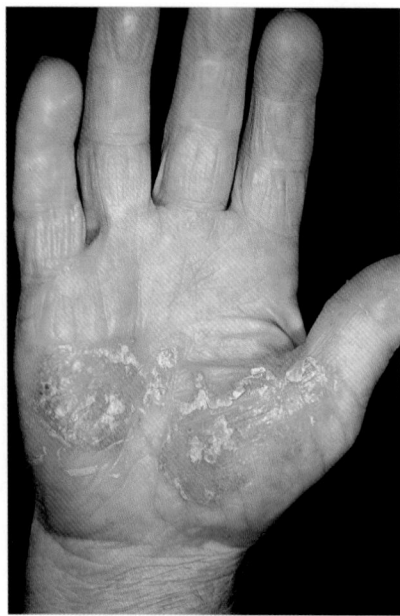

Figure 6-15 Subacute eczematous inflammation. Acute vesicular eczema has evolved into subacute eczema with redness and scaling. (From Habif TP: *Clinical dermatology: a color guide to diagnosis and therapy,* ed 3, St Louis, 1996, Mosby.)

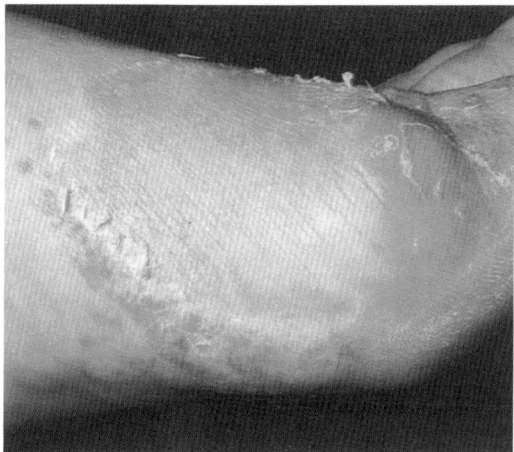

Figure 6-16 Tinea infection. Active border, which contains vesicles that indicate acute inflammation. (From Habif TP: *Clinical dermatology: a color guide to diagnosis and therapy,* ed 3, St Louis, 1996, Mosby.)

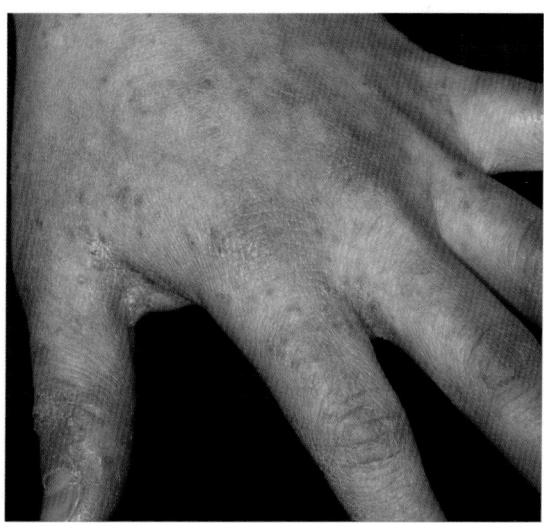

Figure 6-17 Scabies. Tiny vesicles and papules in the finger webs and back of the hand. (From Habif TP: *Clinical dermatology: a color guide to diagnosis and therapy,* ed 3, St Louis, 1996, Mosby.)

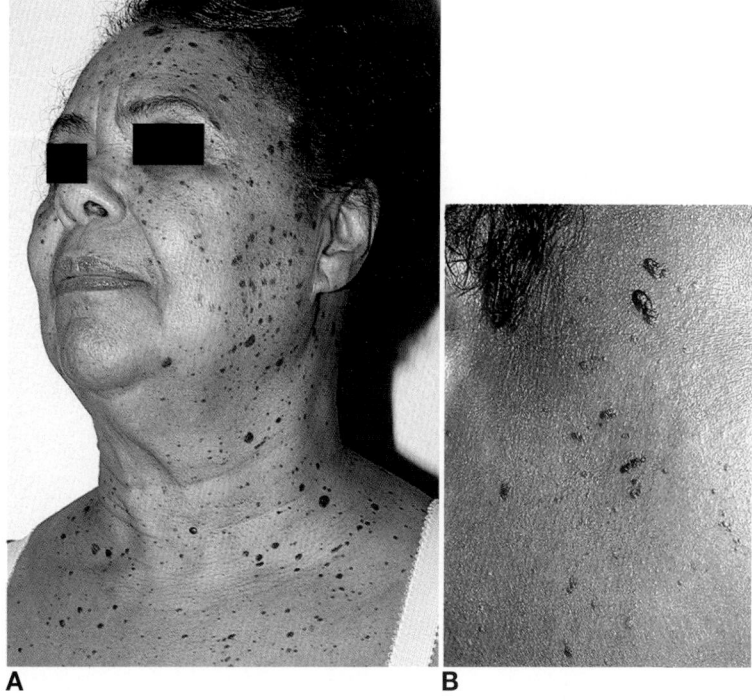

A

B

Figure 6-18 Dermatosis papulosa nigra. (From Johnson BL, Moy RL, White GM: *Ethnic skin: medical and surgical,* St Louis, 1998, Mosby.)

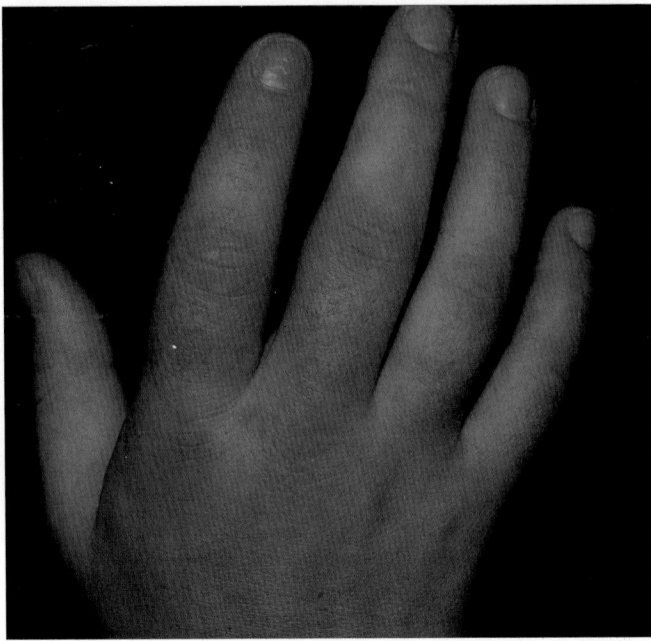

Figure 6-19 Erysipeloid. Approximately 3 days after animal or fish contact, a dull red erythema appears at the inoculation site and extends centrifugally. (From Habif TP: *Clinical dermatology: a color guide to diagnosis and therapy,* ed 3, St Louis, 1996, Mosby.)

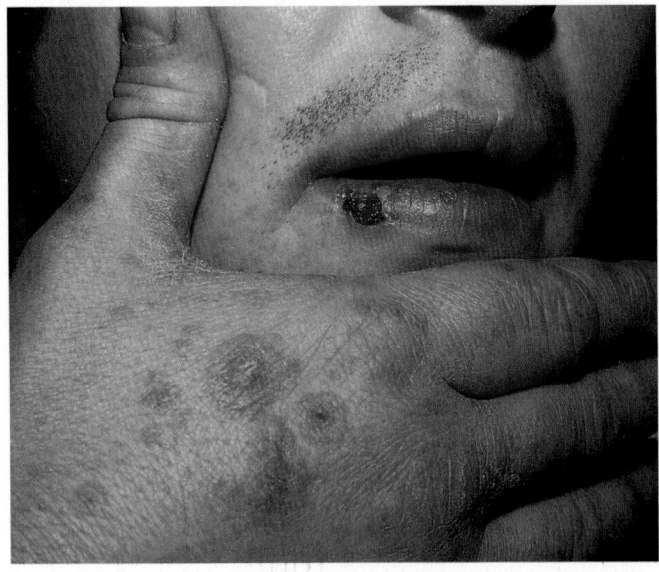

Figure 6-20 Erythema multiforme. An episode may be precipitated by herpes simplex infection. (From Habif TP: *Clinical dermatology: a color guide to diagnosis and therapy,* ed 3, St Louis, 1996, Mosby.)

tests. Tests for the presence of glucose in the urine and, if warranted, guaiac stools, should be performed. If symptoms are unresponsive to treatment, abrupt in onset, and severe, thorough examination and evaluation are necessary.

XEROSIS

Xerosis (dry skin) is the most common geriatric dermatosis and also the most frequent etiology of pruritus (Palmissano and Norman, 2000). Dry skin is most common in the winter months, usually when humidity decreases indoors secondary to heating. Also, exposure to outdoor cold and windy conditions contributes to xerosis. The skin appears scaly, and the areas most involved are the hands, lower legs, and forearms. The process begins when the stratum corneum barrier is compromised by fissure or excoriations that expose this layer to environmental irritants.

Treatment includes home humidification and avoidance of strong soaps, rubbing alcohol, and detergents. Bathing should be kept to a minimum, and mild soap should be used. Avoidance of irritating materials such as wool should also be practiced. Emollients or creams containing lactic acid or urea can be used frequently and liberally, especially following bathing. Petrolatum jelly is an excellent, inexpensive option. If a patient's skin is eczematous, a topical corticosteroid ointment with an occlusive dressing once or twice a day is helpful.

Infectious Diseases

Infections in the skin occur more often as a person ages. Aging produces a slower healing process, compromised circulation, edematous extremities, and the overall decline of the skin's immune function. Thus bacterial infections have a greater tendency to develop. Skin infections can be bacterial, fungal, viral, yeast, or parasitic in origin. It is important to try to establish the causative organism, exclude other cutaneous disorders, and identify precipitating factors (Laube and Farrell, 2002).

BACTERIAL

Staphylococcal Scalded Skin Syndrome

Lyell's syndrome, or staphylococcal scalded skin syndrome (SSSS) is a severe, extensive bullous condition caused by a staphylococcal infection of the skin. The epithelium lifts off in sheets, leaving a large denuded area. It is common in young children and immunocompromised adults. Staphylococci are cultured from the skin or blood. This syndrome often leads to septicemia and ultimately death. A differential diagnosis of toxic epidermal necrolysis (TEN) should also be considered. Both diagnoses are life threatening, and hospitalization is necessary. Differentiation is done by skin biopsy or scraping. The difference is that SSSS presents with cleavage in the epidermis and TEN presents with subepidermal blisters. Patients with SSSS are immediately treated with penicillinase-resistant antistaphylococcal antibiotics. Treatment also includes fluid and electrolyte replacement, topical silver sulfadiazine cream for prevention of cutaneous infection, and systemic antibiotics. Both SSSS and TEN have a poor prognosis. This disorder is further discussed in the section on drug-induced skin reactions.

Erysipelas

Erysipelas is an infection of the skin caused by group A or group C hemolytic streptococci that enter the skin by wounds, insect bites, or minor cuts. Erysipelas presents as an area of erythema and swelling, with lesions having well-defined margins that may spread. In addition to the vesicles or bullae that can be seen in older adults, hemorrhage may occur. Development of malaise, lethargy, and lymphadenopathy is not uncommon. Treatment consists of oral erythromycin, 250 to 500 mg four times a day for 14 days. If erysipelas is seen on the face, treatment with intravenous antibiotics is needed because spreading will continue for the first 24 to 48 hours and sinus involvement is possible.

Cellulitis

Cellulitis, a common occurrence in older adults, is a deep skin infection usually caused by group A streptococci. Gram-negative organisms have been seen. Cellulitis usually manifests as a complication of an open wound or a venous ulcer. It may also appear in intact skin, usually a lower extremity that is edematous; however, sites such as the parotid gland have also become involved. The area appears erythematous, warm, tender, and swollen. Lymph involvement is possible. Treatment with oral erythromycin or penicillin 250 to 500 mg four times a day for 14 days is the treatment of choice. It is important to continue to assess the patient for response to therapy. Cellulitis should be clinically distinguished from erysipelas and necrotizing fasciitis (Laube and Farrell, 2002).

FUNGAL

Older adults commonly have fungal infections of the skin, which may be partially related to the decreased immunologic response of the skin as people age. The word *tinea* refers to a fungal class, dermatophytes, that are present in the dead outer layer of the nail beds or stratum corneum.

Tinea Pedis

Tinea pedis, or athlete's foot, is an infection caused by dermatophytes *Trichophyton mentagrophytes* and *T. rubrum*. It usually begins between the toes and spreads to the toenails and plantar surfaces. Patients often complain of itching and scaly skin. Maceration of the interdigital spaces is common. Because of the potential for cellulitis to develop, careful examination is needed. Diagnosis is done by scrape biopsy and visualizing under a microscope with potassium hydroxide (KOH) solution, which reveals green fungal hyphae.

Treatment is with miconazole or clotrimazole 1% to 2% creams. Several months of application may be needed to prevent recurrence. Nail beds are treated with griseofulvin, which can cause gastrointestinal upset, leukopenia, vertigo, and headaches. Foot care should include full drying of the interdigital spaces, proper footwear, and medicated powder or cotton between the toes for moisture absorption.

Tinea Unguium

This infection is seen on the toenails and occasionally the fingernails and is caused by *T. rubrum* or *T. mentagrophytes*. Nails may appear thickened and enlarged, impeding shoe wearing. Treatment is with griseofulvin 500 to 1000 mg/day for 6 to 9 months for fingernails and 12 to 18 months for toenails. Recurrence is common, especially within the first year. Management such as nail trimming and clipping by podiatry is also recommended.

Tinea Cruris

This cutaneous skin infection of the groin is commonly seen in older persons. At-risk patients are those who are obese, wear nonbreathable clothing, and are immobile. A common complaint is itching, and examination reveals an erythematous scaly area with well-defined margins. Common complications include maceration, lichenification, and secondary bacterial or candidal infections. Diagnosis is confirmed by KOH smear. Treatment two or three times a day with miconazole cream 2% or clotrimazole 1% to the affected area is recommended. Good hygiene to the area and moisture prevention are important.

YEAST

Candidiasis

The definition of candidiasis is an infection caused by yeast. *Candida albicans*, the responsible microorganism, grows in warm, moist areas, usually the groin, axilla, and below the breasts. This infection is common among those receiving antibiotic therapy, the immunocompromised older adult, and patients with diabetes. Sites such as the vagina, mouth, and bowel may carry this organism asymptomatically, creating sources of reinfection. The three types of *Candida* infections follow.

Candidal Vulvovaginitis. This infection presents as a milky vaginal discharge, with examination revealing vulvar erythema and edema. Patients often complain of vaginal itching. It may also be due to the presence of glycosuria, and testing is encouraged.

Oral Candidiasis. Oral candidiasis, or thrush, appears on the tongue as white, creamy plaques. It is often seen in patients after prolonged use of inhaled glucocorticoids. It can be prevented by gargling with water after treatment or using a spacer connected to the inhaler. It is also seen in those with poorly fitting dentures, those with deep skin folds in that area, and those who are saliva and food retainers. For local irritation to the skin, nystatin or miconazole cream three times a day for a week is helpful.

Intertrigo. This infection is caused by yeast and is seen between two skin folds. It is most frequently between the buttocks, the thighs, or the scrotum and the thigh. Intertrigo appears as a moist, reddened rash that may have some flaky, itchy areas at the creases. Itching is a common complaint. It occurs most commonly in persons who do not practice adequate personal hygiene, are obese, or wear tight-fitting clothing that does not provide adequate ventilation.

Treatment for intertrigo is antifungal cream applied to clean dry skin. Nystatin cream does not work effectively against dermatophytes and thus is not useful for treatment. If inflammation is present, a low-dose corticosteroid cream may be used.

VIRAL

Herpes Zoster

Herpes zoster is an acute vesicular eruption caused by an infection of the varicella-zoster virus. Shingles or herpes zoster can occur at any age but is most common in persons 50 to 70 years of age. In older adults postherpetic neuralgia is more common, and the severity and duration are more severe. Pain in the infected area usually precedes the outbreak by 48 hours or longer.

The first sign of herpes zoster is usually a 1- to 4-day period of malaise, fever, headache, and localized pain, burning, itching, or paresthesia. The nerve dysfunction can result in hyperesthesia (increased skin sensitivity), hypoesthesia (diminished sensitivity), dysesthesia (unusual sensations), and allodynia (pain as the result of innocuous stimuli, such as clothing touching the affected skin). This prodromal phase usually precedes the cutaneous eruption. Forty percent of patients have pain more than 4 days before a vesicular rash develops, and 35% have pain fewer than 48 hours before the rash. Rare cases of zoster sine herpes, or acute zoster without the rash, have been documented. The characteristic rash begins as erythematous macules and papules that progress to vesicles within 24 hours, then to pustules (in 3-4 days), and finally to crusts (7-10 days). The lesions erupt over 4 to 7 days and usually are in a unilateral distribution over the area of one or two dermatomes closely grouped together. When crusting of the lesions occurs, the patient is no longer contagious. Lesions resolve during a 2- to 3-week period (Lee and Simpkins, 2000). An underlying lymphoma or immune disease should be suspected if the vesicles spread outside the dermatome area. Herpes zoster may appear in the eyes again because of nerve root involvement affecting the ophthalmic portion of the trigeminal nerve. An ophthalmologic consult is appropriate; conjunctivitis, iridocyclitis, and keratitis may occur. If the nose tip has a lesion, the nasociliary and ophthalmic nerves are involved. Diagnosis is done by cytologic smear with the appearance of multinucleate giant cells.

Acute herpes zoster is a self-limiting condition, and the primary treatment goals are to reduce and manage acute pain, modify the duration of the rash and inflammation, and minimize the development of postherpetic neuralgia. Treatment is with antivirals (acyclovir 800 mg orally five times daily for 7 days or valacyclovir 1 g orally three times daily for 7 days or famciclovir 500 mg orally every 8 hours for 7 days) to accelerate healing and reduce acute pain. Patients with reduced renal function must be monitored closely, and all patients should be advised to maintain good hydration.

Postherpetic neuralgia (PHN) is pain that persists after the rash has resolved. Studies have found that the pain symptoms last about 8 weeks for 45% of patients and less than a year in 78% of cases. In 22% of patients, PHN continued for longer than a year and, in some cases, as long as 20 years. The average age of persons with PHN is 67 (Lee and Simpkins, 2000). The most commonly used drugs for the management of PHN are various tricyclic antidepressants, such as amitriptyline or desipramine, or anticonvulsants such as carbamazepine (Tegretol) and gabapentin (Neurontin). The use of narcotics for chronic neuropathic pain is somewhat controversial because of unclear effectiveness and the risk of dependency. Numerous other interventions are sometimes helpful. Transcutaneous electrical nerve stimulation, regional nerve blocks, cold packs, and acupuncture all have been used successfully in some patients. Because PHN is predominantly a problem for older persons, the choice of therapies often is complicated by coexisting medical conditions, interactions with other medications, and underlying frailty. An individualized approach is important.

PARASITIC

Scabies

Scabies is an eruption caused by a mite, the *Sarcoptes scabiei* var hominis. The female mite deposits eggs beneath the skin, and the eggs hatch into larvae in days. Transmission is skin-to-skin contact, especially among persons living together (families, nursing homes, shelters). It is important to inquire about other household members and animal contact in the history.

The chief complaint is usually unrelenting pruritus, usually at night. The skin is excoriated, and the telltale sign of the burrow mark is from the mite. It appears as a linear ridge, and the mite is usually at one end, where a vesicle is also located. Areas commonly affected include the interdigital webs, umbilicus, wrists (especially the flexor aspect), genitalia, buttocks, and areola. Erythematous nodules or papules in these areas are also common. Among older person scabies is sometimes confused with eczema or exfoliative dermatitis because of the presence of crusted lesions. Evaluation for erythroderma or a generalized lymphadenopathy should be done, especially if scabies goes undetected for a prolonged period.

Examination of the mite under a microscope is possible by removing the mite with a scalpel. Locating one is often difficult, however, especially if the area is widespread. Presumptive diagnosis is often the best option.

Treatment with permethrin 5% cream is the first-line choice. Lindane (Kwell) was formerly the choice for treatment; however, resistance and neurotoxicity have downgraded it to an alternative treatment. It is important to apply the cream to the entire body, from the neck down. Thorough application is important, and assistance is recommended. This treatment kills the mite and ova, but the burrow and its sensitization remain until the skin naturally sheds. Reapplication 1 to 2 weeks apart may be needed. Treatment of all household members is recommended. Prevention of reinfestation by washing bed linens and underwear in hot water is usually effective.

Pediculosis (Lice)

Lice affect different areas: the body, the head, or the genitals. The problem is caused by different organisms. It is often seen among older persons who practice poor hygiene or live in an overcrowded environment. Grandparents of school-aged grandchildren may also be affected by outbreaks in schools. Lice are wingless, dorsoventrally flattened, blood-sucking insects.

Pediculosis capitis, or head lice, can be transmitted by hairbrushes, hair accessories, and close contact. Scalp itching is seen usually in conjunction with secondary eczematous and impetiginization. Small, gray-white ova (nits) are present on examination. The occipital portion of the scalp and sometimes the postauricular area are affected.

Pediculosis corporis (body lice) are responsible for generalized itching. Bacterial infections, eczematous changes, and excoriated areas are often a consequence of body lice. The seams of the patient's clothing should be inspected for nits.

Pediculosis pubis is caused by the crab louse and is sexually transmitted. Transmission by towels or clothing is possible but unlikely. Inspection of the pubic hair is necessary; however, the eyelashes, leg hairs, axillae, and chest hairs may also be involved.

Treatment for head lice is a permethrin 1% cream rinse applied to the hair, left on for 10 minutes, and rinsed. Lindane shampoo is effective, but its neurotoxicity has called for stricter guidelines for use by pregnant women and younger populations. Treatment, like that for scabies, involves all household members and washing all bed linens, hair utensils, and accessories in warm water.

Body lice are treated by dry cleaning the patient's clothing or washing them in hot water. Using a hot iron on clothing seams will kill any nits. Use of a medicated powder with malathion 1% on the clothing may help. Malathion lotion 0.5% may also be effective, but it does have an unpleasant odor. If eyelashes are involved, treatment with petrolatum jelly will suffocate any lice. Physostigmine ophthalmic ointment 0.25% to lashes four times a day for 3 days also helps.

Pubic lice are treated like head lice, and any sexual partners should also be treated. Patient and family education is important, especially for preventive measures.

Dermatitis

Also referred to as eczema or eczematous dermatitis, atopic dermatitis and contact dermatitis are superficial inflammations of the skin secondary to allergen exposure, irritant exposure, or a genetic predisposition. The patient presents with pruritus, edema, and erythema. If vesiculation, oozing, or crusting is present, the process has been longstanding.

Atopic dermatitis is thought to have a genetic component as an important factor. Many patients also have family members with asthma, hay fever, or atopic dermatitis. Contributing factors include stressful events; extremes in temperature or humidity; and allergies to cosmetics, rubber, and *Rhus* plant (e.g., poison ivy, oak). Age is not a diagnosing factor; however, in older adults, it may be more severe and generalized than in younger persons. It manifests with extreme itching, lichenification, and eczematous changes. The neck, wrists, postauricular area, and popliteal and antecubital areas are often involved. Patch testing is sometimes done to identify the precipitating irritant. A variant, termed *nummular dermatitis* or *discoid eczema,* manifests as itchy, scaly, coin-shaped lesions, usually on the posterior trunk, buttocks, and limbs. The lesions may become purulent after oozing and crusting. The precipitating cause is unknown.

Contact Dermatitis

Contact dermatitis can be a challenging diagnosis to make. The area may be chronically irritated (dishpan hands) and appear vesiculated or pustular. In older persons a common diagnosis is dermatitis of unknown origin. Complaints of pruritus, excoriation, and dry scaling skin are common. The location of the affected area may lead to the responsible irritant. Contact dermatitis results when an irritant penetrates and disrupts the stratum corneum, causing an inflammatory reaction within the underlying epidermis. Common irritants include acids, detergents, and solvents. Lichen simplex chronicus or neurodermatitis is a possible diagnosis. This is a localized pruritic area characterized by extreme itching. The area appears well circumscribed or lichenified, with scaling and papulation. It is common in older persons, especially women. The usual sites include the occipital area, wrists, thighs, and lower limbs. Improvement is seen when the itching ceases.

Management is multifaceted. Elimination of all irritants is vital. If the lesion is wet, dry it; if it is dry, hydrate it; and if it is inflamed, apply corticosteroid cream. Drying can be accomplished with Burow's solution compresses. For chronic cases, patients must avoid drying detergents, frequent showers, and irritants. Use of topical steroids of moderate to strong potency may control symptoms. Use of an Unna's boot, especially on affected limbs, is helpful in breaking the itch-scratch cycle.

Stasis dermatitis is inflammation secondary to venous hypertension, usually in the lower limbs. Edema, venous stasis skin changes, and dilation of superficial venules around the ankles are seen. It is affected by edema, contact dermatitis secondary to medicated preparations such as neomycin, and scratching. The etiology is unknown. Management that includes controlling the edema with elastic stockings, elevation, and hydrocortisone 1% may alleviate some symptoms.

Seborrheic Dermatitis

Seborrheic dermatitis is an inflammatory benign disease with an unknown cause. A relationship to the yeast *Pityrosporum ovale* has not been confirmed. It is common in the adult population and difficult to cure because of its chronic and recurrent nature. It appears as scaly, erythematous patches that are slightly papular. It is often asymptomatic, but itching may occur. The scalp is often involved, and dandruff must be ruled out as a possibility. Other areas commonly affected include the postauricular and beard areas, nasolabial folds, eyelids, and eyebrows. Blepharitis or conjunctivitis may occur with eyelid involvement. It is associated with Parkinson's disease, phenylketonuria, zinc deficiency, and epilepsy.

Treatment consists of applying ketoconazole (Nizoral) cream topically to the affected areas. It is also available in a shampoo. For milder cases, daily use of a dandruff shampoo with 1% selenium or 2% pyrithione zinc may be effective, with weekly use of Nizoral shampoo. Maintenance therapy may be needed once or twice a week indefinitely. This treatment often becomes costly, and for maintenance use of an OTC dandruff shampoo is adequate. For the erythema, a topical steroid may be used; however, a spray or gel may be best for hairy areas. Eyelid involvement is treated with baby shampoo applied to the affected area with a cotton swab. Patient education includes reassurance that it is not contagious; however, the chronicity of this disease must be stressed.

Exfoliative Dermatitis

Exfoliative dermatitis or erythroderma is a generalized, severe dermatitis, most often the result of eczema, psoriasis, a drug reaction, or an undetected malignancy. Erythroderma occurs quickly and has a thick, scaly appearance. The exfoliation process creates cutaneous heat loss, which may lead to rigors. In addition, the patient should be examined for lymphadenopathy. Shedding of hair and nails is seen in extreme cases.

The treatment depends on the severity of the disease. Hospital admittance is necessary for severe cases because of the extensive heat, fluid, and protein loss. Topical use of an emollient cream is recommended. Prednisone (40-60 mg a day) is used when it is first diagnosed and then gradually tapered.

Scaling Diseases
PSORIASIS

Psoriasis is a skin disorder that manifests with shiny, silver-tinted, scaly plaques. A family history is usually positive because it is transmitted genetically. Also, the health care professional should inquire about use of beta-blockers, which are known to exacerbate psoriasis. Psoriasis is seen usually in the third and eighth decades of life and more commonly in whites than in African Americans. Psoriasis may appear throughout the body but is most commonly seen on bony areas (knees, elbows, scalp, buttocks). It may also affect the palms, soles, and nails; nail pitting is a common nail abnormality in chronic cases.

In the older adult the signs of psoriatic arthritis are fusiform swelling and tenderness of the distal interphalangeal joint. The rheumatoid factor is negative, although other forms of arthritis may develop. Other sequelae include exfoliative dermatitis and pustular psoriasis.

Treatment includes assessment of the patient's mobility and ability to comply with instructions. Coal tar ointments work well, but they stain, have a distinct odor, and are difficult to work with because of their gluelike texture. Anthralin is a cream or paste that is used on thick, scaly plaques. It comes in varying strengths (0.1%-1%) and is applied to the plaque for a limited time (20 minutes to overnight), depending on strength. In conjunction with these methods, corticosteroids are effective, especially under an occlusive dressing. If plaques appear on the skin, a tar-based shampoo can be used. For more resistant, widespread cases, phototherapy is effective, as is natural sunlight with proper precautions. Other alternatives include photochemotherapy, which involves a photoactive drug (methoxsalen). Finally, methotrexate is helpful in pustular and exfoliative psoriasis. Low doses of 2.5 to 5 mg a week are common doses for older adults. Dermatology evaluation is recommended, as is monitoring of hepatic and renal function for agents such as methotrexate.

Bullous Disorders
BULLOUS PEMPHIGOID

Bullous pemphigoid presents as a localized or generalized bullous eruption. It appears often in the older adult on either normal or erythematous skin. About half of the cases have involvement of the mucous membranes. It is a chronic condition that affects men and women equally. On histologic examination, subepidermal bullae are seen with complement (C3) present after immunofluorescent staining and immunoglobulin G on the dermal-epidermal border. If the disease is active, the bullous pemphigoid antigen may be present in some patients.

Treatment for bullous pemphigoid differs, depending on its presentation. For a mild, localized infection, treatment is high-dose topical corticosteroids. More generalized cases may require hospitalization and systemic administration of prednisone. Older patients should be closely monitored for complications such as upper gastrointestinal bleeding, fluid retention, hypertension, and confusion. Tapering of the steroid therapy begins once the lesions have resolved. It may take several months of systemic therapy for patients to achieve total remission.

PEMPHIGUS VULGARIS

This disorder is uncommon and occurs most often in middle age; however, many patients are 60 years of age or older. Pemphigus vulgaris presents as intraepidermal bullae on the skin or mucous membranes. The bullae easily rupture and can lead to erosions on the abdomen, extremities, and mucous membranes. A common complaint is a painful mouth lesion, which is common in the early stages of the disease. If the disease progresses, widespread blistering and the risk of sepsis and secondary infection may occur. The diagnosis may be difficult to make and confused with bullous pemphigoid, benign mucous membrane pemphigoid, TEN, a drug-induced reaction, or erythema multiforme.

Hospitalization is necessary if it is widespread, and prednisone is used to control the disease. For milder cases prednisone is used and close follow-up is warranted in the older patient. Once the skin lesions have cleared, the prednisone is tapered, and topical or intralesional corticosteroid therapy is used on resistant lesions. Management is similar to bullous pemphigoid, and close monitoring of the elderly patient for steroid complications is again stressed.

Drug-Induced Eruptions

Severe skin adverse drug reactions can result in death. TEN has the highest mortality (30%-35%) (Ghislain and Roujeau, 2002). Older persons are at higher risk for suffering the annoying and hazardous skin reactions that are associated with drug therapy. If a serious reaction occurs, older persons are also at higher risk for major morbidity and mortality compared with younger individuals (Sullivan and Shear, 2002). Drug-induced eruptions usually present as a pruritic, symmetric, maculopapular rash, 1 to 10 days after initiation of a new medication. The rash may last up to 14 days after the drug is stopped. The most common culprits are penicillins, sulfonamides, gold, phenylbutazone, and gentamicin. OTC and new hygiene products may also cause a reaction. Treatment precautions include a careful review of all medications (prescribed, OTC, herbal remedies), a detailed history of possible environmental factors, and any medication changes.

ERYTHEMA MULTIFORME

Erythema multiforme presents as symmetric, edematous, erythematous lesions of the skin or mucous membranes. It is an inflammatory eruption, and the lesions may have a bullous appearance. Its cause is believed to be hypersensitivity reaction to a drug or infection, commonly herpes simplex. Disease severity varies from lesions with a red circumference and a cyanotic middle to clusters on the extremities to widespread erosion with bullae on the mucous membranes (Stevens-Johnson syndrome). Corneal ulceration may occur in severe cases.

Treatment involves removal of all susceptible agents. If the disease is severe, hospitalization is needed. Localized areas are treated symptomatically, and the use of systemic corticosteroids is debatable and not routine.

TOXIC EPIDERMAL NECROLYSIS

Toxic epidermal necrolysis is a severe condition that presents with lethargy, general malaise, skin erythema, and tenderness, which quickly progress to blistering and erosion of the skin. The classic sign of this disease is the shearing off of the overlying epidermis when force is applied laterally, which is termed Nikolsky's sign. This disorder is life threatening and has a high mortality rate.

The pathophysiology of TEN is not clear. Currently three theories exist: an inappropriate immune response that is cell-mediated by the T lymphocytes, an antigen-antibody response to the causative drug, and a genetic predisposition to drug sensitivity (Pirrung, 2001).

Some researchers suggest that the cell-mediated immune response is based on the abnormal metabolism of the causative drug. The metabolites are thought to resemble a hapten, which is a small organic molecule that attaches to a body protein and becomes antigenic. Once introduced into the body it creates a toxin and can produce an inappropriate immune response. Histologic analysis shows necrotic keratinocytes at the epidermal-dermal junction but rarely in the dermal layer. CD8 T cells and antigen-primed cytotoxic T cells are seen commonly in the blister fluid (Pirrung, 2001).

It is not clear how or why medications would cause this type of reaction; however, many different drugs have been found to cause TEN. The most offensive drugs have been sulfonamides, nonsteroidal antiinflammatory drugs, anticonvulsants, allopurinol, and barbiturates. Research shows that when TEN is from a drug reaction it is not related to dose. Other causes of TEN include infections, malignancies, and graft-versus-host reactions. The pathophysiology of malignancies and graft-versus-host reactions is difficult to pinpoint. The many complicating factors include the primary underlying disease, prior chemotherapy, radiation toxicity, and delayed hypersensitivity reactions and infections, which make the diagnosis of TEN difficult (Pirrung, 2001).

Treatment for TEN includes hospitalization on a burn unit and use of a biologic dressing. An ophthalmologist is recommended for management of eye care.

Primary and Secondary Skin Lesions

Skin lesions are divided into primary and secondary lesions, although some experts would include a third special category. The classification is flexible, with overlap, and should serve only as a guide.

PRIMARY (ELEMENTARY) LESIONS

A primary lesion is the first grossly recognizable or most characteristic structural change of skin disease.
- Flat lesions
  Macule: Flat, circumscribed change in color, ordinarily less than 2 cm in diameter
    Hypopigmentation
    Hyperpigmentation
    Transient or permanent (telangiectasia) vascular dilation
  Patch: Larger flat, circumscribed color change
- Solid lesions
  Papule: Circumscribed elevation no more than 1 cm in diameter
  Nodule: Circumscribed larger (> 1 cm) and deeper elevation
  Tumor: Circumscribed elevation larger and deeper than a nodule; also refers to neoplastic elevations of any size

Plaque: Elevation greater than 1 cm with relatively large surface area compared with height (often confluent papules)
- Wheal (hive): Distinctive elevation, usually white to pink, due to localized transient tissue edema
- Fluid-filled lesions (blisters)
Vesicle: Sharply circumscribed collection of free fluid no more than 0.5 cm in diameter
Bulla: Large vesicle (> 0.5 cm)
- Pus-filled lesions
Pustule: Circumscribed elevation containing free pus
   Folliculitis: Pustule of a hair follicle
Abscess: Localized deeper and larger accumulation of pus
   Furuncle: Abscess of hair follicle
   Carbuncle: Coalescent furuncles
- Purpura: Discoloration of skin or mucous membrane due to intracutaneous or subcutaneous bleeding
Petechia: Purpura less than 3 mm in diameter
Ecchymosis (bruise): Large area of purpura (borders indistinct)
Hematoma: Large area of purpura producing swelling
- Comedo (pl. comedones): Sebum and keratin that occlude pilosebaceous ostium
Open comedo: "Blackhead," darkened sebum and keratin that shows at pilosebaceous ostium
Closed comedo: "Whitehead," undarkened sebum and keratin in pilosebaceous apparatus that does not show at narrow ostium
- Burrow: Tunnel or channel in stratum corneum of variable size and shape containing a parasite, such as scabies, creeping eruption

SECONDARY LESIONS

Secondary lesions evolve from primary lesions, either naturally or from adventitious events such as scratching, secondary infection, and treatment:
- Pus-filled lesions
Pustule: Circumscribed elevation containing free pus
Abscess: Localized deeper and larger accumulation of pus
- Crust (scab): Dried exudate (blood, serum, pus)
- Scale: Accumulation of loose, horny fragments of stratum corneum
- Scar (cicatrix): Permanent fibrotic skin change following damage to dermis
- Localized loss of substance from surface downward
Erosion: Superficial denudation of part or all of epidermis
Excoriation: Superficial loss of skin (often linear or punctate) because of scratching or picking
Fissure: Linear cleavage in the skin
Ulcer: Localized loss of substance extending into dermis and sometimes subcutaneous tissue
- Atrophy: Loss of or lack of full development of tissue
Epidermal: Thin, translucent epidermis with fine wrinkling (cigarette paper); may actually reflect histologic changes in papillary dermis
Dermal: Depression of the skin without changes in color or surface markings
- Maceration: Changes secondary to prolonged wetting of skin
- Lichenification: A lichen-like thickening of the skin, with accentuation of skin markings resulting from chronic rubbing

Summary

Many older people view skin problems as a normal part of the aging process. They often hesitate to mention skin problems to their health care provider. It is important for the provider to ask the older person about changes in pigmentation or any skin problems so that assessments can be made and any necessary treatment can take place.

Resources

American Society for Dermatologic Surgery
www.asds-net.org/scfactsheet.html

Dermatology Journals and Publications
tray.dermatology.uiowa.edu

Skin Cancer Zone
www.melanoma.com

References

Elias PM, Ghadially R: The aged epidermal permeability barrier: basis for functional abnormalities, *Clin Geriatr Med* 18(1):103-120, 2002.

Ghislain PD, Roujeau JC: Treatment of severe drug reactions: Stevens-Johnson syndrome, toxic epidermal necrolysis and hypersensitivity syndrome, *Dermatol Online* J 8(1):5, 2002.

Jackson R: Elderly and sun-affected skin: distinguishing between changes caused by aging and changes caused by habitual exposure to sun, *Can Fam Physician* 47:1236-1243, 2001.

Laube S, Farrell AM: Bacterial skin infections in the elderly: diagnosis and treatment, *Drugs Aging* 19(5):331-342, 2002.

LeeVK, Simpkins L: Herpes zoster and postherpetic neuralgia in the elderly, *Geriatr Nurs* 21(3):132-136, 2000.

Palimissano C, Norman R: Geriatric dermatology in chronic care and rehabilitation, *Dermatol Nurs* 12(2):116-123, 2000.

Pirrung MK: Management of toxic epidermal necrolysis, *J Intravenous Nursing* 24(2):107-112, 2001.

Presland RB, Jurevic RJ: Making sense of the epithelial barrier: what molecular biology and genetics tell us about the functions of oral mucosal and epidermal tissues, *J Dent Educ* 66(4):564-574, 2002.

Sullivan JR, Shear NH: Drug eruptions and other adverse drug effects in aged skin, *Clin Geriatr Med* 18(1):21-42, 2002.

7

Pressure Ulcers

Pressure ulcers are a serious and common problem for older persons; they affect about one million adults in the United States (Cobbs, Duthie, and Murphy, 2002). Each pressure ulcer can cost as much as $15,000 in health care costs and can add more than 16 days to a hospital stay. Estimated annual cost reached $1.5 billion in the United States. More alarming is the rise of mortality rates associated with pressure ulcers. In addition, pressure ulcers have evolved to the status of being a synonym for neglect or abuse, especially in the nursing home setting (Meehan and Hill, 2002). Recently, government agencies have become much more aggressive in citing institutions for the development of pressure ulcers in their patients. A few government institutions have concluded that in some cases the development of ulcers with resultant death is so grievous that there should be criminal prosecution of the persons or institutions providing care. A leader in this concept has been the state of Hawaii. In November 2000 the state of Hawaii convicted a person of manslaughter in the death of a patient at an adult residential care home for permitting the progression of pressure ulcers without seeking medical help and for not bringing the patient back to a physician for treatment of the ulcers (Di Maio and Di Maio, 2002). With scrutiny from survey agencies (Centers for Medicare and Medicaid Services and state agencies) and potential litigation increasing, health care (especially long-term care), facilities must implement aggressive pressure ulcer prevention programs (Lyder et al, 2002). There is, however, ongoing discussion regarding whether pressure ulcers are always preventable, and there is a call for further definition of the role of regulations and litigation regarding this matter (Brandeis, Berlowitz, and Katz, 2001). Unfortunately, there is no easy answer to the prevention of pressure injury and ulcers.

Pressure ulcers, the result of ischemic damage and subsequent necrosis affecting the skin, subcutaneous tissue, and often muscle, are caused primarily by intense pressure exerted for a short time or pressure exerted for a longer time.

When tissues are compressed, usually over a bony prominence, the average pressure of the vascular bed may be exceeded. The blood supply to the affected area and its lymphatic drainage is then reduced. The normal capillary blood pressure at the arteriole end of vascular bed averages 32 mm Hg. When sitting, compared with lying down, only a small surface area of the body is providing support, predominantly the buttocks, thighs, and feet. Therefore interface pressures are much greater in a sitting than in a lying position (Collins, 2002). At times, in a sitting position, pressures greater than 300 mm Hg can be measured at the ischial tuberosities, a common site for skin breakdown in persons who sit for long periods or who are confined to a wheelchair.

The most common sites for pressure ulcers are the sacrum, greater trochanters, ischium, medial and lateral condyles, malleoli, and heels. Less common sites are the elbows, scapulae, vertebrae, ribs, ears, and the back of the head.

Age-related Changes

Normal age-related changes that increase an older person's risk for pressure ulcers include the following:

- Thinning and flattening of the epidermis, which increases skin permeability and reduces the effectiveness of barrier functions
- Decreases in cell replacement to less than half that of a young adult
- Decreases in vascularity and elasticity
- Decreases in subcutaneous tissue, particularly over joints and bony prominences
- Decreases in sebaceous and sweat gland activity
- Decrease in local blood supply (Cobbs, Duthie, and Murphy, 2002)

Assessment and Prevention of Risk

Two validated assessment tools are available for identifying patients at risk for developing pressure ulcers: the Braden Scale and the Norton Scale. These tools allow the clinician to evaluate accurately the potential risk of pressure ulcer development and then take appropriate steps to decrease the risks. The risk factors contained in these scales are measures of physical and mental condition, nutrition, mobility, and continence. Patients with scores of 16 or less on the Braden Scale and 14 or less on the Norton Scale are considered to be at high risk (Tables 7-1 and 7-2).

NUTRITIONAL ASSESSMENT

An association has been observed between pressure ulcers and malnutrition, and several studies have identified malnutrition as a risk factor for pressure ulcer formation (Cobbs, Duthie, and Murphy, 2002). Low levels of protein, hemoglobin, and total lymphocyte count (TLC) contribute to skin breakdown and prevent healing. A nutritional assessment should include height, weight, biochemical data, dietary habits, and preferences. Patients who are not properly nourished are at high risk for skin breakdown, and wounds that occur are extremely difficult to heal.

LABORATORY TESTS

A serum albumin measurement of 3.3 g/dl or less is associated with protein malnourishment and increased morbidity and mortality. Hypoproteinemia leads to edema because of changes in osmotic pressures, which in turn decreases oxygenation of tissue and creates an environment for tissue breakdown. Adequate protein is necessary for healing.

Levels of hemoglobin below 11.1 g/dl increase the risk for the development of pressure ulcers and greatly increase the healing time of existing ulcers. A TLC of 800 or lower is considered severe malnutrition. Levels from 800 to 1200 suggest moderate malnutrition. TLC can be calculated by multiplying the percent of lymphocytes by the total white blood count and dividing by 100. Nursing home patients with serum cholesterol levels below 120 to 150 mg/ml demonstrate a higher mortality rate. There is strong evidence that low levels in any or all of these areas are predictive of increased risk for pressure ulcer development and decreased healing ability. The cost of obtaining these laboratory values should be taken into consideration when using these tools in an assessment.

HYDRATION ASSESSMENT

Hydration is an important factor in the prevention and healing of pressure ulcers. The skin of an older person often appears to hang loosely on bony frames as a result of the loss of elasticity, underlying adipose tissue, and years of gravitational pull. Tenting is often the result when testing for skin turgor; thus turgor may not be a reliable or valid estimate of the hydration status of an older patient. The most reliable assessment of hydration is blood urea nitrogen and creatinine studies.

Prevention

The best line of treatment for at-risk patients is the prevention of pressure to body surfaces that could result in ulceration. Prevention intervention options include the following:
- Support surfaces: pressure-relief or pressure-reduction surfaces
- A turning and positioning schedule
- Protective films or real sheepskins
- Maintenance of range of motion and ambulation
- Maintenance of clean and appropriately dry skin
- Maintenance of good nutrition

SUPPORT SURFACES

Pillows and rubber rings (donuts) should not be used because they cause compression and decrease further blood supply to the area. Two types of support surfaces can be used: pressure-relief surfaces and pressure-reduction surfaces. Pressure-relief surfaces are the various mattresses designed to reduce interface pressures below 25 mm Hg (i.e., below capillary closure). Pressure-reduction surfaces are less expensive and are designed to lower pressure but not below the 25 to 35 mm Hg threshold. These devices include alternating pressure pads, foam, and gel pads. It is important to remember that pressure is an issue in wheelchairs and other chairs for those patients who spend time out of bed and a special surface cushion may be required to prevent ischial breakdown. Table 7-3 reviews available support surfaces.

Convoluted Polyurethane Egg Crate Foam Mattress

This high-density foam is made of plastic or silicone and has the advantage of being inexpensive, lightweight, and comfortable. Its disadvantages are that it provides minimal pressure relief and causes retention of body heat, which potentiates perspiration and maceration. Many consider this product a fire hazard. Although the popular 2-inch egg crate pads do not provide any real pressure reduction, they do provide a comfortable surface.

Alternating Pressure Mattress

This vinyl, air-filled mattress is designed to inflate and deflate small air cells at regular intervals by means of an electric pump. Some models also have vents that allow the air to circulate between the mattress and the patient. This type of mattress should be placed on top of a bed mattress. Its advantages are that it mechanically alters the points of pressure against the body, provides a moderate degree of protection against pressure, can decrease maceration (when the model with the air vents is used), is lightweight, and is easy to clean if soiled. Its disadvantages are that it minimizes but does not completely reduce pressure, it may be uncomfortable because it feels lumpy, and it is more costly because an electric pump is needed. The indications for use are patients who are at high risk for skin breakdown or patients who have stage I or stage II pressure ulcers.

Water Mattress

A heavy vinyl mattress filled with water can be placed on top of a bed mattress. Its advantages are that it evenly distributes the patient's weight over the greatest possible surface; it provides a moderately high degree of protection against pressure; and it is comfortable, easy to maintain, and easy to clean if soiled. Its disadvantages are that it minimizes but does not prevent pressure, it is heavy when filled, and it costs about the same as an air mattress. The indications are for patients who are at high risk or who already have stage I, II, or III pressure ulcers.

TABLE 7-1	Braden Scale for Predicting Pressure Ulcer Risk

Patient's Name _____

Sensory perception Ability to respond meaningfully to pressure-related discomfort	1. Completely Limited: Unresponsive (does not moan, flinch, or gasp) to painful stimuli, due to diminished level of consciousness or sedation or limited ability to feel pain over most of body surface.	2. Very Limited: Responds only to painful stimuli. Cannot communicate discomfort except by moaning or restlessness or has a sensory impairment which limits the ability to feel pain or discomfort over $\frac{1}{2}$ of body.
Moisture Degree of which skin exposed to moisture	1. Constantly Moist: Skin is kept moist almost constantly by perspiration, urine, etc. Dampness is detected every time patient is moved or turned.	2. Moist: Skin is often but not always moist. Linen must be changed at least once a shift.
Activity Degree of physical activity	1. Bedfast: Confined to bed	2. Chairfast: Ability to walk severely limited or nonexistent. Cannot bear own weight and/or must be assisted into chair or wheelchair.
Mobility Ability to change and control body position	1. Completely Immobile: Does not make even slight changes in body or extremity position without assistance.	2. Very Limited: Makes occasional slight changes in body or extremity position but unable to make frequent or significant changes independently.
Nutrition Usual food intake pattern	1. Very Poor: Never eats a complete meal. Rarely eats more than $\frac{1}{3}$ of any food offered. Eats 2 servings or less of protein (meat or dairy products) per day. Takes fluids poorly. Does not take a liquid dietary supplement or is NPO and/or maintained on clear liquids or IVs for more than 5 days.	2. Probably Inadequate: Rarely eats a complete meal and generally eats only about $\frac{1}{2}$ of any food offered. Protein intake includes only 3 servings of meat or dairy products per day. Occasionally will take a dietary supplement or receives less than optimum amount of liquid diet or tube feeding.
Friction and smear	1. Problem: Requires moderate to maximum assistance in moving. Complete lifting without sliding against sheets is impossible. Frequently slides down in bed or chair, requiring frequent repositioning with maximum assistance. Spasticity, contractures, or agitation leads to almost constant friction.	2. Potential Problem: Moves feebly or requires minimum assistance. During a move skin probably slides to some extent against sheets, chair, restraints, or other devices. Maintains relatively good position in chair or bed most of the time but occasionally slides down.

Continued

TABLE 7-1	Braden Scale for Predicting Pressure Ulcer Risk—cont'd					
Evaluator's Name_____ **Date of Assessment**						

3. Slightly Limited: Responds to verbal commands but cannot always communicate discomfort or need to be turned or has some sensory impairment which limits ability to feel pain or discomfort in 1 or 2 extremities.	4. No Impairment: Responds to verbal commands. Has no sensory deficit which would limit ability to feel or voice pain or discomfort.				
3. Occasionally Moist: Skin is occasionally moist, requiring an extra linen change approximately once a day.	4. Rarely Moist: Skin is usually dry; linen requires changing only at routine intervals.				
3. Walks Occasionally: Walks occasionally during day but for very short distances, with or without assistance. Spends majority of each shift in bed or chair.	4. Walks Frequently: Walks outside the room at least twice a day and inside room at least once every 2 h during waking hours.				
3. Slightly Limited: Makes frequent though slight changes in body or extremity position independently.	4. No Limitations: Makes major and frequent changes in position without assistance.				
3. Adequate: Eats over half of most meals. Eats a total of 4 servings of protein (meat, dairy products) each day. Occasionally will refuse a meal, but will usually take a supplement if offered or is on a tube feeding or TPN regimen which probably meets most of nutritional needs.	4. Excellent: Eats most of every meal. Never refuses a meal. Usually eats a total of 4 or more servings of meat and dairy products. Occasionally eats between meals. Does not require supplementation.				
3. No Apparent Problem: Moves in bed and in chair independently and has sufficient muscle strength to lift up completely during move. Maintains good position in bed or chair at all times.					
	Total Score				

| TABLE 7-2 | Norton Risk Assessment Scale |

	Physical Condition	Mental Condition	Activity	Mobility	Incontinent	
	Good 4 Fair 3 Poor 2 Very Bad 1	Alert 4 Apathetic 3 Confused 2 Stupor 1	Ambulant 4 Walk/help 3 Chairbound 2 Bed 1	Full 4 Sl. limited 3 V. limited 2 Immobile 1	Not 4 Occasional 3 Usually/Urine 2 Doubly 1	Total score
Name	Date					

From Norton D, McLaren R, Exton-Smith AN: *An investigation of geriatric nursing problems in hospital*, Edinburgh, 1962, reissue 1975, Churchill Livingstone.

| TABLE 7-3 | Support Surfaces for Persons at Risk for Pressure Ulcers |

Type	Examples	Support Area	Low Moisture Retention	Reduced Heat Accumulation	Shear Reduction	Pressure Reduction	Cost per Day
Static surfaces	Foam	Yes	No	No	No	Yes	Low
	Standard mattress	No	No	No	No	No	Low
	Static flotation—air or water	Yes	No	No	Yes	Yes	Low
Dynamic surfaces	Air fluidized	Yes	Yes	Yes	Yes	Yes	High
	Low-air-loss	Yes	Yes	Yes	?	Yes	High
	Alternating air	Yes	No	No	Yes	Yes	Moderate

Source: Adapted from Bergstrom N et al: *Treatment of pressure ulcers. Clinical Practice Guideline No. 15.* Rockville, MD: US Department of Health and Human Services, Public Health Service, Agency for Health Care Policy and Research. December 1994:38. AHCPR Pub. No. 95-0652.3

Air-Fluidized Bed

This type of bed consists of a mattress filled with ultrafine silicone-coated beads and warm air flowing through a compressor. A loose polyester sheet separates the patient from the beads, which allows the air to circulate and body fluids to drain into the bed. When the compressor is turned off, the beads firmly mold around the patient to facilitate positioning for dressing changes, transfers, or cardiopulmonary resuscitation.

Its advantages are the support of the patient at a subcapillary closing pressure (< 15-33 mm Hg) and provision of a high degree of protection against pressure, friction, shearing, and maceration. Its disadvantages are the physical size and weight of the bed, and the circulating warm air may have a dehydrating effect on the patient and the wounds. In addition, patient repositioning (unless the bed does it automatically) is difficult because of the motion and molding. The rental fee is expensive, and new Medicare rules may make reimbursement more problematic for certain nursing home residents. Indications for use include patients with any stage of skin breakdown (particularly stages III and IV pressure ulcers), patients undergoing graft or flap surgery, patients with intractable pain, and patients who fail to improve with pressure-reduction surface treatment.

TURNING AND POSITIONING

The patient's position should be changed every 2 hours, but turning may need to be more frequent for some patients. When positioning, use multiple pillows, positioning wedges, or towels or other rolls to prevent a patient's bony prominences from rubbing together.

Techniques for Positioning

- Keeping the head of the bed elevated less than 30 degrees prevents shearing forces and reduces pressure on the greater trochanter.
- When positioning patients in the supine position, place pillows at the lateral aspect of each buttock to decrease pressure on the sacrum.
- Heels should never rest on the surface of the bed. A pillow placed under the patient's legs or a towel roll superior to the patient's heel eliminates this source of risk.
- For bed-bound patients or patients with pressure ulcers on their feet or lower legs, use of a bed cradle prevents the bedclothes from exerting pressure on these sensitive areas.
- Placing pillows at the end of the bed gives the feet something to rest or push against and decrease the incidence of footdrop

Change of Position in the Wheelchair or Gerichair

Pressure on the sacrum is at its highest when a person is sitting above a 45-degree angle. Many patients are unable to change position by themselves, and therefore turning schedules and pressure-relieving devices are imperative. Consultation with a physical or occupational therapist can ensure that each person is using proper wheelchair and pressure-relieving devices.

USE OF PROTECTIVE FILMS OR REAL SHEEPSKIN

Protective films are effective because they reduce both friction and injury. They are also effective protection against incontinence. This type of dressing may be used to protect against friction can be used on the heels and elbows. Lubricants can be used to protect unbroken skin from friction.

Real sheepskin can be useful to reduce friction and shear. Real skins work well and are good for controlling perspiration. Polyesters should not be used except for comfort.

MAINTAINING RANGE OF MOTION AND AMBULATION

Improving mobility and patient activity helps to keep the pressure off areas at risk. The use of exercise bars or a trapeze over the bed may reduce the risk for bedfast patients. Range-of-motion exercises and ambulation are important to prevent contractions and improve circulation.

MAINTAINING CLEAN AND APPROPRIATELY DRY SKIN

The suggested procedure for cleaning an older patient is to cleanse the affected area gently with a skin cleaner, plain water, or a minimal amount of mild soap and water. After cleaning, a thin layer of moisturizing lotion can be applied, taking care to massage gently around rather than over the reddened area. Vigorous massage increases tissue damage by creating shearing forces. This treatment should be followed by the application of a thin layer of a petroleum-based product. Petroleum products are water resistant, provide a protective barrier against urine and feces and protect denuded skin. A mixture of 30% petroleum jelly with zinc oxide provides protection for fecal incontinence or episodes of diarrhea.

The placement of indwelling catheters is not necessary to protect the skin of an incontinent patient. A catheter puts a patient at increased risk for developing a urinary tract infection and sepsis.

Pressure Ulcer Staging

Once a pressure ulcer has developed, it must be staged to classify the degree of tissue damage. Staging is used as a tool for assessment and communication between health care professionals. The stagings were devised by National Pressure Ulcer Advisory Panel Consensus Development Conference after consultation with the Wound Ostomy and Continence Nurses Society. Ulcers are staged as follows:

- *Stage I:* Nonblanchable erythema of *intact* skin, the herald lesion of skin ulceration. In persons with darker skin, skin discoloration, increased warmth, edema, induration, and hardness may also be indicators.
- *Stage II:* Partial-thickness skin loss involving the epidermis, dermis, or both. The ulcer is superficial and presents clinically as an abrasion, blister, or shallow crater. The wound base is moist, pink, and free of necrotic tissue. An intact blister over a bony prominence is a stage II ulcer. If possible, the blister should be kept intact to promote healing. This stage is reversible with appropriate treatment and care.
- *Stage III:* Full-thickness skin loss that involves damage to or necrosis of subcutaneous tissue and may extend down to, but not through, underlying fascia. The ulcer presents clinically as a deep crater with or without undermining of adjacent tissue. Serous or purulent drainage is usually present. This stage may be life threatening without appropriate treatment and care.
- *Stage IV:* Full-thickness skin and subcutaneous tissue loss with extensive destruction or necrosis of tissue, which exposes muscle, bone, or supporting structures (e.g., tendon, joint capsule). Serous or purulent drainage is usually present. Sinus tracts and widely undermined areas may be present. The wound base itself is not painful, but the sides of the wound may be.

Without appropriate treatment and care, osteomyelitis or septic arthritis in adjoining joints resulting from an infection of this wound type may be fatal without appropriate treatment and care. Osteomyelitis is second only to soft-tissue infection as the most important musculoskeletal infection. Acute osteomyelitis is usually acquired hematogenously, and the most common pathogen is *Staphylococcus aureus*. Acute osteomyelitis can usually be cured with antimicrobial therapy alone. In contrast, chronic osteomyelitis may be caused by *S. aureus* but is often due to gram-negative organisms. The causative organism of chronic osteomyelitis is identified by culture of aseptically obtained bone biopsy specimens. Because of the presence of infected bone fragments without a blood supply (sequestra), cure of chronic osteomyelitis with antibiotic therapy alone is rarely, if ever, possible. Adequate surgical debridement is the cornerstone of therapy for chronic osteomyelitis, and cure is not possible without the removal of all infected bone (Cunha, 2002).

The following limitations are inherent in these definitions:

- Because the skin remains intact in stage I pressure ulcers, these lesions are not ulcers in the usual sense. In addition, stage I pressure ulcers are not always reliably assessed, especially in patients with darkly pigmented skin. Despite these limitations, identification of a stage I pressure ulcer is critical for indicating the need for more vigilant assessment and preventive care.

- Assessing stage I ulcers in persons with darker skin tones requires careful observation for (1) any change in the feel of the tissue; (2) any change in the appearance of the skin in a high-risk area, such as the orange-peel look; (3) a subtle purplish hue; and (4) extremely dry, crustlike areas that, on close examination, are found to cover a break in the tissue.
- An ulcer cannot be accurately staged until the eschar, if present, is removed. Eschar is a black, leather-like layer of dry necrotic cells and debris in the wound. It is either level with the epidermis or somewhat concave.
- Pressure ulcers should be staged to classify the degree of tissue damage observed. It may be difficult to assess pressure ulcers in patients with casts, other orthopedic devices, or support stockings. Routine assessment to check for adequate circulation, movement, and sensation may fail to detect pressure ulcers beneath casts. Be sure to (1) assess the skin under the edges of casts, (2) be alert to patient complaints of pressure-induced pain, (3) determine whether casts need to be altered or replaced to relieve pressure, and (4) remove support stockings to assess the skin.

Documentation

Accurate assessment and documentation are essential to proper staging of a pressure ulcer. At a minimum, pressure ulcer assessment should include the location; the stage or grade of the wound; the quality of the circulation; the dimensions (size); the presence or absence and estimated amount of necrotic tissue; the condition of the wound base; the condition of the periwound skin; the amount, quality, and nature and the presence or absence of exudate; an estimate of the presence or absence of infection; and the presence of healed pressure ulcers.

A Polaroid picture is excellent for documentation purposes. The pictures should be placed in the patient's chart with the date of the pictures written on the back. A simple diagram of the wound with areas of tunneling, undermining, or sinus tracts also is included. Staging, showing progression of the ulcer, can go from I to II to III to IV; however, a healing ulcer should be referred to as "healing stage III" (with measurements) rather than upstaging (i.e., "now stage II"). The only exception to this type of staging is the minimum data set, the federally mandated reporting system in use in nursing homes. Because of reimbursement issues, healing ulcers are coded in the healed stage. Slough and eschar prevent accurate staging and should be documented as such. Consistency in documentation is of great importance for any health care situation, especially in wound care because of the number of staff and caregivers who are observing and treating the wound. Table 7-4 describes a systematic approach to the assessment and management of pressure ulcers.

Elements of a Wound
WOUND SIZE

Measurement of the wound includes length, width, and depth. Depth can be measured by observing how far a saline-moistened sterile cotton tip can be inserted into the wound; a double-gloved finger can also be used. To a great extent, the staging of a wound is an estimate of its depth.

WOUND EDGES

Wound edges are good indicators of the healing process. A sloped edge with epithelium around the wound is a good sign. Rolled under or punched out edges may be a sign that the wound is deteriorating or enlarging. Wounds with rolled edges will not heal, and it is wise to debride them. Rolled edges can be a sign of undermining that was not detected or documented.

NECROTIC TISSUE

The presence of necrotic tissue in a wound indicates that it is at least a full-thickness wound (stage III or IV). Documentation includes the percent of the wound covered with necrotic tissue and the color and consistency of the tissue. The removal of necrotic tissue does not often cause bleeding.

TABLE 7-4	A Systematic Approach to the Management of Pressure Ulcers

Evaluate and Document	*Consider These Strategies:*
Location	Examine other high-risk sites; develop targeted pressure-relieving strategies (e.g., positioning and repositioning, padding, seat cushions, and heel elevation); limit shearing forces by special attention to positioning when the head of bed is elevated; lift rather than slide the patient; cleanse and dry regularly if wetted frequently.
Stage	Differentiate between minor stage I lesions (nonblanchable erythema related to extravasation of red blood cells into the interstitium) and deep tissue injuries that can progress to full-thickness lesions; discuss with caregivers and families the possibility of significant pressure-ulcer development when deep tissue injury is identified.
Area	Record diameter for circular lesions; record lengths of largest perpendiculars for irregular lesions.
Depth	Measure depth from plane of skin; probe and measure extent of undermining or depth of sinus tracts.
Drainage	Estimate amount; identify degree of odor and purulence; monitor hematocrit if more than minor blood loss with dressing changes occurs; monitor serum albumin if volume of ulcer drainage is large.
Necrosis	Consider simple blunt debridement of small amounts of necrotic tissue; involve general or plastic surgeons for extensive debridement; monitor damage to healthy tissue whenever using blunt, enzymatic, or wet-to-dry dressings for debridement; monitor use of pressure dressings (which can cause necrosis) after blunt debridement.
Granulation	Identify granulation as an indication that wound healing is occurring; look for regression when other infections (e.g., urinary tract infection or pneumonia) occur; develop strategies to protect and enhance growth of granulation tissue (e.g., nourishment, vitamins, and minerals; use of dressings to ensure moist wound surfaces); avoid damage with dressing changes.
Cellulitis	Differentiate from a thin rim of erythema surrounding most healing wounds; look for tender, warm redness, particularly if there is progression; consider treatment with systemic antibiotics active against gram-positive cocci.

Source: Bennett RG. Pressure ulcers. In Cobbs EL, Duthie EH Jr, Murphy JB. *Geriatrics review syllabus: a core curriculum in geriatric medicine*, ed. 4, Dubuque, Iowa, 1996, Kendall Hunt Publishing Company for the American Geriatrics Society.

WOUND BASE

A description of the wound base includes any tunneling or undermined edges. The base of the wound should be probed to assess it completely. Granulation tissue should be evident in the wound bed, and the percentage of the wound covered with red granulation tissue should be documented.

WOUND EXUDATE

Wound exudate contains growth factors that actively promote healing. Problems occur when there is too much or too little exudate. Too little exudate creates a desiccated wound; too much overwhelms the dressing and can flood the surrounding skin, causing maceration of the periwound tissues.

CONTAMINATION OR INFECTION

A wound will not heal until any infection is resolved. Infected wounds have the same types of organisms that are present in chronic open wounds, but they are present in much larger numbers. Infection may be signaled by the presence of one or more of the following: induration, fever or a feeling of general malaise, erythema, edema, and purulent, foul-smelling drainage, particularly when accompanied by an elevated white blood count. Infected wounds are usually painful to the patient.

WOUND CULTURES

Routine wound culturing of pressure ulcers in the absence of clinical symptoms and signs of infection is of questionable value. The growth of common pathogens (e.g., *Staphylococcus* organisms, *Escherichia coli*) in such cultures does not necessarily imply the presence of infection that requires antibiotic therapy. If there are signs and symptoms of bacterial or systemic infection or if the healing of the pressure ulcer is delayed, a wound culture and a sensitivity test are indicated.

The guidelines of the Centers for Disease Control and Prevention and the Agency for Health Care Policy and Research (AHCPR) recommend needle aspiration culture or tissue biopsy cultures because swab cultures have no diagnostic value. Bacterial counts of 100,000 organisms per gram of tissue (determined by biopsy) represent the critical value for wound infection and correlate with the inability of the wound to heal normally.

All chronic wounds are contaminated. They will heal, they do not need to be sterilized, and they cannot be sterilized. Adequate cleaning and debridement usually prevent colonization from progressing to infection.

Wound Healing

Healing of a pressure ulcer usually involves three phases: granulation, contraction, and reepithelialization.

FIRST PHASE

The first phase of healing takes place during the first 4 days after a break in skin integrity. During this time the body prepares the wound bed by removing dead tissue. The presence of foreign material or necrotic tissue prevents the wound from progressing. Observation of the wound at this time shows warm, reddened skin and increased serosanguineous fluid and exudate. The exudate is composed of phagocytized bacteria, neutrophils, and living bacteria. During this phase, the exudate or wound drainage is at a peak.

SECOND PHASE

The second phase of healing occurs from day 4 through day 21. Healing activities involve the formation of granulation tissue, contraction of the wound, and the final epithelialization. A new vascular bed is formed, and granulation tissue fills the wound bed to provide the base for the migration of the epithelial cells. The process is a contraction of the wound edges, with a filling in from the bottom. The wound is rough and red; this is the area that must be kept moist to facilitate the mobility of granulation tissue cells. These cells are very fragile and can be easily damaged by dressings. The second phase ends when the edges of the wound are white with epithelialization cells. As might be anticipated for older persons, this phase can take longer; it may take twice the usual time.

THIRD PHASE

The third and last phase of healing can be as short as 3 weeks or as long as 2 to 3 years. The tensile strength of the scar tissue begins to increase. The wound now consists of scar tissue covered by new epithelium from the wound edges. The scar consists of granulation tissue covered by thin epithelial tissue. Ultimately all healed pressure ulcers have only 70% to 75% of their original strength. Further injury is problematic, and these skin areas are at high risk.

The three phases of healing overlap, and various parts of the wound are at different phases at different times. At any specific point in time it is sometimes difficult to determine what is occurring in the wound in terms of healing phases.

FACTORS THAT AFFECT WOUND HEALING

Wound healing depends on a normal blood supply; anything that impedes circulation influences healing of the wound. Intrinsic factors include the following:
- Advanced age
- Nutritional and hydration status
- Diabetes mellitus
- Other comorbidity

Extrinsic factors include the following:
- Mechanical stress (pressure, friction, and shear)
- Medications
- Nonsteroidal antiinflammatory drugs, long-term steroid use
- Debris in the wound
- Infection
- Temperature
- Desiccation (lack of moisture in the wound bed)
- Maceration (abundance of fluid in the wound bed)
- Chemical stress

Temperature

Frequent dressing can alter the temperature of a wound enough to interfere with healing. High fevers, diapers that trap body heat, and high ambient temperature in the patient's environment can alter wound temperature. Applications of ice packs or heating pads for any reason may cause damage to the local circulation and thus affect wound healing.

Chemical Stress

Chemical stress results from the use of many traditional treatments, such as Dakin's solution, peroxide, acetic acid, povidone iodine (Betadine), iodine, hexachlorophene, alcohol, or hypochlorites. These agents are cytotoxic and delay wound healing. They are excellent bacteriostatic agents, but they also kill maturing endothelial cells in a healing wound.

Treatment
STAGE I

The first step is to assess and modify the risk factors. Cleaning the wound with normal saline solution alone is safe and effective. The selection of a dressing may be determined by the location of the wound. A transparent vapor-permeable dressing, a liquid barrier, or an opaque hydrocolloidal occlusive barrier may be used. All decrease friction, shearing, and maceration.

Heat lamps are not recommended for this or any other stage of skin breakdown. In addition to being a source of potential injury to the patient, heat lamps dry and dehydrate wounds and inhibit the healing process. The use of tincture of benzoin on reddened areas is discouraged because it has a high alcohol content and becomes sticky when dry and thus can pull and damage fragile skin.

STAGE II

The first step is to assess and modify the risk factors. Cleansing is the same as in stage I. The dressing may be a transparent vapor-permeable dressing, an opaque hydrocolloidal occlusive barrier, or enzymatic spray, which has a mild debriding action and improves epithelialization by stimulating the vascular bed. Wet-to-dry dressings may also be used but require more frequent changes, tend to be less comfortable, and inhibit inspection of the wound. Dry sterile dressings are not recommended because they dry out a wound at this stage and inhibit healing.

STAGE III

The first step is to assess and modify the risk factors. At this stage, it is easy to become so focused on local care that the risk factors are overlooked. For healing to occur, the wound must be free of infection and necrotic tissue. Wound debridement is necessary if necrotic tissue is present. Culture and sensitivity studies should be performed if there are signs of infection (elevated temperature, malodorous exudate, inflamed tissue surrounding the wound). In addition, wound and skin precautions should be taken until the results are known.

Local care of a wound that is free of necrotic material consists of three basic components: irrigation, packing, and outer dressings. For irrigation, normal saline is recommended in clean wounds. With aseptic technique, a catheter-tipped syringe may be used to direct the flow of the irrigant into the wound. Packing material should be appropriate to the depth and size of the wound. If wet-to-dry techniques are used, the dressing should be plain gauze without cotton filling because it is more absorbent. Using aseptic technique, the dressing should be gently packed to conform to the wound without extending onto the intact skin, which may cause tissue irritation or maceration. Care must be taken not to pack the wound too tightly, which inhibits the absorption capability of the dressing and applies pressure to the area.

Other absorption dressings may be used. The outer dressing should be applied over the packed wound to prevent contamination from the external environment. The dry sterile dressing should be of a size appropriate for the wound and secured with hypoallergenic tape or other methods (e.g., Montgomery straps or a stockinette). Care must be taken to protect the surrounding skin. Care of a stage III ulcer is costly and labor intensive.

STAGE IV

The first step is to assess and modify the risk factors. The procedures for care are similar to those for stage III. Variations may be indicated by the presence of sinus tracts or exposed bone. Irrigation should be performed with aseptic technique. If sinus tracts are present, the flow of the irrigant needs to be appropriately directed. All exudate and necrotic debris must be removed from these narrow pathways. The wound should be packed. Packing should be loosely directed into all crevices and sinuses, with no dead or empty spaces. If used, rolled gauze (available in various widths) should be kept in one piece to permit easy removal and prevent the possibility of dressing material being left in the wound. If more than one roll is used, the rolls should be tied together. Exposed bone should be covered with a wet, normal saline dressing and changed every 4 hours to avoid drying and to maintain viability of the bone tissue. An outer dressing should be applied, as in stage III.

PRESSURE ULCER TREATMENT: DEBRIDEMENT OF NECROTIC TISSUE

The three methods of debridement are mechanical, surgical, and chemical. Chemical is best used in conjunction with one of the other two methods. All three are intended to assist the natural process of autolytic debridement.

For mechanical debridement, normal saline is used to irrigate a wound that has purulent drainage or necrotic debris. A whirlpool bath is often used as well. A wet-to-moist dressing consisting of plain gauze moistened with normal saline is then gently packed into the wound. Loose necrotic tissue and wound drainage are absorbed into the dressing and removed with each dressing change. These dressings are usually changed every 8 hours. Wet-to-moist gauze dressings changed three or four times daily remove necrotic debris, but mechanical debridement is minimally effective on eschar. It is slower, time-consuming, and uncomfortable for the patient. There is also the problem of removing viable tissue along with the necrotic tissue. Care must be taken when removing a dry dressing to avoid damaging new cell growth and destroying viable tissue.

Surgical debridement is the fastest way to remove necrotic tissue and the only effective method of removing eschar. Although effective surgical debridement may add the risks of hemorrhage, infection, increased wound size, and pain, the advantages of surgical debridement are speed and completeness for patients who have large, thick, necrotic debris. When sepsis threatens, the best method is to remove the necrotic tissue surgically. Removal can be performed with laser surgery, which reduces some risks. Surgical debridement for thorough excision of infected or necrotic tissue usually is followed by a musculocutaneous flap procedure. Postoperative care includes monitoring the patient for infection and keeping pressure off the flap.

Chemical debridement is accomplished with enzymatic agents. Debriding enzymes are proteolytic or fibrinolytic agents that act against devitalized tissue. They are most useful on superficial wound layers because they must be in contact with the substrata of the wound. They are ineffective on dense, dry eschar. These agents should be used as an adjunct to mechanical or surgical debridement.

Enzymatic Agents

Enzymes are recommended in the AHCPR pressure ulcer treatment guidelines as an effective method for debriding pressure ulcers. Enzymes are useful when a patient's inflammatory response is suppressed. The manufacturer's written recommendations should be followed carefully and fully. The enzymes are designed to liquefy necrotic tissue and can be somewhat unpleasant when used. The use of enzymes should be discontinued as soon as the wound is free of necrotic tissue. These products are generally available to Medicaid beneficiaries under the prescription drug benefit but are not covered under Medicare Part B. Autolytic debridement is the process by which the normal enzymes contained in the wound exudate are retained in the wound. The collected moisture and enzymes act to liquefy and rehydrate the eschar and slough. Creating a moist environment by using films, hydrocolloids, or gels has been shown to remove effectively necrotic debris in 7 to 10 days. The advantage is that only necrotic debris is removed. It is relatively inexpensive compared with other debriding modalities, and it is easy for the patient because there is less pain. The wound must be cleaned with each dressing change. Daily dressing changes are usually required when the wound undergoes autolytic debridement because the liquefied debris should be irrigated from the wound. The daily use of hydrogel covered with transparent film is recommended for yellow, stringy slough.

Important Considerations. All hardened or dry eschar should be removed or crosshatched so the enzyme can come in contact with the wound. The use of antibacterials and antiseptics (povidone-iodine, hexachlorophene, silver nitrate, hydrogen peroxide, benzalkonium chloride) is discouraged because they may inhibit the action of some enzymes. Because some preparations become inactive in 24 hours, they must be freshly reconstituted so that each use is optimally effective. They may also require refrigeration. Enzymatic sprays are easy-to-use, economic products for home use or on superficial wounds. When necessary, silver nitrate can be used to debride rolled wound edges. Wounds with rolled edges are slow to heal.

PRESSURE ULCER TREATMENT: COMMONLY USED DRESSINGS AND TOPICAL AGENTS

At least 3000 products for wound care are on the market. Table 7-5 reviews common dressings, indications, and contraindications. The care products used for long-term care residents are often based on corporate decisions that have nothing to do with the individual but everything to do with cost savings through contracts. It is important to remember that no single product meets all needs situ-

TABLE 7-5	Common Dressings for Treating Pressure Ulcers		
Dressing	**Indication**	**Contraindications**	**Example**
Transparent film	Stage I ulcer Protection from friction	Skin tears Draining ulcers	Bioclusive Tegaderm Op-site
	Superficial scrape Autolytic debridement of slough Apply skin prep to intact skin to protect from adhesive	Suspected skin infection or fungus	
Foam island	Stage II, III Low to moderate exudate Can apply as window to secure transparent film	Excessive exudate Dry, crusted wound	Alleyn Lyofoam
Hydrocolloids	Stage II, III Low to moderate drainage Good peri-wound skin integrity Autolytic debridement of slough Left in place 3-5 days Can apply as window to secure transparent film Can apply over alginate to control drainage Must control maceration Apply skin prep to intact skin to protect from adhesive	Poor skin integrity Infected ulcers Wound needs packing	Duoderm Extrathin film Duoderm Tegasorb Replicare
Petroleum-based nonadherent	Stage II, III Graft sites		Vaseline gauze Xerofoam Adaptic
Alginate	Stage II, III, IV Excessive drainage Apply dressing within wound borders Requires secondary dressing Must use skin prep Must control for maceration	Dry or minimally draining wound Superficial wounds with maceration	Sorbsan Kaltostat Algosteril Algiderm
Hydrogel (amorphous gels)	Stage II, III, IV Needs to be combined with gauze dressing Stays moist longer than saline gauze Changed 1-2 times/day Used as alternative to saline gauze for packing deep wounds with tunnels, undermining	Macerated areas Wounds with excess exudate	Intrasite gel Solosite gel

Continued

| TABLE 7-5 | Common Dressings for Treating Pressure Ulcers—cont'd | | |

Dressing	Indication	Contraindications	Example
(gel sheet)	Reduces adherence of gauze to wound Must control for maceration Stage II Skin tears Needs to be held in place with topper dressing	Macerated areas Wounds with moderate to heavy exudate	Vigilon
Gauze packing (moistened with saline)	Stage III, IV Wounds with depth, especially those with tunnels, undermining Must be remoistened often to maintain moist wound environment		square 2X2s, 4X4s Fluffed Kerlix Plain Nugauze

Source: Copyright © 1999 by Rita Frantz. Reprinted from Reuben DB et al: *Geriatrics at tour fingertips.* 2001 ed, Belle Mead, NJ, 2001, Excerpta Medica, Inc. for the American Geriatrics Society. Reprinted with permission.

ations; the location of the wound influences the type of dressing that is chosen, and dressing choices may change from week to week.

The goal is a wound that is neither too dry nor too wet. The choice of dressing should meet this goal. When wounds are moist, there is less pain, faster healing, a cleaner appearance, and the dressing changes are faster.

The recommendations from AHCPR are that the best choice of a wound dressing is one that will keep the wound bed moist and the periwound skin dry. There is a rule of thumb regarding dressing a wound: If it is wet, absorb it; if it is dry, moisten it.

Traditional gauze dressings are still in use for chronic wound care. Although the cost may be less, they are more time consuming in many instances, and the frequent dressing changes cause the patient additional pain and discomfort. In contrast, modern dressings can often be changed every 2 to 3 days versus two or three times each day for gauze. Moist dressings cost more per piece than gauze, but less personnel time is involved because the dressing is not changed as frequently.

Dressing choices are films, hydrocolloids, gels and gel sheets, foams, alginates, and exudate absorbers. Films, hydrocolloids, and gels and gel sheets are excellent for autolytic debridement. Foams, alginates, and exudate absorbers are excellent for exudate management.

Therapeutic ultrasound has been used to enhance healing of pressure ulcers; however, limited clinical research is available, and no consensus exists regarding the efficacy of ultrasound for treating pressure ulcers, particularly full-thickness pressure ulcers, in the elderly (Selkowitz et al, 2002).

Films

Liquid barrier film dressings contain plasticity agents that provide a protective waterproof coating over affected areas to reduce maceration and shearing. Application is by spray, wipes, or a roll-on method. These dressings are generally nonirritating and are not affected by urine, perspiration, or digestive acids. Although insoluble in water, they can be dissolved by a soap solution.

Transparent vapor-permeable dressings are made from polyurethane that is permeable to oxygen and moisture vapor but not to fluids. These dressings allow oxygen to reach the healing tissues while preventing the entrance of fluids that would contaminate the wound. The dressing stays in place for 3 to 5 days, creates a moist environment that keeps the wound exudate against the wound surface, and promotes migration of epithelial cells across the wound. The exudate that collects under the dressing varies in color and consistency from thin, clear, and serous to thick, cloudy, and brown. This range is considered normal, and the exudate should not be drained. The dressing may need to be changed if the exudate leaks from its edges. If a wound infection is suspected, the dressing should be changed daily. As the amount of exudate decreases, the wound becomes darker and begins to dry. When healing is complete, the dressing may be removed or left on to protect the new skin by reducing shearing, friction, and maceration.

Important Considerations. The wound should be cleaned, and the surrounding skin must be completely dry for the dressing to adhere. This dressing should cover at least a 1-inch margin around the wound and should not be tightly stretched over the wound, which causes shearing forces against the tissues. Dressings may be cut or overlapped without reducing their effectiveness.

Films cannot absorb wound exudate and cause a collection of fluid under the dressing if used to dress a draining wound. *They are not considered a good choice for draining a wound.* If excessive exudate threatens to loosen and pull the dressing off the drainage, the exudate may be aspirated through the dressing with a small-bore needle. The dressing may seal itself or may need to be patched with another piece of dressing. A film is an excellent dressing for wounds in the later stages of healing when there is little drainage because it will not stick to moist wound tissue. It is now widely used as a secondary dressing for gauze, alginates, and gels.

Films are also used as protective dressings over skin that is at risk for breakdown. These are removed with care with the lateral pull technique: Support the dressing with one hand while pulling the edges laterally away from the center and parallel to the skin surface with the other hand, thus removing it slowly from the sides.

Hydrocolloids

Hydrocolloids are the most popular group of moist wound-healing dressings. Like films, they are also waterproof and bacteria-proof, but they have the advantage of being able to absorb moderate amounts of wound exudate. Hydrocolloids are easy to apply and are versatile.

Opaque hydrocolloid occlusive barriers are occlusive dressings made of inert hydrophobic polymers containing fluid-absorbent hydrocolloid particles. When these particles come in contact with the wound exudate, they swell to form a moist gel that promotes debridement, granulation, and cell migration. The product works on the principle that optimal wound healing occurs in a closed, moist environment. The lack of atmospheric oxygen is not thought to prevent healing when the wound is superficial.

Important Considerations. Hydrocolloids can be used on most wound types but are best on a light to moderately exuding wound. This dressing is only really good with small to moderate amounts of exudate. It is a good idea to warm the dressing in your hands before putting it on because it adheres better if warmed. It is also a good idea to tape it in place as if placing it in a picture frame.

The wound and surrounding skin should be cleaned before to application. The surrounding skin should be completely dry so the dressing can adhere. This dressing should completely cover the wound and extend at least 1 to 2 inches beyond the wound edges. Care must be taken because it is easy to get macerated skin around the wound with this type of dressing. The dressing may be left in place up to 7 days unless leakage of exudate necessitates a change. If the wound becomes infected, the dressing must be changed more frequently. *This dressing is not recommended for wounds that show clinical signs of infection;* an infected wound must be looked at daily. Hydrocolloids are almost totally occlusive. When this dressing is removed from the wound, there is some gelled residue to clean up, and the odor is often unpleasant.

Gels and Gel Sheets

Gels are absorption dressings that use hydrophilic beads, grains, or flakes designed to absorb excess wound exudate and necrotic debris that may inhibit tissue regeneration. At the same time, they keep the wound moist enough to encourage healing, and they hydrate eschar and necrotic tissue. Wound gels high in water content can donate water from the gel to desiccated eschar and slough and thus help to liquefy necrotic tissue. These dressings also deodorize the wound.

Gels and gel sheets are amorphous hydrogels and create a hydrophilic environment over the wound. The gel sheets are transparent and conformable, similar to a soft contact lens. They are soothing when initially applied because of the cool nature of the dressing. The gel can absorb a small amount of exudate and permit evaporation from the upper surface of the gel. In this way, the gels wick watery exudate from the wound surface through the hydrophilic gel. The moisture is then allowed to evaporate without drying the wound surface. Gels can also run out of the wound, however, and allow it to dry out if exposed.

Important Considerations. These types of dressings usually require changing once or twice a day. The products should be reconstituted according to the manufacturer's instructions and then gently packed into the wound and covered with a dry outer dressing.

Hydrogel sheets are best for dressing lightly to moderately draining wounds because the gel sheets do not absorb a large amount of drainage. Gels require a secondary dressing, and gauze and non-woven tape are the best combinations for such a dressing. The gel sheet may be cut to the shape of the wound, which assists in returning moisture to dry wounds; however, there is a tendency for fluid to collect under the gel sheets, which leads to maceration.

Foams

Foams are made from polyurethane and are ideal for more heavily draining wounds. Some are now available in easy-to-apply adhesive versions, which make the foam more versatile. Foams do not leave any dressing residue in the wound and generally provide clean, moist healing environments.

Important Considerations. *Foams are best used for moderately to heavily draining wounds and for those with friable skin surrounding the wound.* The nonadhesive foams do not damage this fragile periwound skin. A roller bandage such as Kerlex is a good covering for these dressings.

Alginates

Alginates are nonwoven absorbent dressings derived from seaweed. They are placed into the wound dry, absorb exudate, and form a gel over the wound, thus maintaining a moist healing environment. The gel is hydrophilic and permits evaporation of excess exudate. This combination of absorption and evaporation allows alginates to handle more exudate than absorption alone. *A wound with little exudate is not a good candidate for alginate dressing* because alginates desiccate wounds with a low volume of exudate, and the dressing then tends to stick to the dried wound edges. Medicare Part B has covered these products in the past, but with new regulations it is wise to check with the fiscal intermediary regarding coverage.

Important Considerations. *Alginates are not good for wounds with sinus tracts or undermining and tunneling because they are difficult to remove.* They should not be used on a dry wound. An alginate goes in dry and comes out like mucus. It should not be wet before use. The dressing should be dated, and the time applied should be included on the dressing. There can be copious drainage through the alginate. It must be monitored regularly or the drainage may soil clothing and bedding. All alginates require secondary dressings. Secondary dressings should be highly permeable to moisture vapor so that the evaporation of exudate from the top surface of the gelled alginate is not inhibited. Gauze, nonwoven tapes, and highly moisture vapor-permeable film dressings are excellent for covering alginates. When the drainage lessens, it is time to change to another product.

Exudate Absorbers

Exudate absorbers are copolymer starch dressings that maintain a moist environment while absorbing exudate from the wound. They are messy to apply but are easily removed from the wound by irrigation. All exudate absorbers require a secondary dressing to keep them in place. *The copolymer starches are best used in heavily draining, cavity-type wounds.*

Important Considerations. It is wise to use a skin preparation before applying an adhesive for the secondary dressing. This practice allows the removal of the dressing but leaves the first level of the skin intact. Because the dressing swells a great deal, the wound is not filled to the top.

Cost consideration is an essential component in planning the management of pressure ulcers. The stage of the ulcer determines the need for more aggressive and thus more expensive treatment. Costly specialty beds, such as the Mediscus and Clinitron, are reserved for extreme cases such as multiple stage III or stage IV nonhealing ulcers.

NUTRITIONAL CONSIDERATIONS

It is important to maximize nutritional and hydration status by maximizing protein and fluid intake. A prescription of 500 mg of vitamin C and 220 mg of zinc sulfate daily has been widely recognized as effective in promoting wound healing.

SURGICAL REPAIR

The use of surgical repair of pressure ulcer is a viable option for stage III and stage IV pressure ulcers. Because many stage III and stage IV pressure ulcers eventually heal over a long period with the use of modern wound-healing principles and also because the rate of recurrence of surgically closed pressure ulcers is high, the practitioner must carefully weigh the benefits of surgery. When the surgical option is exercised, the most common type of surgical repairs include direct closure, skin grafting, skin flaps, musculocutaneous flaps, and free flaps (Cobbs, Duthie, and Murphy, 2002).

Pain

For many years it was thought that pressure ulcers did not cause pain, but this belief has been disproved. It is now widely accepted that most patients with pressure ulcers experience pain and that most patients never receive analgesia. Many patients studied were unable to respond; therefore clinicians failed to consider whether these wounds were painful.

Chronic wound pain is a complex subjective phenomenon of extreme discomfort experienced by a person in response to skin or tissue injury. Pain assessment for pressure ulcers should be no different. The clinician should question the patient about the quality, quantity, onset, duration, and type of pain. If a patient is unable to respond, the clinician should look for nonverbal signs and symptoms of pain, including restlessness, grimacing, and agitation. When pain is assessed, the wound is treated with analgesics. The clinician should ensure that the analgesic has been given before changing the dressing. As with any chronic pain, an around-the-clock pain control regimen should be considered.

Summary

The importance of a true team approach to the care of a patient with a pressure ulcer cannot be overstressed. Education of all staff and family, especially if they are caregivers, is essential to providing even minimal effective care. Consultation with knowledgeable clinicians in nutrition and physical and occupational therapy, plus the involvement of all paraprofessional staff, is critical. Prevention of tissue damage to the debilitated patient for whom adequate nutrition and hydration are no longer possible is challenging. Despite of the difficulty, these patients deserve no less than the best effort to heal the ulcer and provide quality of life that is pain free. For all other patients, pressure ulcers are preventable with proper assessment and care.

Resources

Tissue Viability Society
www.tvs.org.uk

Wound Care Community Network
www.woundcarenet.com

References

Brandeis GH, Berlowitz DR, Katz P: Are pressure ulcers preventable? A survey of experts, *Adv Skin Wound Care* 14(5):244, 2001.

Cobbs EL, Duthie EH, Murphy JB, editors: *Geriatrics review syllabus: a core curriculum in geriatric medicine*, ed 5, Malden, Mass, 2002, Blackwell Publishing for the American Geriatrics Society.

Collins F: Use of pressure reducing seats and cushions in a community setting, *Br J Community Nurs* 7(1): 15-22, 2002.

Cunha BA: Osteomyelitis in elderly adults, *Clin Infect Dis* 1(3):287-293, 2002.

Di Maio VJ, Di Maio TG: Homicide by decubitus ulcers, *Am J Forensic Med Pathol* 23(1):1-4, 2002.

Lyder CH et al: A comprehensive program to prevent pressure ulcers in long-term care: exploring costs and outcomes, *Ostomy Wound Manage* 48(4):52-62, 2002.

Meehan M, Hill WM: Pressure ulcers in nursing homes: does negligence litigation exceed available evidence? *Ostomy Wound Manage* 48(3):46-54, 2002.

Selkowitz DM et al: Efficacy of pulse low-intensity ultrasound in wound healing: a single-case design, *Ostomy Wound Manage* 48(4):40-44, 46-50, 2002.

8

Oral Health

Oral health is integral to general health, well-being, and quality of life. Diet, nutrition, sleep, psychological status, and social interactions are all affected by impaired oral health (U.S. Department of Health and Human Services, 2000). The word *oral* refers to the mouth and includes not only the teeth and the gums (gingiva) and their supporting tissues, but also the hard and soft palate, the mucosal lining of the mouth and throat, the tongue, the lips, the salivary glands, the chewing muscles, and the upper and lower jaws. Equally important are the branches of the nervous, immune, and vascular systems that animate, protect, and nourish the oral tissues (U.S. Department of Health and Human Services, 2000).

At the turn of the twentieth century, most Americans could expect to lose their teeth by middle age. More persons are retaining their natural teeth over their lifetime as a result of education, improved hygiene, and better, more accessible dental care. About 30% of adults 65 years of age and older are edentulous, compared with 46% twenty years ago, although this figure is higher for those living in poverty (U.S. Department of Health and Human Services, 2000). Although this is certainly good news, it carries with it an increased incidence of dental decay and a steadily increasing prevalence of gum and periodontal disease.

Although great strides have been made in oral health for most of the nation, disparities exist in the oral health among certain populations. Those who suffer the worst oral health are found among the poor of all ages; poor children and poor older Americans are particularly vulnerable. Members of racial and ethnic minority groups also experience a disproportionate level of oral health problems. Persons who are medically compromised or who have disabilities are at greater risk for oral diseases, and in turn oral diseases further jeopardize their health (U.S. Department of Health and Human Services, 2000).

The reasons for disparities in oral health are complex. Issues include socioeconomic factors, lack of resources to pay for care, lack of community programs such as fluoridated water supplies, and lack of transportation to a dental clinic. Many older adults lose their dental insurance when they retire. The situation may be worse for older women, who generally have lower incomes and may never have had dental insurance. Medicaid funds dental care for low-income and disabled older adults in some states, but reimbursements are low. Medicare is not designed to reimburse for routine dental care.

Physical disability or other illness may also limit access to services. At any given time, 5% of Americans 65 years of age and older are living in a long-term care facility (currently some 1.65 million people), where dental care is problematic (U.S. Department of Health and Human Services, 2000). In addition, a lack of public understanding and awareness of the importance of oral health is a major barrier to seeking and obtaining professional oral health.

Altered food choices (such as reduction in dietary fiber, fruits, and vegetables) as a result of reduced chewing ability might be placing persons at increased risk of medical conditions such as atherosclerosis or cancer. A person with reduced chewing ability may overprepare (e.g., removing the skin from fruits and vegetables) or overcook fresh foods in an effort to facilitate consumption.

People who have ill-fitting dentures, those who experience pain while wearing them, and people who need dentures but do not have them are at an increased risk of experiencing malnutrition. Even well-fitting partial dentures may increase a person's risk of developing oral diseases. Patients with removable partial dentures are more likely to have untreated root caries than are patients without partial dentures because of the lack of routine removal and cleaning (Slavkin, 2000).

Oral Health Issues

Older adults are more likely to have chronic conditions that can affect oral health, but they are less likely to visit a dental care provider than are younger adults (Slavkin, 2000). Frail and functionally dependent older adults historically have high levels of oral complications; yet they are even less likely to receive adequate dental care. In a survey of more than 250 functionally dependent adults (44% percent of whom were older than 80 years of age) nearly three fourths reported difficulty in chewing in the previous 4 weeks, one fifth reported oral pain, and more than 70% reported some incident of oral discomfort (Slavkin, 2000). It is thought that many older adults expect their oral health to deteriorate and believe that they must "live with the pain." Health care providers can help dispel these myths and help all people understand that regular visits for oral preventive care can contribute immensely to overall quality of life.

Poor oral health can increase the risk of systemic disease and conditions or may result from systemic diseases. In frail older adults poor oral health increases the risk of developing a respiratory tract infection and may increase the risk of developing pneumonia and other systemic infections. Evidence suggests that oral bacteria can be aspirated into the lungs, leading to pneumonia (Slavkin, 2000). The primary care practitioner plays a critical role in promoting oral health as an integral aspect of overall health.

Expenditures for dental services alone made up 4.7% of the nation's health expenditures in 1998 ($53.8 billion of $1.1 trillion). This figure is underestimated, however, because data are unavailable to determine the extent of expenditures and services provided for craniofacial health by other health providers and institutions (U.S. Department of Health and Human Services, 2000).

Oral Health Conditions
PERIODONTAL (GUM) DISEASE

An estimated 80% of American adults currently have some form of periodontal disease, and 23% of persons 65 to 74 years of age have severe periodontal disease (U.S. Department of Health and Human Services, 2000). Risk factors include smoking, hormonal changes in women, diabetes, stress, medications, poor nutrition, illnesses such as cancer and human immunodeficiency virus (HIV), and genetic susceptibility.

Periodontal diseases range from simple gum inflammation to serious disease that results in major damage to the soft tissue and bone that support the teeth. In worst cases, teeth are lost. Slight gingival recession and minimal degenerative gingival changes are considered a normal part of aging; however, recession in excess of 1 to 2 mm is likely a result of past or present periodontal disease activity.

Periodontal disease is caused by bacteria, mucus, and other particles that combine to form plaque on the teeth. Plaque that is not removed by brushing and flossing can harden and form bacteria-harboring tartar that cannot be removed by brushing. The persistence of the bacteria within the plaque and tartar on the teeth causes inflammation of the gums (gingivitis), which can be reversed by professional cleaning by a dental professional and daily oral care. Gingivitis does not include any loss of bone and tissue that hold teeth in place.

When gingivitis is not treated, it can progress to periodontitis ("inflammation around the tooth"), in which the gums pull away from the teeth and form pockets that are infected. Bacterial toxins and infection fighting enzymes cause deterioration of the bone and connective tissue and, if not treated, lead to loosening and possible loss of teeth.

Patient education should focus on oral hygiene (brushing at least twice daily with a fluoride toothpaste and flossing daily), routine visits to a dental professional, a well-balanced diet, and avoidance of tobacco products.

DENTAL CARIES

The word *caries* comes from the Latin for "rotten." By the twentieth century caries came to describe the condition of having holes in the teeth: cavities. A cavity is actually a late manifestation of a bacterial infection (U.S. Department of Health and Human Services, 2000). The bacteria colonizing the mouth are known as *oral flora*. They adhere to the tooth surfaces, forming a gelatinous mat or "biofilm," commonly called *dental plaque*. A cariogenic biofilm at a single tooth site may contain one-half billion bacteria. These bacteria are able to ferment sugars and other carbohydrates to form lactic and other acids. Repeated cycles of acid generation can result in the microscopic dissolution of minerals in tooth enamel and the formation of an opaque white or brown spot under the enamel surface.

If the caries infection in enamel goes unchecked, the acid dissolution can advance to form a cavity that can extend through the dentin (the component of the tooth located under the enamel) to the pulp tissue, which is rich in nerves and blood vessels. This leads to significant pain, and treatment requires endodontic (root canal) therapy. If untreated, the pulp infection can lead to abscess, destruction of the bone, and spread of the infection via the bloodstream.

Dental caries pose a significant risk to older adults with natural teeth. Everyone is vulnerable to dental caries throughout life, with 85% of adults aged 18 and older affected (U.S. Department of Health and Human Services, 2000). Studies indicate that dental caries is the most significant risk for tooth loss in persons 50 years of age and older (Bray and Williams, 2000).

The gingival tissues tend to recede over time, exposing the tooth root to cariogenic bacteria that can cause root caries. The prevalence of root surface caries increases dramatically among institutionalized or chronically ill individuals (up to 90% prevalence). The increased prevalence is thought to be due to the increase in the number and severity of risk factors, including loss of periodontal attachment, increased use of xerostomic medications, poor oral hygiene levels, and lack of access to preventive dental services.

Caries prevention and therapeutic strategies should focus on plaque control, topical fluoride, dietary counseling, and prevention of gum recession. Literature suggests that root caries be managed as an infection with a combination of an antimicrobial agent (such as 0.12% chlorhexidine) to control the bacteria and topical fluoride to protect exposed root surfaces (Bray and Williams, 2000). Obviously, routine care by a dentist is imperative in the effort to combat tooth decay; however, the primary care provider plays an important role in education and primary prevention. Examinations of older patients should include not only the patient's oral health but also his or her ability to perform oral hygiene (Reynolds, 1997). Patients who have arthritis or other conditions that make it difficult to hold a toothbrush may benefit from a specially adapted toothbrush or strapping the toothbrush to a larger object such as tennis ball. An electric toothbrush may also help.

XEROSTOMIA

Saliva aids in digestion, mastication, oral microbial defense, gustation (taste), lubrication, speech, deglutition (swallowing), and preservation of mineralized and mucosal tissues. These functions are essential for the maintenance of oral and pharyngeal health and a comfortable quality of life. Salivary dysfunction has been associated with an increased rate of caries, fungal infections, dysphagia, dysgeusia (impaired taste), impaired denture use, altered mastication, and sialadenitis (salivary gland infection) (Astor, Hanft, and Ciocon, 1999; Chavez et al, 2000). Dryness of the oral mucosa increases susceptibility to microbial colonization, and infections of the oral cavity can rapidly lead to systemic disease in older, medically compromised patients.

Xerostomia, or dryness of the mouth, is frequently reported in the geriatric population, but evidence is strong that aging itself does not lead to salivary hypofunction (Chavez et al, 2000). Until recently, dry mouth was considered a normal consequence of aging, but now it is known that healthy older adults produce as much saliva as younger adults; however, saliva does seem to undergo chemical changes with aging. For example, as the amount of ptyalin (alpha-amylase) decreases and mucin increases, saliva can become thick and viscous (Astor, Hanft, and Ciocon, 1999).

Xerostomia and salivary gland hypofunction in older adults may be due to an increased prevalence of a variety of medical problems. The inhibition of salivary flow increases the risk for oral disease because saliva contains antimicrobial components as well as minerals that can help rebuild tooth enamel after attack by acid-producing, decay-causing bacteria. The list of causes includes medications, diseases such as Sjögren syndrome, diabetes, radiation therapy or chemotherapy, nerve damage caused by injury to the head and neck, and chronic breathing through the mouth. One of the most common types of causative medications is anticholinergic drugs, such as psychotropic agents, antihistamines, and diuretics.

Symptoms include a sticky, dry feeling in the mouth; difficulty chewing, swallowing, tasting, or speaking; a burning sensation in the mouth; a dry feeling in the throat; cracked lips; a dry, tough tongue; mouth sores; and an infection in the mouth.

Because the treatment for dry mouth depends on what is causing the problem, a careful assessment of possible etiologies is the first step. Medications may be adjusted or changed if they are suspected to be the cause. Artificial saliva products or saliva stimulants such as pilocarpine may be helpful. Patients should be educated to drink plenty of water and to avoid sweets, tobacco, alcohol, caffeine, and acidic beverages. Sour lemon drops and cinnamon- or mint-flavored candies can help to stimulate saliva production. Commercial mouthwashes should be avoided because they can further dry and irritate the mouth. A soft toothbrush should be used and the mouth rinsed with a mild mouthwash such as plain water with salt and baking soda twice a day. A cool-mist humidifier in the bedroom can enhance comfort by adding moisture to the air. In addition, the patient with dry mouth needs to visit a dentist at least twice a year for evaluation and preventive care.

ORAL CANCER

Cancers of the oral cavity are malignancies arising in the lip, tongue, floor of the mouth, gingivae, palate, buccal mucosa or vestibule, and salivary glands. *Pharyngeal cancer* is a term that describes cancers developing in the tonsillar fossa, oropharynx, nasopharynx, and hypopharynx. Nearly 90% of these cancers are carcinomas. Oral and pharyngeal cancers represent about 3% of all cancers in the United States. In 2001, it was estimated that these cancers would account for 30,100 new cases and 7800 deaths. The 5-year relative survival rate is low: 58% for whites and 34% for African-Americans (Silverman, 2001). These numbers have remained relatively unchanged despite advances in surgery and radiation. In addition, for those who survive, there is a large risk of developing a new primary head or neck cancer; this risk varies between 10% and 30%. The risk is greater among smokers (Silverman, 2001). Box 8-1 outlines the primary risk factors for oral and pharyngeal cancers (Silverman, 2001).

Risk factors for oral and pharyngeal cancers include tobacco and alcohol use (which are estimated to account for 75% of these cancers in the United States), exposure to human papillomavirus, and use of marijuana. Age is also a risk factor, with 90% of oral cancers occurring in people older than the age of 45 years (Silverman, 2001). The consumption of fresh fruits and vegetables, however, seems to be associated with a decreased risk of developing these cancers.

Box 8-1

Risk Factors for Oral and Pharyngeal Cancers

Use of any kind of tobacco product
Heavy use of alcohol
Certain viruses (Such as Human Papillomavirus)
Low consumption of fruits and vegetables
Marijuana use
Age Older than 45 yr
Black face
Male sex

From Silverman S: Demographics and occurrence of oral and pharyngeal cancers: the outcomes the trends, the challenge, *J Am. Dental Assoc* 132:75-80, 2001.

Unfortunately, early detection of oral cancers has not improved over three decades. *Early detection* is defined as diagnosis at stage I or II. In these stages the oral tumor does not exceed 4 cm in its largest diameter and has not spread to adjacent structures or tissues; no metastasis has occurred to regional cervical lymph nodes or to other organs.

A comprehensive oral cancer examination takes about 90 seconds and includes a review of the patient's medical and dental history, extraoral and intraoral inspections of the head and neck, and manual palpation of related specific sites. Box 8-2 outlines The World Health Organization's recommended procedure for a comprehensive oral cancer examination (remove all removable prostheses before starting the examination).

DIABETES

Type 2 diabetes is prevalent among older adults and often results in systemic complications such as hypertension, neuropathies, and vascular and renal disease. Older persons with diabetes frequently complain of xerostomia. Multiple physiologic factors could contribute to compromised salivary function in an older adult with poorly controlled diabetes. Diabetes frequently leads to hormonal, microvascular, and neuronal changes as a result of metabolic dysregulation, which often compromises the ability of multiple organ systems to function. It has been suggested that the same pathologic mechanisms underlying diabetes-related organ deterioration might lead to salivary gland hypofunction in the person with poorly controlled diabetes (Chavez et al, 2000).

Oral complications of diabetes can in turn interfere with overall diabetes management, potentially undermining blood glucose control and impairing the chewing of nutritionally appropriate foods. Oral complications typically observed in patients with diabetes include an increased susceptibility to and accelerated onset of periodontal disease, increased caries rate, unusually prolonged fungal and bacterial infections, xerostomia, delayed wound healing, numbness, burning sensations, oral pain, parotid (salivary) gland enlargement, and altered taste sensations (Martin, 1999). Special considerations must be given to the diabetic patient receiving dental care, such as appointment scheduling, dietary intake, stress management, choice of local anesthesia, pain control, oral infections and antibiotic therapy, and diabetic emergency management in the dental office. Again, good communication between the primary health team and the dental care team is essential in ensuring optimal outcome for the patient.

DEMENTIA

The progression of dementia is accompanied by a gradual inability to perform self-care, including adequate oral hygiene, because of self-neglect and a loss of cognitive and motor skills. It has been

Box 8-2

Recommended Procedure for a Comprehensive Oral Cancer Examination

1. The extraoral examination includes inspection of the face, head, and neck. Note any asymmetry or lesions on the skin such as crusts, fissuring, and growths. The regional lymph nodes in the submandibular and neck areas should be palpated to detect any enlarged nodes.
2. Observe the lips with the patient's mouth both closed and open. Note the color, texture, and any surface abnormalities of the vermilion borders.
3. Visually inspect the labial mucosa and sulcus of the maxillary vestibule and frenum as well as the mandibular vestibule. Note the color, texture, and any swelling or other abnormalities.
4. Retract the buccal mucosa, examining both sides for change in pigmentation, color, texture, and other abnormalities. Pay special attention to the commissures.
5. Examine the buccal and labial aspects of the gingival and alveolar ridges by starting with the right maxillary posterior gingiva and alveolar ridge and then move around the arch to the left posterior area. Then examine the left mandibular posterior gingiva and alveolar ridge moving around the arch to the right posterior area. Then examine the palatal and lingual aspects on the maxillary and mandibular aspects.
6. With the patient's tongue at rest and mouth partially open, inspect the dorsum of the tongue for any swelling, ulceration, or variation in size, color, or texture. Ask the patient to protrude the tongue and examine for any abnormality of mobility or positioning. Grasp the tongue with a piece of gauze to assist in full protrusion of the tongue. Use a mouth mirror to assess visually the more posterior aspects of the tongue's lateral borders and to retract the cheek. Run your finger along the lateral borders of the tongue to feel for any hard tissues. Then examine the ventral surface. Palpate the tongue to detect growths.
7. With the tongue still elevated, inspect the floor of the mouth for changes in color, texture, swellings or other surface abnormalities.
8. With the patient's mouth wide open and head tilted back, gently depress the base of the tongue with a mouth mirror. Inspect the hard and soft palates.

Data from the World Health Organization and Alice M. Horowitz, PhD, senior scientist, National Institute of Dental and Craniofacial Research, National Institutes of Health, Building 45, Room 3AN-44B, Bethesda, MD, 20892-6401.

demonstrated that persons with dementia have impaired oral health (gingival plaque, bleeding, calculus and caries) as a result of poor oral hygiene (Ghezzi and Ship, 2000). In addition, dentures tend to be less well maintained. The dental management of these patients requires a great deal of understanding and patience, coupled with background knowledge of the disease and proficiency in providing behavior modification techniques. The five major areas that need to be considered before providing dental care for patients with dementia (or other neurologic impairments) are the presence or absence of pain, presenting dental condition, stage of the disease, the concerns of the caregiver, and the capabilities of the dental professional (Henry, 1999). Specially adapted items and equipment can make the treatment of these patients easier. In addition, sedation may be required to treat the very difficult or late stage Alzheimer's patient who requires dental care.

CRANIAL ARTERITIS

Cranial arteritis (CA) is a vascular disease that affects mostly older adults. CA frequently mimics temporomandibular joint, myofascial, or odontogenic pain; initial symptoms include gradual onset of fatigue, anorexia, weight loss, mental confusion, or depression. Classic symptoms are temporal headaches, scalp tenderness, and jaw claudication (which has been shown to be the strongest predictor of CA) (Kleinegger and Lilly, 1999). CA may coexist with polymyalgia rheumatica, which involves pain and stiffness of the shoulders and pelvic girdle, accompanied by fever, night sweats and malaise. Diagnosis is confirmed by temporal artery biopsy and treatment includes systemic steroids.

ENDOCARDITIS PROPHYLAXIS

Endocarditis is caused by bacteria that adhere to damaged or otherwise receptive surfaces of the endocardium. Dental and other surgical procedures may predispose susceptible patients to infective endocarditis by inducing bacteremias.

Blood-borne bacteria may lodge on damaged or abnormal heart valves or on the endocardium or the endothelium near anatomic defects, resulting in bacterial endocarditis or endarteritis. Although bacteremia is common following many invasive procedures, only certain bacteria commonly cause endocarditis. It is not always possible to predict which patients will develop this infection or which particular procedure will be responsible (Dajani et al, 1997). In addition, bacteremias from oral infections that occur frequently during normal daily activities, coincidental even with chewing food, toothbrushing, and flossing, contribute more substantially to the risk of infective endocarditis (U.S. Department of Health and Human Services, 2000).

Oral organisms are common etiologic agents of infective endocarditis. Infective endocarditis occurs with different incubation periods, which differ in causative bacteria and signs and symptoms. For example, *Staphylococcus aureus* endocarditis may have a rapid onset and fatal course if it affects the left side of the heart. With a more indolent course, patients often are unaware of infection and may experience fever, night chills, myalgia, and arthralgia for a considerable time before diagnosis. The infection is often curable if diagnosed and treated early (U.S. Department of Health and Human Services, 2000).

Persons at highest risk are those who have prosthetic heart valves, a previous history of endocarditis (even in the absence of other heart disease), complex cyanotic congenital heart disease, or surgically constructed systemic pulmonary shunts or conduits. These patients are at a much higher risk for developing severe endocardial infection, which is often associated with high morbidity and mortality rates.

Persons with certain other underlying cardiac defects are at moderate risk for severe infection. Congenital cardiac conditions listed in the moderate-risk category include the following uncorrected conditions: patent ductus arteriosus, ventricular septal defect, primum atrial septal defect, coarctation of the aorta, and bicuspid aortic valve. Acquired valvular dysfunction (e.g., due to rheumatic heart disease or collagen vascular disease) and hypertrophic cardiomyopathy are also moderate-risk conditions. See Table 8-1 for recommendations for prophylaxis (Dajani et al, 1997).

Mitral valve prolapse (MVP) is common, and the need for prophylaxis for this condition is controversial. Only a small percentage of patients with documented MVP develop complications at any age (Dajani et al, 1997). Mitral valve prolapse represents a spectrum of valvular changes and clinical behavior. Patients with prolapsing and leaking mitral valves, evidenced by audible clicks and murmurs of mitral regurgitation or by Doppler-demonstrated mitral insufficiency, should receive prophylactic antibiotics. In patients of any age, myxomatous mitral valve degeneration with regurgitation is an indication for antibiotic prophylaxis. See Figure 8-1 for a suggested approach to the determination of the need for prophylaxis for patients with suspected MVP (Dajani, 1997).

Antibiotic prophylaxis for at-risk patients is recommended for dental and oral procedures likely to cause bacteremia (Table 8-2). In general, prophylaxis is recommended for procedures associated with significant bleeding from hard or soft tissues, periodontal surgery, scaling, and professional teeth cleaning.

Edentulous patients may develop bacteremia from ulcers caused by ill-fitting dentures. Denture wearers should be encouraged to have periodic examination or to return to the practitioner if discomfort develops. If a series of dental procedures is required, it may be prudent to observe an interval between procedures both to reduce the potential for the emergence of resistant organisms and to allow repopulation of the mouth with antibiotic susceptible flora. Various studies have suggested an interval of 9 to 14 days. If possible, a combination of procedures should be planned within the

TABLE 8-1	Cardiac Conditions Associated with Endocarditis

Endocarditis Prophylaxis Recommended	*Endocarditis Prophylaxis Not Recommended*

High-risk category
  Prosthetic cardiac valves, including
    bioprosthetic and homograft valves
  Previous bacterial endocarditis
  Complex cyanotic congenital heart disease
    (e.g., single ventricle states, transposition of
    the great arteries, tetralogy of Fallot)
  Surgically constructed systemic pulmonary
    shunts or conduits
Moderate-risk category
  Most other congenital cardiac malformations
    (other than above and below)
  Acquired valvar dysfunction (e.g., rheumatic
    heart disease)
  Hypertrophic cardiomyopathy
  Mitral valve prolapse with valvar regurgitation
    or thickened leaflets
	Negligible-risk category (no greater risk than
	  the general population)
	  Isolated secundum atrial septal defect
	  Surgical repair of atrial septal defect, ventricular
	    septal defect, or patent ductus arteriosus
	    (without residua beyond 6 mo)
	  Previous coronary artery bypass graft surgery
	  Mitral valve prolapse without valvar regurgitation
	  Physiologic, functional, or innocent heart murmurs
	  Previous Kawasaki disease without valvular
	    dysfunction
	  Previous rheumatic fever without valvular
	    dysfunction
	  Cardiac pacemakers (intravascular and
	    epicardial) and implanted defibrillators

From Dajani A et al: Prevention of bacterial endocarditis: recommendations by the American Heart Association, *JAMA* 277(22): 1794-1801, 1997.

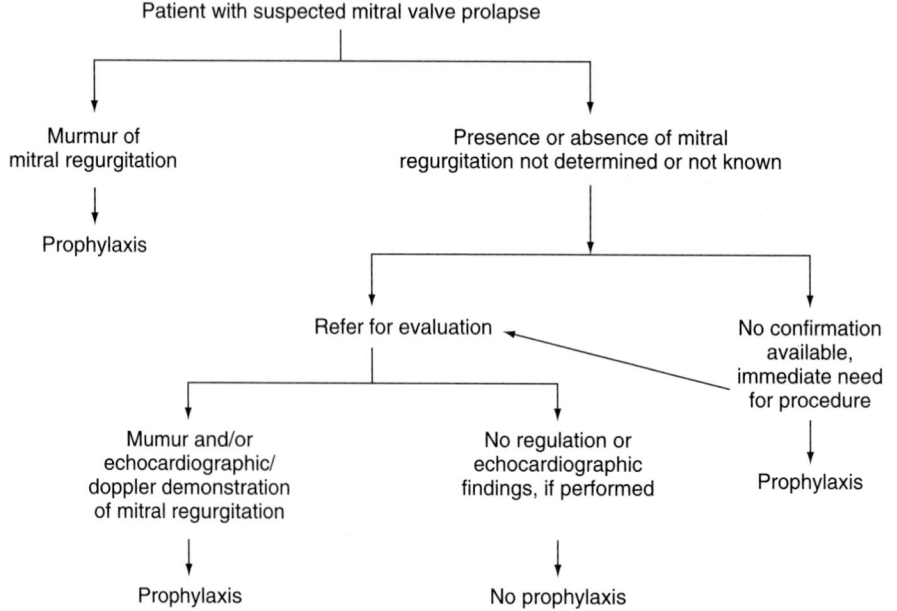

Figure 8-1   Clinical approach to determination of the need for prophylaxis for patients with suspected mitral valve prolapse. (From Dajani A et al: Prevention of bacterial endocarditis: recommendations by the American Heart Association, *JAMA* 277(22):1794-1801, 1997.)

same period of prophylaxis (Dajani et al, 1997). See Table 8-3 for recommended prophylactic regimens (Dajani et al, 1997).

Oral-Facial Pain

Oral-facial pain can greatly reduce quality of life and restrict major functions. Pain is a common symptom for many of the conditions affecting oral-facial structures. Dental pain is among the most prevalent of all pain complaints, and pain is frequently given as a common reason for both avoiding and seeking dental care. Pain is frequently an essential component in the differential diagnosis of many diseases; however, in older adults, diagnosis is more difficult because of the greater frequency of multiple chronic diseases and an altered pain response (Cox, 2000). A variety of painful oral syndromes that occur in the older adult include aphthous ulcers, herpes zoster, toothache pain, burning mouth syndrome, and trigeminal neuralgia (Table 8-4). As with other types of pain, the assessment may include pain scales or open- and closed-ended questions regarding the pain. Careful and appropriate but adequate use of analgesics is often necessary.

APHTHOUS ULCERS

Recurrent aphthous ulcers (RAU) or recurrent aphthous stomatitis, more commonly known as *canker sores,* is the most common mild oral mucosal disease. Between 5% and 25% of the general population is affected. The disease takes three clinical forms: RAU minor, RAU major, and herpetiform RAU. The minor form accounts for 70% to 87% of cases. The sores are small, discrete, shallow ulcers surrounded by an erythematous halo appearing at the front of the mouth or the tongue.

TABLE 8-2	**Dental Procedures and Endocarditis Prophylaxis**

*Endocarditis Prophylaxis Recommended**	*Endocarditis Prophylaxis Not Recommended*

Dental extractions
  Periodontal procedures including
  surgery, scaling and root planing, probing, and
  recall maintenance
Dental implant placement and reimplantation
  of avulsed teeth
Endodontic (root canal) instrumentation or
  surgery only beyond the apex
Subgingival placement of antibiotic
  fibers or strips
Initial placement of orthodontic bands
  but not brackets
Intraligamentary local anesthetic injections
Prophylactic cleaning of teeth or implants
  where bleeding is anticipated
	Restorative dentistry[†] (operative and
	  prosthodontic) with or without retraction cord[‡]
	Local anesthetic injections (nonintraligamentary)
	Intracanal endodontic treatment; post placement
	  and buildup
	Placement of rubber dams
	Postoperative suture removal
	Placement of removable prosthodontic or
	  orthodontic appliances
	Taking of oral impressions
	Fluoride treatments
	Taking of oral radiographs
	Orthodontic appliance adjustment
	Shedding of primary teeth

*Prophylaxis is recommended for patients with high- and moderate-risk cardiac conditions.
[†]This includes restoration of decayed teeth (filling cavities) and replacement of missing teeth.
[‡]Clinical judgment may indicate antibiotic use in selected circumstances that may create significant bleeding.
From: Dajani A et al: Prevention of bacterial endocarditis: recommendations by the American Heart Association, *JAMA* 277(22): 1794-1801, 1997.

TABLE 8-3	Prophylactic Regimens for Dental, Oral, Respiratory Tract, or Esophageal Procedures	
Situation	**Agent**	**Regimen***
Standard general prophylaxis	Amoxicillin	Adults: 2.0 g; children: 50 mg/kg orally 1 h before procedure
Unable to take oral medications	Ampicillin	Adults: 2.0 g intramuscularly (IM) or intravenously (IV); children: 50 mg/kg IM or IV within 30 min before procedure
Allergic to penicillin	Clindamycin *or*	Adults: 600 mg; children: 20 mg/kg orally 1 h before procedure
	Cephalexin[†] or cefadroxil[†] *or*	Adults: 2.0 g; children; 50 mg/kg orally 1 h before procedure
	Azithromycin or clarithromycin	Adults: 500 mg; children: 15 mg/kg orally 1 h before procedure
Allergic to penicillin and unable to take oral medications	Clindamycin *or*	Adults: 600 mg; children: 20 mg/kg IV within 30 min before procedure
	Cefazolin[†]	Adults: 1.0 g; children: 25 mg/kg IM or IV within 30 min before procedure

From Dajani A et al: Prevention of bacterial endocarditis: recommendations by the American Heart Association, *JAMA* 277(22): 1794-1801, 1997.
*Total children's dose should not exceed adult dose.
†Cephalosporins should not be used in individuals with immediate-type hypersensitivity reaction (urticaria, angioedema, or anaphylaxis) to penicillins.

The ulcers, which usually last up to 2 weeks, are painful and may make eating or speaking difficult. About half of patients experience recurrences every 1 to 3 months; as many as 30% report continuous recurrences (U.S. Department of Health and Human Services, 2000). RAU major accounts for 7% to 20% of cases and usually appears as 1 to 10 larger coalescent ulcers at a time, which can persist for weeks to months. Herpetiform RAU occurs in 7% to 10% of RAU cases. These ulcers

TABLE 8-4	Estimated Number of U.S. Adults with > 1 episode of Orofacial Pain Within the Past 6 Months		
Entity	**No. per 100,000**	**Rate (%)**	**Estimated No. in Population**
Oral sores	15,066	8.4	9,648,000
Jaw joint pain	9,465	5.3	4,364,000
Face pain	2,541	1.4	593,000
Burning mouth	1,270	0.7	303,000
Combination of above	4,518	2.6	1,101,000
Totals	32,860	18.4	16,009,000

From Miller CS et al: Changing oral care needs in the United States: the continuing need for oral medicine, *Oral Surg Oral Med Oral Pathol Oral Radiol Endod* 91(1): 34-44, 2001.

appear in crops of 10 to 100 at a time, concentrating at the back of the mouth and lasting for 7 to 14 days (U.S. Department of Health and Human Services, 2000).

An association has been made between RAU and genetics as well as with hypersensitivities to some foods, food dyes, and food preservatives. Nutritional deficiencies—especially iron, folic acid, and various B vitamins—have also been reported, and the condition may improve with suitable dietary supplements. The most strongly associated factors, however, are immunologic abnormalities and trauma. RAU can also occur in a number of systemic diseases, including HIV infection, ulcerative colitis, Crohn's disease, and Behçet disease (U.S. Department of Health and Human Services, 2000).

Although RAU does not cause other illnesses, it is uncomfortable. Symptomatic treatment includes analgesics, antibacterial rinses, and topical corticosteroids. Dentists may prescribe other medications (oral corticosteroids, Aphthasol, Levamisole) to help to reduce pain and healing time (U.S. Department of Health and Human Services, 2000).

HERPES ZOSTER

Herpes zoster (HZ), caused by reactivation of the varicella-zoster virus, can affect the cheek, tongue, gingiva or palate. HZ of the maxillary division of the trigeminal nerve causes vesicles of the uvula and tonsillar area. Involvement of the mandibular branch produces vesicles on the floor of the mouth, buccal membranes, and the anterior part of the tongue. This condition can be very painful both during and after the occurrence, with postherpetic neuralgia being a common sequela. Older persons generally suffer more acute pain and experience a longer course. Chapter 6 discusses the diagnosis and management of acute HZ.

Postherpetic neuralgia (PHN) is pain that persists after the rash has resolved. Studies have found the pain symptoms last about 8 weeks for 45% of patients and less than a year in 78% of cases. In 22% of patients, however, PHN continued for longer than a year and, in some cases, as long as 20 years. The average age of persons with PHN is 67 years (Lee and Simpkins, 2000).

The most commonly used medications for the management of PHN are various tricyclic antidepressants, such as amitriptyline or desipramine, or anticonvulsants carbamazepine (Tegretol) and gabapentin (Neurontin). The use of narcotics for chronic neuropathic pain is somewhat controversial because of unclear effectiveness and the risk of dependency. Numerous other interventions are sometimes helpful. Transcutaneous electrical nerve stimulation, regional nerve blocks, cold packs, and acupuncture all have been used successfully in some patients.

Because PHN is predominately a problem for older persons, the choice of therapies often is complicated by coexisting medical conditions, interactions with other medications, and underlying frailty. An individualized approach is important.

TRIGEMINAL NEURALGIA

Tic douloureux, or trigeminal neuralgia, is a painful disease of unknown etiology, which generally occurs in later life (although it may occur earlier in patients with multiple sclerosis). The condition affects one, two, or all three branches of the trigeminal nerve. The pain is highly intense and stabbing in nature, with attacks that occur every few minutes or several hours. Sometimes no precipitating factor is found, or it may occur in response to a gentle touch or a soft breeze. This condition, allodynia, is a feeling of pain in response to a normally nonpainful stimulus. At times, however, a specific trigger zone is found. Spontaneous remissions may last weeks or months but are rarely permanent, often leading to an overwhelming fear of recurrent pain (U.S. Department of Health and Human Services, 2000).

Medical treatment of trigeminal neuralgia primarily consists of carbamazepine (Tegretol). Chronic or severe sufferers should be referred to a neurologist for further evaluation. Surgical removal of a small vein or artery that may be exerting pressure on the nerve root or the selective destruction of the nerve fibers using chemical or electrical methods often provides permanent relief.

Medication Issues

Most older Americans take both prescription and over-the-counter drugs. In all probability, at least one of the medications will have an oral side effect, usually dry mouth. Table 8-5 identifies the percent of people taking drugs by age and dental implication (Miller et al, 2001). Persons in long-term care facilities are prescribed an average of eight drugs (U.S. Department of Health and Human Services, 2000).

It is critical that the dental provider be informed of all medications that the older patient is taking, both prescribed and over-the-counter medications. Patient should be encouraged to carry a current, written list of all medications and to share this with all medical and dental providers. Otherwise, the primary care provider should contact the dentist directly to discuss medications as well as medical conditions that can impact dental care. This facilitates preparation for potential complications in the dental office (Paunovich, Sadowsky, and Carter, 1997).

Special Concerns for Older Women

In the course of aging, significant numbers of women experience compromised functional status, physical confinement, medical conditions, and cognitive impairments. These factors place women's oral health at risk while also limiting a woman's ability to maintain oral hygiene self-care regimens, seek professional dental services, and tolerate dental treatment (U.S. Department of Health and Human Services, 2000).

Women who are menopausal or postmenopausal may experience changes in their mouths, especially as a result of loss of bone and structural tissues in the jaw. Estrogen deficiency could place postmenopausal women at higher risk for severe periodontal disease and tooth loss (U.S. Department of Health and Human Services, 2000). Hormonal changes in older women may result in discomfort in the mouth, including dry mouth, pain and burning sensations in the gum tissue, and altered taste, especially salty, peppery, or sour. In addition, osteoporosis may lead to tooth loss when the density of the bone that supports the teeth is decreased.

Issues Surrounding Anesthesia

Oral sedatives and nitrous oxide analgesia are frequently and successfully used for dental treatments in medically, behaviorally, cognitively, and physically impaired older adults. Many compromised older adults, however, cannot safely tolerate dental treatment with these sedative techniques in an

---

TABLE 8-5	Percent of People in the United States Who Take Prescription Medication by Age and Dental Implications, 1980				

		Age (yr)			
Drug Type	Dental Effect	<25	25-44	45-64	65+
Class I*	Direct	22%	31%	44%	47%
Class II†	Indirect	44%	43%	37%	34%
Class III	No effect	34%	24%	18%	19%

From Miller CS et al: Changing oral care needs in the United States: the continuing need for oral medicine, *Oral Surg Oral Med Oral Pathol Oral Radiol Endod* 91(1):34-44, 2001.
*Includes such drugs as antihistamines, tricyclics, and phenothiazines.
†Includes such drugs as coumadin and steroids.

outpatient setting. Coordinated with medical and anesthesia specialists, general anesthesia is a viable, safe, and effective treatment tool for providing comprehensive dental and oral surgical treatment for the older patient. Not every older adult is eligible, however, usually because of underlying medical conditions. Therefore a careful assessment including medical, dental, nutritional, social, and behavioral factors must be performed by an interdisciplinary health care team, and the patient must satisfy acceptance criteria for general anesthesia (Ghezzi Chavez, and Ship, 2000).

Summary

Oral health has evolved from a narrow focus on teeth and gingiva to the recognition that the mouth is the center of vital tissues and functions that are critical to total health and well-being across the life span. The mouth is a mirror of health or disease, a sentinel or early warning system, and a potential source of pathology affecting other systems and organs (U.S. Department of Health and Human Services, 2000). Most changes in oral health in the older population are consequences of comorbid conditions, pharmacotherapy, functional disabilities, or cognitive impairment and their results: reduced self-care, reduced access to preventive services, or both (Slavkin, 2000). The primary care provider plays a critical role in educating patients about preventive practices and ensuring that all persons receive timely and appropriate professional dental care.

Resources

National Institute of Dental and Craniofacial Research
www.nidr.nih.gov

National Oral Health Information Clearinghouse Web Site
www.nohic.nidr.nih.gov

References

Astor FC, Hanft KL, Ciocon JO: Xerostomia: a prevalent condition in the elderly, *Ear Nose Throat J* 78(7): 476-479, 1999.
Bray KK, Williams K: Epidemiology of oral diseases in older adults, *Periospective, Oral-B Laboratories,* Chicago, 2000, ADHA.
Chavez EM et al: Salivary function and glycemic control in older persons with diabetes, *Oral surg Oral Med Oral Pathol Oral Radiol Endod* 89(3):305-311, 2000.
Cox MO: Issues and challenges of orofacial pain in the elderly, *Special Care in Dentistry* 20(6):245-249, 2000.
Dajani A et al: Prevention of bacterial endocarditis: recommendations by the American Heart Association, JAMA 277(22):1794-1801, 1997.
Ghezzi EM, Chavez EM, Ship JA: General anesthesia protocol for the dental patient: emphasis for older adults, *Special Care in Dentistry* 20(3):81-108, 2000.
Ghezzi EM, Ship JA: Dementia and oral health, *Oral Surg Oral Med Oral Pathol Oral Radiol Endod* 89(1):2-5, 2000.
Henry RG: Alzheimer's disease and cognitively impaired elderly: providing dental care, *J California Dent Assoc* 27(9):709-717, 1999.
Horowitz AM: Perform a death-defying act: the 90-second oral cancer examination, *J Am Dent Assoc* 132, S36-40, 2001.
Kleinegger CL, Lilly GE: Cranial arteritis: a medical emergency with orofacial manifestations, *J Am Dent Assoc* 130(8):1203-1209, 1999.
Lee VK, Simpkins L: Herpes zoster and postherpetic neuralgia in the elderly, *Geriatric Nursing* 21(3):132-136, 2000
Martin WE: Oral health and the older diabetic, *Clin Geriatr Med* 15(2):339-350, 1999.
Miller CS et al: Changing oral care needs in the United States: the continuing need for oral medicine, Oral Sur *Oral Med Oral Pathol Oral Radiol Endod* 91(1):34-44, 2001.

Paunovich ED, Sadowsky JM, Carter P: Most frequently prescribed medications in the elderly and their impact on dental treatment, *Dental Clin North Am* 41(4):699-726, 1997.

Reynolds MW: Education for geriatric oral health promotion, *Special Care in Dentistry* 17(1):33-36, 1997.

Silverman S: Demographics and occurrence of oral and pharyngeal cancers: the outcomes, the trends, the challenge, *J Am Dental Assoc* 132:75-80, 2001.

Slavkin HD: Maturity and oral health: live longer and better, *J Am Dent Assoc* 131:805-808, 2000.

U.S. Department of Health and Human Services: Oral health in America: a report of the Surgeon General—executive summary. Rockville, MD, 2000, U.S. Department of Health and Human Services, National Institute of Dental and Craniofacial Research, National Institutes of Health.

9

Sensory Impairment

VISION

Vision is an amazing process that happens so quickly and easily that many take it for granted until it is threatened by the slow but predictable process of aging. Vision impairment is one of the most dreaded disabilities because the quality of life is significantly threatened. *Vision impairment* is defined as 20/40 or worse in the better eye with glasses. *Legal blindness* is an artificial designation that defines eligibility for federal-government benefits, typically defined as visual acuity with the best correction in the better eye worse or equal to 20/200 or a visual-field extent of less than 20 degrees in diameter. An estimated 3.5 million Americans have visual impairments and one million have blindness. Corrective eyewear with either glasses or contact lens or both is used by 150 million Americans at a cost of 150 billion dollars per year (National Eye Institute and Prevent Blindness America [NEI/PBA], 2002).

The prevalence of vision impairment increases with age. Seventeen percent (3.1 million) of Americans 65 to 69 years of age report some form of vision impairment, as do 26% (4.3 million) of those 75 years of age and older (Lighthouse International, 2002). The leading causes of blindness in the United States are cataracts, diabetic retinopathy, glaucoma, and macular degeneration. The primary care practitioner is in an excellent position to institute early intervention and rehabilitation because many older people with vision impairment have conditions that are amenable to treatment.

Age-related Changes

External changes result from a loss of orbital fat, a loss of elastic tissue, and decreases in muscle tone. The primary result is lid laxity, which can lead to senile *entropion* (a condition in which the lid margin turns inward) or senile *ectropion* (a condition in which the eyelid margin turns outward).

Other age-related changes of the eye include the following:

- Xanthomas, cutaneous deposits of lipid material, sometimes appear at the inner portion of the lid; they may indicate elevated blood lipid levels.
- Arcus senilis, a gray-yellow ring around the iris, may begin on the upper portion of the eye and develop until the entire iris is encircled. It is caused by a fatty invasion of the corneal margin, which blurs demarcation between the cornea and the sclera. It is common but has no known pathologic or functional implications.

- Tear viscosity and production decrease, which predisposes the eye to infections of the conjunctiva.
- The cornea tends to flatten, which reduces its refractory power and limits its protective function.
- The sclera tends to take on a yellow coloration because of fatty deposits.
- The pupil becomes smaller, and the response to different levels of illumination is lessened because of the loss of range of pupil dilation and constriction.
- The retina receives only one third the amount of light, which necessitates a higher level of illumination for reading.
- The lens increases in density and elasticity, which leads to impairment in accommodation; therefore glare increases as a severe adaptive problem for older people.
- Decreased contrast sensitivity and increased sensitivity to glare increase impairments in driving and detailed near-vision tasks.
- Adaptation to dark occurs more slowly and to a lesser total extent.
- Color perception, especially the blue-green distinctions, becomes more difficult.
- *Floaters,* opacities occurring in the vitreous humor, may appear in the older person's field of vision. Although floaters can be considered a normal process of the aging eye, they may be a harbinger of a serious problem in some instances, such as retinal detachment. Therefore the patient should see an ophthalmologist if floaters are observed (Burke, 1997).

Conditions Affecting Vision

REFRACTIVE ERRORS

Blurred vision is a common problem for older persons experiencing visual problems. Many times this complaint is the result of ineffective glasses or contact lenses. At times the transient problem may be caused by erratic control of diabetes or an adverse response to a drug, such as a motion sickness patch of scopolamine. Treatment is focused on the causal agent and on referral to an ophthalmologist if appropriate (Riordan-Eva and Vaughan, 1997).

Laser in situ keratomileusis (LASIK) refractive surgery is a relatively new technology that has become the subject of intense commercialization. The benefits of the procedure are emphasized to the exclusion of the significant risks. At times patients seek advice from their primary care practitioner. At present we recommend extreme caution; the risks to intact vision are not to be minimized. It is prudent for health care providers to read current professional literature to provide appropriate information to their patients (Melki and Azar, 2001).

KERATOCONJUNCTIVITIS SICCA (DRY EYES)

Complaints of dryness, redness, or a scratchy feeling of the eyes are usual in mild cases of dry eyes; marked discomfort with photophobia and excessive secretions of mucus accompany severe cases. This condition occurs primarily in older adults because of the age-related loss of tear production and viscosity. Other causes to consider are systemic disease (autoimmune conditions), drugs, and environmental factors (hot climates or high winds). Treatment depends on cause. Tear deficiency can be treated with artificial tears. Most preparations have no side effects and can be used three or four times a day or more often if the patient finds them helpful. If the condition worsens after treatment, it is prudent to refer to an ophthalmologist.

CATARACTS

The risk factors for development of cataracts are advanced age, female gender, sunlight exposure, brown irides, myopia, cigarette smoking, alcohol intake, diabetes (McCarty, 2002). The World Health Organization (WHO) reports cataracts as the leading cause of blindness in the world, but in the United States cataracts are considered a conquered disease, although some citizens still do not have access to treatment. The cost of surgical treatment for the Medicare program is 3.4 billion dollars each year (NEI/PBA, 2002).

History

The process of lens opacification develops over time, with formation of the cataract beginning at the periphery of the eye.

- Diminished ability to see detail because of a reduction in the amount of light available to the retina
- Increased difficulty adjusting to glare
- Significant problems in adjusting between light and dark environments, creating a major safety problem
- Blurred vision that is progressive over time
- No report of pain or redness
- Screening for all unusual problems, which includes asking the questions listed in Box 9-1

Focused Physical Examination

- As the cataract matures, the retina becomes increasingly difficult to visualize.

Treatment

Referral to Ophthalmologist. When cataracts interfere significantly with vision and with the patient's quality of life, surgery may be appropriate. Lens extraction surgery improves visual acuity in 95% of patients (Riordan-Eva and Vaughan, 1997).

Health Promotion

- Risk-reduction education
- Decision-making consultation, with the following factors for review:
  Degree of correctable visual acuity in each eye
  Physical and psychological ability to withstand the stress of the surgery
  Type of work or leisure activities
  Social support system available to provide immediate monitoring and care, if necessary
- Dark sunglasses to protect from glare
- Visual rehabilitation (Box 9-2)

Box 9-1

Screening for Visual Problems

1. What is different now about your vision?
2. When did you last see an ophthalmologist about your vision?
3. When was the last time the prescription for your glasses was changed?
4. When did you last purchase glasses? (Providers need to consider that Medicare does not reimburse patients for their purchase of prescribed glasses.)
5. Are you experiencing any difficulty in driving or watching television?
6. Are you experiencing any difficulty in seeing at night?
7. Do you see rings around lights?
8. Is your vision blurred?
9. Have you changed any of your activities because of your vision?
10. Have you experienced loss of vision in one eye?
11. Have you experienced lack of tears or any minor irritations of your eyes?
12. Have you experienced eye pain?
13. Have you taken any medicines or other treatments to correct any eye problem you have experienced?
14. Are you concerned about your vision?
15. Is there anything else you can tell me about your vision?

Glaucoma

Glaucoma is caused by a gradual degeneration of cells that make up the optic nerve; as nerve cells die vision is slowly lost. The cause of this change is uncertain. Risk factors for glaucoma include increased age, race, positive family history, eye trauma, and long use of steroid medication (Gordon et al, 2002; NEI/PBA, 2002). Black Americans are affected four to five times more frequently than are white Americans (Coleman and Brigatti, 2001).

The triad of signs that characterize the disease is elevated intraocular pressure, optic disc cupping, and visual field loss. Two of the three signs are necessary for a diagnosis (NEI/PBA, 2002). The two major types of glaucoma are *primary open-angle glaucoma,* which occurs in people over 40 years of age and constitutes 90% of glaucoma cases, and *acute (angle-closure) glaucoma.* Glaucoma is a treatable disease, but left untreated it will lead to blindness. Treatment slows the decline in vision but does not restore any vision that has been lost (Coleman and Brigatti, 2001). About 2.2 million Americans, or 1.9% of the population, are affected with glaucoma.

Primary Open-angle Glaucoma
HISTORY

- Insidious onset without symptoms in early stages
- Peripheral visual loss in late stages
- Halo effect around lights
- Risk factors: increased age, first-degree family history, and steroid therapy

FOCUSED PHYSICAL EXAMINATION

- Slight cupping of optic disc
- Gradual constriction of visual fields

OPHTHALMOLOGIST EXAMINATION

- Testing for an increase in intraocular pressure
- Visualization of optic nerve for damage
- Testing of central and visual field

TREATMENT

- Medications
  Eyedrops
  Beta-blockers (e.g., timolol) should not be used for patients with heart failure or reactive airway disease.
  Parasympathomimetics (pilocarpine) and epinephrine must be used carefully with cataracts because vision may be constricted.
- Laser treatment and surgery are used to lower intraocular pressure (NEI&PBA, 2002).

HEALTH PROMOTION

- Recommendation of an annual examination by an ophthalmologist if the patient is at risk for glaucoma
- Follow-up on adherence to eye-drop schedule and monitoring for side effects
- Visual rehabilitation (Box 9-2)

Acute (Angle-Closure) Glaucoma
HISTORY

Acute glaucoma presents in older adults as follows:
- Rapid onset of severe pain and loss of vision
- Possible nausea and vomiting

FOCUSED PHYSICAL EXAMINATION

- Eye is red.
- Cornea is steamy.
- Pupil may be dilated and nonreactive to light.

TREATMENT

- Medical emergency
- Referral to an ophthalmologist
- Possibility of severe vision loss in 2 to 5 days if left untreated

Age-related Macular Degeneration (AMD)

Age-related macular degeneration (AMD) is a condition that occurs over time and leads to a loss of central vision. About 1.6 million Americans are afflicted with AMD, one of the most common causes of legal blindness in older adults (NEI/PBA, 2002). Risk factors supported by scientific measures are advanced age (i.e., 70 years of age; most patients are over 80 years of age), genetic makeup, white race, and cigarette smoking. Risk factors that need further evidence are alcohol consumption, estrogen replacement therapy, and lifetime exposure to light (Evans, 2001; la Cour, Kiilgaard, Nissen, 2002). The two types of AMD are dry AMD (nonexudative), which constitutes 90% of cases, and wet AMD (exudative).

Dry

Dry AMD is the most common type of AMD. The causative factor found early in the disease is the presence of drusen fatty deposits under light-sensing cells in the retina. Late development may also be caused by atrophy of the supporting layer, causing further deterioration of the light-sensing cells of the retina. Vision loss early in the disease is usually moderate and progresses slowly. Significant loss can result.

Wet

Wet AMD is less common than dry AMD, but it is more threatening to vision. The causative factor is the growth of tiny new blood vessels under the retina that leak fluid that distorts vision and causes scar tissue.

HISTORY

It is most important for the primary care practitioner to ask older patients (especially those over 75 years of age) if they have encountered any vision changes, such as the following:
- Gradual progressive bilateral loss: dry AMD
- Rapid onset of greater severity of loss, with eyes affected sequentially: Wet AMD
- Distortion of the center of the visual field (the usual first symptom)
- Deficits in form recognition and light sensitivity

TREATMENT

Referral to an ophthalmologist is essential, and the importance of having the patient seen as quickly as possible needs to be stressed. No generally accepted treatment modality for dry AMD exists at present. Laser therapy to destroy leaking blood vessels can help to reduce the risk of loss of vision in some cases of wet AMD. Bressler, of Johns Hopkins Medical School, reported on vertiform therapy, a new treatment option for neovascular AMD. This treatment involves photodynamic therapy, which was recently shown to be relatively safe and effective in reducing the risk of vision loss in selected cases (Bressler, 2002).

The use of antioxidants and mineral supplements was postulated to prevent cellular damage to the retina by reacting with harmful free radicals. Evans, in a review of the extant research literature, found no evidence that patients with early signs of the disease should take supplements (Evans, 2002). Furthermore, in two randomized placebo-controlled studies, one with a supplement of vitamin E only and the other with high-dose supplements of vitamin C, E, and beta carotene, reported that each treatment arm found no evidence for any effect either in the development or prevention of progression of early or late-stage AMD (Age-Related Eye Disease Study Research, 2001; Taylor et al, 2002).

HEALTH PROMOTION

- Education on progression of disease
- Visual rehabilitation: central field magnification to minimize loss; peripheral vision remains intact

Diabetic Retinopathy

Diabetic retinopathy is a complication of diabetes. According to the Centers for Disease Control and Prevention, about 10.3 million diagnosed diabetic patients and an estimated five million undiagnosed persons with diabetes are currently living in the United States. The longer a person has the disease, the more likely it is that he or she will develop diabetic retinopathy (NEI/PBA, 2002), which occurs at a rate of 7% in persons who have had diabetes for less than 10 years, 26% in those who have had diabetes for 10 to 14 years, and 63% in those who have had diabetes for at least 15 years (Infield and O'Shea, 1998). Progression of the diabetes affects the tiny blood vessels of the retina, and these retinal blood vessels break down, leak, or become blocked, thereby impairing vision over time. Yearly dilated fundus examination by an eye specialist along with aggressive control of blood glucose and blood pressure combined with aggressive use of laser photocoagulation can prevent or slow the progression of vision loss from diabetes (Skyler, 2001).

HISTORY

- Transient blurring
- Significant shifts in vision

FOCUSED PHYSICAL EXAMINATION
- Funduscopic examination: small, irregular hemorrhages and yellow-white exudates in retina

TREATMENT
- Optimal control of blood glucose
- Laser photocoagulation

HEALTH PROMOTION
- Annual ophthalmology examination
- Education by diabetic educator if possible
- Visual rehabilitation (Box 9-2)

Visual-acuity Screening

SNELLEN CHART

Each line of the Snellen chart is marked with a fraction (i.e., 20/20, 20/30, 20/40, up to 20/200). Visual acuity is recorded as a fraction, with the numerator 20 indicating the distance of the patient from the chart. The distance at which a person with normal vision would see the line is the number assigned to the denominator. This is the significant number because it indicates the degree of vision loss. The higher the denominator, the more impaired the vision.

In situations such as bedside evaluation in a nursing home, in which no Snellen chart is available or the patient is unable to cooperate, a suggested method to test gross vision is as follows: Ask the patient to count the number of fingers held up within his or her field of vision; test each eye separately. After checking the patient's literacy level, have the patient read from printed material such as a newspaper. This allows assessment of the ability to read different sizes of type, such as headlines, headings, and regular newspaper print. In addition, ask the patient to describe your appearance (what color is my shirt?). This assessment provides a rough estimate of visual acuity and is readily available at all times and in all settings (Burke, 1997).

HEARING

The prevalence of hearing impairments in the older population in the United States is significant but not universal:
- People 65 to 74 years of age: 25% have hearing loss
- People 75 to 84 years of age: 39% have hearing loss
- People 85 years of age and older: 65% have hearing loss
- Nursing home residents: 70% have hearing loss

For too many older people, a hearing loss goes unrecognized by the older person and undetected by primary care practitioners, which leads to an unnecessary loss of self-confidence and quality of life for the older patient. For a large majority of patients, the hearing loss can be corrected or at least ameliorated. Not addressing the problem is an unethical professional practice.

Age-related Changes

As with many conditions ascribed to aging, age-related hearing loss is multifactorial in nature. In both men and women of advanced age (i.e., 80 years of age and older) it is associated with rapidly deteriorating auditory function (Martini et al, 2001; Megighian, 2000). Some causes of hearing loss attributable to aging are due in part to a loss of cochlear hair cell function; severe hearing loss is generally due to cochlear hair loss combined with age-related diseases (Gates and Rees, 1997). Exposure to occupational or leisure activities that include loud noise as a frequent and continued aspect of the activity are associated with significant hearing loss (Dalton et al, 2001). Primary practitioners need to assess past and present history of the older person to understand present loss and to prevent further loss. Two aspects of hearing are affected by biologic aging:

- Loss of high-frequency sensitivity
- Reduction in ability to understand speech

The loss is insidious. Most patients do not report hearing loss but instead complain of not being able to understand what was said. Contributing factors to hearing loss in older adults include the following:

- Cerumen impaction
- Otosclerosis, otitis media, head trauma
- Disease: Paget, Ménière, acoustic neuroma
- Intense noise exposure
- Certain ototoxic drugs
- Salicylates
- Aminoglycosides
- Vancomycin
- Furosemide
- Cisplatin

Classification of Hearing Impairments
PRESBYCUSIS

Associated with normal aging, presbycusis includes the following:
- Impairment for high-frequency tones
- Impairment of frequency discrimination
- Impairment of sound localization
- Impairment of speech discrimination

TINNITUS

Tinnitus is a continuous or intermittent sound that is not attributable to external sources. It is a common symptom that accompanies hearing loss.

CONDUCTIVE HEARING LOSS

With conductive hearing loss, normal sound waves are not transmitted through the external auditory canal, the tympanic membrane, or the ossicles.

SENSORINEURAL HEARING LOSS

Dysfunction of the inner ear, the eighth cranial nerve, or the auditory pathway produces sensorineural hearing loss.

MIXED HEARING LOSS

Mixed hearing loss is a combination of both conductive and sensorineural losses.

History

The symptoms of hearing loss include gradual loss of auditory sensitivity, with the perception of high-frequency sounds diminishing first. In addition, there is difficulty in localizing signals and a problem in understanding speech in unfavorable situations. This loss leads to a distortion of words, and sounds become jumbled. The resultant effect is poor speech discrimination, characterized by an often-heard remark of the hearing-impaired person: "I can hear you, but I cannot understand what you are saying."

Hearing loss is not uniform; some sounds are heard, and others are not. For example, hearing loss is worse for high than for low frequencies and is greater for consonants than for vowels. This loss makes word discrimination extremely difficult. The sentence "The thinner cat is red" may be heard as "The dinner hat is red," leading to an inappropriate response, ensuing embarrassment, and perhaps social withdrawal for the older person who is hard of hearing.

One form of hearing loss is referred to as "loudness recruitment." With this type of hearing loss, the sounds of normal speech cannot be understood and must be made more intense to be heard; however, the sounds are heard with disturbing loudness if they exceed the individual's hearing threshold.

Psychosocial complications that need to be assessed during the history include the following:

- Depression
- Isolation
- Fatigue
- Irritability
- Loss of confidence in abilities
- Negativism
- Paranoia
- Diminished quality of life

Social reasons for the increased denial of hearing loss may be attributed to the negative stereotypes of older people not hearing well, a loss of social status, and an inability to compensate for hearing problems. This image persists despite the many successful persons who are hard of hearing. The older patient who experiences a hearing loss has lost a significant sensory ability that often goes unrecognized by both the patient and the patient's family. Providing screening and early detection of hearing loss is an opportunity to contribute to the quality of life for many older adults. Box 9-3 lists suggested screening questions.

Hearing Assessment
EXAMINATION

The first step in the hearing assessment is to examine each ear for cerumen impaction, a common and often overlooked problem.

Spoken Word Test

By simply standing behind the patient and saying, once at close range and then at arm's length, two series of numbers in a normal and then in a whispered voice, one can test both ears. Patients who are unable to decipher whispered numbers from 2 feet will benefit from formal audiometric evaluation.

Box 9-3

Screening for Hearing Loss

1. Is there any specific problem you are experiencing that is related to your hearing loss?
2. Have you changed in any way your communications with family or friends?
3. Are you having difficulties listening on the telephone or listening to the radio, television, or movies?
4. At times, does your hearing problem cause you to avoid groups of people?
5. Do you feel a loss of self-confidence because of your hearing problem?
6. At times, does your hearing problem cause you to feel depressed?
7. Is there any information you need to help you live with your hearing problem?
8. Is there anything that I have not covered that you would like to tell me about concerning your hearing?

Weber's Test

People with sensorineural hearing loss hear the sound in the better ear, those with conductive loss hear the sound in the impaired ear, and those with normal hearing hear the sound equally in both ears.

Rinne's Test

With conductive hearing loss, the sound of the vibrating tuning fork is heard louder and longer at the mastoid process.

Screening Audiometer Housed Within an Otoscope

This test can identify hearing impairment with high rate of accuracy.

Treatment

Some cases of hearing loss can be treated by cochlear implants, but the main treatment modality remains the hearing aid. New technology in hearing aids allows accommodation to different listening situations. Some aids are better suited to decreasing background noise levels automatically, whereas others work better in decreasing loud levels of high-pitched background noise. Digital hearing aids can perform operations on signals to remove some background noise. Multiple choices are available when selecting a hearing aid. These choices are influenced by the type of loss, personal choice, and financial considerations (Box 9-4).

A referral to an audiologist is appropriate. Hearing-aid fitting, instruction in use, hearing tactics, and lip reading are components of a successful auditory rehabilitation program for persons using a hearing aid for the first time. A study at a Veterans Administration clinic demonstrated that effectiveness and satisfaction with hearing aids is influenced by the type of hearing loss, the type of hearing aid, and socioeconomic factors. The group in the study that used a programmable hearing aid with a directional microphone reported the highest level of effectiveness (Yueh et al, 2001). The economic status of the older patient has a significant impact on the ability to purchase and maintain a hearing aid because the current Medicare program does not cover hearing aids.

Advances in hearing aid technology hold great promise for improving ease of adaptability and increased efficiency in correcting for each individual's hearing loss.

OTHER ASSISTIVE LISTENING DEVICES

Some older adults are unable to use a hearing aid successfully because of physical, cognitive, or social conditions. Common reasons for not purchasing or using hearing aids include an inability to manipulate the hearing aid successfully because of arthritis, an inability to understand instructions because of dementia, an inability to afford the high cost of the hearing aid, or even an unwillingness

---

Box 9-4

Hearing Aid Choices

Case style
  Behind the ear
  In the ear
  Half shell
  Canal
  Completely in the canal
Circuit types
  Linear

Noise processor
Digitally programmed
Digital signal processor
Multiple channels
Directional microphones
And any combination
  Cost of hearing aid
  Approximate range from $450 to $4000

to accept the necessity of wearing a hearing aid. Another reason may be that the hearing aid is not effective in particular situations, such as listening to the television or listening in noisy environments.

Assistive listening devices (ALDs) can be used either in addition or as an alternative to hearing aids. These devices enhance the ability of the older person to understand speech in difficult situations. An inexpensive and easy-to-use ALD is a hardwire system that includes (1) a microphone that is held close to the sound source, (2) an amplifier, (3) a transducer, and (4) a headphone. The ALD (hardwire) system can be used to facilitate interviews and history taking for hearing-impaired older adults who may have chosen not to use a conventional hearing aid. The low cost and the commercial availability of these devices make them an attractive alternative for some older persons.

Follow-up

The efficacy and use of the hearing aid should be assessed during all subsequent visits.

Summary

Vision and hearing are senses that are often taken for granted, with little attention given to them until they begin to fade. For the most part, older adults experience some sensory loss and make a successful accommodation. This chapter alerts the practitioner to the vigilance necessary for the recognition of signs and symptoms, methods of treatment, and risk factors of common disorders that affect these senses.

Resources

American Academy of Audiology
www.audiology.org

American Academy of Ophthalmology
www.eyenet.org

The Hearing and Speech Center
www.hearingcenter.com

National Eye Institute
www.nei/nih.gov

References

Age-related Eye Disease Study Research: A randomized placebo controlled clinical trial of high dose supplementation with vitamin C and E and beta carotene for age-related cataract and vision loss: AREDS no. 9, *Arch Ophthalmol* 119(10):1439-1452, 2001.

Bressler NM: Early detection and treatment of neovascular age-related macular degeneration, *J Am Board Fam Pract* 15(2):142-152, 2002.

Burke M: Sensation. In Burke M, Walsh M, editors: *Gerontologic nursing: wholistic care of the older adult*, ed 2, St Louis, 1997, Mosby.

Coleman AL Brigatti L: Glaucomas, *Minerva Med* 92(5):365-379, 2001.

Dalton DS et al: Association of leisure-time noise exposure and hearing loss, *Audiology* 40(1):1-9, 2001.

Evans JR: Antioxidant vitamins and mineral supplements for age-related macular degeneration, *Cochrane Database Syst Rev* CD 000254 (2):2002.

Evans JR: Risk factors for age related macular degeneration, *Prog Retin Eye Res* 20(2):227-253, 2001.

Gates GA, Rees TS: Hear ye? Hear ye! Successful auditory aging, *West J Med* 16(4):247-252, 1997.

Gordon MO et al: The Ocular Hypertension Treatment Study: baseline factors that predict the onset of primary open-angle glaucoma, *Arch Ophthalmol* 120(6):714-720, 2002.

Infield DA, O'Shea JG: Diabetic retinopathy, *Postgrad Med J* 74(869):129-133, 1998.

la Cour M, Kiilgaard JF, Nissen MH: Age-related macular degeneration: epidemiology and optimal treatment, *Drugs Aging* 19(2):101-133, 2002.

Lighthouse International: Prevalence of vision impairment: statistics on vision impairment, 2002.

Martini A et al: Hearing in the elderly: a population study, *Audiology* 4096:285-293, 2001.

McCarty CA: Cataract in the 21st century: lessons from previous epidemiological research, *Clin Exp Optom* 85(2):91-99, 2002.

Megighian D: Audiometric and epidemiological analysis of elderly in Veneto region, *Gerontology* 4694:199-204, 2000.

Melki SA, Azar DT: LASIK Complications: etiology, management, and prevention, *Surv Ophthalmol* 46(2): 95-111, September/October 2001.

National Eye Institute and Prevention Blindness America: Vision problems in U.S.: prevalence of adult vision impairment and age-related eye diseases in America, ed 4, Washington, DC, 2002, National Institutes of Health.

Riordan-Eva P, Vaughan DG: Eye. In Tierney LM, McPhee SJ, Papadakis MA, editors: *Current medical diagnosis and treatment*, 1997, ed 36, Stamford, Conn, 1997, Appleton & Lange.

Skyler JS: Microvascular complications: retinopathy and nephropathy, *Endocrinol Metab Clin North Am* 30(4):833-856, 2001.

Taylor HR et al: Vitamin E supplements and macular degeneration: randomized controlled trial, *BMJ* 6:325(7354):1-2, 2002.

Yueh B et al: Randomized trial of amplification strategies, *Arch Otolaryngol Head Neck Surg* 127(10): 1197-1204, 2001.

10

Respiratory System

Age-related Changes

There is a gradual age-related decline in pulmonary function beginning at about 40 years of age. The elastic recoil of the lungs decreases as a result of changes in elastin and collagen. The lung weight is decreased by about one fifth; the bronchi harden, and the bronchial epithelium and mucous glands degenerate. The alveolar ducts and bronchioles enlarge, with an accompanying decrease in the depth of the alveolar sacs. The number of alveoli decreases, and the cilia become less active. With inhalation, the lung bases of older adults do not inflate well, and secretions are not expelled. Resistance to airflow increases because of narrowing of the bronchioles. The vital capacity decreases, and the residual volume increases because of loss of elastic recoil. Additional age-related respiratory system changes in older adults include the following:

- The thoracic muscles of inspiration and expiration grow weaker, leading to incomplete lung expansion and decreased elastic recoil.
- Pulmonary function test changes are reduced respiratory function, reduced vital capacity, reduced breathing capacity, and increased residual lung volume.
- Poor ciliary function, reduced cough reflex, and decreased T-cell immunity develop.
- The number of functioning alveoli decreases.
- The number of beta-receptors decreases.
- Concerning the arterial blood gases (ABGs), partial pressure of oxygen (Pao_2) decreases with age; Pao_2 corrected for age equals 109 minus 0.43 times (patient's age); Pao_2 in an 80-year-old is 75 mm Hg.
- $Paco_2$ and pH may be outside the normal range, and the response to change may be blunted.
- There is decreased oxygen uptake by cells.
- The incidence of sleep apnea and sleep disorders increases. The anteroposterior chest diameter increases, the thoracic transverse measurement decreases, and kyphosis ensues.
- Costal cartilage calcifies, and the ribs become less mobile.

The clinical implications of the age-related changes are as follows (Witta, 1997):
- Barrel-shaped chest or senile emphysema
- Bibasilar crackles at baseline; increased risk for respiratory muscle fatigue
- Increased risk for pneumonia and aspiration; increased risk for reactivation of tuberculosis
- Decreased reserve (patients are more susceptible to disease)
- Decreased response to beta-agonists

219

- Possible normal hypercapnia (therefore oxygen should be titrated cautiously to prevent impairment of hypercapnia-driven respiration.)
- Delayed symptoms of hypoxemia and hypercapnia
- Decreased response to exercise, stress, and disease
- Increased risk for nocturnal hypoxemia
  The older population may present with a number of clinical entities in the primary care setting.

CHRONIC COUGH

Cough is the host defense mechanism to clear the airway of secretions and inhaled particles. A chronic cough is one that lasts at least 3 weeks. Psychogenic cough should be considered in an adult patient who presents with a chronic cough with no obvious basis and for whom therapy has failed for postnasal drip, asthma, and gastroesophageal disease (GERD) (Mastrovich and Greenberger, 2002).

In adults, chronic bronchitis resulting from cigarette smoking or inhaled irritants and postnasal drip from chronic sinusitis or allergic rhinitis may be contributors. Additional illnesses that can cause chronic cough include viral infections, bacterial infections, asthma, GERD, foreign-body aspiration, tuberculosis, medications such as beta-blockers or angiotensin converting enzyme (ACE) inhibitors, and psychogenic factors. Worrisome causes of chronic cough include mediastinal masses and chronic lymphadenopathy.

Conditions

- Chronic bronchitis: A dry, hacking cough is present and is worse in the morning.
- Postnasal drip: 41% of patients with a chronic cough complain of a clear nasal discharge, nasal congestion, and frequent throat clearing (Uphold and Graham, 1994).
- Asthma: Patients have a cough at bedtime or after exercise, laughing, or exposure to cold air. Cough occurs seasonally and with a strong family history. Cough may be nonproductive or productive but not purulent. Associated symptoms may include wheezing and intercostal retraction, but cough may be the sole manifestation.
- GERD: Patients describe a history of heartburn, dysphagia, or a sour taste in the mouth, which may be relieved by sitting up.
- Viral infections: Symptoms often occur in the winter, with a nonproductive cough, rhinitis, and nasal congestion.
- Bacterial infections: Cough may be productive or purulent, accompanied by fever, respiratory distress, or both.
- Aspiration of a foreign body: The cough may persist for weeks or months, and there is a fixed, localized wheezing on auscultation that suggests a distinct affected area.
- Tuberculosis: Initially, patients describe minimal production of yellow-green mucus on arising, but with progressive disease, the cough becomes more productive. Associated symptoms include fever, night sweats, dyspnea, and hemoptysis.
- Tumor: Characteristics of the cough depend on the location of the primary tumor.
- Psychogenic factors: The cough disappears during sleep; it is worse when attention is brought to it and when the patient is under stress; it lacks associated symptoms.

BRONCHITIS

Bronchitis is an inflammatory condition of the tracheobronchial tree characterized by hyperemic, edematous bronchi, heightened bronchial secretions, impaired mucociliary activity, and destruction of the epithelium. Bronchitis may be acute or chronic and may result from infections with rhinoviruses, pneumococci, *Mycoplasma*, *Chlamydia*, or *Moraxella catarrhalis*. A secondary bacterial infection may result from *Streptococcus pneumoniae* or *Haemophilus influenzae*.

History

- Onset and duration of symptoms
- Associated symptoms: fever, pharyngitis, dyspnea, chest pain
- Other household members with infectious illness
- History of respiratory illnesses
- Past and current smoking history
- Quality and nature of sputum production
- Drug or environmental allergies
- Current medications, including over-the-counter drugs (OTCs)

Symptoms

- Cough is the hallmark symptom
- Fever (unless infected with rhinovirus or coronavirus)
- Chest pain
- Bronchospasm with wheezing (uncommon in nonsmokers)

Focused Physical Examination

The physical examination should include vital signs; a mental status examination; an eyes, ears, nose, and throat (EENT) examination; a lymph node examination; and a heart and lung examination. Pay particular attention to fever, edematous turbinates or pharynx, enlarged lymph nodes, wheezing, and tachycardia.

Differential Diagnoses

Acute bronchitis and pneumonia are extremely difficult to differentiate. Patients with pneumonia often have high fevers, rigors, pleuritic chest pain, rusty or bloody sputum, focal crackles, and x-ray abnormalities. Older adults, however, may present atypically, without evidence of high fever or with less severe constitutional symptoms.

- Pneumonia
- Tuberculosis
- *Pneumocystis carinii* pneumonia
- Asthma
- Exposure to airborne irritants
- Congestive heart failure
- Drug-related: beta blockers, ACE inhibitors, acetylsalicylic acid (ASA), nonsteroidal antiinflammatory drugs (NSAIDs), particularly naproxen
- Foreign-body obstruction
- Paroxysmal nocturnal dyspnea as a complication of chronic sinusitis
- Allergic rhinitis
- GERD: glottic dysfunction
- Tumors
- Psychogenic

Diagnostic Tests

Bronchitis is a diagnosis of exclusion. A complete blood cell count (CBC) with differential, sputum culture, and chest x-ray examination are necessary only if the patient has worsening symptoms despite management. Consider a purified protein derivative (PPD) test if the patient is at risk for tuberculosis.

Treatment
THERAPEUTICS

Because most cases are viral in origin, antibiotics are generally not needed. Treatment should include increased fluids and rest, and discontinuation of cigarette smoking. Cough suppressants, antihistamines, and sedatives should be used sparingly, based on the severity of symptoms. Expectorants have not proven helpful.

Clearance of secretions should be promoted with postural drainage and therapeutic doses of bronchodilators (e.g., albuterol [Proventil] metered-dose inhaler, 9 µg per puff, two puffs every 4 to 6 hours, with an onset of action in 5 to 15 minutes, peak effect in 60 to 90 minutes, and duration of 3 to 6 hours).

If a bacterial infection complicates the viral infection, treat with *one* of the following:
- Erythromycin 250 mg to 500 mg four times a day for 10 days *or*
- Trimethoprim sulfamethoxazole (TMP/SMX) twice a day for 10 days *or*
- Doxycycline 100 mg twice a day for 10 days

For patients with coexisting chronic obstructive pulmonary disease (COPD), treat with antibiotics when there is a change in the color, consistency, and amount of sputum production.

EDUCATION

The patient should be instructed to avoid persons with upper respiratory infections, to increase fluid intake, to rest, to monitor temperature daily, and to notify his or her health care provider if symptoms do not improve within 3 days. Medications must be taken as instructed.

FOLLOW-UP

If symptoms last longer than 14 days, a 10-day course of antibiotic therapy should be begun. If there is no improvement within an additional 2 weeks, it is time to consider referral to a specialist. Chronic cough resolves completely within 1 month in half of the patients who are motivated by an acute illness to discontinue cigarettes permanently (Barker, Burton, and Zieve, 2003).

CHRONIC OBSTRUCTIVE PULMONARY DISEASE

Chronic obstructive pulmonary disease is a complex syndrome of airway obstruction or airflow limitation. The two components of COPD are emphysema and chronic bronchitis.

Emphysema is a pathologic diagnosis based on a permanent, abnormal dilation and obstruction of alveolar ducts and air spaces distal to the terminal bronchioles. It is characterized by airway obstruction, hyperinflation, loss of elastic recoil, and destruction of the alveolar-capillary interface, which impairs gas exchange.

Chronic bronchitis is a clinical diagnosis based on the presence of cough and sputum production that occurs on most days of a 3-month period during 2 consecutive years. It is characterized by thickened bronchial walls; hyperplasia and hypertrophied mucous glands; and mucosal inflammation in the bronchial walls, large central airways, and, later, smaller airways.

The sequelae of emphysema or chronic bronchitis may be chronic hypoxemia, which causes pulmonary hypertension, and cor pulmonale; both conditions are associated with poor survival if untreated (Barker, Burton, and Zieve, 2003).

History

- Onset and duration of symptoms
- Occupational and environmental exposures to dusts (e.g., grain, wood, cotton, mineral, or polyurethane) and chemical fumes
- Cigarette smoking (number of packs times number of years equals pack-year smoking history)
- Number of attempts to quit smoking and duration of cigarette-free time
- Shortness of breath (Ask the patient whether he or she has trouble keeping up with peers doing routine activities such as walking, sports, or work activities. More advanced dyspnea is roughly quantified by distance walked or flights of stairs walked before stopping.)
- Quantity and characteristics of sputum production
- Drug or environmental allergies
- Current medications, including OTC

Alpha$_1$-antitrypsin deficiency (α_1-antitrypsin) is an uncommon genetic disorder, found in about 1 in 2500 whites, in which the circulating levels of antiproteases are less than 10% of normal. A DNA-base substitution causes an amino acid substitution that prevents secretion of antiproteases from liver cells. Serum levels are less than 15% of normal, which leads to the development of premature emphysema in deficient persons. Although affected persons seek medical care with severe emphysema in the third and fourth decades, many persons with α_1-antitrypsin deficiency have normal or only mildly abnormal lung function if they do not smoke (Barker, Burton, and Zieve, 2003).

Symptoms

- Chronic cough
- Wheezing
- Weight changes
- Recurrent respiratory infections
- Progressive exertional dyspnea
- Lack of libido
- Tachypnea
- Sputum production
- Fatigue
- Insomnia
- Limitation of activities of daily living from shortness of breath

Focused Physical Examination

1. Check vital signs. Be alert for fever, tachypnea, tachycardia, and irregular pulse.
2. Check for increase in resting chest anteroposterior diameter, flattening of the angle of the clavicle and trapezius, widening of the xiphocostal angle, and increase in the intercostal spaces.
3. Check for diminished muscle mass in the thighs and legs.
4. The characteristic seating posture is leaning forward with both hands on the knees to elevate the shoulders.
5. Note purse-lipped breathing and prolonged expiration.
6. Note cyanosis and clubbing of the nails.
7. Note tobacco staining of the fingers.
8. Chest percussion reveals increased resonance and a low diaphragm.
9. Auscultation shows diminished transmission of breath sounds and early inspiratory crackles.
10. Wheezing may be elicited with forced expiration.
11. Systemic findings include neck-vein distention, peripheral edema, hepatomegaly, tricuspid regurgitation, and a ventricular heave.

Differential Diagnoses

- Emphysema
- Chronic bronchitis
- Congestive heart failure
- Asthma
- Pneumonia
- Lung cancer
- Tuberculosis

Diagnostic Tests

Chest x-ray film is abnormal only in advanced disease. There is hyperinflation with flattening of the diaphragm, increased retrosternal air space on the lateral view, narrow cardiac silhouette, and a paucity and tapering of peripheral blood vessels. The electrocardiogram (ECG) shows a vertical or indeterminate heart axis and low voltage. Enlarged P waves, right-axis deviation, or right ventricular hypertrophy is present with cor pulmonale (Barker, Burton, and Zieve, 2003). It is important to administer a PPD and to obtain a CBC with differential and chemistries, in particular, liver function tests (LFTs) and to consider Gram stain and culture of sputum if infection is suspected.

SPIROMETRY

As a general rule, forced expiratory volume at 1 second (FEV_1) measurements greater than 2 liters indicate mild obstruction; 1 to 2 L, moderate obstruction; and less than 1 L, severe obstruction.

BRONCHODILATOR TESTING

Bronchodilator testing can reveal reversible bronchospasm, and the postbronchodilator measure of FEV_1 is the best overall predictor of life expectancy in COPD (Barker, Burton, and Zieve, 2003).

CARBON MONOXIDE DIFFUSING CAPACITY TEST

The carbon monoxide diffusing capacity test is a test done to evaluate the amount of functioning pulmonary capillary bed in contact with functioning alveoli. It is helpful in distinguishing emphysema from asthma. Cigarette smokers without emphysema have mild reductions in diffusing capacity because of the accumulation of carbon monoxide in the blood, which is only partially reversible with smoking cessation. A diffusing capacity below 70% of the predicted value is present with emphysema but may also be found with interstitial fibrosis and pulmonary vascular diseases. In chronic asthmatic bronchitis, the diffusing capacity tends to be preserved. Consider ABGs and pulse oximetry as conditions warrant.

Treatment
THERAPEUTICS

The recommended stepped-treatment approach to COPD is to start with anticholinergic agents, then beta-adrenergic agents, followed by theophylline and corticosteroids. Response to treatment is judged by symptomatic improvement and spirometry.

Drug treatment should use the minimum number of agents and the least frequent dosing schedule, starting with the agents having the greatest benefit and least toxicity (Barker, Burton, and Zieve, 2003) (Table 10-1).

Oxygen Therapy

Oxygen therapy prolongs survival and improves physical and psychological functioning in hypoxemic patients with COPD. Proven benefits of home oxygen include longer survival, reduced hospi-

TABLE 10-1	Pharmacologic Therapy for Chronic Obstructive Pulmonary Disease		
Name of Drug	**Dosage**	**Side Effects**	**Other Clinical Pearls**
Inhaled Anticholinergic Ipratropium (Atrovent)	2 puffs t.i.d. to 6 puffs q.i.d.	Mouth irritation and cough	Side effects may be decreased by use of a spacer.
Beta-adrenergic Agonists Albuterol (Proventil)	2-4 puffs 2-4 times daily	Hypokalemia and occasional tachycardia or tremor	Supplemental potassium may be needed. Avoid over-the-counter inhalers, as many contain epinephrine.
Theophylline	200 mg q12 hr; actual dose based on drug levels	Tremors, potential for drug-drug interactions	Thought to be the most useful drug for the prevention of nocturnal symptoms.
Oral Corticosteroids Prednisone	40 mg daily for 2 weeks	Weight gain, appetite increase, increased risk of infection, fluid and electrolyte imbalance	An improvement in spirometry of 15% indicates a positive response. Taper to lowest possible dose.
Inhaled Steroids Triamcinolone (Azmacort)	2 puffs t.i.d. to q.i.d.	Oral candidiasis; rinse mouth well and use spacer	Benefit is mainly in nonsmokers or those with asthmatic bronchitis.

talization needs, and improved quality of life. Requirements for Medicare coverage for home use of oxygen and oxygen equipment are listed in Table 10-2. The monthly cost of home oxygen therapy ranges from $300 to $500, with Medicare paying 80% of the cost (Chestnutt and Prendergast, 2002).

Survival in hypoxemia patients with COPD treated with supplemental O_2 is directly proportionate to the number of hours per day O_2 is administered. Oxygen by nasal cannula given 15 hours a day leads to 65% survival rate, whereas those treated only at night with O_2 have a 45% survival rate. Portable liquid oxygen systems allow mobility out of the home and should be used whenever possible. The danger of smoking in the presence of oxygen must be stressed.

EDUCATION

It is crucial to educate the patient about the disease process, prevention of disease progression, treatment of complications, drug treatment to maximize lung function, and rehabilitation to optimize activity levels. The patient should be given realistic expectations about the long-term

TABLE 10-2	Home Oxygen Therapy: Requirements for Medicare Coverage.[1]

Group I (any of the following):
1. $Pao_2 \leq 55$ mm Hg or $Sao_2 \leq 88\%$ taken at rest breathing room air, while awake.
2. During sleep (prescription for nocturnal oxygen use only):
   a. $Pao_2 \leq 55$ mm Hg or $Sao_2 \leq 88\%$ for a patient whose awake, resting, room air Pao_2 is ≥ 56 mm Hg or $Sao_2 \geq 89\%$,

   or

   b. Decrease in $Pao_2 > 10$ mm Hg or decrease in $Sao_2 > 5\%$ associated with symptoms or signs reasonably attributed to hypoxemia (e.g., impaired cognitive processes, nocturnal restlessness, insomnia).
3. During exercise (prescription for oxygen use only during exercise):
   a. $Pao_2 \leq 55$ mg Hg or $Sao_2 \leq 88\%$ taken during exercise for a patient whose awake, resting, room air Pao_2 is ≥ 56 mm Hg or $Sao_2 \geq 89\%$.

   and

   b. There is evidence that the use of supplemental oxygen during exercise improves the hypoxemia that was demonstrated during exercise while breathing room air.

Group II:[2]
$Pao_2 = 56-59$ mm Hg or $Sao_2 = 89\%$ if there is evidence of any of the following:
1. Dependent edema suggesting congestive heart failure.
2. P pulmonale on ECG (P wave > 3 mm in standard leads II, III, or aVF).
3. Hematocrit $> 56\%$.

From Chestnutt M, Prendergast T: Lung. In Tierney LM et al, editors: *Current medical diagnoses and treatment: adult ambulatory and in-patient management*, New York, 2002, Lange Medical Books/McGraw Hill.
[1]Health Care Financing Administration, 1989.
[2]Patients in this group must have a second oxygen test 3 months after the initial oxygen set-up.

progressive course of the disease, tempered by the understanding that temporary worsenings are treatable. Achievement of maximum social and physical functioning may be assisted by simple measures, such as special parking areas for the disabled, use of wheelchairs and motorized carts in shopping malls, and portable oxygen and oxygen supplementation during air travel. Patients and their families should understand that the dyspnea that occurs with exertion is not harmful to the lung and that with the appropriate pacing of activities a certain level of dyspnea is actually desirable to achieve and maintain functioning (Barker, Burton, and Zieve, 2003). Inquiries about sexual functioning should be encouraged. Education of the patient's bed partner about proper techniques and the use of prophylactic bronchodilators and oxygen can establish more normal sexual functioning, even with severe disease. Discussions with the patient and the family can cover issues surrounding advance directives and mechanical ventilation as treatment for acute respiratory failure. Educating the patient about smoking cessation should include cigarettes, cigars, marijuana, and cocaine. Patients should avoid respiratory irritants. Pneumococcal vaccination every 6 years is recommended, and influenza vaccination is recommended annually. During an influenza epidemic, amantadine prophylaxis for persons who have not been immunized can prevent or attenuate this potentially fatal infection. The patient needs to be instructed to contact health care providers at the onset of any symptoms of an upper respiratory tract infection. The patient should be encouraged to become involved in a pulmonary rehabilitation program and support group.

If a bacterial infection ensues, treatment is with *one* of the following:
- Erythromycin 250 mg to 500 mg four times a day for 10 days *or*
- TMP/SMX twice a day for 10 days *or*
- Doxycycline 100 mg twice a day for 10 days

FOLLOW-UP

After an acute exacerbation, follow-up by phone should be done in 24 to 48 hours. After beginning oral theophylline, follow-up for drug level should occur 2 weeks after initiation of therapy. Stable patients can be followed up every 3 to 6 months. Patients should consult with their health care provider immediately if any signs and symptoms of respiratory infection or distress develop.

PNEUMONIA

Pneumonia is a lower respiratory tract infection accompanied by systemic symptoms and evidence of consolidation on chest x-ray film. Bronchitis and pneumonia represent a continuum of lower respiratory infection. Aspirated pathogens, including bacteria, *Mycoplasma*, and viruses, invade the bronchial epithelium, causing inflammation, edema, and leukocyte infiltration. X-ray examination findings depend on the extent of involvement of adjacent lung parenchyma. It may take 24 hours or longer to visualize x-ray film changes that support clinical findings. Patients seen early and those with emphysema may fail to show any infiltrate or may show a patchy infiltrate on their chest films despite considerable inflammation. Pneumonia is increasingly common among older patients and in persons with coexisting illnesses. Patients 65 years of age and older are at increased risk for mortality from bacteremic pneumococcal disease.

The most commonly cultured organisms in people 65 of age and older are *S. pneumoniae*, *H. influenzae*, and other gram-negative bacilli. In the absence of laboratory analysis and documentation of a causative organism, consideration should be given to where the patient lives. If the patient is living at home, the most common pathogens in community-acquired pneumonia should be considered and any suspicions about causative organisms expanded if the patient resides in a long-term care facility or was recently hospitalized. Aspiration pneumonia results from upper airway obstruction that may be caused by food. This type of pneumonia is associated with old age, dementia, and the need for long-term care (Chestnutt and Prendergast, 2003).

History

- History of previous pneumonia
- Frequency of upper respiratory tract infections (URIs)
- Fever
- Shortness of breath
- Quality and nature of sputum production
- Cough
- Constitutional symptoms
- Wheezing
- Rhinorrhea
- Weight changes
- Rigors
- Nausea or diarrhea
- Smoking history
- Tuberculosis history and recent exposure
- Travel history (especially recent travel)

- Comorbid illness (e.g., diabetes, hypertension, cancer or chronic illnesses such as rheumatoid arthritis or lupus, asthma, COPD, emphysema)
- Alcohol intake
- Drug and environmental allergies
- Current medications, including OTCs

Symptoms

Bacterial pneumonias are commonly preceded by a viral-like prodrome of headache, myalgias, and malaise. Also, there may be some of the following:
- Abrupt onset of shaking chills
- Fever
- Pleuritic chest pain
- Cough productive of purulent or rusty sputum
    Nonbacterial pneumonias (atypical pneumonia) are distinguished by a prodrome of headache and myalgia before the respiratory symptoms. The onset is a flu-like illness (Table 10-3).
- Fever
- Headache
- Sore throat
- Myalgia and malaise
- Nonproductive hacking cough at onset or several days later
- Substernal chest pain
- Dyspnea and respiratory distress
    When caring for older patients, a clinician must be alert for subtle changes in behavior. Two common indicators of illness in this age group are tachycardia and tachypnea. Patients who live at home are more likely to have classic symptoms, whereas residents of long-term care facilities may exhibit mental status changes, falls, anorexia, and new behavioral problems. Early recognition of subtle changes in this population, leading to early interventions, decreases morbidity and mortality.

Focused Physical Examination

- Check vital signs.
- Consider weight if the patient has coexisting illness.
- Inspect and observe respiratory rate, ability to speak in sentences, use of pursed-lip breathing, jugular venous distention (JVD), use of accessory muscles, positioning to relieve shortness of breath, cyanosis, tachypnea, grunting, nasal flaring, and mental status changes.
- Auscultation: Crackles may be an age-related change.
    Crackles that do not clear with cough are suggestive of pneumonia of either type. Signs of consolidation (bronchial breath sounds, dullness to percussion, and egophony) are more common in bacterial pneumonia.
    In early stages of pneumonia the examination may be normal, despite an infiltrate on x-ray film; however, crackles and rhonchi may indicate pneumonia before the appearance of an infiltrate.
    Palpation and percussion may show tactile fremitus and dullness over the area of consolidation.

Diagnostic Tests

In a patient with classic symptoms, diagnostic studies serve only to confirm the diagnosis. In an older patient with an atypical presentation, a broader workup may be required to determine an etiology and therefore better focus case management. An appropriate diagnostic workup should be focused and cost effective.

TABLE 10-3	Pneumonia-Producing Organisms	
Organism	**Symptoms**	**Statistics of Interest**
Pneumococcus: may occur in previously healthy adults or after URI.	Presents abruptly High fever Shaking chills Productive cough of purulent or rusty sputum Headache Prostration Pleuritic chest pain	Bacteremia occurs in 15%-30% of cases.
H. influenzae: predilection for elderly or patients with COPD or preexisting illnesses but may affect healthy persons. Often occurs after a period of influenza.	Symptoms are similar to other bacterial pneumonias	
Staphylococcus: often occurs in patients with specific risk factors: nursing home residents, alcohol abusers, or individuals with chronic disease. Also occurs after an influenza epidemic.	Symptoms are similar to other bacterial pneumonias	
M. catarrhalis: consider in individuals with chronic illness or underlying COPD.	Symptoms are mild, no myalgias, chills, pleuritic chest pain or extreme prostration	
Gram-negative bacilli: rare in previously healthy adults. High risk: old age, nursing home residents, immobilization, lack of independence for some portion of ADLs, incontinence, stroke, severe underlying illness, alcohol abusers, malnutrition.		There is a high risk for complications. There is a 20%-30% mortality rate.
M. pneumoniae: close contact is necessary for transmission. Epidemics have occurred in cramped housing areas and in the military.	Symptoms: Mild and course is self-limited. There is an insidious onset, with hacking cough, fever, malaise, headache.	Only 3%-10% of all community-acquired pneumonias are from this organism. In individuals age 30-60, symptoms may last up to 6 weeks despite treatment.
Chlamydia pneumonia	Symptoms are similar to *M. pneumoniae*	
Legionella pneumonia	Symptoms are more severe than other atypical pneumonias. Unique characteristics include	There is a 10%-30% mortality rate.

Continued

TABLE 10-3	Pneumonia-Producing Organisms—cont'd	
Organism	**Symptoms**	**Statistics of Interest**
	hyponatremia, neurologic symptoms of confusion, headache, nausea, diarrhea, hematuria, and elevated serum transaminase.	
Viruses are not a common cause of pneumonia in adults except in the immunocompromised.	Symptoms are fever, chills, dry hacking cough, and pharyngitis.	
RSV is increasingly being recognized as a cause of pneumonia in adults.	Patients with viral pneumonias have more prolonged prodromal illness, milder	
CMV and herpes simplex viruses in immunocompromised patients cause pneumonias that are treatable.	symptoms and less elevated white blood cells than patients with bacterial pneumonias. Chest x-ray films do not reveal lobar infiltrates with pleural effusions as in bacterial pneumonias.	
Pneumocystis	Symptoms are insidious onset of fever, cough, and dyspnea in an immunocompromised patient.	

From Uphold CR, Graham MV: *Clinical guidelines in adult health*, Gainesville, Fla, 1994, Barmarrae.

Chest x-ray examination is helpful in the differential diagnosis of cough, shortness of breath, or chest pain. It may also be helpful in revealing other underlying conditions, such as cardiomegaly, lung abscess, tuberculosis, obstruction, tumor, and multilobar involvement. Although the x-ray is essential for the firm diagnosis of pneumonia, a normal x-ray does not necessarily rule out pneumonia, and subsequent films may actually reveal a progression of pulmonary infiltrates. One reason for this change may be that older patients tend to be dehydrated at initial consultation, and rehydration causes the infiltrate to appear. A 24-hour lag time between the clinical presentation and x-ray changes often occurs.

Sputum microbiology and chest x-ray film are appropriate. Consider pulse oximetry if it is available and blood gases if O_2 saturation is less than 90. The O_2 saturation and ABGs should be used to assist in determining the severity of illness. Severe hypoxemia is an indicator of poor outcome and may require admission to an intensive care unit. The spirometry change is that FEV_1 is decreased. The ECG shows atrial changes.

A blood chemistry 20 (Chem 20) and a CBC with differential are appropriate if the patient is older than 60 years of age or has coexisting illnesses. In a classic scenario the CBC reveals a marked leukocytosis with a left shift; this phenomenon can be absent or delayed in older patients. PPD should be considered, as should sputum acid-fast bacilli (AFB) each morning for three mornings if history indicates. Blood cultures are done if bacteremia is suspected.

Treatment

Hospitalization compared with outpatient management is based on a number of factors, including physical parameters, social support, insurance issues, and the ease of treatment for the probable causative organism. Hospitalization should be strongly considered for patients with the risk factors listed in Box 10-1, especially if multiple risk factors are present.

THERAPEUTICS

Antipyretics can be provided for general comfort. Guaifenesin should be considered for tenacious secretions and dextromethorphan avoided because it suppresses cough reflex. Outpatient treatment for patients 60 years of age or older is based on the presumptive diagnosis from the signs and symptoms exhibited. The most common pathogens include S. *pneumoniae,* respiratory viruses, *H. influenzae,* aerobic gram-negative bacilli, *Staphylococcus aureus, M. catarrhalis, Legionella* organisms, *Mycobacterium tuberculosis,* and endemic fungi.

Antimicrobial therapy in older adults should provide broad-spectrum activity and therapy initiated with a third-generation cephalosporin or multiple antibiotics. Before the results of microbiologic analysis, ceftriaxone (Rocephin), 250 to 500 mg administered intramuscularly, allows the clinician to treat the patient in the office setting, the long-term care facility, or the hospital. Other choices for treatment include second-generation cephalosporins, TMP/SMX, beta-lactam or beta-lactamase inhibitors, and macrolides. Fluoroquinolones such as sparfloxacin (Zagam) and levofloxacin (Levaquin) occasionally cause skin rashes or gastrointestinal disturbances. Central nervous system toxicity, including dizziness, insomnia, confusion, hallucinations, and seizures, can occur, particularly in older patients. Tendinitis or tendon rupture has occurred with sparfloxacin, as it has with other fluoroquinolones, and will probably occur with levofloxacin as well. Fluoroquinolones have been associated with cartilage damage in high doses in the pediatric population, but there is no indication that similar effects could occur in adults (Stahlmann and Lode, 2003).

When microbes have been identified, *H. influenzae, Staphylococcus* species, *M. catarrhalis,* and gram-negative bacilli can be treated with *one* of the following:

- Augmentin 250 to 500 mg every 8 hours for 10 days *for everything except gram-negative bacilli or*
- Ceftin 250 to 500 mg every 12 hours for 10 days for all organisms *or*

Box 10-1

Risk Factors Associated with Hospitalization and Increased Mortality Rate

Increased age over 50 years
Male gender
Nursing home resident or lack of home care support
Coexisting illness:
  Neoplastic disease
  Liver disease
  Congestive heart disease
  Cerebrovascular disease
  Renal disease
Absence of pleuritic pain
Hypothermia

Examination findings:
  Altered mental status
  Pulse rate > 125 beats/min
  Respiratory rate > 30 breaths/min
  Systolic blood pressure < 90 mm Hg
  Temperature < 35° C (95° F) or > 40° C (104° F)
Laboratory findings
  Arterial pH < 7.35
  Blood urea nitrogen > 30 mg/dl
  Hematocrit < 30%
  Pleural effusion

Adapted from Fiebach NH, Rastegar DA: Respiratory tract infections. In Barker LR et al, editors: *Principles of ambulatory medicine,* ed 6, Philadelphia, 2003, Lippincott Williams & Wilkins.

- TMP/SMX twice a day for 7 to 14 days *or*
- Ciprofloxacin 200 mg twice daily for 10 days for gram-negative organisms

S. pneumoniae can be treated with *one* of the following:

- Procaine penicillin 300,000 U intramuscularly for the first dose *then*
- Penicillin VK 250 to 500 mg four times a day for 7 to 10 days *or*
- Erythromycin 250 to 500 mg three or four times a day for 7 to 10 days

Mycoplasma and *Chlamydia* species can be treated with *one* of the following:

- Doxycycline 100 mg twice daily for 10 to 14 days *or*
- Erythromycin 250 to 500 mg three or four times daily

For *Legionella* species, the patient is hospitalized and administered *one* of the following:

- Erythromycin intravenously *or*
- Doxycycline 100 mg twice daily for 14 days *or*
- Ciprofloxacin 200 mg twice daily for 10 to 14 days

    Pneumocystis carinii can be treated with TMP/SMX twice a day for 21 days and suspected aspiration pneumonia with either clindamycin 0.3 g administered orally four times daily for 10 to 14 days or cephalosporin (Rocephin) 1 g administered intramuscularly once or twice daily for 10 to 14 days. Tequin (Gatifloxacin) administered orally or intramuscularly has been clinically effective for patients with recurrent aspiration pneumonia. Viral infections can be treated with symptomatic treatments.

EDUCATION

- Stop smoking.
- Take deep breaths: 10 each hour.
- Increase hydration and nutritional intake.
- Educate about the importance of antibiotic therapy. The patient should finish all medication.
- Instruct the patient about what to do for missed doses.
- Avoid other persons with upper respiratory infections.
- Patient and family members should practice good hand-washing techniques.
- Instruct the patient to schedule activities with rest periods.
- Establish practice mechanisms to ensure that older patients receive pneumococcal vaccines every 6 years and influenza vaccine yearly.

FOLLOW-UP

A telephone contact with the patient within 24 hours of the initial visit provides a check on antibiotic compliance, side effects, and the status of symptoms. This contact also reassures ill patients that the health care provider is available if their condition worsens. A follow-up visit to the office 3 to 4 days later can assess the response to therapy. Symptoms of pneumococcal pneumonia in the uncompromised patient abate dramatically within 48 to 72 hours of initiation of penicillin therapy. If substantial response has not occurred, switching to erythromycin or hospitalizing the patient should be considered.

    Early follow-up chest x-ray films are mandatory for patients who do not show clinical improvement by 5 to 7 days of therapy or who have a later relapse. Old age, COPD, and alcoholism may delay radiologic clearing for an additional 2 to 6 weeks (Barker, Burton, and Zieve, 2003).

ASTHMA

According to the National Heart, Lung, and Blood Institute of the National Institutes of Health, the following is the current, accepted, working diagnosis of asthma: Asthma is a chronic, inflammatory disorder of the airways in which many cells and cellular elements play a role. In part, mast cells, eosinophils, T-lymphocytes, macrophages, neutrophils, and epithelial cells are involved. In susceptible persons, this inflammation causes recurrent episodes of wheezing, breathlessness, chest tightness, and coughing, particularly at bedtime or in the early morning. These episodes are usually associated with widespread, but variable airflow obstruction that is often reversible, either spontaneously or with therapy. The inflammation also causes an associated increase in the existing bronchial hyperresponsiveness to a variety of stimuli.

The highest rate of asthma-related deaths occurs in persons 55 years of age and older. The prevalence, severity, and death rate have increased in the past decade, particularly in blacks and Hispanics. An estimated 15 million patients have asthma.

History

The clinician should determine whether symptoms worsen in association with the following specific factors:
- Airborne chemicals or dust
- Animals with fur or feathers
- Changes in weather
- Exercise
- House dust mites in mattresses, upholstered furniture, and carpets
- Menses
- Mold
- Nighttime
- Pollen
- Smoke: tobacco or wood
- Strong emotional expression: laughing or crying hard
- Viral infection
- Medications: acetylsalicyclic acid, ACE inhibitors, nonsteroidal antiinflammatory drugs (NSAIDs), beta-blockers

Ask about the following factors:
- Family history
- Impact of disease
- Previous therapies and responses
- Drug and environmental allergies
- Current medications, including OTCs

Symptoms

- Cough, especially nocturnal
- Recurrent wheeze
- Recurrent dyspnea
- Chest tightness

Occupational asthma should be considered in all patients with adult-onset asthma and in patients with asthma that worsens in adulthood. Roughly 200 chemicals have been implicated in occupational asthma (Table 10-4).

The total duration of exposure, duration of symptoms, and severity of symptoms at diagnosis are important determinants of outcome. Early diagnosis and early withdrawal from exposures to offending chemicals are the keys to recovery.

Focused Physical Examination

- Check vital signs.
- Observe general appearance, noting distress or decreased responsiveness.
- Note accessory muscle use, retraction, posture, nasal flaring, diaphoresis, and cyanosis.

TABLE 10-4	Examples of Occupational Hazards Implicated in Asthma

Chemical	*Occupation*
Grain dust	Grain store workers
Henna	Hairdressers
Coffee beans	Coffee roasters
Penicillin	Pharmacists and health care workers
Oil mists	Tool setters
Cobalt dust	Metal grinders
Flour	Bakers

Source: Richman E: Asthma diagnosis and management: new severity classifications and therapy alternatives, *Clin Rev* 7(8):76-78, 83-84, 86-90, 96-97, 101-102, 107-109, 112, 1997. Data extracted from Venables KM, Chan-Yeung M: Occupational asthma, *Lancet* 349:1465-1469, 1997.

- Examine skin for eczema and atopy.
- EENT examination: nasal discharge, allergic shiners, nasal polyps, postnasal drip, frontal tenderness.
- Pulmonary examination: note adventitious sounds, particularly prolonged expiratory phase and wheezing. Unilateral wheezing suggests an aspirated foreign body.

Differential Diagnoses

- Obstructed airway, foreign body, tumor, or anatomic changes
- Chronic bronchitis or emphysema
- Pneumonia
- Pulmonary infiltrates with eosinophilia
- Congestive heart failure
- Allergic reaction
- Laryngeal dysfunction
- Cough secondary to drugs
- Vocal cord dysfunction

Diagnostic Tests

If infection is suspected, chest x-ray film or CBC with differential should be considered, and pulse oximetry or ABGs are considered if the patient's condition warrants. Perform peak expiratory flow with a peak flow meter. Spirometry evaluation may be considered. For patients with persistent asthma despite taking appropriate daily medication, allergen exposure should be identified, sensitivity to seasonal allergies assessed with a thorough history, and sensitivity to perennial indoor allergens assessed with skin or in vitro testing.

Treatment
THERAPEUTICS

According to the Second Expert Panel, the goals of asthma therapy are (Richman, 1997) as follows:
- Prevent chronic and troublesome symptoms, such as coughing or breathlessness at night, in the morning, or after exertion
- Maintain nearly normal pulmonary function
- Maintain normal activity levels (including exercise)

- Prevent recurrent exacerbations and minimize the need for emergency care and hospitalization (Table 10-5)
- Provide optimal pharmacotherapy with minimal or no adverse effects
- Meeting the patient's and family's expectations of, and satisfaction with, asthma care

The goals can be met by the following measures:

- Prescribing daily antiinflammatory therapy to provide the most effective control
- Following the stepped-care approach by initiating therapy at higher levels and stepping down as stability is achieved (Table 10-6)
- Performing office-based assessment at intervals ranging from 1 to 6 months
- Considering referral to an asthma specialist when control of asthma cannot be maintained or the patient requires step 4 care

Pharmacologic Therapy

The most effective medications continue to be those with antiinflammatory actions, inhaled steroids, mast cell stabilizers, and leukotriene modifiers. The next step includes medications that provide relief from acute symptoms, such as short-acting beta adrenergics, anticholinergics, and systemic glucocorticoids.

Asthma treatment is based on a stepped approach. Guidelines for treatment should be initiated at higher levels or steps rather than higher doses of medications.

| **TABLE 10-5** | **Management of Asthma Exacerbations/Severity** |

Assess Severity

Measure PEFR: A value <50% of personal best or of the predicted value suggests a severe exacerbation. Note signs and symptoms: degree of cough, breathlessness, wheeze, and chest tightness correlate imperfectly with severe exacerbation. Accessory muscle use and suprasternal retractions suggest severe exacerbation.

Initial Treatment

Inhaled short-acting β_2-agonist: up to three treatments of 2-4 puffs by metered-dose inhaler at 20-minute intervals or single nebulizer treatment

Good Response	*Incomplete Response*	*Poor Response*
Mild Exacerbation	**Moderate Exacerbation**	**Severe Exacerbation**
PEFR >80% predicted or personal best. No wheezing or shortness of breath. Response to β_2-agonist sustained for 4 hours. • May continue β_2-agonist every 3-4 hours for 24-48 hours • For patients on inhaled glucocorticoid, double dose for 7-10 days	PEFR 50% to 80% predicted or personal best. Persistent wheezing and shortness of breath. • Add oral glucocorticoid • Continue β_2-agonist	PEFR <50% predicted or personal best. Marked wheezing and shortness of breath. • Add oral glucocorticoid • Repeat β_2-agonist immediately • If distress is severe and nonresponsive, consider calling ambulance or 911

Source: Richman E: Asthma diagnosis and management: new severity classifications and therapy alternatives, *Clin Rev* 7(8):76-78, 83-84, 86-90, 96-97, 101-102, 107-109, 112, 1997. Data extracted from Expert Panel Report II: *Guidelines for the diagnosis and management of asthma*, NIH Publication 97-4051, Bethesda, Md, 1997, National Asthma Education and Prevention Program.
PEFR, Peak expiratory flow rate.

TABLE 10-6 Classification and Stepped Care in Asthma Therapy		
Step	**Daily Medication for Long-Term Control**	**Medication for Quick Relief**
Step 4: Severe Persistent Symptoms: Continual Limited physical activity Frequent exacerbations Frequent nocturnal symptoms Pulmonary function: FEV_1/PEFR is no greater than 60% of predicted PEFR variability exceeds 30%	Antiinflammatory agent (high-dose inhaled glucocorticoid) **and** long-acting bronchodilator (inhaled or oral β_2-agonist or theophylline) **and** oral glucocorticoid	Short-acting inhaled β_2-agonist. Daily use or increasing use indicates need for additional long-term therapy.
Step 3: Moderate Persistent Symptoms: Daily Daily use of inhaled short-acting β_2-agonist Exacerbations affect activity Exacerbations at least twice weekly and may last for days Nocturnal symptoms more frequent than once weekly Pulmonary function: FEV_1/PEFR exceeds 60% but is less than 80% of predicted PEFR exceeds 30% variability	Antiinflammatory agent (medium-dose inhaled glucocorticoid) **and/or** medium-dose inhaled glucocorticoid plus long-acting bronchodilator	Short-acting inhaled β_2-agonist. Daily use or increasing use indicates need for additional long-term therapy.
Step 2: Mild Persistent Symptoms: more frequent than twice weekly but less than once a day Exacerbations may affect activity Nocturnal symptoms more frequent than twice monthly Pulmonary function: FEV_1/PEFR is at least 80% of predicted PEFR variability is between 20%-30%	**One daily medication:** antiinflammatory agent (low-dose inhaled glucocorticoid, cromolyn, or nedocromil) or sustained-release theophylline	Short-acting inhaled β_2-agonist. Daily use or increasing use indicates need for additional long-term therapy.
Step 1: Mild Intermittent Symptoms: no more frequent than twice weekly	**No daily medication**	Short-acting inhaled β_2-agonist. Use more than twice weekly

Source: Richman E: Asthma diagnosis and management: new severity classifications and therapy alternatives, *Clin Rev* 7(8):76-78, 83-84, 86-90, 96-97, 101-102, 107-109, 112, 1997. Data extracted from Expert Panel Report II: *Guidelines for the diagnosis and management of asthma*, NIH Publication 97-4051, Bethesda, Md, 1997, National Asthma Education and Prevention Program.
FEV_1, Forced expiratory volume (in one second); PEFR, peak expiratory flow rate.

TABLE 10-6	Classification and Stepped Care in Asthma Therapy—cont'd

Step	Daily Medication for Long-Term Control	Medication for Quick Relief
Step 1: Mild Intermittent—cont'd Asymptomatic and with normal PEFR between exacerbations Exacerbations brief (hours to days) Intensity of exacerbations varies Nocturnal symptoms no more frequent than twice monthly Pulmonary function: FEV_1/PEFR is at least 80% of predicted PEFR variability is less than 20%		may indicate need to initiate long-term therapy.

- Antiinflammatory drugs
  Corticosteroids
  Beclomethasone (Beclovent, Vanceril metered-dose inhaler [MDI]) two
  puffs four times a day or four puffs twice a day
  Flunisolide (AeroBid MDI) two to four puffs twice a day
  Triamcinolone acetonide (Azmacort MDI) two puffs three or four times a day or four
  puffs twice a day
  Fluticasone (Flovent MDI) two to four puffs twice a day
  Prednisone or prednisolone tablets for acute treatment, up to 80 mg per day, for 7 to 14
  days; for chronic treatment, up to 40 mg every other day
  Cromolyn (Intal MDI) two to four puffs four times a day
- Bronchodilators
  B_2 adrenergics
    Albuterol (Proventil, Ventolin MDI) two puffs every 4 to 6 hours as needed
    Ipratropium plus albuterol (Combivent MDI) two puffs four times a day
  Long-acting agents:
    Salmeterol (Serevent MDI) two puffs every 12 hours
- Anticholinergics
  Ipratropium (Atrovent MDI) two puffs four times a day
- Leukotriene receptor antagonist
  Zafirlukast (Accolate tablet) 20 mg twice a day 1 hour before or 2 hours after meals
- 5-Lipoxygenase inhibitor
  Zileuton (Zyflo tablet) 600 mg four times a day

Management of URI symptoms is an integral component of asthma management. Coexisting rhinitis, sinusitis, and GERD require treatment.

EDUCATION

Patient education is key in the management of chronic asthma and acute exacerbations. Education is a partnership between patients and clinicians.

The asthma education program should include five components:

1. Basic asthma facts: Review pathophysiology.
2. Roles of asthma medications: See previous instructions.
3. Skills for use of inhaler, spacer, and peak flow meter.
4. Office spirometry should be performed at the initial assessment and diagnosis of asthma, after the patient's condition has stabilized after the initiation of therapy, and at least every 1 to 2 years thereafter.
5. Peak expiratory flow rates (PEFRs) should be recorded by patients two to four times daily for 2 to 3 weeks during initial medication therapy. After removing the two high results and two low results, the morning and afternoon scores are averaged. These values show the patient's personal best before medication (morning value) and after medication therapy (afternoon value). After maximum medical therapy has occurred and the patient's medical condition has stabilized, the patient should perform PEFRs in the early afternoon. Patients should contact their health care provider if the PEFR falls to less than 80% of their personal best.

Because predicted values vary across racial and ethnic populations, the personal best PEFR is a better choice for individual monitoring than population-based normative values.

Environmental Control and Avoidance Measures

- Avoid exposure to tobacco smoke and allergens to which the patient is sensitive.
- Avoid pets. If pets cannot be removed from the home, have designated pet-free living areas. Close bedroom doors, use air filters, and remove carpets or upholstery from pet-free areas.
- Avoid exertion when pollution levels are high.
- Avoid foods and beverages containing sulfites, including wine.
- Avoid nonselective beta-blockers for patients with cardiovascular disease, ophthalmologic indications, migraines, or stage fright.
- Mattresses and pillows should be encased in allergen-free cases. Sheets and blankets should be washed weekly in water hotter than 140° F.
- Vacuums with HEPA filters may help to reduce symptoms in the home.
- Consider allergy testing and immunotherapy when the connection between symptoms and exposure to allergens is unavoidable. Skin or in vitro testing may also be considered when patients are perennially exposed to indoor allergens.

When and How to Take Rescue Steps

The clinician should provide written signs and symptoms, in appropriate language, of acute exacerbations and treatment plan changes (such as when to use short-acting bronchodilators). Also, he or she educates patients to recognize the symptoms and changes in symptom patterns that herald a diminution of asthma control and the need for stepping up the therapy.

FOLLOW-UP

- For acute exacerbations requiring a nebulizer or corticosteroids, see the patient within 24 hours and reevaluate in 3 to 5 days. After the exacerbation has resolved completely, follow-up visits are every 1 to 3 months.
- For patients taking theophylline, take serum drug levels after 2 weeks of initiating therapy and every 4 to 6 months thereafter.
- Schedule a yearly influenza vaccine (if the patient is not allergic to eggs).
- Consider pneumococcal vaccine every 6 years.

INFLUENZA

Influenza is an infection of the respiratory tract caused by the influenza virus. The three types of virus are labeled A, B, and C. The proteins that coat the flu virus change constantly, making it difficult for the immune system to recognize and fight new strains. The virus is spread mainly by airborne transmission versus direct contact as in the common cold. Therefore people with lung disease, older patients, or those with weakened immunity are susceptible to severe and possibly fatal complications from the flu.

During flu epidemics, up to 40% of people in a given community may develop flu symptoms during the time span of a few weeks. Flu season is usually November through February. Illness is severe for 3 to 14 days, and convalescence lasts for 1 to 4 weeks.

History

- There is an abrupt onset of systemic symptoms.
- Headache and myalgias that involve the back, arms, legs, and occasionally the eyes are the predominant symptoms.
- Temperature may rise up to 106° F for 3 days and may persist for 5 to 7 days.
- Respiratory symptoms such as cough, nasal discharge, hoarseness, and sore throat appear as systemic symptoms wane.
- Cough and weakness usually subside after 2 weeks but may persist longer.
- Drug or environmental allergies
- Current medications, including OTCs

Symptoms

Symptoms include sudden onset of fevers, chills, muscle aches, malaise, cough, and sore throat and usually are self-limiting.

Focused Physical Examination

Check vital signs, for example, whether the patient appears constitutionally ill; has a flushed face, hot skin, watery red eyes, clear nasal discharge, tender cervical lymph nodes, or occasionally localized crackles in the chest; signs of anorexia, nausea, vomiting, or diarrhea. The WBC and differential counts usually demonstrate mild neutropenia and relative lymphocytosis because of absolute granulocytopenia.

Differential Diagnoses

- Common cold
- Pneumonia
- Allergic rhinitis
- Sinusitis
- Streptococcal pharyngitis
- Otitis media

Diagnostic Tests

Doing a CBC should be considered if bacterial infection is suspected. Generally, diagnostic tests are not indicated.

Treatment
THERAPEUTICS

Treatment is entirely symptomatic. Acetaminophen or NSAIDs can be given for aches and fever. Combination products with decongestants, such as pseudoephedrine or phenylephrine (care must be exercised in hypertensive patients), for congestion, cough, and nasal discharge. Nasal sprays should not be used for longer than 3 days to decrease the chance of rebound nasal congestion. Other medications that can be used are antihistamines, such as diphenhydramine, chlorpheniramine, or clemastine, or cough suppressants, such as dextromethorphan.

Two antiviral agents that may be helpful in treating symptoms of influenza A infection **when started within 48 hours** are amantadine (Symmetrel) and rimantadine (Flumadine). These drugs attenuate clinical disease in all patients with influenza A by reducing fever by 50% and by shortening the duration of illness by 1 or 2 days. Side effects include insomnia, nervousness, dizziness, and difficulty in concentrating and may occur in about 7% of adults. Dose is 100 mg twice a day for 7 days. In frail older patients and those with an elevated creatinine clearance, 100 mg daily should be given.

EDUCATION

- Advise patients that if they develop dyspnea, hemoptysis, wheezing, purulent sputum, fever persisting more than 7 days, dark urine, or severe muscle pain or tenderness, prompt medical attention is needed.
- Encourage bed rest. Return to full activity should be delayed until symptoms are gone.
- Supportive measures, including increased nutrition, are important, and symptoms should be managed as previously discussed with combination products.

INFLUENZA VACCINE

For maximum protection, patients should receive the vaccine between the beginning of October and mid-November. The vaccine should be administered anytime symptoms are present in the community, however. People 65 years of age and older should also receive the pneumococcal vaccine every 6 years. Both vaccines can be given at the same time without increasing the risk of vaccine side effects. Older patients and certain patients with chronic disease may develop lower postvaccination titers and remain susceptible to infection. Vaccinated persons develop antibody titers that are protective against illnesses caused by strains similar to those in the vaccine. Related variants may emerge during outbreak periods.

Persons who are allergic to eggs should never be vaccinated. Patients who have an acute illness with fever should not be vaccinated until the illness has subsided.

FOLLOW-UP

Because this illness is usually self-limited, follow-up is dictated by persistent symptoms beyond 7 to 10 days or if signs and symptoms of bacterial infection ensue.

SEVERE ACUTE RESPIRATORY SYNDROME

Severe acute respiratory syndrome (SARS) is a global, contagious viral illness first recognized in China in November of 2002. In May of 2003 33 countries had reported cases of SARS. Significant outbreaks have occurred in China, Hong Kong, Singapore, and Toronto, Canada (WHO, 2003) (Table 10-7). The causative agent has been identified as a Coronavirus, one that has not been recognized before this outbreak. At the time of this writing, no definite diagnostic test has been developed. Therefore the Centers for Disease Control and Prevention (CDC) have issued an Interim Case Definition of SARS (CDC, 2003) (Box 10-2).

The spread of SARS primarily appears to be through close person-to-person contact, although there have been cases in an apartment building in China that seem to question this assumption. The spread of cases seems to be from people who have traveled to Asian countries that are most affected. The World Health Organization (WHO) estimates the incubation period to be 10 days. Health care workers were at extreme risk during the first wave of cases. Of the 144 patients in Toronto, 111 (77%) were exposed to SARS in the hospital setting (Booth et al, 2003). Strict isolation precautions are now a significant aspect of prevention and management of persons who may be exposed to SARS (Figure 10-1). Quarantine laws have been

TABLE 10-7 Cumulative Number of Reported Probable Cases of Severe Acute Respiratory Syndrome (SARS)

From: 1 Nov 2002[1] To: 12 May 2003, 17:00 GMT+2
SARS Travel Recommendations Summary Table 12 May 2003

Country	Cumulative number of case(s)[2]	Number of new cases since last WHO update[2,3]	Number of deaths	Number recovered[4]	Date last probable case reported	Date for which cumulative number of cases is current
Australia	6	2	0	6	12/May/2003	12/May/2003
Brazil	2	0	0	2	10/Apr/2003	24/Apr/2003
Bulgaria	1	0	0	0	24/Apr/2003	28/Apr/2003
Canada	143	0	22	98	4/May/2003	11/May/2003
China	5013	144	252	1693	12/May/2003	12/May/2003
China, Hong Kong Special Administrative Region[5]	1683	9	218	1066	12/May/2003	12/May/2003
China, Macao Special Administrative Region	1	0	0	0	9/May/2003	12/May/2003
China, Taiwan	184	12	20	26	11/May/2003	11/May/2003
Colombia	1	0	0	1	5/May/2003	5/May/2003
Finland	1	0	0	0	7/May/2003	9/May/2003
France	7	0	0	4	9/May/2003	9/May/2003
Germany	9	0	0	9	9/May/2003	12/May/2003
India	1	0	0	0	5/May/2003	9/May/2003
Indonesia	2	0	0	1	23/Apr/2003	6/May/2003
Italy	9	0	0	8	29/Apr/2003	12/May/2003
Kuwait	1	0	0	1	9/Apr/2003	20/Apr/2003
Malaysia	7	0	2	4	9/May/2003	11/May/2003
Mongolia	9	0	0	6	6/May/2003	9/May/2003
New Zealand	1	0	0	1	30/Apr/2003	12/May/2003
Philippines	10	0	2	3	7/May/2003	11/May/2003
Poland	1	0	0	0	1/May/2003	5/May/2003
Republic of Ireland	1	0	0	1	21/Mar/2003	12/May/2003
Republic of Korea	2	1	0	1	12/May/2003	12/May/2003
Romania	1	0	0	1	27/Mar/2003	22/Apr/2003
Singapore	205	0	28	156	9/May/2003	12/May/2003
South Africa	1	0	1	0	9/Apr/2003	3/May/2003

Continued

Country	Cumulative number of case(s)[2]	Number of new cases since last WHO update[2,3]	Number of deaths	Number recovered[4]	Date last probable case reported	Date for which cumulative number of cases is current
Spain	1	0	0	1	2/Apr/2003	5/May/2003
Sweden	3	0	0	2	18/Apr/2003	23/Apr/2003
Switzerland	1	0	0	1	17/Mar/2003	9/May/2003
Thailand	7	0	2	5	12/Apr/2003	11/May/2003
United Kingdom	6	0	0	6	29/Apr/2003	9/May/2003
United States	64	0	0	34	10/May/2003	11/May/2003
Vietnam	63	0	5	58	14/Apr/2003	4/May/2003
Total	**7447**	**168**	**552**	**3195**		

From the World Health Organization.

Notes: Cumulative number of cases includes number of deaths.

As SARS is a diagnosis of exclusion, the status of a reported case may change over time. This means that previously reported cases may be discarded after further investigation and follow-up.

[1]The start of period of surveillance has been changed to 1 November 2002 to capture cases of atypical pneumonia in China that are now recognized as being cases of SARS.

[2]A decrease in the number of cumulative cases and discrepancies in the difference between cumulative number of cases of the last and current WHO update are attributed to the discarding of cases.

[3]The number of new cases since last WHO update includes new cases reported for 11 and 12 May 2003, when these reports have been recieved.

[4]Includes cases who are "discharged" or "recovered" as reported by the national public health authorities.

[5]One death attributed to Hong Kong Special Administrative Region of China occurred in a case medically transferred from Vietnam.

Box 10-2

Updated Interim U.S. Case Definition for Severe Acute Respiratory Syndrome (SARS)

The previous CDC SARS case definition (published April 20, 2003) has been updated as follows:
- Laboratory criteria for evidence of infection with the SARS-associated coronavirus (SARS-CoV) have been added.
- Clinical criteria have been revised to reflect the possible spectrum of respiratory illness associated with SARS-CoV.
- Epidemiologic criteria have been retained. Taiwan has been added to the areas with current documented or suspected community transmission of SARS; Hanoi, Vietnam is now an area with recently documented or suspected community transmission of SARS.

Clinical Criteria
- Asymptomatic or mild respiratory illness
- Moderate respiratory illness
  - Temperature of $> 100.4°$ F ($> 38°$ C)*, and

---

*A measured documented temperature of $> 100.4°$ F ($> 38°$ C) is preferred. However, clinical judgment should be used when evaluating patients for whom a measured temperature of $> 100.4°$ F ($> 38°$ C) has not been documented. Factors that might be considered include patient self-report of fever, use of antipyretics, presence of immunocompromising conditions or therapies, lack of access to health care, or inability to obtain a measured temperature. Reporting authorities might consider these factors when classifying patients who do not strictly meet the clinical criteria for this case definition.

Box 10-2

Updated Interim U.S. Case Definition for Severe Acute Respiratory Syndrome (SARS)—cont'd

Clinical Criteria—cont'd
- One or more clinical findings of respiratory illness (e.g., cough, shortness of breath, difficulty breathing, or hypoxia).
- Severe respiratory illness
  - Temperature of > 100.4° F (> 38° C)*, and
  - One or more clinical findings of respiratory illness (e.g., cough, shortness of breath, difficulty breathing, or hypoxia), and
  - radiographic evidence of pneumonia, or
  - respiratory distress syndrome, or
  - autopsy findings consistent with pneumonia or respiratory distress syndrome without an identifiable cause

Epidemiologic Criteria
- Travel (including transit in an airport) within 10 days of onset of symptoms to an area with current or recently documented or suspected community transmission of SARS[†], or
- Close contact[‡] within 10 days of onset of symptoms with a person known or suspected to have SARS infection

Laboratory Criteria[§]
- Confirmed
  - Detection of antibody to SARS-CoV in specimens obtained during acute illness or > 21 days after illness onset, or
  - Detection of SARS-CoV RNA by RT-PCR confirmed by a second PCR assay, by using a second aliquot of the specimen and a different set of PCR primers, or
  - Isolation of SARS-CoV
- Negative
  - Absence of antibody to SARS-CoV in convalescent serum obtained > 21 days after symptom onset
- Undetermined: laboratory testing either not performed or incomplete

Case Classification[‖]
- Probable case: meets the clinical criteria for severe respiratory illness of unknown etiology with onset since February 1, 2003, and epidemiologic criteria; laboratory criteria confirmed, negative, or undetermined
- Suspect case: meets the clinical criteria for moderate respiratory illness of unknown etiology with onset since February 1, 2003, and epidemiologic criteria; laboratory criteria confirmed, negative, or undetermined

---

For more information, visit http://www.cdc.gov/ncidod/sars or call the CDC public response hotline at (888) 246-2675 (English), (888) 246-2857 (Español), or (866) 874-2646 (TTY).
[†]Areas with current documented or suspected community transmission of SARS include mainland China and Hong Kong Special Administrative Region, People's Republic of China; Singapore; Taiwan; and Toronto, Canada. Hanoi, Vietnam is an area with recently documented or suspected community transmission of SARS.
[‡]Close contact is defined as having cared for or lived with a person known to have SARS or having a high likelihood of direct contact with respiratory secretions and/or body fluids of a patient known to have SARS. Examples of close contact include kissing or embracing, sharing eating or drinking utensils, close conversation (< 3 feet), physical examination, and any other direct physical contact between persons. Close contact does not include activities such as walking by a person or sitting across a waiting room or office for a brief period of time.
[§]Assays for the laboratory diagnosis of SARS-CoV infection include enzyme-linked immunosorbent assay, indirect fluorescent-antibody assay, and reverse transcription polymerase chain reaction (RT-PCR) assays of appropriately collected clinical specimens (Source: CDC. Guidelines for collection of specimens from potential cases of SARS. Available at http://www.cdc.gov/ncidod/sars/specimen_collection_sars2.htm). Absence of SARS-CoV antibody from serum obtained ≤21 days after illness onset, a negative PCR test, or a negative viral culture does not exclude coronavirus infection and is not considered a definitive laboratory result. In these instances, a convalescent serum specimen obtained > 21 days after illness is needed to determine infection with SARS-CoV. All SARS diagnostic assays are under evaluation.
[‖]Asymptomatic SARS-CoV infection or clinical manifestations other than respiratory illness might be identified as more is learned about SARS-CoV infection.

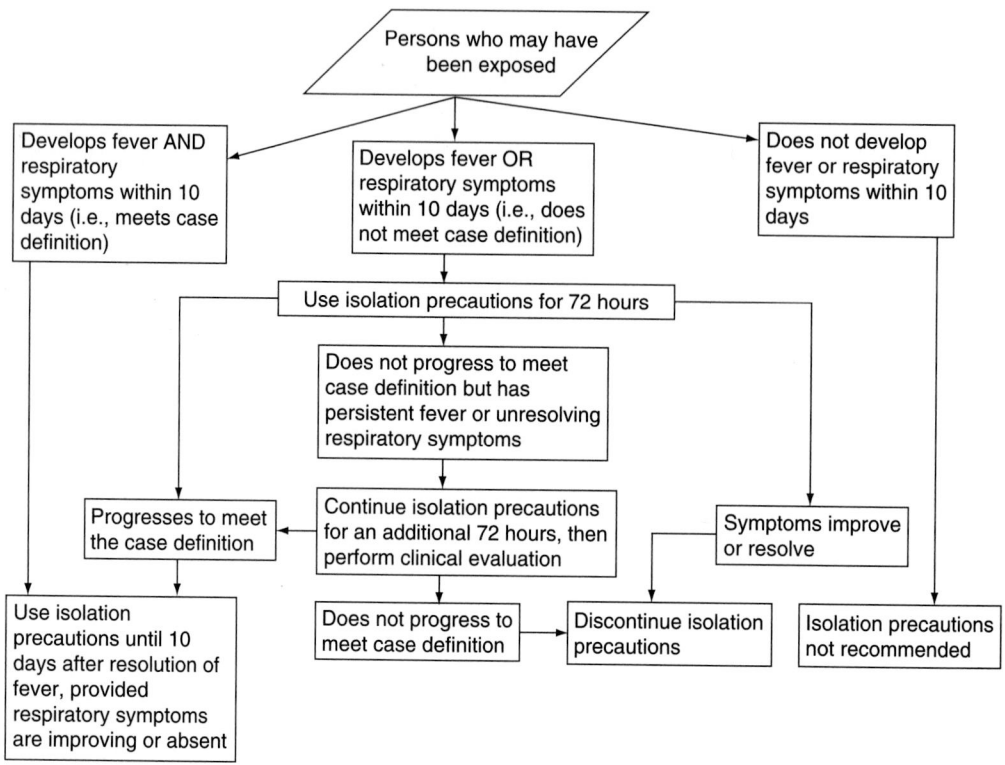

Figure 10-1   Management of persons who may have been exposed to SARS. (Available at www.cdc.gov/ncidod/sars. Accessed May 2003.)

strengthened in case of an increase in the number of cases within any area of the United States, although health officials appear optimistic that the epidemic is being brought under worldwide control.

The mortality rate for SARS is quite high. The first reports cited a 4% to 5% death rate, but that has risen due to more extensive epidemiologic research and better data. Older persons with diabetes and other comorbid conditions are at greater mortality risk than others (Booth et al, 2003). The mortality rate for those younger than 60 years of age is between 6.8% and 13.2% but for those 60 years of age and older is between 43.3% and 55% (Stein, 2003). Clinicians need to stay abreast of the latest developments and be vigilant in obtaining travel history from any suspect patient.

COMMON COLD

The common cold is a minor infection of the nose and throat that causes symptoms that last from a few days to a few weeks. Five different families of viruses cause colds. Rhinoviruses are the etiologic agent in 25% to 30% of colds, with seasonal peaks in the early fall and mid to late spring. Nearly 100 strains of rhinovirus have been found to date. Coronaviruses account for another 10% to 15% of annual colds, with a seasonal peak in midwinter. Multiple cases occur in family, work, and school settings. The virus is commonly spread via hand-to-hand contact and infrequently via droplet infection. Infectious material can survive on the hand for as long as 4 hours. Adults average two to four colds per year.

History

- Presence of facial, ear, throat, or chest pain
- Number and seasonal patterns of colds for the previous year
- Exposure to others with similar symptoms
- Drug or environmental allergies
- Current medications, including OTCs

Symptoms

Symptoms develop 1 to 3 days after the virus enters the body. Illness is characterized by one or more of the following symptoms:

- General malaise
- Low-grade or no fever
- Nasal discharge, obstruction, or congestion
- Sneezing, coughing, sore throat, and hoarseness
- Conjunctivae that may be watery and inflamed

Patients can readily make the correct diagnosis of the common cold. The challenge for health care providers is to identify patients with complicating secondary bacterial sinusitis and otitis media, for whom antimicrobial drugs will be beneficial.

Focused Physical Examination

- Check vital signs. Physical examination should include the pharynx, nasal cavity, ears, and sinuses.
- Watery red eyes and clear nasal discharge may be the only objective signs unless bacterial infection complicates the clinical picture.

Differential Diagnoses

- Influenza
- Pneumonia
- Allergic rhinitis
- Sinusitis
- Streptococcal pharyngitis
- Otitis media

Diagnostic Tests

If bacterial infection is suspected, CBC should be considered. Generally, diagnostic tests are not indicated.

Treatment
THERAPEUTICS

Treatment is entirely symptomatic. Acetaminophen or NSAIDs can be given for aches and fever, and combination products with decongestants, such as pseudoephedrine or phenylephrine, can be used for congestion, cough, and nasal discharge. Caution is recommended when using decongestants in hypertensive patients. Nasal sprays are not to be used for more than 3 days to decrease the chance of rebound nasal congestion. Other medications that can be used are antihistamines such as diphenhydramine, chlorpheniramine, and clemastine and cough suppressants such as dextromethorphan. Patients should be advised about the side effects of all these drugs.

EDUCATION

Supportive measures are important, including increased nutrition and symptom management as described previously with combination products. Because transmission of colds occurs chiefly by physical contact, it is reasonable to counsel patients, and those around them, that transmission can be minimized by hand washing, reduced finger-to-nose contact, and reduced exposure to the cold sufferer. The prophylactic and therapeutic properties of large doses of vitamin C have been examined in a number of trials, and no consistent beneficial effect has been found.

FOLLOW-UP

Because this illness is usually self-limited, follow-up is dictated by persistent symptoms beyond 7 to 10 days or if signs and symptoms of bacterial infection ensue.

SINUSITIS

Sinusitis is inflammation of the mucosal lining of the paranasal sinuses, which leads to stasis, obstruction, and subsequent infection. Factors that may induce a response include allergens and environmental irritants such as nicotine or other air pollutants. The sinuses are air-filled bony cavities that produce and drain up to 2 pints of mucus every day. Self-cleaning occurs by movement of the mucus, propelled by cilia, through the ostia, which are located behind the turbinates. Acute sinusitis is a bacterial infection of one or more paranasal sinuses, which occurs when the normal drainage is impaired because of blockage of one or more ostia. Up to 10% of cases of acute sinusitis are extensions of dental abscess. Nursing home or homebound patients with nasogastric tubes occasionally have occult sinusitis as a cause of persistent fever (Barker, Burton, and Zieve, 2003).

Sinusitis is subdivided by duration into *acute sinusitis*, with symptoms lasting up to 3 weeks; *subacute sinusitis*, with symptoms lasting from 3 weeks to 3 months; and *chronic sinusitis*, with symptoms occurring longer than 3 months. Allergy is the most common underlying cause of chronic sinusitis. Colds are the most common cause of acute sinusitis.

History

- Recent URI
- Allergies
- Recent swimming or diving
- History of nasal polyps
- Dental abscess
- Adenoidal hypertrophy
- Foreign body
- Immune deficiency

Symptoms

ACUTE SINUSITIS

- Dull pain over maxillary sinuses that becomes throbbing pain in later stages
- Fever
- Congestion
- Green nasal discharge
- Postnasal drip
- Cough
- Fatigue
- Congested ears or nose unresponsive to oral decongestants

- Headache
- Toothache
- Facial fullness
- Coughing, dependency, and percussion over the involved sinus exacerbate the pain
- Early morning periorbital swelling

CHRONIC SINUSITIS

- Nasal discharge, nasal congestion, or cough lasting more than 30 days
- Hallmark sign: dull ache or pressure across midface or headache
- Thick postnasal drip
- Popping ears, eye pain, halitosis, and fatigue

Focused Physical Examination

- Check vital signs.
- Examination should include the pharynx, nose, and ears. Transillumination of the sinuses can be attempted but is often unreliable.
- Examine teeth and gingiva for caries and inflammation; tap maxillary teeth with tongue blade because 5% to 10% of maxillary sinusitis is caused by dental root infection.
- Auscultate heart and lungs.

Differential Diagnoses

- Dental abscess
- Cluster headache
- Migraine headache
- Allergic rhinitis
- Vasomotor rhinitis
- Nasal polyp
- Tumor
- Uncomplicated upper respiratory infection

Diagnostic Tests

Radiologic examination of the sinuses is not necessary for patients with typical signs and symptoms. Acute sinusitis can be treated without culture. Nasopharyngeal swabs are usually contaminated with normal flora and are of no use. CBC with differential should be considered if patient exhibits constitutional signs.

Treatment
THERAPEUTICS

Of acute infections, 60% are caused by *S. pneumoniae* and *H. influenzae*. *S. aureus* causes fewer than 5% and tends to be associated with pansinusitis and general toxicity:

- Ampicillin or amoxicillin 250 to 500 mg four times a day for 14 days *or*
- TMP/SMX two tablets twice daily for 14 days *or*
- Augmentin 500 mg every 12 hours for 14 days, with the dose based on the patient's creatinine clearance, if known, *or*
- Cefuroxime 250 to 500 mg twice a day for 14 days

For treatment of chronic sinusitis, the same antimicrobial therapy is used. However, extend therapy for a total of 3 to 4 weeks:

- Topical decongestants (e.g., phenylephrine 0.25% or 0.5%) one or two sprays every 3 to 4 hours for 2 to 4 days
- Oral decongestants (e.g., pseudoephedrine 30 to 60 mg) every 4 to 6 hours
- Topical corticosteroids (beclomethasone) one to two sprays each nostril twice daily
- Guaifenesin (Robitussin 100 mg/5 ml) 10 to 20 ml every 4 hours
- Nasal sinus irrigation daily with saline solution
  Pain relief is important, and codeine may be required.

EDUCATION

The patient is instructed to return for further evaluation if symptoms are not improved within 48 hours and to increase fluids. Steam inhalation and warm compresses may relieve pressure. Allergens, excessively dry heat, swimming, and diving must be avoided during acute sinusitis. Also, the patient should avoid the use of antihistamines, which slow the movements of secretions out of the sinuses. Smoking cessation is important and should be encouraged, and air travel during the acute phase is best avoided.

FOLLOW-UP

Patients whose symptoms worsen during the first 48 hours of vigorous ambulatory therapy should be referred to an EENT specialist. Tender periorbital swelling associated with proptosis (downward or outward displacement of the eyes) and chemosis (scleral edema) represents orbital cellulitis and requires immediate referral to an EENT specialist.

ALLERGIC RHINITIS

Allergic rhinitis, the most common of all allergic disorders, is inflammation of the mucous membranes of the nose, usually accompanied by edema of the nasal mucosa and nasal discharge. It is estimated that 17% of Americans suffer from acute and chronic conditions generally considered to be allergic in origin. Allergic rhinitis alone accounts for 7% of common allergic conditions in the general population. Most office visits to health care providers are for conditions known to be mediated by antibodies of the immunoglobulin E (IgE) class or for conditions that resemble IgE-mediated allergy. The most common form of allergic rhinitis is seasonal and is caused by ragweed pollen. The perennial form of allergic rhinitis occurs year round and is usually related to house dust mites, mold, cockroaches, and animal dander. This form of rhinitis is more difficult to diagnose and treat. The onset of symptoms is most common between the ages of 10 and 20 and rarely begins before age 4 or after age 40. Atrophic or geriatric rhinitis is a perennial nonallergic rhinitis resulting from progressive degeneration and atrophy of nasal mucous membranes and bones of the nose.

History

- Age of onset of symptoms
- Recent use of nasal decongestants
- History of allergies
- History of nasal polyps or deviated septum
- Seasonal versus perennial symptoms

Symptoms

- Triad of symptoms: nasal congestion, sneezing, and clear rhinorrhea
- Cough, sore throat, pruritic, edematous eyelids
- Obstructed airflow

Focused Physical Examination

- Check vital signs.
- Palpate lymph nodes.
- Assess allergic shiners or dark discoloration beneath both eyes.
- Verify that nasal mucosa is pale and boggy, with thin, clear secretions. Turbinates are enlarged, and the edematous membranes may be difficult to differentiate from nasal polyps, which may resemble peeled green grapes in the nasal cavity.
- The conjunctiva have a cobblestone appearance that is due to concurrent allergic conjunctivitis.
- Transverse nasal crease is present because of chronic upward wiping of the nose.
- Tonsils and adenoids are enlarged.
- Speech is nasal or breathing is through the mouth.
- Examine the heart and lungs.

Differential Diagnoses

- Upper respiratory infection
- Sinusitis
- Otitis media
- Foreign body if blockage is unilateral
- Deviated septum if blockage is unilateral
- Nasal polyps
- Hypothyroidism
- Pregnancy
- Drug related: oral contraceptives, hormonal replacement therapy

Diagnostic Tests

Diagnosis and treatment are based on history and physical examination. CBC with differential is considered if the patient exhibits signs and symptoms of infection.

Treatment
THERAPEUTICS

Antihistamines or H_1-receptor antagonists are the primary sources of symptomatic relief. It may be necessary to try several antihistamines before an effective one is found. Also, it may be necessary to switch medications occasionally to avoid tolerance:
- Diphenhydramine (Benadryl) 12.5 to 50 mg three or four times a day (dose based on symptom relief versus somnolence; use caution in older adults because of the risk of confusion)
- Clemastine (Tavist) one or two tablets twice daily *or*
- Chlorpheniramine (Chlor-Trimeton) 4 mg four times a day *or*
- Hydroxyzine (Atarax, Vistaril) 10 to 25 mg three or four times a day *or*
- Brompheniramine (Dimetane) 4 mg four times a day *or*
- Loratadine (Claritin) 10 mg daily

Many of these medications come in combination preparations:
- Topical decongestants (phenylephrine 0.25% or 0.5%) one or two sprays every 3 to 4 hours for 2 to 4 days
- Oral decongestants (pseudoephedrine 30 to 60 mg) every 4 to 6 hours (use with caution in patients with hypertension)
- Topical corticosteroids
- Beclomethasone one or two sprays each nostril twice daily
- Mometasone furoate (Nasonex) two sprays each nostril once daily

- Guaifenesin (Robitussin 100 mg/5 ml) 10 to 20 ml every 4 hours
- Nasal sinus irrigation daily with saline solution

ENVIRONMENTAL CONTROL AND AVOIDANCE MEASURES

- Avoid exposure to tobacco smoke and allergens to which patients are sensitive.
- Avoid pets. If pets cannot be removed from the home, have designated pet-free living areas. Close bedroom doors, use air filters, and remove carpets or upholstery from pet-free areas.
- Avoid exertion when pollution levels are high.
- Avoid foods and beverages containing known allergy triggers.
- Mattresses and pillows should be encased in allergen-free cases. Sheets and blankets should be washed weekly in water hotter than 140° F.
- Consider allergy testing and immunotherapy when the connection between symptoms and exposure to allergens is unavoidable. Skin testing or in vitro testing may also be considered when patients are perennially exposed to indoor allergens.
- Reduce humidity in the home.
- Stay inside with closed doors and windows while running the air conditioner during times of peak pollen exposure.

FOLLOW-UP

Consider referral to an EENT specialist or allergist if symptoms are not well controlled with adequate trial of environmental control and medications.

HEMOPTYSIS

Hemoptysis is expectoration of both blood-tinged and grossly bloody sputum. Inflammation of the tracheobronchial mucosa is the causative factor in many cases of hemoptysis. Minor mucosal erosion can occur from UTIs, bronchitis, bronchiectasis, tuberculosis, and endobronchial inflammation due to sarcoidosis. Bronchogenic cancer may injure the mucosa, whereas metastatic lung cancer rarely results in hemoptysis. Lung tumors account for about 20% of the cases of hemoptysis. In addition, there may be injury to the pulmonary vasculature via necrotizing pneumonia (e.g., *Klebsiella* organisms), lung abscesses, aspergillomas, and pulmonary infarction secondary to embolization. Hemoptysis may also occur because of elevations in the pulmonary capillary pressure as in pulmonary edema, multiple sclerosis, Wegener syndrome, Goodpasture syndrome, and arteriovenous malformations. Patients with mitral stenosis and pulmonary vascular congestion are susceptible to hemoptysis with any source of lung irritation. Additional causes may be bleeding disorders, excessive coagulant therapy, or chest trauma (Table 10-8).

TABLE 10-8	Differentiation		
	pH	Color	Characteristics
Blood-streaked sputum			Common and may occur in nonthreatening conditions
Hemoptysis	Alkaline	Bright red and frothy	Blood is mixed with sputum
Hematemesis	Acid	Darker brown	Blood may be mixed with food particles

Conditions

- Bronchitis and bronchiectasis: occasionally blood-tinged sputum; patient usually has chronic cough and dyspnea, which may be worse in the morning.
- Lung tumors: occur most frequently in persons over 40 years of age and in smokers; a change in the cough pattern occurs; chest ache may be an accompanying symptom.
- Pneumonia: sputum appears red-brown or red-green and is mixed with pus; fever, pleuritic chest pain, or malaise may develop.
- Pulmonary infarction secondary to pulmonary embolus: sudden onset of pleuritic chest pain in conjunction with hemoptysis; patient has diaphoresis and syncope, dyspnea, and anxiety. Frequently, the patient has a history of calf pain, deep venous thrombosis, or phlebitis.
- Pulmonary edema: pink frothy sputum, diaphoresis, tachypnea, tachycardia, anxiety; jugular venous distension (JVD), hepatomegaly, or ankle edema may be present.

History and Symptoms

Question the patient about the onset of hemoptysis:
- Ask whether this is a first-time episode or a recurrent problem. Explicitly determine whether the bleeding is coming from the lungs or from expectorated blood from the nasopharynx.
- Describe the color, consistency, and characteristics of sputum.
- Quantify the amount of bleeding.
- Inquire about associated symptoms: weight loss, fatigue, persistent cough, dyspnea, wheezing, fever, night sweats, or excessive bruising.
- What is the past medical history, particularly regarding lung, cardiac, hematologic, or immunologic disorders?
- Inquire about recent respiratory infection or exposure to tuberculosis, environmental exposures (e.g., asbestos), use of anticoagulants, history of chest trauma, cigarette smoking, family history of hemoptysis, last chest x-ray or PPD, drug or environmental allergies, and current medications, including OTCs.

Focused Physical Examination

- Check vital signs, particularly noting fever or tachypnea.
- Observe skin for ecchymoses and telangiectasias and nails for clubbing.
- Examine nose and pharynx for signs of bleeding. Differentiate hemoptysis from epistaxis.
- Inspect neck for JVD, and check for lymphadenopathy.
- Perform a complete lung and cardiovascular examination.
- Assess for ankle edema.

Differential Diagnoses

- Bronchitis or bronchiectasis
- Lung tumors
- Pneumonia
- Pulmonary infarction secondary to pulmonary embolus
- Pulmonary edema

Diagnostic Tests

- Perform chest x-ray examination.
- Consider Gram stain for suspected infection.

- Consider AFB for suspected tuberculosis.
- Consider cytology for suspected malignancy.
- Consider PPD.
- Consider ventilation-perfusion (V/Q) scan or angiography when pulmonary embolus is suspected.
- Consider bronchoscopy for patients who smoke and are over 40 years of age or who have an abnormal chest x-ray and recurrent hemoptysis.
- Consider prothrombin time, partial thromboplastin time, and platelet count studies.

Treatment
THERAPEUTICS

First, any underlying illness or infection must be treated. Judicious use of mild cough suppressants should be encouraged. Patients with blood-tinged or blood-streaked sputum who have an upper respiratory infection or bronchitis that does not resolve in 2 to 3 days should be reevaluated or referred to a specialist.

EDUCATION

- Explain that blood is irritating to the tracheobronchial tree and mucus should be expectorated, not swallowed.
- Have patient record the number of episodes of hemoptysis and collect the blood that is expectorated.
- Have patient return to the clinic or emergency room if the amount of blood increases or becomes filled with clots or if the patient develops respiratory distress, diaphoresis, chest pain, or tachypnea.

FOLLOW-UP

Because hemoptysis is usually self-limited, follow-up is indicated with persistence or recurrence of symptoms or with suspicion of neoplastic process or coagulopathy.

TUBERCULOSIS

Tuberculosis is a necrotizing bacterial infection most commonly affecting the lungs. Primary or initial infection occurs by inhalation of the etiologic agent, *Mycobacterium tuberculosis,* which is dispersed as microdroplet nuclei by a person who is positive for tuberculosis. Of primary tuberculosis infections, 90% to 95% remain in a latent or dormant infection stage. It is estimated that 10 to 15 million Americans have latent tuberculosis infections. Active TB may develop during periods of stress, when the body is going through change or fighting off a disease such as human immunodeficiency virus (HIV) or diabetes, with use of corticosteroids, during adolescence, and during old age. Apical areas of the lungs are the most common sites, but tuberculosis is a systemic disease that may result in pleural effusion, disseminated tuberculosis, or infections in the lymphatic or genitourinary systems.

From 1985 to 1991, annually reported cases increased by 18% because of a variety of issues, including an increase in diagnosis of HIV disease, deterioration of the medical infrastructure, an increase in adverse social and economic conditions, and an increase in foreign-born persons who have emigrated to the United States and are infected with tuberculosis (U.S. Department of Health and Human Services, 1994). In the United States the highest incidence, except for people with HIV disease, is in people over 65 years of age. Efforts to control the spread of tuberculosis have been confounded by the emergence of strains of that are resistant to multiple drugs. Tuberculosis control in the United States depends on screening populations at high risk and providing preventive therapy to those who are most likely to develop active disease (Box 10-3).

Box 10-3

Individuals at High Risk for Tuberculosis

- Racial or ethnic minority populations as defined locally.
- Foreign-born individuals, especially children, who arrive from countries with a high incidence of TB (African, Asian, and Latin American nations). In 1995, 63% of new cases of TB were in individuals from the following countries: Haiti, India, Mexico, Philippines, People's Republic of China, and Vietnam.
- Domestic or occupational contacts of infectious TB cases.
- Alcoholic and injection drug users.
- Residents and staff of acute and long-term facilities (hospitals, nursing homes, correctional and mental health institutions).
- Individuals with chronic disease such as HIV, diabetes, ESRD, hematologic disease, history of intestinal bypass or gastrectomy, chronic malabsorption syndromes, silicosis, cancer of the upper gastrointestinal tract or oropharynx, prolonged steroid use and immunosuppressive therapy, and being 10% or more *below* the ideal body weight.

From U.S. Department of Health and Human Services: *The clinician's handbook of preventive services*, McLean, Va, 1994, International Medical.
TB, Tuberculosis; *ESRD*, end-stage renal disease.

History

- Onset and duration of symptoms
- Exposure at home, school, social occasions
- Previous history of tuberculosis infection
- Review of risk factors (e.g., chronic disease)
- Review of dates of skin tests and chest x-ray examination
- Recent travel to countries where tuberculosis is prevalent
- Drug or environmental allergies
- Current medications, including OTCs

Symptoms

Symptoms vary but may include the following:
- Increasing fatigue
- Malaise
- Anorexia
- Weight loss
- Periodic fever
- Night sweats
- Hemoptysis
- Productive, prolonged cough lasting longer than 3 weeks

Focused Physical Examination

- Note the patient's vital signs. The physical examination often may be entirely negative, even with obvious evidence of pulmonary disease on the chest x-ray film. The following positive findings, when present, may be of considerable help in supporting the diagnosis:

- Crackles localized to the upper posterior chest or auscultatory evidence of pulmonary cavitation (bronchovesicular breath sounds and whispered pectoriloquy)
- Evidence of pleural effusion
- Supraclavicular and infraclavicular retraction
- Lymphadenopathy
- Skin pallor
- Evidence of weight loss and fever

Differential Diagnoses

- Malignancy
- Silicosis
- COPD
- Asthma
- Bronchiectasis
- Pneumonia

Diagnostic Tests

The incubation period is 2 to 10 weeks from the time of exposure to the development of a positive reaction to a tuberculosis test. The response to PPD may wane with age and can be restored with repeat testing. Because of this booster effect, patients (particularly those over 55 years of age) who undergo repeated testing may be falsely classified as new converters and unnecessarily treated with isoniazid. Some authorities advise initial screening of adults in institutional and hospital settings with a two-step PPD testing procedure. If the first Mantoux test is negative, a second should be performed in 1 to 2 weeks. Reaction to the booster test usually indicates old, not new, infection. The Centers for Disease Control and Prevention also recommend this two-step procedure for the initial screening of residents and employees of long-term care facilities such as nursing homes, adult foster care homes, and board and care homes (U.S. Department of Health and Human Services, 1994) (Figure 10-2). Consultation with an infection control nurse or the community public health department will be helpful in determining the need for testing of others in the household, nursing home, or other contacts.

The Mantoux test should be read 48 to 72 hours after placement by palpating the margin of induration and measuring the diameter transverse to the long axis of the forearm. It may be helpful to outline the margin of induration with a ballpoint pen. Erythema surrounding the induration should not be considered in evaluating test results. Providers should always record the actual millimeters of induration. Simply recording positive or negative is not precise enough and may lead to improper treatment.

Absence of tuberculin reaction does not exclude a diagnosis of tuberculosis infection, especially when symptoms suggest active disease. Induration of less than 5 mm may occur early in the course of infection or in patients with altered immune function. Anergy testing with at least two other delayed-type hypersensitivity skin tests (i.e., *Candida,* mumps, or tetanus toxoid) should be used in conjunction with PPD testing in adults with decreased cell-mediated immune function (including those with HIV infection).

Adverse reactions to tuberculosis skin testing are uncommon. Reactions described include pain, fever, ulceration, vesiculation, and regional adenopathy. Because of the potential for adverse reactions, it is not advisable to retest patients who have a documented history of a positive Mantoux test.

Although bacillus Calmette-Guérin (bCG) vaccine can cause false-positive Mantoux reactions, this response decreases with time and rarely causes reactions 15 mm or greater. In general, bCG-vaccinated persons with positive Mantoux tests should be considered to have true infection with tuberculosis and given appropriate follow-up care (Table 10-9).

ADMINISTERING

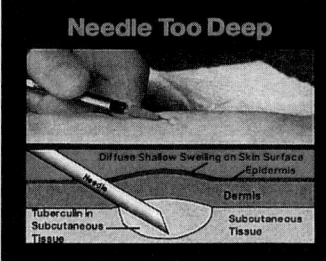

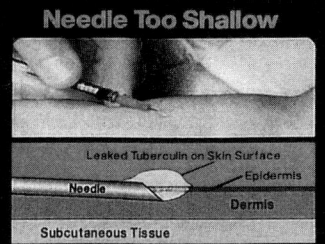

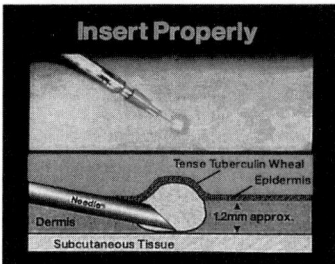

Give 0.1 cc of 5 Tuberculin Units PPD intradermally.

All tests should be read between 48-72 hours. If more than 72 hours has elapsed and there is not an easily palpable positive reaction, repeat the test on the other arm and read at 48-72 hours.

Measure induration - not erythema.

Measure and report results in millimeters of induration.

READING

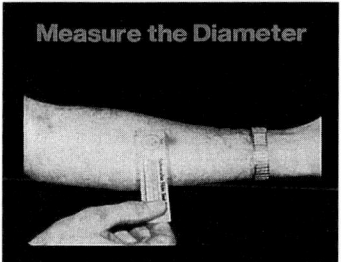

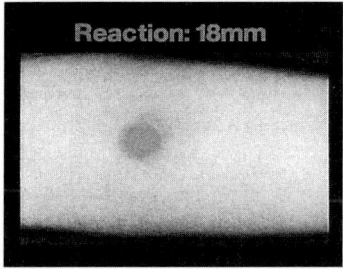

All persons with positive reactions should be evaluated for preventive therapy, once TB disease has been ruled out.

5 or more millimeters induration is considered positive for the highest risk groups, such as:

• Persons with HIV infection;

• Persons who have had close contact with an infectious tuberculosis case;

• Persons who have chest radiographs consistent with old, healed tuberculosis;

• Intravenous drug users whose HIV status is unknown.

10 or more millimeters induration is considered positive for other high risk groups, such as:

• Foreign-born persons from high prevalence areas (such as Asia, Africa, and Latin America);

• Intravenous drug users known to be HIV seronegative;

• Medically-underserved low income populations, including high-risk racial or ethnic minority populations (especially blacks, Hispanics, and Native Americans);

• Residents of long-term care facilities (such as correctional institutions, nursing homes, mental institutions);

• Persons with medical conditions which have been reported to increase the risk of tuberculosis such as silicosis, being 10 percent or more below ideal body weight, chronic renal failure, diabetes mellitus, high dose corticosteroid and other immunosuppressive therapy, some hematologic disorders (such as leukemias and lymphomas), and other malignancies;

• Locally identified high risk populations;

• Children who are in one of the high risk groups listed above; and

• Health care workers who provide services to any of the high risk groups.

15 or more millimeters induration is considered positive for persons with no risk factors for tuberculosis.

Negative Reactions - For each of the categories, reactions below the cutting point are considered negative.

  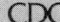

U.S. DEPARTMENT OF HEALTH & HUMAN SERVICES
Public Health Service
Centers for Disease Control and Prevention
National Center for Prevention Services
Division of TB Elimination
Atlanta, Georgia 30333

Please use this wall chart in conjunction with the CDC skin test video

Figure 10-2 The Mantoux tuberculin skin test. (Courtesy U.S. Department of Health and Human Services, Public Health Service, Centers for Disease Control and Prevention, National Center for Prevention Services, Division of TB Elimination, 1999, Atlanta, Ga.)

TABLE 10-9	Criteria for Determining Need for Preventive Therapy with Positive PPD	

Category	<35	≥35
With risk factor	Treat all ages if reaction to 5 TU PPD is ≥10 mm (or ≥5 mm and recent TB contact, HIV infected or has radiographic evidence of old TB)	
Without risk factor High-incidence group*	Treat if PPD is ≥10 mm	Do not treat
Without risk factor Low-incidence group	Treat if PPD is ≥15 mm	Do not treat

From U.S. Department of Health and Human Services: *The clinician's handbook of preventive services*, McLean, Va, 1994, International Medical.
*High-incidence groups include foreign-born persons, medically underserved low-income populations, and residents of long-term care facilities.

A chest x-ray examination and sputum culture should be taken. A positive culture is essential to confirm the diagnosis. Three sputum samples should be examined for AFB smear and culture. Culture results may take from 3 to 6 weeks.

Baseline laboratory tests include LFTs and CBC with differential. Baseline drug susceptibility of the first isolate is determined and repeat drug susceptibility testing in patients whose isolates do not convert to negative is done within 3 months. Urinalysis should be obtained routinely; if sterile pyuria is found, it is suggestive of renal TB, and cultures should be sent.

If clinical features suggest infection outside the lung, smears and cultures of other body fluids such as cerebrospinal fluid are appropriate.

Treatment
THERAPEUTICS

Option 1 is to administer daily isoniazid, rifampin, and pyrazinamide for 8 weeks, followed by 16 weeks of isoniazid and rifampin daily or two to three times per week. *All regimens administered two to three times per week should be monitored by directly observed treatment for the duration of therapy:*
- Isoniazid: 5 mg/kg up to 300 mg for everyday dosing *or* 15 mg/kg up to 900 mg for two to three times weekly dosing
- Rifampin: 10 mg/kg up to 600 mg for all dosing schedules
- Pyrazinamide: 15 to 30 mg/kg up to 2 g for daily dosing *or* 50 to 70 mg/kg up to 3 g for two to three times weekly dosing

In areas where resistance to isoniazid is documented, ethambutol or streptomycin can be added for at least 6 months as well as 3 months beyond culture conversion:
- Ethambutol: 15 to 25 mg/kg for daily dosing *or* 25 to 30 mg/kg up to 2.5 g for two to three times weekly dosing
- Streptomycin: 15 to 20 mg/kg up to 1 g intramuscular for daily dosing *or* 25 to 30 mg/kg up to 1 g for two to three times weekly dosing

Option 2 is to administer daily isoniazid, rifampin, pyrazinamide, and streptomycin or ethambutol for 2 weeks, followed by twice weekly administration of the same drugs for 6 weeks by directly observed treatment. Subsequent administration is twice weekly with isoniazid and rifampin for 16 weeks by directly observed treatment.

Option 3 is directly observed treatment three times per week with isoniazid, rifampin, pyrazinamide, and ethambutol or streptomycin for 6 months (Uphold and Graham, 1994).

Liver function tests should be checked before initiation of therapy and then monthly throughout the course of treatment, and the patient should be monitored for signs of hepatic toxicity. *Consult a tuberculosis medical expert if the patient continues to remain symptomatic or if the smear* **or** *culture remains positive after 3 months.*

EDUCATION

Teach patient the possible side effects of medications, including the following:
- Peripheral neuritis from isoniazid
- Multiple drug interactions
- Orange urine and tears that may stain contact lenses with rifampin
- Possible eighth cranial nerve damage with streptomycin: have hearing tested
- Hyperuricemia with pyrazinamide
- Optic neuritis with ethambutol: have vision, especially color sensitivity, tested
  All antitubercular medications have possible liver damage as a side effect. *No alcohol is allowed.*
- Teach proper disposal of secretions and tissues as well as the mode of transmission, and reinforce the need to cover mouth with coughing.
- Have patients take pyridoxine (vitamin B_6) 25 mg daily while on isoniazid.
- Patients are usually back to their usual state of health in 1 to 2 months.

FOLLOW-UP

The patient's role in successful treatment of tuberculosis, daily self-administration of drugs for a period of 6 to 9 months, and return for regular follow-up schedules is crucial. After treatment has been initiated, the patient should be seen or contacted at least once per month, chiefly to ensure drug compliance and to monitor for drug side effects. Sputum cultures should be obtained monthly for the first 3 months. At 3 months and between 6 and 12 months, chest x-ray films should be obtained. Sputum cultures should be negative after 3 months of therapy, although occasionally nonculturable acid-fast organisms can be seen on smear for longer periods. A test-of-cure culture should be done on all patients at 5 or 6 months.

At the cessation of traditional chemotherapy regimen (9 months), prolonged follow-up is not necessary. After short-course (6 months) chemotherapy, it is recommended that follow-up be continued for another 12 months to detect relapses by symptoms and sputum culture.

Summary

Age-related changes in the respiratory system are significant, as are the number of potential acute and chronic diseases of the lungs and airways. The practitioner must be able to distinguish between acute, self-limiting, life-threatening, and chronic lung diseases and to treat each appropriately to minimize discomfort and loss of function. It is important to know the risk factors for lung disease so that prevention and appropriate screening can be started early. This point is important whether the concern is COPD, cancer of the lung, or infectious concerns such as tuberculosis, a resurgent and significant threat.

Resources

American Lung Association
www.lungusa.org

National Coalition for Adult Immunization
www.nfid.org/ncai

New York Online Access to Health (NOAH)
COPD Website
www.noah.cuny.edu

References

Abramowicz M, editor: Sparfloxacin and levofloxacin, *Med Lett Drugs* Ther 39:41-43, 1997.

American Thoracic Society: Guidelines for the initial management of adults with community-acquired pneumonia: diagnosis, assessment of severity, and initial antimicrobial therapy, *Am Rev Respir Dis* 148: 1418-1426, 1993.

Barker LR, Burton JR, Zieve PD: *Ambulatory medicine*, ed 6, Baltimore, 2003, Lippincott Williams & Wilkins.

Booth CM et al: Clinical features and short-term outcomes of 144 patients with SARS in the greater Toronto area, *JAMA* May 6, 2003 (epub ahead of print).

Centers for Disease Control and Prevention: *Severe acute respiratory distress syndrome.* Available at www.cdc.gov/ncidod/sars. Accessed May 8, 2003.

Chestnutt M, Prendergast T: Lung. In Tierney LM et al, editors: *Current medical diagnosis and treatment: adult ambulatory and in-patient management*, New York, 2002, Lange Medical Books/McGraw Hill.

Mastrovich JD, Greenberger PA: Psychogenic cough in adults: a report of two cases and a review of the literature. *Allergy Asthma Proc* 23 (1):27-33, 2002.

Richman E: Asthma diagnosis and management: new severity classifications and therapy alternatives, *Clin Rev* 7:76-112, 1997.

Stahlmann R, Lode H: Fluoroquinolone in the elderly: safety considerations, *Drugs Aging* 20(4):289-302, 2003.

Stein R: Death rate from SARS is expected to increase, *Washington Post,* May 6, 2003.

Uphold CR, Graham MV: *Clinical guidelines in adult health*, Gainesville, Fla, 1994, Barmarrae.

U.S. Department of Health and Human Services: *The clinician's handbook of preventive services,* McLean, Va, 1994, International Medical.

U.S. Department of Health and Human Services: *Core curriculum on tuberculosis: what every clinician should know*, ed 3, Atlanta, 1999, Centers for Disease Control and Prevention.

Witta KM: COPD in the elderly: controlling symptoms and improving quality of life, *Adv Nurse Pract* 5:18-27, 1997.

World Health Organization: *Cumulative number of reported probable cases of severe acute respiratory syndrome (SARS)*. Available at www.who.int/csr/sarscountry/2003. Accessed May 12, 2003.

11

Cardiovascular System

Epidemiology

Eight of every 10 people 65 years of age or older have at least one chronic medical problem, but 60% of those over 65 years of age are without any functional or physical limitations from their conditions. When illness or disability occurs in the older population, however, cardiovascular disease is still the most frequent cause. Congestive heart failure (CHF) is the most common medical problem necessitating hospitalization in older patients. More than half of patients hospitalized annually for acute myocardial infarction (MI) are more than 65 years of age. Finally, coronary artery disease (CAD) is the most common cause of death in persons 65 years of age and older (Cobbs, 2002). Therefore proper diagnosis and treatment of cardiovascular diseases can help both to maintain the health of the large number of functionally independent older adults and to reduce morbidity and mortality rates in older patients in acute and chronic care settings.

Changes in the cardiovascular system occur with aging. Some of these changes can be considered natural in an aging organism. Others occur with the onset of a disease process in the cardiovascular system itself. Still other changes are the result of coexisting medical conditions. Anatomic changes occur in the blood vessels, the heart itself, the heart valves, and the conducting systems; physiologic and functional changes also may occur.

Much evidence exists for identifying certain risk factors, such as hypertension, diabetes, raised cholesterol levels, smoking, obesity, hormone changes, and sedentary lifestyle, to reduce the incidence of cardiovascular disease (Gladdish and Rajkumar, 2001).

Age-related Changes in the Vasculature

With aging, atherosclerotic plaque builds up in the vascular tree throughout the body. The *plaques* are complex aggregates of necrotic cells, mostly smooth muscle cells, connective tissue such as collagen and elastin, and lipid deposits. Often deposition of calcium in and around these plaques develop, resulting in a hardened, irregular vessel wall and a narrowing of the lumen of the vessel, with obstruction or partial obstruction of blood flow. Commonly referred to as "hardening of the arteries," this process probably begins in late adolescence and advances with aging. During the Korean War, autopsies done on soldiers who were war casualties revealed that atherosclerotic

259

Box 11-1

Risk Factors for the Development of Atherosclerosis

- Cigarette smoking
- Diabetes
- Hypertension
- Hyperlipidemia
- Obesity
- Genetic factors

changes had already begun in some soldiers who were as young as 18 years of age. Of course, other factors influence the rate at which atherosclerosis progresses. Known risk factors for development of atherosclerosis are listed in Box 11-1.

Other changes in the vascular tree occur as a natural consequence of aging, and these changes take place regardless of the presence or rate of atherosclerosis. The cells of the arterial walls become more and more irregular in size and shape with aging. Their usual orderly layering becomes deranged, with the orientation of the cells one to another irregular and disorderly. The subendothelial layer thickens because of increased connective tissue production and increased calcium and lipid deposition. In the medial layer are thickened smooth muscle layers. The smooth muscle cells have more protein and calcium deposition. The surrounding elastin or connective tissue is prone to fragmentation. Loss of the integrity of elastin means poor elasticity in the vessel wall. In the intimal layer are similar fragmentation of elastin and increased collagen content. The intimal surface becomes irregular, leaving more pits and crevices in which lipids can deposit. All these changes result in thicker, less distensible, less pliable arterial walls. With any atherosclerotic change, the stiffening is even worse. These aged arteries cannot distend when blood flow increases, effectively increasing the peripheral "resistance" to flow. An aorta affected by these aging changes has decreased compliance or resistance to the systolic ejection, affecting the percentage of the blood volume pumped by the left ventricle (LV) during systole that actually is ejected into the peripheral circulation *(ejection fraction)*. At some point, when circulatory demand increases, these stiff, noncompliant blood vessels cannot expand to accommodate the demand, leading to higher pressures within the arterial tree.

In the coronary arteries these aging changes tend to affect the proximal part of the artery first and the left coronary artery before the right. Autopsy studies consistently find changes in persons as young as middle adulthood, whereas changes in the right coronary artery are noted in persons in their fifties.

Changes also occur in the function of the blood vessel walls. With aging the usual constriction response of the vascular smooth muscle to alpha-adrenergic stimulation is unchanged. However, the usual relaxation response of the vascular smooth muscle to beta-adrenergic stimulation declines with age, another factor in the aged blood vessel's decreased ability to relax. This response to alpha-adrenergic input, without a corresponding response to beta-adrenergic input, may be part of the etiology of isolated systolic hypertension in older adults, in addition to the increase in the level of plasma catecholamines in older adults.

Changes in the Heart Muscle

The age-related changes in the myocardium include enlargement of the cardiac muscle cells: the *myocytes.* Inside the cell are lipid and lipofuscin deposits; the tubules dilate, and there is decreased mitochondrial activity, resulting in abnormal products of oxidation, such as malonaldehyde, which irreversibly denatures deoxyribonucleic acid. This leads to a larger cell with impaired cellular functions that does not get replaced by replication when cell death occurs. At about 75 years of age, a body has only 10% as many sinus node cells as it had at 20 years of age. This change may account for the increased incidence of sinus node disease, such as sick sinus syndrome (SSS) or supraventricular tachyarrhythmias, in older patients.

Around the myocytes, as in the blood vessel walls, deposition of elastic tissue, fat, and collagen occurs; multiple foci of fibrosis and calcification may occur. The result is a stiff, inelastic, noncompliant myocardium. Deposition of amyloid, especially in the LV, also may occur. The LV thickens slightly, but in general the overall size of the LV remains the same with aging changes alone. Within the myocardium capillaries are obliterated because of the deposition of lipids, connective tissue, and calcium. Therefore the myocardium can actually be relatively ischemic, with inadequate blood flow, because of this small-vessel disease, even with the major coronary arteries open. Small-vessel ischemic disease occurs with increased frequency in patients with diabetes.

These changes have a functional consequence for the myocardium. The stiffer the myocardial wall becomes, the more time is required for this stiff heart muscle to relax, and the relaxation phase requires more energy and uses more oxygen. The first result is that decreased relaxation of the myocardial wall impedes diastolic filling and therefore effectively reduces cardiac output. With severe impairment to diastolic filling, reduced forward flow or cardiac output can occur. The result can be left-sided CHF, leading to pulmonary vascular congestion and systemic congestion and edema. Second, with increased myocardial oxygen demand, there can be a relative hypoxia or ischemia in the heart muscle, even when the major coronary arteries are not diseased. Compounding this effect is the fact that as people age arterial oxygen tension decreases by 4 mm Hg per decade, from an average of 90 mm Hg at 30 years of age to 75 mm Hg at 80 years of age.

Changes in the Heart Valves and Conducting System

Again, the changes effected by aging in the heart valves and the conductive system are largely deposition of calcium; an increase in connective tissue, with fragments of degenerated connective tissue and cells remaining or deposited within the normal tissue; and fibrosis. In the heart valves calcium deposition has the largest effect. Calcium deposits below the mitral valve, in the space between the posterior leaflet of the mitral valve and the adjacent myocardial wall, effectively decrease the motion of the valve leaflets and prevent complete opening of the valve. Calcium deposits in the mitral annulus likewise decrease excursion of the valve leaflets. The physiologic result is mitral stenosis, decreased LV filling, and eventual left atrial strain and enlargement. Atrial fibrillation with submitral calcium deposits and frequently associated conduction defects develop (Duncan and Vittone, 1996).

In the conducting system, similar aging changes occur, with predictable effects. In addition, a loss of conducting cells occurs. As described earlier, a 90% loss of the number of cells in the sinus node occurs by 75 years of age. The atrioventricular (AV) node and bundle of His show a decrease in the number of both cells and conducting fibers. From the AV node the bundle of His emerges as a main bundle and then branches into the left and right bundles. Proximally fewer fascicles are connecting the main bundle with the left bundle. Also, fewer distal conducting fibers are present. Predictably, conduction disorders such as left or right bundle branch blocks (RBBB) and AV node blockade increase with aging. Box 11-2 lists the structural and functional changes in the aging heart.

Changes in Cardiovascular Physiology

The structural changes described translate into specific cardiovascular problems, such as hypertension, decreased cardiac output, CHF, valvular dysfunction, and cardiac arrhythmias or conduction disturbances. Other changes in cardiovascular physiology compound these problems. Already mentioned is the decreased arterial oxygen tension, which can aggravate any vascular problem and make older patients with circulatory compromise (coronary artery or peripheral artery insufficiency) have more severe symptoms than they would otherwise based on their anatomic vascular disease alone. Older patients also have an increased resting heart rate, perhaps related in part to an increased level of catecholamines. Nonetheless, when increased heart rate or contractility is needed, in the case of

Box 11-2

Age-related Changes in Cardiovascular Structure and Function

Structure	Function
Myocardial	Heart rate
Increased myocardial mass	Decreased heart rate at rest
Increased LV wall thickness	Decreased maximal heart rate during exercise
Increased deposition of collagen	Decreased heart rate variability
Valvular	Decreased sinus node intrinsic rate
Increased thickness of aortic and mitral leaflets	LV systolic
Increased circumference of all four valves	Unchanged cardiac output
Calcification of mitral annulus	Increased stroke volume index
Arterial	LV diastolic
Increased intimal thickness	Decreased LV compliance
Increased collagen content	Increased early diastolic LV filling
	Myofibril
	Unchanged peak contractile force
	Increased duration of contraction
	Decreased Ca^{++} uptake by sarcoplasmic reticulum
	Decreased β-adrenergic-mediated contractile augmentation
	Vascular
	Decreased compliance
	Increased pulsed-wave velocity

From Duncan A, Vittone JM: Cardiovascular disease in elderly patients, *Mayo Clin Proc* 71:184-196, 1996.
LV, Left ventricular.

physiologic stress, there is a decrease in responsiveness to beta-adrenergic stimulation. Thus maximum heart rate and the ability to increase the ejection fraction are lower.

Older patients are also much more sensitive to small changes in plasma volume. The natural changes of aging in the kidneys, coupled with changes in the function of the renin-angiotensin axis, actually make the older person more susceptible to dehydration. There is a decreased thirst drive. Vasopressin secretion is decreased in response to decreased plasma volume. There is also decreased renin production, and therefore decreased angiotensin, and ultimately decreased aldosterone production. In addition, when plasma volume is decreased, the older person may be more symptomatic because compensatory mechanisms such as the baroreceptor reflex are also less responsive. Thus the older person with small decreases in plasma volume might be light headed, dizzy, or even syncopal.

One study found a substantial drop in arterial blood pressure (BP) in older patients after a meal. This group also experiences significant increases in postprandial symptoms, including syncope, angina, and MI. The mechanism of postprandial hypotension is thought to be the diversion of blood flow to the gut, resulting in a relatively reduced intravascular volume elsewhere in the vascular tree. Other relatively mild hemodynamic changes occur with defecation, urination, and postural changes. The incidence of symptoms associated with such mild hemodynamic changes is negligible in young persons but significant in older adults. The frequency of falls increases dramatically in older adults, and although falls are often multifactorial, no doubt many are related to events such as those described, which can cause small but eventful hemodynamic changes in older adults. Add to that diuretic therapy for hypertension or CHF, and the older adult is at even more risk.

As an illustration of the impact of aging in the older heart and vascular system, imagine the older adult facing a physiologic stress, such as surgery, acute illness, or perhaps pneumonia. In either instance the heart now needs to increase its cardiac output to generate a greater circulatory flow to vital organs. First, the LV early (passive) diastolic filling is less because of a stiffened, less compliant ventricle. Less volume is delivered to the aorta in systole. Therefore an increase in systolic contraction may be required. The LV is slightly thickened, but unless an MI or ischemia occurs, contractile strength should be preserved. Yet the maximum increase possible in ejection fraction is lower in older adults. Increased heart rate can compensate for decreased filling volume, but the maximum heart rate attainable is lower in older adults. In addition, because of aging changes in the arterial tree, the peripheral resistance is higher. The systolic contraction must overcome afterload. The blood volume delivered to the peripheral circulation is therefore less, despite the increased demand. Add to that any decrease in plasma volume, and the situation is compounded. Beta-adrenergic stimulation is present, but the aging heart responds less to this stimulus. If aging coronary arteries are also affected by atherosclerotic changes, ischemia and increased risk for MI occur. All of this, plus decreased arterial oxygen tension and decreased efficiency of oxygen extraction, can make an aging cardiovascular system unable to deliver increased cardiac output on demand.

Age-related changes in the cardiovascular system are a combination of changes natural to aging, the presence of cardiovascular disease, and comorbid conditions that affect the cardiovascular system. Overall, the natural history of heart disease is that it increases with aging. The manifestations of heart disease, the treatments, and the outcomes may all differ in older persons compared with younger adults. Yet older people can improve their cardiovascular function with exercise. With regular cardiovascular exercise such as a gradual program of brisk walking for 30 minutes at least three times a week, exercise tolerance improves through increased arterial oxygen tension but chiefly through increased efficiency of oxygen uptake and extraction (air to blood to tissue). As a result, resting heart rate and BP fall. Body fat percentage can be decreased, and muscle strength and joint flexibility can be increased, resulting in better mobility, balance, and gait. Therefore the aging cardiovascular system, like the aging musculoskeletal system, can still be conditioned.

Cardiac Examination of the Older Patient

The cardiac examination of the older person contains the same elements as that of any other patient. Cardiac disease increases with age, however, and findings may be encountered that are seen comparatively infrequently in young persons. First, BP and heart rate are measured and the heart rhythm assessed for regularity and ectopic beats. For BP measurement of all patients, even more pertinent in older patients, the cuff should be inflated initially to 200 mm Hg or slightly greater. Failure to do so may result in a falsely low reading. Another method is to palpate the brachial artery as the cuff is inflated to at least 20 mm Hg above the point at which the artery ceases to be palpable (the palpable systolic BP [SBP]). The cuff is deflated slowly. If Korotkoff's sounds are heard immediately as deflation begins, chances are the cuff was not inflated to a high enough pressure, and the patient's SBP could be higher than measured. (This caution applies even if the cuff was initially inflated to 200 mm Hg or above.) The measurement should be repeated on the other arm and inflated to a higher level. In evaluating older patients for hypertension, it is prudent to take a series of BP readings and to measure BP while the patient is both sitting and standing.

Orthostatic Hypotension

The increased incidence of orthostatic hypotension in older persons is due to a number of normal aging structural and physiologic changes that have already been discussed. Older adults have a lower resting heart rate and are less able to increase cardiac output with demand. They have lower plasma renin activity, a decreased vasopressin response to thirst, and decreased renal conservation of salt with decreased volume. Thus they may have a relatively decreased intravascular volume. As a result, BP may fall significantly with change from a lying or sitting posture to a standing position, a phenomenon called *orthostatic blood pressure change*. If that change causes abnormally low BP or symptoms such as light-headedness, dizziness, or syncope, the diagnosis is orthostatic or postural hypotension. The BP criterion for a diagnosis of orthostatic hypotension is a drop of more than 20 mm Hg in SBP or a drop of more than 10 mm Hg in DBP on change of position. Orthostatic hypotension can be a result of volume depletion, as in fluid or blood loss, or it can be from other causes, such as autonomic nervous system dysfunction. Alternately, a rise in pulse of more than 20 beats per minute on change of position can be considered a sign more specific for volume depletion. The presence of symptomatic orthostatic hypotension can have important therapeutic implications for older patients.

Auscultation of the Heart
BRUITS

First, the clinician listens for carotid bruits. Asymptomatic carotid bruits are indicative of diffuse atherosclerotic disease. Asymptomatic carotid bruits can be predictors of increased stroke risk, but the incidence of stroke in these patients is contralateral as often as ipsilateral. Totally occluded carotid arteries are silent and do not produce a bruit.

HEART SOUNDS

The clinician listens for the heart sounds and physiologic splitting of the second heart sound, S2. It should be split in inspiration because of delayed pulmonic closure, which occurs from increased filling of the right side of the heart. It should be heard best at the left sternal border. As one listens toward the apex, the splitting should disappear; the pulmonic component of S2 should be so faint as to be inaudible there. A reversed split, called a *paradoxic split* (i.e., a splitting or two-component sound in expiration and no split in inspiration) can occur. It accompanies LV conduction delay as in left bundle branch block (LBBB). Pacemaker patients have paradoxic splitting because pacemakers activate the right side of the heart before the left side. The delay in the closing of the aortic valve makes the second heart sound a one-component sound in inspiration because both pulmonic closure and aortic closure are delayed. In RBBB, the pulmonic valve closure is delayed in both inspiration and expiration, and so the second heart sound is constantly split. See Table 11-1 for the normal occurrence of heart sounds.

Although a fourth heart sound is common in older patients, a third heart sound represents disease. A third heart sound is common in CHF, but it is not found exclusively in CHF. In CHF rapid passive (early) diastolic filling is associated with a gallop if there is increased end-systolic volume. If the systolic ejection fraction is lower than normal, there is increased residual volume in the left ventricle after systole. In other words, the ventricle does not empty well with systole. The flow of blood into that residual pool of blood is one of the conditions that cause an S3 gallop.

MURMURS

Perhaps the most common murmur heard in the older heart is the murmur of aortic sclerosis, a calcified valve with an irregular orifice that causes turbulent flow but without a hemodynamically significant decrease in the dimensions of the valve orifice. It is a systolic murmur that can be heard in the second intercostal spaces, radiating to the neck over both carotids; depending on intensity, it may radiate to the base or the apex. The presence or absence of symptoms or evident hemodynamic compromise helps to make the important distinction between benign aortic sclerosis and aortic valve stenosis.

Usually in aortic stenosis, palpable carotid upstrokes are diminished (pulsus parvus et tardus), but a palpable systolic thrill over the carotids may be present. Delayed aortic closure can result in paradoxic splitting of the second heart sound. Usually low to normal BP is present with a narrowed pulse pressure (SBP is not much higher than diastolic blood pressure [DBP]), but in older patients noncompliant arteries may result in normal or even hypertensive BP, even in the face of significant aortic stenosis. In tight stenosis the reduced flow through the valve may result in a softer murmur than in benign aortic sclerosis. More important than these signs may be symptoms. Any older person with an aortic outflow murmur and symptoms suggestive of angina or CHF needs evaluation of the aortic valve by echocardiogram.

TABLE 11-1 Relative Differences of Heart Sounds

	Cause	End-piece	Location	Pitch	Respirations	Position	Variables
S_1	Closure of tricuspid and mitral valves	Diaphragm	Entire precordium (apex)	High	Softer on inspiration	Any position	Increased with excitement, exercise, amyl nitrate, epinephrine, and atropine
S_2	Closure of pulmonary and aortic valves	Diaphragm	A_2 at 2nd RICS; P_2 at 2nd LICS	High	Fusion of A_2P_2 on expiration; physiologic split on inspiration	Sitting or supine	Increased in thin chest walls and with exercise

	Aortic	Pulmonic	Second Pulmonic	Mitral	Tricuspid
Pitch	$S_1 < S_2$	$S_1 < S_2$	$S_1 < S_2$	$S_1 < S_2$	$S_1 < S_2$
Loudness	$S_1 < S_2$	$S_1 < S_2$	$S_1 < S_2$*	$S_1 > S_2$†	$S_1 > S_2$
Duration	$S_1 > S_2$	$S_1 > S_2$	$S_1 > S_2$	$S_1 > S_2$	$S_1 > S_2$
S_2 split	> inhale < exhale	> inhale < exhale	> inhale < exhale	> inhale‡ < exhale	> inhale < exhale
A_2	Loudest	Loud	Decreased		
P_2	Decreased	Louder	Loudest		

*S_1 is relatively louder in second pulmonic area than in aortic area.
†S_1 may be louder in mitral area than in tricuspid area.
‡S_2 split may not be audible in mitral area if P_2 is inaudible.

Respiratory Examination

On a lung examination of an older patient, crackles at the lung bases are not an infrequent finding. Crackles often reflect mild fibrotic pulmonary changes that can be a part of the natural aging process. They may not represent congestion, as in CHF. In fact, CHF in older patients can manifest with no crackles or rales at all, but with "cardiac asthma," a wheezing that mimics bronchospastic disease, or simply with persistent cough. Severe pulmonary vascular congestion might manifest with cough productive of rusty, blood-tinged sputum. The significance of crackles heard on the examination of the lungs of the older patient must be determined by other related findings such as jugular venous distention, edema, or productive cough.

Abdominal Examination

Palpating the abdomen for silent, asymptomatic abdominal aortic aneurysms has diagnostic sensitivity in thin persons but not in obese patients.

Peripheral Vascular Examination

First, the clinician checks the pulses: femoral, popliteal, dorsalis pedis, and posterior tibial. Asymmetry of pulses, skin lesions, dryness, hair loss, duskiness, and edema should be noted. An absence of pulses without symptoms and with intact skin that is appropriately warm, with good capillary filling, is usually no cause for alarm. Then history should be taken, looking especially for history that suggests claudication with exercise. In that case, and certainly if there is ulceration of the skin, arterial Doppler studies and vascular surgery evaluation should be considered.

HYPERTENSION IN THE OLDER ADULT

Hypertension affects about 50 million Americans and 1 billion individuals worldwide. As the population ages, the prevalence of hypertension will continue to increase unless effective prevention measures are implemented. The Framingham Heart Study suggests that people who have normal blood pressure at 55 years of age have a 90% lifetime risk for developing hypertension (NIH, 2003). To meet this challenge, the National Heart, Lung, and Blood Institute (NHLBI) released new clinical practice guidelines for the prevention, detection, and treatment of high blood pressure in May 2003. The guidelines, called the "Seventh Report of the Joint National Committee on Prevention, Detection, Evaluation, and Treatment of High Blood Pressure" include a new "prehypertension" level and merging of other categories. The new report changes the former blood pressure definitions to normal, less than 120/less than 80 mm Hg; prehypertension, 120-139/80-89 mm Hg; stage 1 hypertension, 140-159/90-99 mm Hg; and stage 2 hypertension, at or greater than 160/ at or greater than 100 mm Hg (Table 11-2). The 1997 categories were optimal, normal, high-normal, and

TABLE 11-2	**Classification and Management of Blood Pressure for Adults***				
				Initial Drug Therapy	
BP Classification	*SBP* (mm Hg)*	*DBP* (mm Hg)*	*Lifestyle Modification*	*Without Compelling Indication*	*With Compelling Indications*
Normal	< 120	and < 80	Encourage		
Prehypertension	120–139	or 80–89	Yes	No antihypertensive drug indicated.	Drug(s) for compelling indications‡
Stage 1 Hypertension	140–159	or 90–99	Yes	Thiazide-type diuretics for most. May consider ACEI, ARB, BB, CCB, or combination.	Drug(s) for the compelling indications‡ Other antihypertensive drugs (diuretics, ACEI, ARB, BB, CCB) as needed.
Stage 2 Hypertension	≥160	or ≥100	Yes	Two-drug combination for most† (usually thiazide-type diuretic and ACEI or ARB or BB or CCB).	

DBP, Diastolic blood pressure; *SBP*, systolic blood pressure.
Drug abbreviations: *ACEI*, Angiotensin converting enzyme inhibitor; *ARB*, angiotensin receptor blocker; *BB*, beta-blocker; *CCB*, calcium channel blocker.
*Treatment determined by highest BP category.
†Initial combined therapy should be used cautiously in those at risk for orthostatic hypotension.
‡Treat patients with chronic kidney disease or diabetes to BP goal of < 130/80 mmHg.

hypertension stages 1, 2, and 3. The 2003 guidelines and related information are available on the Internet at http://www.nhlbi.nih.gov/guidelines/zhypertension/index.htm.

Isolated Systolic Hypertension

There is new emphasis on control of systolic blood pressure in those 50 years of age and older. Systolic hypertension is a more important cardiovascular risk factor than diastolic hypertension in later years and is also more common and harder to control.

Because of increased arterial stiffness or decreased compliance, there is probably an exaggerated rise in hypertension in older adults in all situations that result in transient BP elevations, such as stress and anxiety, increased heart rate, or increased stroke volume with exercise. As a result, it is unwise to make a diagnosis of hypertension based on one reading. Unless BPs require urgent intervention, such as systolic readings above 200 mm Hg or diastolic readings above 115 mm Hg, it is preferable to have the patient get a series of readings before instituting treatment. Without this precaution, hypertension in older adults may be overdiagnosed, with significant side effects when patients who are really usually normotensive are treated.

Ambulatory blood pressure monitoring (ABPM) provides BP measurements as people go about their daily activities and during sleep. ABPM is helpful to assess if there is a white coat phenomenon causing unreliable high office readings of BP. Also it provides the extent of BP sleep reduction, which normally decreases 10% to 20% (NIH, 2003).

Pseudohypertension

Occasionally a phenomenon called pseudohypertension is encountered. When an older adult has a brachial artery with walls so thickened, calcified, and sclerosed that the artery is essentially noncompressible by the standard BP cuff, an inaccurately high BP may result. To rule out pseudohypertension, first palpate the pulsating brachial artery, and then inflate the cuff and listen for Korotkoff's sounds. When these sounds disappear, palpate the arm for the brachial artery again. If the pulseless artery can still be palpated, this indicates a stiff, noncompressible artery, and an elevated systolic reading under these circumstances may represent pseudohypertension. This procedure is known as Osler's maneuver. Pseudohypertension is actually rare. If needed, an accurate reading in this circumstance would require an intraarterial line.

Evaluation of Hypertension
HISTORY

A medical history should include the following (NIH, 2003):
- Known duration and levels of elevated BP
- Patient history or symptoms of CAD, heart failure, cerebrovascular disease, peripheral vascular disease, renal disease, diabetes, dyslipidemia, other comorbid conditions, gout, or sexual dysfunction
- Family history of high BP, premature CAD, stroke, diabetes, dyslipidemia, or renal disease
- Symptoms suggesting causes of hypertension
- History of recent changes in weight, leisure time physical activity, and smoking or other tobacco use
- Dietary assessment, including intake of sodium, alcohol, saturated fat, and caffeine
- History of all prescribed and over-the-counter medications, herbal remedies, and illicit drugs, some of which may raise BP or interfere with the effectiveness of antihypertensive drugs
- Results and adverse effects of previous antihypertensive therapy
- Psychosocial and environmental factors (e.g., family situation, employment status, and working conditions) that may influence hypertension control

PHYSICAL EXAMINATION

The initial physical examination should include the following (NIH, 2003):

- Two or more BP measurements (persons should be seated quietly for at least 5 minutes in a chair [rather than on an exam table] with feet on the floor and arm supported at heart level [NIH, 2003]) and verification in the collateral arm
- Measurement of height, weight, and waist circumference
- Funduscopic examination for hypertensive retinopathy (e.g., arteriolar narrowing, focal arteriolar constrictions, arteriovenous crossing changes, hemorrhages and exudates, disk edema)
- Examination of the neck for carotid bruits, distended veins, or an enlarged thyroid gland
- Examination of the heart for abnormalities in rate and rhythm, increased size, precordial heave, clicks, murmurs, and third and fourth heart sounds
- Examination of the lungs for rales and evidence of bronchospasm
- Examination of the abdomen for bruits, enlarged kidneys, masses, and abdominal aortic pulsation
- Examination of the extremities for femerol bruits, diminished or absent arterial pulsations, bruits, and edema
- Neurologic assessment

LABORATORY ASSESSMENT

Routine laboratory tests recommended before initiating therapy determine the presence of target organ damage and other risk factors. These routine and optional tests are listed in Table 11-3.

Treatment

Fortunately, treatment of hypertension can make a difference in the patient's outcome. In studies of people over 60 years of age, treatment of hypertension, including isolated systolic hypertension, has shown a reduction in strokes of up to 32% in some series. Although the number of nonfatal MIs did not decrease, the number of fatal MIs and the number of deaths from CHF did decrease. In fact, the number of cardiac deaths from all causes was decreased by 38% in older adults whose hypertension was treated.

| TABLE 11-3 | Tests and Procedures in Evaluating Hypertension |

Routine	Optional
Urinalysis	Creatinine clearance
CBC	Microalbuminuria
Electrolytes	24-hour urinary protein
Renal function tests	Blood calcium
Glucose	Uric acid
Total cholesterol and HDL	Fasting triglycerides/LDL
12-lead electrocardiogram	Glycosylated hemoglobin
	TSH
	Echocardiography

From National Institutes of Health: The sixth report of the Joint National Committee on prevention, detection, evaluation, and treatment of high blood pressure, Bethesda, Md, 1997, International Medical.
CBC Complete blood count; *HDL*, high-density lipoprotein; *LDL*, low-density lipoprotein; *TSH*, thyroid-stimulating hormone.

The new guidelines do not recommend drug therapy for those with prehypertension unless it is required by another "compelling" condition, such as heart disease, diabetes, or chronic kidney disease. However, the report does advise lifestyle changes, including losing excess weight, becoming physically active, limiting alcoholic beverages, and following a heart-healthy eating plan, including cutting back on salt and other forms of sodium. The report also recommends smoking cessation for overall cardiovascular health (Table 11-4).

As in the 1997 guidelines, the new report recommends that Americans follow the DASH (Dietary Approaches to Stop Hypertension) eating plan, which is rich in vegetables, fruit, and nonfat dairy products. Clinical studies have shown that DASH significantly lowers blood pressure. The decreases are often comparable to those achieved with blood-pressure–lowering medication.

PHARMACOLOGIC TREATMENT

If pharmacologic treatment is required, several agents are available, including diuretics, angiotensin-converting enzyme (ACE) inhibitors, beta blockers, adrenergic inhibitors, and calcium channel blockers. See Figure 11-1 for information regarding guidelines for treatment of hypertension and Tables 11-5 and 11-6 for lists of single and combination hypertensive drugs. According to the new guidelines, many persons will need two, and at times, three or more medications to lower blood

| TABLE 11-4 | Lifestyle modifications to manage hypertension[*†] | |

Modification	Recommendation	Approximate SBP Reduction (Range)
Weight reduction	Maintain normal body weight (body mass index 18.5–24.9 kg/m^2).	5–20 mm Hg/10 kg weight loss
Adopt DASH eating plan	Consume a diet rich in fruits, vegetables, and lowfat dairy products with a reduced content of saturated and total fat.	8–14 mm Hg
Dietary sodium reduction	Reduce dietary sodium intake to no more than 100 mmol per day (2.4 g sodium or 6 g sodium chloride).	2–8 mm Hg
Physical activity	Engage in regular aerobic physical activity such as brisk walking (at least 30 min per day, most days of the week).	4–9 mm Hg
Moderation of alcohol consumption	Limit consumption to no more than 2 drinks (1 oz or 30 mL ethanol; e.g., 24 oz beer, 10 oz wine, or 3 oz 80-proof whiskey) per day in most men and to no more than 1 drink per day in women and lighter weight persons.	2–4 mm Hg

From National Institutes of Health: *The seventh report of the Joint Committee on Prevention, Detection, Evaluation, and Treatment of High Blood Pressure,* NIH Publication No. 03-5233, Bethesda, Md, May 2003.
DASH, Dietary Approaches to Stop Hypertension.
*For overall cardiovascular risk reduction, stop smoking.
†The effects of implementing these modifications are dose and time dependent, and could be greater for some individuals.

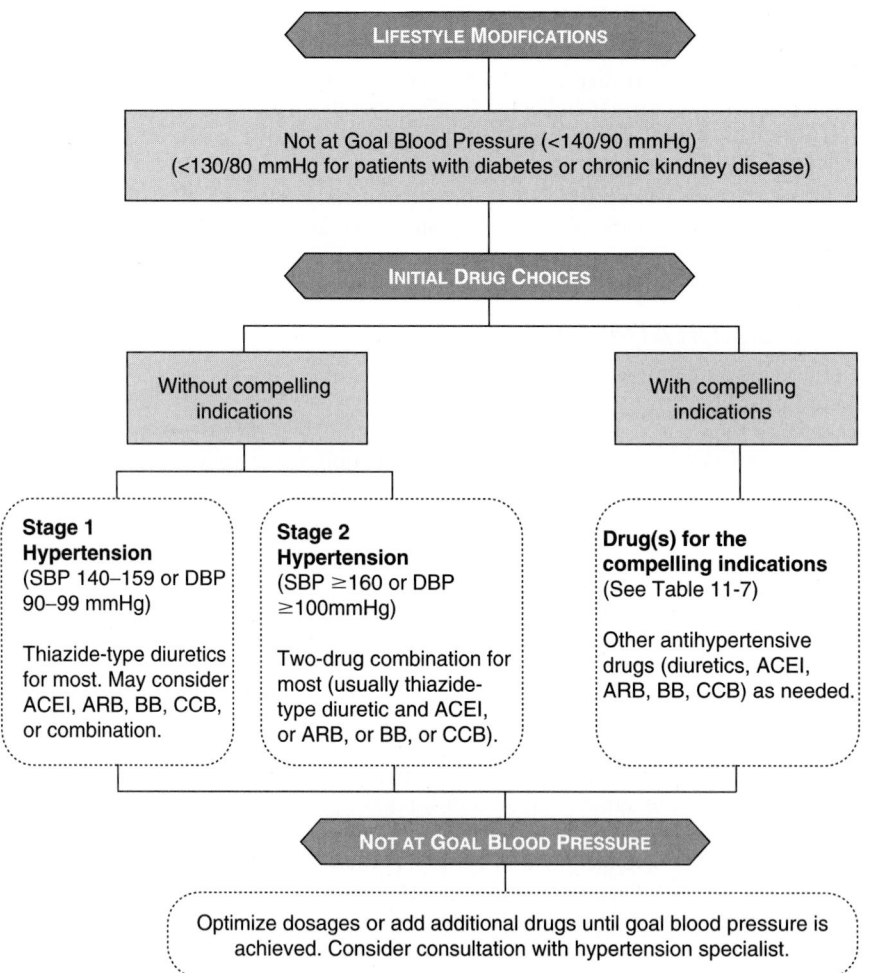

DBP, Diastolic blood pressure; SBP, systolic blood pressure.
Drug abbreviations: ACEI, Angiotensin converting enzyme inhibitor; ARB, angiotensin receptor blocker;
BB, beta-blocker; CCB, calcium channel blocker.

Figure 11-1 Algorithm for the treatment of hypertension. (Modified from National Institutes of Health: *The seventh report of the Joint National Committee on Prevention, Detection, Evaluation, and Treatment of High Blood Pressure*, NIH Publication No. 03-5233, Bethesda, Md, May 2003.)

pressure to the desired level (NIH, 2003). Table 11-7 provides recommendations for classes of drugs to be used for patients with comorbid "compelling" conditions.

Diuretics

The physiologic mechanisms that leave older adults with relatively lower plasma volumes and at risk for dehydration have been discussed. Although the new guidelines do recommend the use of diuretics (especially thiazide-type) as part of the drug treatment plan for high blood pressure in most patients, it is prudent to use caution when prescribing diuretics in high-risk older adults. Diuretics lower both systolic and diastolic BPs, but in addition to the risk for volume depletion or dehydration, diuretics also affect potassium, glucose, and lipid metabolism. However, hypokalemia can be critical, and patients who are also taking digoxin must be closely monitored to avoid arrhythmia.

TABLE 11-5	Oral Antihypertensive Drugs*

Class	Drug (Trade Name)	Usual Dose Range in mg/day (Daily Frequency)
Thiazide diuretics	chlorothiazide (Diuril)	125–500 (1)
	chlorthalidone (generic)	12.5–25 (1)
	hydrochlorothiazide (Microzide, HydroDIURIL†)	12.5–50 (1)
	polythiazide (Renese)	2–4 (1)
	indapamide (Lozol†)	1.25–2.5 (1)
	metolazone (Mykrox)	0.5–1.0 (1)
	metolazone (Zaroxolyn)	2.5–5 (1)
Loop diuretics	bumetanide (Bumex†)	0.5–2 (2)
	furosemide (Lasix†)	20–80 (2)
	torsemide (Demadex†)	2.5–10 (1)
Potassium-sparing diuretics	amiloride (Midamor†)	5–10 (1–2)
	triamterene (Dyrenium)	50–100 (1–2)
Aldosterone receptor blockers	eplerenone (Inspra)	50–100 (1–2)
	spironolactone (Aldactone†)	25–50 (1–2)
Beta-blockers	atenolol (Tenormin†)	25–100 (1)
	betaxolol (Kerlone†)	5–20 (1)
	bisoprolol (Zebeta†)	2.5–10 (1)
	metoprolol (Lopressor†)	50–100 (1–2)
	metoprolol extended release (Toprol XL)	50–100 (1)
	nadolol (Corgard†)	40–120 (1)
	propranolol (Inderal†)	40–160 (2)
	propranolol long-acting (Inderal LA†)	60–180 (1)
	timolol (Blocadren†)	20–40 (2)
Beta-blockers with intrinsic sympathomimetic activity	acebutolol (Sectral†)	200–800 (2)
	penbutolol (Levatol)	10–40 (1)
	pindolol (generic)	10–40 (2)
Combined alpha- and beta-blockers	carvedilol (Coreg)	12.5–50 (2)
	labetalol (Normodyne, Trandate†)	200–800 (2)
ACE inhibitors	benazepril (Lotensin†)	10–40 (1–2)
	captopril (Capoten†)	25–100 (2)
	enalapril (Vasotec†)	2.5–40 (1–2)
	fosinopril (Monopril)	10–40 (1)
	lisinopril (Prinivil, Zestril†)	10–40 (1)
	moexipril (Univasc)	7.5–30 (1)
	perindopril (Aceon)	4–8 (1–2)
	quinapril (Accupril)	10–40 (1)
	ramipril (Altace)	2.5–20 (1)
	trandolapril (Mavik)	1–4 (1)
Angiotensin II antagonists	candesartan (Atacand)	8–32 (1)
	eprosartan (Tevetan)	400–800 (1–2)

*These dosages may vary from those listed in the "Physicians' Desk Reference."   *Continued*
†Are now or will soon become available in generic preparations.

TABLE 11-5	Oral Antihypertensive Drugs*—cont'd	

Class	Drug (Trade Name)	Usual Dose Range in mg/day (Daily Frequency)
Angiotensin II antagonists—cont'd	irbesartan (Avapro)	150–300 (1)
	losartan (Cozaar)	25–100 (1–2)
	olmesartan (Benicar)	20–40 (1)
	telmisartan (Micardis)	20–80 (1)
	valsartan (Diovan)	80–320 (1)
Calcium channel blockers–non-Dihydropyridines	diltiazem extended release (Cardizem CD, Dilacor XR, Tiazac†)	180–420 (1)
	diltiazem extended release (Cardizem LA)	120–540 (1)
	verapamil immediate release (Calan, Isoptin†)	80–320 (2)
	verapamil long acting (Calan SR, Isoptin SR†)	120–360 (1–2)
	verapamil-Coer (Covera HS, Verelan PM)	120–360 (1)
Calcium channel blockers–non-Dihydropyridines	amlodipine (Norvasc)	2.5–10 (1)
	felodipine (Plendil)	2.5–20 (1)
	isradipine (Dynacirc CR)	2.5–10 (2)
	nicardipine sustained release (Cardene SR)	60–120 (2)
	nifedipine long-acting (Adalat CC, Procardia XL)	30–60 (1)
	nisoldipine (Sular)	10–40 (1)
Alpha₁-blockers	doxazosin (Cardura)	1–16 (1)
	prazosin (Minipress†)	2–20 (2–3)
	terazosin (Hytrin)	1–20 (1–2)
Central alpha₂-agonists and other centrally acting drugs	clonidine (Catapres†)	0.1–0.8 (2)
	clonidine patch (Catapres-TTS)	0.1–0.3 (1 wkly)
	methyldopa (Aldomet†)	250–1,000 (2)
	reserpine (generic)	0.05‡–0.25 (1)
	guanfacine (generic)	0.5–2 (1)
Direct vasodilators	hydralazine (Apresoline†)	25–100 (2)
	minoxidil (Loniten†)	2.5–80 (1–2)

‡A 0.1 mg dose may be given every other day to achieve this dosage.

Administration of potassium supplements necessitates close monitoring of potassium levels for hyperkalemia. The risk of hyperkalemia is increased if the patient is on ACE inhibitors, which conserve potassium. Loop diuretics such as furosemide (Lasix) and bumetanide (Bumex) are in general more effective in treating edema and CHF but give even less BP control. They are generally not good choices as single-agent antihypertensives because of their short duration of action. Because of their rapid onset of action and rapid progression to peak action, some older adults experience urge or functional incontinence with these agents. They may frequently delay or deliberately omit these medications if they have a social engagement. *Compliance must always be considered when choosing a medication.*

Angiotensin-converting Enzyme Inhibitors

For some patients, an alternative to diuretics may be ACE inhibitors. The ACE inhibitors decrease sodium and water retention by interfering with the conversion of angiotensin I to angiotensin II,

TABLE 11-6	Combination Drugs for Hypertension

Combination Type*	Fixed-Dose Combination, mg†	Trade Name
ACEIs and CCBs	Amlodipine/benazepril hydrochloride (2.5/10, 5/10, 5/20, 10/20)	Lotrel
	Enalapril maleate/felodipine (5/5)	Lexxel
	Trandolapril/verapamil (2/180, 1/240, 2/240, 4/240)	Tarka
ACEIs and diuretics	Benazepril/hydrochlorothiazide (5/6.25, 10/12.5, 20/12.5, 20/25)	Lotensin HCT
	Captopril/hydrochlorothiazide (25/15, 25/25, 50/15, 50/25)	Capozide
	Enalapril maleate/hydrochlorothiazide (5/12.5, 10/25)	Vaseretic
	Lisinopril/hydrochlorothiazide (10/12.5, 20/12.5, 20/25)	Prinzide
	Moexipril HCl/hydrochlorothiazide (7.5/12.5, 15/25)	Uniretic
	Quinapril HCl/hydrochlorothiazide (10/12.5, 20/12.5, 20/25)	Accuretic
ARBs and diuretics	Candesartan cilexetil/hydrochlorothiazide (16/12.5, 32/12.5)	Atacand HCT
	Eprosartan mesylate/hydrochlorothiazide (600/12.5, 600/25)	Teveten/HCT
	Irbesartan/hydrochlorothiazide (150/12.5, 300/12.5)	Avalide
	Losartan potassium/hydrochlorothiazide (50/12.5, 100/25)	Hyzaar
	Telmisartan/hydrochlorothiazide (40/12.5, 80/12.5)	Micardis/HCT
	Valsartan/hydrochlorothiazide (80/12.5, 160/12.5)	Diovan/HCT
BBs and diuretics	Atenolol/chlorthalidone (50/25, 100/25)	Tenoretic
	Bisoprolol fumarate/hydrochlorothiazide (2.5/6.25, 5/6.25, 10/6.25)	Ziac
	Propranolol LA/hydrochlorothiazide (40/25, 80/25)	Inderide
	Metoprolol tartrate/hydrochlorothiazide (50/25, 100/25)	Lopressor HCT
	Nadolol/bendrofluthiazide (40/5, 80/5)	Corzide
	Timolol maleate/hydrochlorothiazide (10/25)	Timolide
Centrally acting drug and diuretic	Methyldopa/hydrochlorothiazide (250/15, 250/25, 500/30, 500/50)	Aldoril
	Reserpine/chlorothiazide (0.125/250, 0.25/500)	Diupres
	Reserpine/hydrochlorothiazide (0.125/25, 0.125/50)	Hydropres
Diuretic and diuretic	Amiloride HCl/hydrochlorothiazide (5/50)	Moduretic
	Spironolactone/hydrochlorothiazide (25/25, 50/50)	Aldactone
	Triamterene/hydrochlorothiazide (37.5/25, 50/25, 75/50)	Dyazide, Maxzide

*Drug abbreviations: *ACEI*, Angiotensin converting enzyme inhibitor; *ARB*, angiotensin receptor blocker; *BB*, beta-blocker; *CCB*, calcium channel blocker.
†Some drug combinations are available in multiple fixed doses. Each drug dose is reported in milligrams.

a step in the overall production of aldosterone. Older patients with hypertension are more likely to be "low-renin" hypertensives; that is, they have low serum renin values. Their hypertension is less likely a volume-dependent hypertension. Therefore ACE inhibitors may be less effective in this type of patient. Some older patients have side effects from ACE inhibitors, such as rash, loss of taste, increase in blood urea nitrogen (BUN) and creatinine, persistent cough, and angioedema. If ACE inhibitors are chosen, they should be started with the smallest therapeutic dose. The initial dose, especially if the patient is already on diuretics or has hyponatremia, can cause marked hypotension within the first 3 hours of dosing. If the patient has renal insufficiency and

TABLE 11-7	Clinical Trial and Guideline Basis for Compelling Indications for Individual Drug Classes

	Recommended Drugs[†]					
Compelling Indication[*]	Diuretic	BB	ACEI	ARB	CCB	Aldo ANT
Heart failure	•	•	•	•		•
Postmyocardial infarction		•	•			•
High coronary disease risk	•	•	•		•	
Diabetes	•	•	•	•	•	
Chronic kidney disease			•	•		
Recurrent stroke prevention	•		•			

*Compelling indications for antihypertensive drugs are based on benefits from outcome studies or existing clinical guidelines; the compelling indication is managed in parallel with the BP.

†Drug abbreviations: *ACEI,* Angiotensin converting enzyme inhibitor; *ARB,* angiotensin receptor blocker; *Aldo ANT,* aldosterone antagonist; *BB,* beta-blocker; *CCB,* calcium channel blocker.

‡Conditions for which clinical trials demonstrate benefit of specific classes of antihypertensive drugs.

is already taking a diuretic, reduced doses of both the diuretic and the ACE inhibitor should be used and renal functions and serum potassium carefully monitored. Potassium-sparing diuretics with ACE inhibitors are to be avoided or serum potassium monitored regularly. The angiotensin II receptor blocker losartan (Cozaar) likewise reduces sodium and water retention. Similar cautions apply.

Beta-Blockers

This class may be less effective in older patients, again because there is decreased renin activity with aging. In addition, the response to beta-adrenergic stimulus decreases. Therefore the elevation of BP in an older person is less likely to involve either of these two mechanisms, or at least these mechanisms are less likely to be the major mechanism at work. The important role of beta-blockade in the treatment of angina and CAD is discussed later; however, as antihypertensives in older patients, they may be less efficacious. In addition, side effects such as lethargy, depression, aggravation of the peripheral vascular disease, and sleep disturbance may be exaggerated in older patients. The high incidence of CHF in older patients is also reason for caution; but recent studies of patients treated with beta-blockers for CAD have shown that even patients with CHF have been able to tolerate beta-blockers in many cases. This tolerance is definitely to their advantage in CAD. By decreasing heart rate and contractility, the beta-blockers decrease the myocardial oxygen demand. Beta-blockers have been shown to be effective in preventing both extension of the infarct after acute MI and repeat MI. For patients with CHF who need an antihypertensive and have no history of MI, however, it is probably desirable to try other antihypertensives first. Nitrates and calcium channel blockers can still be used if CAD is suspected or if there are anginal symptoms.

Adrenergic Inhibitors

Centrally acting adrenergic inhibitors decrease sympathetic output from the brain and central nervous system to the peripheral vascular system. Decreased sympathetic stimulation results in decreased vasoconstriction, smooth muscle in the vessel walls relaxes, and peripheral resistance falls. Alpha-methyldopa (Aldomet), clonidine (Catapres), guanabenz (Wytensin), guanadrel sulfate

(Hylorel), and guanfacine hydrochloride (Tenex) are some of the products available. These agents work in various ways on the alpha-adrenergic system. They may stimulate these receptors as false transmitters, effectively blocking the reception of the true neurotransmitters that would, in turn, trigger the release of adrenergic agents such as norepinephrine from neuronal storage sites. They may stimulate alpha-adrenergic inhibitory receptors. Some may even prevent norepinephrine reuptake by the nerve once it is released from the neuronal stores. The net result is decreased tissue concentration of norepinephrine and other sympathetic stimulants.

More peripherally acting alpha-blockers such as prazosin (Minipress) and terazosin (Hytrin) stimulate alpha-adrenergic receptors, acting as false transmitters in the postsynaptic or peripheral site. These medications avoid the sedation or drowsiness of the more centrally acting drugs, but orthostatic hypotension is still a potential problem. Also, the profound drop in BP that can occur with first exposure to these drugs makes it prudent to give the first dose to the patient at bedtime; if a profound drop in pressure occurs, the patient is in the supine position. Labetalol (Normodyne, Trandate) has some beta-blockade properties but is primarily an alpha-blocker. Centrally or peripherally, alpha-blockade is generally an effective approach to treatment of hypertension in the elderly. Although older adults have reduced responsiveness to beta-adrenergic stimuli, they have normal alpha-adrenergic responsiveness and increased circulating norepinephrine levels.

Calcium Channel Blockers

Calcium channel blockers are usually a good choice for BP control in older patients. As a class, they are vasodilators. They have effectiveness in vasodilation of the coronary artery bed and therefore are effective antianginals. Thus when hypertension and CAD coexist, calcium channel blockers are an excellent therapeutic choice. The different products available do have different properties in terms of their negative inotropism and effect on AV node conduction. Verapamil, diltiazem (Cardizem) and nifedipine do depress LV contractility, probably in that order, and have to be used carefully or avoided in CHF on account of systolic dysfunction. Nifedipine is prone to provoking reflex tachycardia, as some of the others can also do to a lesser extent. Verapamil and diltiazem depress AV node conduction and may be used for that purpose to control ventricular rate in supraventricular tachyarrhythmias such as atrial fibrillation. They are usually used in conjunction with digitalis in this setting but can be effective alone, particularly diltiazem. They may, however, have an adverse effect in the presence of conduction defects or any degree of heart block. Amlodipine (Norvasc) has the advantage of little or no effect on LV contractility or on AV node conduction. In treating hypertension, amlodipine may require 2 to 3 weeks before its maximum effect is shown, and it may provoke reflex tachycardia. As a class, calcium channel blockers can cause edema, and orthostatic hypotension can be a problem.

ADVERSE EFFECTS OF ANTIHYPERTENSIVE THERAPY

Older patients are more likely to suffer side effects, both from prescribed medications and from the effects of reduced intraarterial pressures. In general, however, reducing the peripheral vascular resistance is compensated for by an increase in cardiac output. The heart is able to circulate a larger blood volume when the force against which it must work (i.e., the peripheral vascular resistance) is lower. That seems to be the case with blood flow to vital organs when high BP is treated. There may be a level of BP below which compensatory increase in cardiac output is compromised; that is, BP can be too low for optimum perfusion of vital organs, especially if that pressure is low because of volume depletion. The perfect BP that is under good control but not too low may be a delicate balance that is difficult to achieve. One easy indication to follow may be renal function, BUN levels, and creatinine levels, which tend to rise when renal perfusion is compromised. On first encountering an older patient with hypertension, it is best to administer a medication regimen that gradually reduces the BP to desired levels. Abrupt, large drops in pressure may cause symptoms such as light-headedness and dizziness, have an adverse effect on gait and balance, put the patient at risk for falls, and contribute to confusion. When BP has been elevated for a time, the cerebral autoregulatory mechanisms have been reset regarding what is normal cerebral blood flow. When BP is lowered slowly and gradually, these autoregulatory mechanisms can reset appropriately. As with any medication in the older person, "start low, and go slow" with dosing is the rule.

EXERCISE

Endurance exercise training can lower BP in older adults with mild (grade I) hypertension; however, the BP-lowering effect of exercise training, compared with antihypertensive medications, is generally modest for both SBP and DBP. Exercise training alone is likely to be ineffective in lowering BP sufficiently in older adults with moderate to severe (grade II and higher) hypertension. Exercise and weight loss, however, may potentiate the effects of antihypertensive medications in these persons. Low-intensity endurance exercise training appears to be most effective in reducing BP in older hypertensive adults. Metabolic adaptations to exercise training can significantly reduce other risk factors for CAD and atherosclerosis, in addition to reducing BP. Endurance exercise training improves exercise capacity and quality of life and can induce a modest but significant regression of LVH in older adults with hypertension (Ehsani, 2001).

CORONARY ARTERY DISEASE

Epidemiology

Coronary artery disease is the most common cause of death in persons 65 years of age and older. Studies show that 70% of persons 70 years of age and older have CAD with 50% or more atherosclerotic obstruction of one or more coronary arteries. More than 30% of persons 65 years of age and older have clinical manifestations of CAD. Eighty percent of deaths from CAD occur in persons 65 years of age and older; 60% of persons hospitalized with acute MI are 65 years of age and older. The prevalence of CAD and the incidence of new coronary events are similar among men and women 75 years of age and older. Eighty-three percent of MIs in women occur after menopause. Women are less likely than men to survive the initial MI (Cobbs et al, 2002). One study estimates that 10% to 12% of the chronic disease limitations in older patients are due to CAD. About 60% of all acute MIs in the United States occur in people 65 years of age or older, and 30% occur in persons over 75 years of age (Tresch and Alla, 2001). Mortality rates from acute MIs are down in older adults, but more patients are suffering the complications of chronic coronary insufficiency (i.e., CHF, systolic and diastolic) from myocardial ischemia.

Certain patient characteristics and clinical conditions may place women at higher risk for CAD development and progression. These factors include depression, race (African Americans are at higher risk), menopausal status, age, type 2 diabetes, and thyroid function. In addition, female gender may adversely influence the relative benefits of cholesterol lowering with borderline high serum cholesterol levels and response to interventions for modifications of sedentary behavior and for smoking cessation (Jairath, 2001).

Modifiable risk factors for CAD should be controlled in older persons. Cessation of cigarette smoking, treatment of hyperlipidemia, treatment of hypertension, ingestion of a diet low in saturated fat and cholesterol, maintenance of ideal body weight, and regular physical activity will lead to a reduction in CAD and new coronary events (Cobbs et al, 2002). Other factors, although modifiable, have not yet been proven to have a beneficial effect on cardiovascular disease, including reduction in fibrinogen levels, apolipoprotein concentrations, homocysteine (an amino acid regulated by nutrient intake particularly vitamins B6, B12, and folic acid) levels, and increasing dietary antioxidant and micronutrient levels, such as vitamin E and folate (Gladdish and Rajkumar, 2001). The risk factors for the development of CAD are listed in Box 11-3.

> **Box 11-3**
>
> *Risk Factors for the Development of Coronary Artery Disease*
>
> - Cigarette smoking
> - Diabetes
> - Hypertension
> - Elevated cholesterol and serum lipids
> - Obesity
> - Sedentary lifestyle
> - Male sex
> - Family history

Atypical Presentation in Older Adults

The diagnosis of CAD in older adults may present a challenge. Like so many other syndromes, presentation of CAD in the older patient may be atypical. Typical angina is less likely to be the initial symptom. Precordial chest pain, pressure, or heaviness that might radiate to the neck, jaw, or shoulder or down the left arm is often completely absent in the older patient. Dyspnea is the most common presenting symptom of CAD in older patients, which can make recognition of early symptoms difficult because often concomitant respiratory disease exists in older adults, and symptoms may be attributed to it. Sometimes CAD in older patients is completely silent.

In general, the incidence of typical precordial chest pressure or pain denoting myocardial ischemia is less common, whereas dyspnea as an anginal-equivalent symptom is frequent. Neurologic symptoms, confusional states, weakness, and worsening heart failure are common clinical presentations of an acute infarction in older patients (Gregorato, 2001). If patients do present with chest pain, pressure, or heaviness, it, too, may have an atypical pattern. Attacks of angina pectoris may vary in frequency from several a day to occasional episodes. They may increase in frequency (crescendo angina) to a fatal outcome or gradually decrease or disappear if an adequate collateral circulation develops, if the ischemic area becomes infarcted, or if heart failure supervenes and limits activity (Cobbs et al, 2002). In older adults the complaint of pain radiating to both shoulders and arms has been a symptom that can confound the diagnosis. When older patients do present with symptoms that suggest new-onset angina, whatever the presentation, the likelihood, compared with younger persons, is that CAD will be confirmed. Therefore it pays to have a lower threshold of suspicion in older adults, and CAD should be considered when any older patient complains of dyspnea.

Although referral to a cardiologist is definitely indicated, strong evidence exists to support admitting for an inpatient evaluation the older patient with convincing symptoms of new-onset angina. In fact, it is justifiable to consider new-onset angina in this age group as "unstable" angina. Certain other findings predict a high likelihood that symptoms represent significant coronary artery stenosis: if the patient is male and over 60 years of age or if the patient if female and over 70 years of age, if there are transient hemodynamic changes during the pain, if there are transient electrocardiogram (ECG) changes associated with the pain, if there are ST segment elevations or depressions equal to or greater than 1 mm, or if there are marked symmetric T-wave inversions in multiple precordial leads. Such findings can help make the decision as to whether the patient needs coronary artery catheterization in the diagnostic workup.

Confirming the Diagnosis

To confirm the suspicion of CAD, noninvasive stress testing is usually the first step. Exercise testing, either alone or with radionuclide or echocardiographic imaging, is a useful tool in older patients capable of performing vigorous treadmill or cycle exercise. Even those without limitations may not be able to accomplish a meaningful exercise stress test. Resting heart rate and maximum achievable heart rate with exercise both decline with aging. Many older adults are not able to reach the 85% maximum predicted heart rate that is the target for interpreting the exercise stress test. Fortunately, for the large older subset incapable of such exercise, pharmacologic stress testing with dypiridamole, adenosine, or dobutamine offers an excellent alternative (Fleg, 2001). For those who can exercise but have baseline ECG abnormalities that would make it difficult to interpret the recordings made during exercise, such as LBBB or ST segment abnormalities, radionucleotide scanning combined with exercise can be used. The rest and stress thallium test uses an injection of thallium to trace or scan perfusion of the heart muscle at rest, during exercise, and after exercise. The radioactive thallium is distributed evenly in the blood, and scanning can then give a pictorial estimate of relative volumes of blood flowing through the heart muscle in different locations. Less thallium activity in an area of heart muscle means less blood flow there. When an area of heart muscle shows decreased blood flow during exercise, this means that the coronary artery supplying that area is not able to increase blood flow or perfusion to meet the increased oxygen demands of exercise. Thus that area of heart muscle would likely be ischemic with exercise. If the flow increases again with rest, the coronary artery supplying that area is not completely obstructed and, with decreased demand, is able to meet the perfusion needs of that segment of muscle. This segment is in jeopardy of ischemic injury or infarction. Coronary angiography would be indicated to visualize directly the coronary artery in question and to determine the degree of stenosis. Any area that is underperfused with rest and exercise and does not reperfuse after exercise is termed a *fixed defect;* the muscle is already permanently damaged by ischemia. If the area also moves abnormally, that is, it is hypokinetic, that fact further suggests prior permanent damage by MI. If the patient has no clinical history of MI, this patient most likely has had a subclinical, unrecognized, or silent MI.

The presence of evidence of prior silent MI, coupled with new symptoms compatible with angina, may be indication enough for coronary angiography to evaluate the degree of CAD.

If an older person cannot exercise at all, radionucleotide scanning of the myocardium can still be done by using dipyridamole (Persantine), dobutamine, or adenosine injections to create a physiologic stress on the heart. These nonexercise thallium scans are valuable and almost noninvasive; however, the agents used to induce the physiologic stress can have side effects. For instance, dipyridamole may cause bronchospasm and aggravate any concomitant pulmonary disease, and it is contraindicated in patients with active pulmonary disease.

Echocardiography with Doppler flow studies is an excellent tool for diagnosing valvular disease; evaluating chamber size; and evaluating LV function, systolic and diastolic. Presence of wall motion abnormality on echocardiogram can also indicate ischemic or scarred myocardium. Exercise echocardiography can be even more specific in demonstrating heart muscle that functions inadequately with exercise, most likely because of ischemia or prior infarct.

Patients found to have significant abnormalities on exercise or nonexercise stress testing are most likely recommended for cardiac catheterization if their overall medical condition and prognosis are good. Knowing the exact anatomy of the coronaries, whether there is diffuse or single-vessel disease, whether the left main coronary artery is diseased, and the extent of stenosis in each vessel is the only way of verifying whether coronary artery bypass grafting is indicated in the patient who is healthy enough to be a surgical candidate. Yet in older patients, multivessel disease is statistically more common than left main CAD alone. The presence of other concomitant illnesses such as severe CHF might make the patient an unacceptable operative risk. Other concomitant conditions such as advanced dementia may make it ethically impossible to pursue major surgery, or surgery may be contraindicated because of overall poor condition or poor prognosis. Nonetheless, even in some patients who are definitely not surgical candidates, by choice or because of overall condition and prognosis, cardiac catheterization can be beneficial by identifying patients with single-vessel disease or other anatomic patterns that are amenable to percutaneous transluminal coronary angioplasty (PTCA).

Therapy for Coronary Artery Disease

As mentioned, modifiable risk factors for CAD should be addressed appropriately. The practitioner should identify and correct reversible factors that can aggravate angina pectoris and myocardial ischemia, such as anemia, infection, obesity, hyperthyroidism, uncontrolled hypertension, arrhythmias such as atrial fibrillation with a rapid ventricular rate, and severe valvular aortic stenosis. Aspirin 160 to 325 mg daily decreased the incidence of MI, stroke, and vascular death (Cobbs et al, 2002).

If hypertension is present, the BP should be lowered to below 140/90 mm Hg. If CAD or other vascular disease is present and the serum low-density lipoprotein (LDL) cholesterol is greater than 100 mg/dL, despite use of the American Heart Association Step II diet, then lipid-lowering drug therapy (preferably statin therapy) should be administered to lower the serum LDL cholesterol to below 100 mg/dL. If a second lipid-lowering drug is used in addition to a statin to achieve this, a bile acid resin such as cholestyramine should be used. The serum LDL cholesterol should also be lowered to below 100 mg/dL if the older person has diabetes mellitus (Cobbs et al, 2002).

Table 11-8 outlines the recommendations of Step I and II diets. The American Heart Association dietary guidelines were updated in October 2000, and although they are no longer called Step I and Step II, they are still commonly referred to in this way. The revised guidelines retain the principles of the Step I and Step II designations; however, they put more emphasis on foods than on percentages of food components, such as fat. For patients who have not yet reduced their fat and

---

TABLE 11-8 **Step I and Step II Diets**

Recommended intake as percent of total calories

Nutrient*	Step I Diet	Step II Diet
Total Fat	30% or less	30% or less
Saturated	7-10%	less than 7%
Polyunsaturated	Up to 10%	Up to 10%
Monounsaturated	Up to 15%	Up to 15%
Carbohydrate	55% or more	55% or more
Protein	Approximately 15%	Approximately 15%
Cholesterol	Less than 300 mg per day	Less than 200 mg per day
Total Calories	To achieve and maintain desired weight	To achieve and maintain desired weight

What are recommended amounts of total fat and saturated fat in grams?

Calorie Level	Total Fat (g)	Step I Diet Saturated Fat (g)	Step II Diet Saturated Fat (g)
1200	40 or less	9-13	less than 9
1500	50 or less	12-17	less than 12
1800	60 or less	14-20	less than 14
2000	67 or less	16-22	less than 16
2200	73 or less	17-24	less than 17
2500	83 or less	19-28	less than 19
3000	100 or less	23-33	less than 23

From American Heart Association website, 2002. http://www.americanheart.org.
Calories from alcohol not included.

cholesterol intake, Step I is the starting point. For those already at the Step I goals, the Step II diet goals are even lower for saturated fat and cholesterol. Also, patients with a high-risk cholesterol level (240 mg/dL and higher) or who have had a heart attack should start with the Step II goals. These dietary changes should be carried out along with regular physical activity in all patients and with weight reduction in those who are overweight (American Heart Association Web Site www.americanheart.org, 2002).

For the older patient with CAD who is not going to undergo coronary artery bypass grafting, the therapy for angina is medication. Medications used in older patients are the same as in other age groups: nitrates, beta-blockers, and calcium channel blockers. These medications and their side effect potential in older patients are discussed under the subject of hypertension. In summary, older patients are more likely to be compromised by the postural hypotension, AV blockade, and negative inotropism that some of these agents cause. Doses of each are lower in older adults in general, but doses still must be titrated to achieve elimination of anginal symptoms, which is the standard for treatment success. It is important to maximize control of concomitant conditions such as hypertension and CHF because decompensation of control of either condition aggravates angina, and a previously well-controlled angina patient may become symptomatic again.

NITRATES

Nitrates are available in many forms and routes of administration. They act primarily as coronary vasodilators by improving myocardial blood flow and decreasing preload. Nitrates are well tolerated and effective, but chronic use can induce tolerance. The degree of tolerance can be limited by prescribing a regimen that includes a minimum 8 to 10 hours without nitrates. Available longer-acting nitrates include isosorbide dinitrate 10 to 40 mg orally twice a day, isosorbide mononitrate 10 to 40 mg orally twice a day, or 60 to 120 mg once a day in a sustained-release preparation; oral sustained-release nitroglycerin preparations 6.25 to 12.5 mg two to four times daily; and transdermal nitroglycerin patches that deliver nitroglycerin at a predetermined rate. Side effects of nitrates include headache, nausea, dizziness, and hypotension.

Therapy for Acute Myocardial Infarction

The older patient who is actually having an acute MI, like the older patient with angina, may present atypically. Most have some chest discomfort, but again dyspnea is more likely to be present than pain or pressure. Older patients are less likely to become diaphoretic. Instead, the presenting symptoms of acute MI in older patients may be acute confusion, peripheral gangrene, claudication, palpitations, restlessness, sweating, syncope, and stroke, if not sudden death (Cobbs et al, 2002). Interestingly, in older patients, the common early complication of acute MI is stroke, and a common complication of acute stroke is acute MI. The rates of in-hospital and long-term mortality from acute MI are greater in older patients than in the younger age group. The mortality rate in those over 70 years of age is four times greater than the average rate. Complications that are more frequent in the older patient with a new acute MI are listed in Box 11-4.

The prevalence of clinically unrecognized Q-wave MI in older persons with MI documented by an ECG is about 40%. The incidence of new coronary events is similar in older men and women with

---

Box 11-4

Complications of Acute Myocardial Infarction

- Stroke
- Atrial arrhythmias
- Conduction disturbances
- Congestive heart failure

clinically recognized or unrecognized Q-wave MI. Non-Q-wave MI is more common in older persons than in younger persons. Because body muscle mass is reduced in older persons, the increased plasma level of the MB isoenzyme of creatine kinase (5% or greater) resulting from acute MI may occur with a normal total creatine kinase level (Cobbs et al, 2002).

Older persons with acute MI are more likely than younger persons to die from the MI and to have pulmonary edema, CHF, left ventricular (LV) systolic dysfunction, cardiogenic shock, conduction disturbances requiring insertion of a pacemaker, atrial fibrillation or flutter, and a rupture of the LV free wall, septum, or papillary muscle (Cobbs et al, 2002). The increase in CHF is due to increased incidence of prior infarction, cardiomyopathy, hypertensive cardiac hypertrophy, and increased frequency of multivessel CAD, meaning more and larger areas of heart muscle already compromised by ischemia. Table 11-9 lists factors indicating a high risk of new coronary events in older persons with a history of myocardial infarction.

Emergency Treatment of Acute Myocardial Infarction

Initial therapy of the patient should include an immediate aspirin 160 to 325 mg, administration of sublingual nitrates (NTG SL 1/150 every 5 minutes × three), and immediate transfer to an emergency room or acute care setting. Aspirin should be continued indefinitely. Ticlopidine 250 mg twice a day or clopidogrel 75 mg daily may be used in persons unable to tolerate aspirin (Cobbs et al, 2002). If available, oxygen administration (carefully noting any history of chronic obstructive pulmonary disease [COPD]), pain relief with morphine as required, and use of nitrates unless the SSBP is below 90 or the heart rate is below 50 or higher than 100 are indicated. Once the patient is in an acute setting, intravenous (IV) heparin is started, as well as thrombolytic therapy if the history and ECG meet the criteria. In the absence of contraindications, older persons with ischemic symptoms of at least 30 minutes' duration occurring within 6 to 12 hours of clinical presentation and with at least 1 to 2 mm of ST-segment elevation in two or more ECG leads or the presence of LBBB should be considered for reperfusion therapy with either thrombolytic therapy or PTCA (Cobbs et al, 2002).

TABLE 11-9   **Factors Indicating a High Risk of New Coronary Events in Older Persons With a History of Myocardial Infarction**
Abnormal LV ejection fraction detected by echocardiography or radionuclide ventriculography
Abnormal signal-averaged ECG
Complex ventricular arrhythmias or silent myocardial ischemia detected by a 24-hour ambulatory ECG
Echocardiographic LV hypertrophy
Exercise-induced hypotension
Exercise-induced ischemic ST-segment depression in both anterior and inferior leads
Exercise-induced marked ischemic ST-segment depression ($\geq$ 2.0 mm)
Inadequate blood-pressure response to exercise
Ischemic ST-segment depression occurring within 6 minutes of exercise
Ischemic ST-segment depression on a resting ECG
Persistence of exercise-induced ST-segment depression past 8 minutes in the recovery period
Poor exercise duration (< 6 minutes using a standard Bruce treadmill protocol)

From Cobbs EL, Duthie EH, Murphy VB, editor: *Geriatrics Review Syllabus: a core curriculum in Geriatric medicine*, ed 5, Malden, Mass 2002, Blackwell Publishing for the American Geriatrics Society.
ECG, Electrocardiogram (-graphy); *LV*, left ventricular.

Oxygenation should be monitored by pulse oximetry and subsequent arterial blood gas measurements if there is significant history of lung disease. If pain is not relieved, narcotics should be administered, starting with 2 to 5 mg of IV morphine if not otherwise contraindicated (e.g., by allergy). If pain persists, the patient is a candidate for IV nitroglycerin drip, for which the starting dose is usually 5 µg per minute and titrated upward to a maximum of 75 to 100 µg per minute, as required to control pain. The patient presenting with symptoms compatible with angina, in whom suspicion of acute MI is high, should also be heparinized, hospitalized on a telemetry unit, and evaluated by a cardiologist.

After the acute perimyocardial infarction period, long-term management should include aspirin therapy, beta-blocker therapy with or without other antianginals (nitrates and calcium channel blockers), and ACE inhibitors. Nonmedical management of cardiac risk factors is equally important. Treatment goals should include maintenance of ideal weight and control of hyperlipidemia. Recent clinical trials have called into question the risk and benefits of estrogen therapy, and it is no longer routinely recommended. (Please refer to the chapter regarding menopause for further discussion of hormone therapy.) Diet should be the American Heart Association Step II diet for most patients. It contains less than 7% saturated fat and 200 mg per day of cholesterol minimally. Smoking cessation is essential to success. Patients who are functionally able should be in a formal rehabilitation program, which should include working up to a goal of 20 minutes of exercise at least three times per week. Such programs have shown a positive benefit in older patients but have been underused.

Coronary Artery Bypass Grafting in Older Patients

Coronary artery bypass grafting (CABG) in older patients can be appropriate for long-term treatment of CAD. If the patient is a good surgical candidate and in the course of evaluation and treatment of angina or acute MI is found to meet the indications for surgery, it should never be avoided or eliminated because of advanced age alone.

Not unexpectedly, the operative mortality for CABG does go up with age, and it increases when the procedure is done as an emergency. Nonetheless, older patients who undergo successful CABG do better than those with medical or even angioplasty treatment in terms of prolonged survival, relief of symptoms, and restoration of an active lifestyle. They have fewer cardiac events, including acute MI and cardiovascular deaths. CABG gives more symptom-free time, therefore enhancing quality of life. This is not to say that CABG in older patients can be approached cavalierly. Indeed, the decision must be approached with great caution. In addition to a greater operative risk of mortality, older surgical patients have greater morbidity rates; they stay in the hospital longer and have significantly higher costs.

In younger patients newer approaches to avoid CABG include coronary artery stents. In older patients the rate of clinical success has been lower with coronary artery stents, and the event-free survival time has been shorter.

COMMON ARRHYTHMIAS

Changes in the conducting system of the heart lead to an increased incidence of arrhythmias and other conduction abnormalities in the older patients. Degeneration and fibrosis occur throughout the conduction system, in the sinus node, in the AV node, and in the bundle of His. As a result, there is a high prevalence of SSS and other atrial arrhythmias in older patients. The incidence of AV node block of all degrees, of LBBB, and of RBBB increase in older patients; however, the internodal tracts do not lose as many muscle cells with aging and do not accumulate as much fibrous tissue as the sinus and AV nodes. Thus, when there is LBBB, CAD usually accompanies it. Likewise, when left anterior hemiblock and RBBB coexist, the combination almost always implies some structural heart disease, such as coronary artery insufficiency or ischemia or previous MI. This degree and type of conduction system disease would be unlikely because of aging changes in the heart alone. Atrial fibrillation, SSS, and AV node blockade such as second-degree or third-degree (complete) heart block can occur solely as a consequence of an aging conductive system.

Atrial Fibrillation

The prevalence of atrial fibrillation increases with age. In one study the prevalence was 16% in older men and 13% in older women. Atrial fibrillation may be paroxysmal (lasting a few seconds to several weeks) or chronic (Cobbs et al, 2002). It is estimated that 2.3 million adults in the United States currently have atrial fibrillation and that this number will increase to 5.6 million by the year 2050 (Go et al, 2001). Increased mortality is most often due to increased incidence of stroke. Other complications of atrial fibrillation include systemic emboli, with embolic infarction in the extremities, or loss of vision from thromboemboli to the ophthalmic branches of the carotid arteries. See Box 11-5 for factors that predispose older adults to atrial fibrillation.

Because the patient is older, acute alcohol excess should not be discounted as part of the differential diagnosis for the cause of new-onset atrial fibrillation. Alcohol can be indicated in both acute and long-term atrial fibrillation, acute from alcohol's toxic effect and long-term from alcoholic cardiomyopathy.

Drugs, particularly stimulants, can also contribute to atrial fibrillation. Drugs that can cause or contribute to atrial fibrillation include caffeine, nicotine, and cough and cold remedies such as decongestants, which are sympathetic stimulants, as well as local anesthetics such as lidocaine (Xylocaine), which are often combined with epinephrine for injection. Some drugs with anticholinergic side effects predispose to tachycardia, palpitations, and tachyarrhythmias as well.

Diagnosis

Atrial fibrillation as diagnosed on the ECG shows a wavy baseline with no, or only occasional, deflections that resemble P-waves and with irregular ventricular contractions. The ventricular rate is rapid, usually in the 100 to 160 range. The primary goal for treatment of atrial fibrillation is to control the ventricular rate. A usual goal is a ventricular rate of 90 or below. Some older patients have atrial fibrillation with a controlled ventricular rate, with no treatment, which indicates that intrinsic AV node disease is already present. With the usual rapid rate, the stiffened, less compliant ventricle, which may not be able to stretch for optimum filling, has even more decreased filling.

Box 11-5

Factors That Predispose Older Persons to Atrial Fibrillation

- Dilation of the atrium
- Sinus node disease (due to muscle cell loss, loss of nodal fibers, fibrosis, deposition of fatty tissue and amyloid in the sinus node)
- Calcification of the mitral valve
- Acute myocardial ischemia or infarct
- Inflammatory or infiltrative diseases that affect the myocardium (e.g., myocarditis from autoimmune disease such as lupus, rheumatoid arthritis)
- Pericarditis

- Cardiac surgery
- Pulmonary diseases
- Hypoxia
- Acute pulmonary embolism
- Hypokalemia
- Hypomagnesemia
- Hypocalcemia
- Hypoglycemia
- Hypothermia
- Alcohol
- Drugs

There is less time for diastolic filling at a faster rate. In addition, the phase of diastolic filling, the atrial contraction, is completely missing. Less diastolic filling means less end-diastolic volume. The systolic function of the LV may be normal, with the heart ejecting the normal 45% to 50% of the end-diastolic volume (i.e., a normal ejection fraction). The volume is smaller, however, so even with a normal ejection fraction, the volume of blood actually pumped into the circulation is smaller (i.e., the cardiac output is smaller). The difference may be enough to result in hypotension and decreased perfusion to the vital organs. CHF and pulmonary vascular congestion may develop, with dyspnea and hypoxia resulting. Acute atrial fibrillation can result in hemodynamic instability based on rapid ventricular rate alone.

Even the patient with AV node disease whose rate with atrial fibrillation is not rapid can be compromised because of the lack of atrial contraction. The atrial contraction is the last phase of diastolic filling. The stiffened ventricle that does not fill well during the passive, or stretch, phase of filling may need the atrial contraction to achieve an effective filling volume. Without the atrial contraction, cardiac output can decrease, even without a rapid rate. Older patients are much more likely to be dependent on this atrial contraction to achieve adequate ventricular filling during diastole. Therefore the ultimate goal is to restore normal sinus rhythm, but rate control must be achieved first. At the same time, giving the patient oxygen after checking pulse oximetry or arterial blood gases, establishing IV access, and other supportive measures are indicated as well. It is wise to presume that acute new-onset atrial fibrillation could be a sign of myocardial ischemia or MI. Therefore treating any chest pain or discomfort with nitrates is indicated while monitoring vital signs. Telemetry should also be instituted.

In the long-term management of atrial fibrillation, the decision must be made whether to pursue a treatment strategy of rate control or rhythm control. Both strategies require use of anticoagulation therapy with warfarin (target international normalized ration of 2.5 with a range from 2 to 3). If a decision is made for rhythm control, the critical therapy is almost always with an antiarrhythmic drug. Before selecting an antiarrhythmic drug for use, it is first necessary to determine the presence or absence of underlying structural heart disease because this will affect the available options for antiarrhythmic drug use (Waldo, 2002).

Diagnostic Testing in New-onset Atrial Fibrillation

Appropriate diagnostic laboratory studies to rule out MI (creatinine phosphokinase, isoenzymes, cardiac troponin levels) should be ordered. A complete blood count to rule out severe anemia, chemistry profiles to look for metabolic disorders, and thyroid function studies to rule out hyperthyroidism should be ordered. When the patient is stable enough, a chest x-ray film to rule out an acute pulmonary process should be done, as well as ECG to look for intraatrial thrombi, pericardial effusion, valvular disease, and abnormality in chamber size or contractility. In the case of intraatrial thrombus or valvular vegetation, some prefer the transesophageal echocardiogram for greater accuracy.

Rate Control in Atrial Fibrillation

The usual first drug used to control a rapid ventricular rate in atrial fibrillation is digoxin. Digoxin slows conduction across the AV node by increasing AV node refractory time. Therefore the number of beats successfully conducted from the rapidly fibrillating atrium, through the AV node, and into the ventricle are fewer, and the ventricle slows down. As a result of a slower ventricular rate and therefore increased time for diastolic ventricular filling, and with the addition of the positive inotropic effect of digoxin on the strength of systolic contractions, cardiac output increases. Often hemodynamic instability is corrected just by slowing the ventricular rate.

Generally, a rate of 90 or less is the target. The usual dosage of digoxin is a total of 1 mg over 24 hours or less if the rate slows sufficiently. Some give digoxin initially in a dose of 0.5 mg IV, followed by 0.25 mg IV another one to two times, about 6 hours apart. If rate is controlled, a daily dose of oral digoxin at 0.125 to 0.25 mg can be started. If the rate is still a problem after a total of 1 mg of digoxin, the practice in the past has been to continue to give additional IV doses at intervals of 6 to 12 hours until the rate was controlled. Of course, this practice increased the possibility that patients would develop signs of digoxin toxicity, including nausea and vomiting and ventricular ectopy.

Calcium channel blockers, some of which have the property of slowing AV node conduction, especially verapamil and diltiazem, provide an adjunct to digoxin for rate control in atrial tachyarrhythmias. Diltiazem is usually chosen because it has less negative inotropic effect (i.e., less depression of ventricular contractility) than verapamil. Therefore diltiazem is better tolerated in the CHF patient and in the patient who has acute CHF because of arrhythmia. Also, diltiazem, unlike verapamil, does not aggravate COPD or bronchospastic disease. In the acute setting it is prudent to use the short-acting form of diltiazem, starting at 30 mg orally three times a day. All patients treated for rate control with atrial fibrillation should be on cardiac monitoring or telemetry. It is always possible that, after multiple doses of digoxin along with verapamil or diltiazem, the patient could develop excessive AV node blockade, varying degrees of heart block, or severe bradycardia, when serum levels of these drugs equilibrate. Digoxin toxicity can contribute to dangerous ventricular arrhythmias. Digoxin does not itself convert atrial fibrillation to normal sinus rhythm. What frequently happens, however, when it does result in a slowing of rate and AV node blockade is spontaneous conversion by the heart back to a normal sinus rhythm.

Beta-blockers can also be used for rate control of supraventricular tachyarrhythmias. Although less useful in atrial fibrillation, they can be effective in paroxysmal atrial tachycardia or for patients with short bursts of, but not sustained, supraventricular tachyarrhythmia. In hyperthyroidism associated with atrial fibrillation, beta-blockers may be quite effective. Of course, beta-blockers are contraindicated in patients with asthma and COPD and can aggravate CHF with their negative inotropy, and even those that are in theory selective for cardiac beta receptors may still show some negative effects on lung function.

On the rare occasion that drugs do not work to control the rapid rate in atrial fibrillation, pacing with electrical destruction of the sinus node, called *ablation* of the sinus node, is a last-choice, last-chance option. Afterward, a pacemaker must be inserted permanently.

Once the rate is controlled, if conversion to sinus rhythm has not occurred spontaneously, other medications can be added to attempt conversion. Quinidine is most commonly added. Other drugs that can convert atrial fibrillation to sinus rhythm are procainamide, flecainide, and amiodarone. None of these drugs lacks potential for serious side effects, which may limit their usefulness in older patients. At times they can be temporary. After conversion occurs and is maintained for a period of 3 or 4 months, it may be possible to taper the drug. Unfortunately, recurrence of atrial fibrillation once the patient is no longer taking antiarrhythmic drugs is more frequent in older patients. Additional factors that seem to affect the likelihood that a patient will or will not remain in sinus rhythm once converted are left atrial size and mitral valve disease. If the left atrium is significantly dilated on echocardiogram, the success rate at maintaining sinus rhythm without antiarrhythmics, and perhaps even with them, is poor.

Atrial Flutter

A variation on atrial fibrillation is atrial flutter. The hallmark of atrial flutter is a regular rhythm. The atria are beating at a rapid but regular rate. Usually the rate is not so rapid as in atrial fibrillation. The rate is slow and regular enough that some of the beats are regularly conducted across the AV node and capture the ventricles in a regular fashion. The result is that the atria may contract at a ratio of 2:1, 3:1, 4:1, or any ratio of atrial to ventricular contractions. In the case of a 3:1 atrial flutter, an ECG shows P-waves in a sawtooth pattern, with every third-wave successfully conducting and resulting in a ventricular contraction and a QRS complex. The degree of block may not be constant. Portions of a rhythm strip from a patient in atrial flutter may show a 3:1 block, another part of the strip may show a 4:1 block, and still another part of the strip may show 2:1 or 6:1 blockade. Each portion shows a regular pattern for a time, until the ratio changes. The treatment of rapid atrial flutter is the same as that for rapid atrial fibrillation. In either case, if the ventricular rate is already 90 or less without treatment, treatment for rate control is not necessary and could cause excessive bradycardia. A rate that is controlled without medication treatment indicates intrinsic AV node disease in the patient. In this case, attention can be turned immediately to determining the underlying cause of the arrhythmia, if possible.

Anticoagulation in Atrial Fibrillation

In older men and women atrial fibrillation is associated with the increased incidence of mortality, death from cardiovascular causes, thromboembolic stroke, and CHF. In a study of 2101 older persons (mean age, 81 years) the 3-year incidence of thromboembolic stroke was 38% in persons with atrial fibrillation and 11% in persons with sinus rhythm; the 5-year incidence of thromboembolic stroke was 72% in persons with atrial fibrillation and 24% in persons with sinus rhythm (Cobbs et al, 2002). Atrial fibrillation is associated with at least 75,000 ischemic strokes each year in North America (Gage, Fihn, and White, 2001). Instead of a clot that forms in the venous circulation, it may be a clot that forms in the right atrium with atrial fibrillation that is responsible for at least some of the pulmonary emboli that occur. The risk for stroke can be dramatically reduced by chronic anticoagulation with warfarin; a reduction of up to 86% of stroke risk for atrial fibrillation in the patient with nonrheumatic heart disease was achieved in one series. Aspirin therapy alone did not show any benefit at low doses; although some benefit with one whole aspirin a day, 325 mg, was shown in one series, it was obtained only in those under 75 years of age. Aspirin at a low dose, 81 mg a day, has been shown effective as a stroke preventive, and many in clinical practice recommend increasing that dose to 325 mg a day for those who have already had one stroke, but these benefits were seen in patients who were not in chronic atrial fibrillation.

To anticoagulate with warfarin or not is a difficult decision to make for some patients. Obviously, the risk of hemorrhagic events with warfarin increases. In some situations warfarin is definitely contraindicated. Patients whose stroke was hemorrhagic should not be anticoagulated. Patients with hypertension should be well controlled before they are anticoagulated to reduce the risk of hemorrhagic stroke. Patients with any active bleeding, with allergy to warfarin, or with recent central nervous system or eye surgery should not be given warfarin. Patients may need to have laboratory tests to monitor the prolongation of prothrombin time, often weekly initially and then sometimes as frequently as every 3 to 4 weeks chronically. If access to regular laboratory monitoring at appropriate intervals is not available, the patient should not be administered warfarin. Also, if the patient is unreliable about following instructions and following up with appointments and there is no remedy for this behavior, the patient should not be given warfarin. If the patient has bleeding dyscrasias, including thrombocytopenia, warfarin should not be used. Relative contraindications to warfarin include high risk for injury from falls, significant dementia, history of gastrointestinal bleeding, or presence of known pathology in any system that predisposes to bleeding. Age alone should not be considered a contraindication to warfarin therapy. For anticoagulation in chronic atrial fibrillation, the therapeutic range of the international normalized ratio (INR) is from 2 to 3. With older patients, the goal should be to keep the INR at the low end of the therapeutic range, if possible. Surprisingly, if properly monitored, warfarin therapy is not associated with an increased rate of spontaneous bleeding except in the central nervous system, where intracranial bleeding in patients over 75 years of age taking warfarin occurred at 1.8% in one series. If a patient taking warfarin does bleed from other sites, there is most likely trauma or another underlying reason. If the patient does not have excessively prolonged prothrombin times, hematuria, hemoptysis, or gastrointestinal bleeding in a patient taking warfarin should prompt an investigation for genitourinary, pulmonary, or gastrointestinal pathology. Excessively prolonged prothrombin times associated with abnormal bleeding can be corrected with parenteral vitamin K or, in emergent cases, with infusions of fresh frozen plasma. There is no doubt that, barring contraindications, patients in chronic atrial fibrillation should be anticoagulated to prevent morbidity and mortality from stroke. It is important to educate the patient and caregiver regarding dietary vitamin K intake while the patient is taking warfarin.

Cardioversion to Achieve Normal Sinus Rhythm

Patients who achieve rate control but remain in atrial fibrillation have such significantly increased risks for stroke and other thromboembolic events that converting them back to normal sinus rhythm is desirable; however, it is not always possible. There are risks to chronic anticoagulation, but most patients who are cardioverted electrically or medically must remain on antiarrhythmic drugs chronically, and these drugs likewise have risks. In which group is outcome better in terms of lifestyle, illness burden, function, and survival? That question has not yet been answered. Older patients, however, do seem more likely to miss their "atrial kick" and suffer reduced cardiac output and, as a result, reduced function. What about electrical cardioversion for older patients?

Electrocardioversion carries a small risk of thromboembolism from the procedure itself. Therefore if the patient has been in atrial fibrillation for more than 1 to 2 days, it is customary to anticoagulate the patient for about 3 weeks before the electrocardioversion and to continue it for about 3 weeks afterward. Another risk to the procedure, particularly in older patients and in those with known sinus node disease, is that the patient can go into sinus arrest as a result of the cardioversion. This event is usually followed by bradycardia and then a return to normal sinus rhythm. When sinus node disease is known, it may be prudent to use temporary pacing before cardioversion. The long-term success of cardioversion depends on the age of the patient and the duration of the atrial fibrillation. Cardioversion is most successful if done within 3 months of onset. In one series of patients who underwent cardioversion early after onset, 70% remained in sinus rhythm after 1 year. Other factors affecting the success of cardioversion are the presence of mitral valve disease, the cardiac functional class of the patient, and left ventricular size. A left atrial dimension of 45 mm or greater is a negative predictor for success. In another series of patients, because of multiple factors, only 30% were still in sinus rhythm at 3 months and only 25% at 1 year, and half of these required antiarrhythmic drugs to maintain sinus rhythm. If there is a clear precipitating cause such as pneumonia or heavy alcohol intake, conversion to and remaining in sinus rhythm are much more successful. Otherwise, older adults are overall less likely to have successful conversion to sinus rhythm. They are also less likely to maintain sinus rhythm, and they are more likely to be among those requiring antiarrhythmic drugs to maintain sinus rhythm. Therefore the decision to attempt cardioversion, medically or electrically, must be weighed carefully.

Sick Sinus Syndrome

Another common arrhythmia in the elderly is SSS, also called *sinus node dysfunction* (SND). Again, idiopathic degeneration of the sinus node occurs with aging. Ischemia can also affect sinus node function. SND occurs in 4% to 45% of patients after CABG. In this setting it is usually temporary, and fewer than 1% of CABG patients have SND that lasts over the long term and requires pacing. When this does occur, however, it is usually in patients over 64 years of age. In fact, in all settings, SSS or SND is primarily a problem of older adults.

Sick sinus syndrome occurs because of abnormal sinus node pulse formation and abnormal sinoatrial conduction. It is characterized by intermittent episodes of both bradycardia and tachyarrhythmia. Most diagnoses of SND are made by 12-lead electrocardiography, which shows severe sinus bradycardia, sinus arrest, or sinoatrial block (Brignole, 2002). The patients have symptoms according to whether the bradycardia episodes or the tachycardia episodes predominate in their presentation. Symptoms may be fatigue or palpitations. Light-headedness and syncope can occur with both bradycardia and tachycardia episodes. Sudden death also can occur. The term *sick sinus syndrome* should be reserved for patients with symptomatic SND (Brignole, 2002).

Ambulatory heart monitoring is a helpful tool in evaluating SND. If symptoms are not frequent enough to demonstrate on 24-hour Holter monitoring, prolonged event monitoring for up to 1 week may be necessary. Patients can trigger the recordings when there is an event, call in, and have the recording transmitted by telephone.

Patients with symptomatic or sustained tachyarrhythmias can be treated medically. Beta-blockers are effective for short, unsustained bursts of supraventricular ectopy from which patients are symptomatic. Beta-blockers are also effective in most episodic paroxysmal atrial tachycardia. For episodes of atrial fibrillation, digoxin is often the choice, but verapamil or diltiazem can be used as first-line therapy or as an adjunct to digoxin, as in atrial fibrillation of any etiology; however, patients documented to have recurrent "in and out" atrial fibrillation should undergo anticoagulation.

The bradycardia associated with SSS is treated only if it is symptomatic (i.e., if it causes light-headedness, dizziness, syncope, or fatigue or is associated with chest discomfort or dyspnea). Sometimes in older patients with a lot of comorbidity, it is difficult to assess whether nonspecific symptoms are due to a relative bradycardia or to other chronic illnesses and disabilities. In this case, monitoring that shows sinus pauses greater than 3 seconds and a heart rate less than 40 should probably lower the threshold for pacemaker insertion. In SSS, the bradycardia may not be symptomatic enough to require pacing; however, an attempt to treat the tachyarrhythmias with medication may worsen the bradycardia to the degree that the patient becomes more symptomatic, and pacemaker implantation is then necessary.

Pacemakers

Pacemakers may be atrial, ventricular, or dual chamber. The mode of pacing does not seem to affect survival in SSS. In fact, pacing at all may not improve survival in SSS. In one series of 50 patients, 5-year mortality was 50% and not significantly influenced by pacemaker implantation. Causes of death are mostly CHF, acute MI, and stroke in SSS patients. In cases of heart block from AV node disease (i.e., AV node block), however, pacing and the mode of pacing do seem to affect survival. Patients with AV node blockade do better with dual-chamber pacemakers. Having the atria and then the ventricles fire in physiologic synchrony seems to effect a hemodynamic benefit. For patients with either atrial or dual-chamber pacing, there is a lower incidence of atrial fibrillation, the advantages of which are obvious.

Ventricular Arrhythmias

In older patients the most common ventricular arrhythmias, premature ventricular contractions (PVCs), increase in frequency with age. There are also increased numbers of "premalignant" PVCs, that is, PVCs with characteristics that portend the possibility of ventricular tachycardia, a life-threatening arrhythmia often responsible for sudden death phenomena. Premalignant characteristics are PVCs that are multifocal or multiform, that occur in pairs (couplets), that fall on the previous T-wave (R on T), or that occur with a frequency greater than 5 per minute. As for every age group, treating these PVCs, whether benign or premalignant in their characteristics, does not decrease mortality but does improve quality of life if the patient is symptomatic from the PVCs. Some of the drugs used to treat ventricular ectopy are themselves associated with increased mortality rates. For a person whose LV function is good, the first approach to treatment should be a trial of a cardioselective beta-blocker. Ventricular tachycardia (V-tach) is defined as a run of PVCs, three or more in a row, at a rate or interval equivalent to 100 per minute or more. The usual rate is 120 to 180 beats per minute. Episodes of V-tach may last from just seconds, to minutes, to hours. Patients may report transient light-headedness or dizziness, weakness, nausea, or faintness, with or without chest discomfort or palpitations, from a few seconds of V-tach. Many patients lose consciousness from V-tach sustained beyond a few seconds because of the poor perfusion capability of a heart whose ventricles are contracting so rapidly that there is literally no time for filling. Many patients have acute pulmonary vascular congestion, which further complicates their hemodynamics. Finally, most patients with sustained V-tach have some underlying structural heart disease, either cardiomyopathy or CAD causing myocardial ischemia.

Antiarrhythmic drugs used to treat ventricular tachyarrhythmias include quinidine, beta-blockers, encainide, flecainide, and amiodarone. The problem with many of the drugs used to treat ventricular arrhythmias is their potential for serious side effects, often including the promotion of ventricular arrhythmias themselves. Acute treatment of sustained ventricular tachycardia is IV lidocaine, sometimes in conjunction with electric shock therapy. Long-term therapy in some patients may include implantable electric defibrillators. When a patient has had life-threatening arrhythmias of any type, electrophysiologic studies are often used to induce the arrhythmia and study its electrophysiology (i.e., its point of origin and the conduction pathways involved). They can help to determine the appropriate therapy (i.e., which drugs versus the need for pacemaker placement or defibrillator implantation). They can also be used to check the effectiveness of drug therapy by testing to determine whether the arrhythmia is still inducible when the patient is receiving the optimum dosage and regimen of a particular drug.

VALVULAR DISEASE

Aortic Stenosis

In the older patient the most common valvular disorder is aortic stenosis. The orifice of the aortic valve is narrowed, and the opening and closing movements of the aortic valve leaflets are inhibited, further decreasing the flow of blood through the valve. These changes occur largely from degenerative changes and calcium deposition in the valve tissue. Aortic stenosis most often becomes a hemodynamically significant problem for patients in their eighties and nineties. In one series of patients undergoing aortic valve replacement, only 18% of those younger than 70 years of age had aortic stenosis purely on the basis of aging and degenerative changes, whereas 48% of those over 70 years of age had purely "senile" aortic stenosis. The others had histories of rheumatic heart disease or congenitally bicuspid valves, where the valve orifice is occluded by the tendency of the valve leaflets to fuse together over time.

Diagnosis is aided by the characteristic aortic systolic ejection type of murmur. The murmur is harsh, crescendo-decrescendo, but peaks late in systole. It is heard best in the second right intercostal space and radiates up over both carotids and to the base of the heart. If the murmur is loud enough, it may be heard at the apex as well. If aortic valve closure is sufficiently delayed, there may be paradoxic splitting of the second heart sound, splitting on expiration and closing to one sound on inspiration. A short early diastolic puff or blow compatible with aortic insufficiency may also be present. So many older patients have some calcium deposition in the aortic valve leaflets, causing turbulent, noisy flow through the valve and loud systolic murmurs, that it can be difficult to differentiate this benign aortic "sclerosis" from significant aortic valve outflow obstruction attributable to aortic "stenosis." Therefore an echocardiogram may be necessary to differentiate between sclerosis and stenosis and to quantify the degree of stenosis.

If the patient is asymptomatic and has normal LV function, periodic repeat echocardiography and close clinical follow-up may be all that is required. The mortality rate from sudden death in this asymptomatic group with no intervention is less than the perioperative mortality rate with aortic valve replacement (Duncan and Vittone, 1996). When angina or CHF develops with aortic stenosis, however, the prognosis for survival falls dramatically. If symptoms such as chest pain or pressure, dyspnea, syncope, evidence of pulmonary vascular congestion on examination or chest x-ray, or evidence of ischemia on ECG with symptoms, are noted, it is time to plan for aortic valve replacement. Echocardiography with Doppler flow studies can give good estimations of valve orifice area and even of the pressure gradient across the aortic valve in addition to estimations of ejection fraction. With surgery planned, however, cardiac catheterization is usually required for exact data and to evaluate the coronary arteries as well. A valve orifice with an area of less than 0.75 cm^2 or a peak systolic pressure gradient over the valve of more than 50 mm Hg is an indicator for surgical valve replacement. Ideally, replacement is done before any significant LV dysfunction develops.

For patients who do not undergo surgery but who have severe aortic stenosis and angina or CHF, prognosis for survival is about 2 years. Balloon valvuloplasty, a less invasive procedure, is available for correction of aortic stenosis. Balloon valvuloplasty has a high rate of restenosis, however, and should not be considered definitive therapy (Duncan and Vittone, 1996). It has been used for patients with severe aortic stenosis who are not candidates for aortic valve replacement surgery but require other surgical procedures and need to have their cardiovascular status improved before surgery. An example would be the older patient with a fractured hip who needs surgery but has a significant increase in risk for perioperative mortality because of tight aortic stenosis.

Up to 10% of patients with aortic stenosis that is noncritical and asymptomatic develop atrial fibrillation. Some may also throw off calcific emboli, which are usually small and rarely cause any clinical sequelae. Subacute bacterial endocarditis (SBE) is not common, but it is common practice to use SBE prophylaxis with patients with aortic stenosis, although it is not necessary with aortic sclerosis (Duncan and Vittone, 1996).

Aortic Insufficiency

Once a disease attributed to either rheumatic heart disease or syphilis, the etiologic factors of aortic regurgitation have changed considerably during the past 50 years. Earlier literature stated that 83% of aortic insufficiency is secondary to rheumatic fever. Subsequent reviews have shown this incidence to be reduced to 30% to 35% of patients, with an increasing incidence of cystic medial necrosis or myxomatous degeneration of the aortic valve being important etiologic factors. Syphilis, one of the original causative agents, is an extremely rare factor in most areas of the world, whereas bacterial endocarditis, ankylosing spondylitis, and trauma are included in a more complete differential diagnosis. Diseases of genetic origin, such as Marfan disease, Ehlers-Danlos syndrome, Hurler syndrome, dissection of the aorta, and ventricular septal defect have all been associated with the development of aortic insufficiency (Hicks and Massey, 2002).

In older patients mild aortic insufficiency may be chronic, and a compensatory increase in ventricular systolic ejection fraction may occur, resulting in little or no hemodynamic compromise. Over time, LV may result. At the point that significant LVH develops, the stiffened, thickened ventricular walls might lend to diastolic dysfunction (i.e., decreased filling), or LV wall hypertrophy could result in outflow tract obstruction, compromising the ability of the heart to increase ejection fraction and compensate for the aortic insufficiency. If there is hypertension that is not optimally controlled, this increased peripheral resistance also negatively affects the ability of the heart to increase ejection fraction and compensate for the aortic insufficiency. In general, the aging heart is less able to increase ejection fraction with exercise.

A medical history of dyspnea, fatigue, palpitations, increasing shortness of breath, and angina can all be part of a symptom complex associated with aortic insufficiency. It is also possible that patients with significant aortic insufficiency have no symptoms and present with subtle findings on physical examination. Clinical symptoms, in most instances, depend on the magnitude of regurgitant flow and the chronicity or acuteness of its onset. Patients with acute, severe aortic insufficiency may have

LV failure, pulmonary edema, and cardiac collapse without evidence of a significant diastolic murmur. The diagnosis in this group by physical examination is difficult, and the use of emergency echocardiography is mandatory. With the exception of the acute-onset group, physical findings, chest radiography, electrocardiography, and color Doppler flow echocardiography constitute the initial evaluation of patients with aortic insufficiency (Hicks and Massey, 2002).

Therefore therapy for aortic insufficiency is focused on preventing LVH or reducing it, optimizing hypertension treatment, and even further decreasing peripheral resistance, if tolerated. Calcium channel blockers are appropriate agents in chronic asymptomatic aortic insufficiency. They may actually decrease LVH and peripheral resistance. Vasodilator drugs also decrease peripheral resistance.

Mitral Regurgitation

Again, degenerative changes in the mitral valve can lead to mitral valve insufficiency with aging. This degeneration may be accompanied by calcification of the mitral valve annulus or calcium deposits in the submitral areas of the LV wall. The latter deposits actually cause more trouble than regurgitation, being implicated in the etiology of atrial fibrillation. In patients with mitral valve calcifications in the submitral area, there is a 12-fold increase in the incidence of atrial fibrillation. In older patients degeneration of valvular components can lead to mitral valve prolapse as a cause of mitral valve insufficiency. Ischemic heart disease can cause papillary muscle dysfunction and subsequent mitral valve insufficiency.

Surgical correction of mitral insufficiency can and should be done before there is irreversible LV dilation and dysfunction, but it carries a higher risk than aortic valve replacement. Procedures to reconstruct rather than replace the valve carry less risk. For older patients, reconstruction procedures with simultaneous CABG are associated with 13% mortality compared with 22% mortality for mitral valve replacement with simultaneous CABG. When the mitral insufficiency is due to calcification of the mitral valve annulus, however, the reconstruction procedure is technically more difficult and carries higher operative risk.

Pericarditis and Endocarditis

Although pericarditis and endocarditis are not frequently seen, they do occur, and the practitioner must be alert to the possibility. In older patients, pericarditis and accompanying pericardial effusion are most commonly secondary to CHF or malignancy. If infectious, pericarditis is less likely viral and more likely to be tuberculosis in an older person. Other causes of pericarditis in older patients include acute MI, acute pulmonary embolus, and uremia.

It is important to be aware of the incidence of bacterial endocarditis in older adults. The source of the bacteria in older patients is likely to be mouth organisms, including viridans streptococci, because of poor dentition, or bacteremia introduced via surgical procedures. Because of the higher incidence of aortic sclerosis and stenosis, the site is usually the aortic valve in the older patient. Chapter 8 (Oral Health) provides detailed information regarding endocarditis prophylaxis.

CONGESTIVE HEART FAILURE

Epidemiology

Congestive heart failure is the end stage of heart disease. The heart is unable to pump enough blood to supply the vital organs and the body tissues with enough oxygen and nutrients to meet their metabolic demands. Most CHF is a result of CAD. The Framingham 32-year follow-up study showed that some 76.4% of the men and 79.1% of the women with long-standing hypertension developed CHF, whereas 45.8% of men and 27.4% of women with CAD developed CHF. Older patients with chronic CHF have a poor prognosis and high mortality rate. There is a high incidence of ventricular arrhythmias leading to sudden death. The 5-year mortality with chronic CHF is greater than 50%, and there is a twofold increase in mortality in persons over 60 years of age. The annual mortality is as high as 50% in those with end-stage (ejection fraction less than 20%) or functional class IV CHF. The prevalence of CHF more than doubles with each decade of age starting in the forties. Heart failure affects more than two million adults in the United States, mainly the older adults, with prevalence rates of up to 10% in patients older than 65 years of age (McConaghy and Smith, 2002). The management of heart failure is responsible for millions of outpatient visits per year, it is the most common discharge diagnosis for Medicare beneficiaries, and it accounts for more than 5% of total health care dollars spent with the cost of treatment ranging from $10 to $30 billion per year (McConaghy and Smith, 2002). At least 50% of those over 65 years of age who are hospitalized for CHF are hospitalized again within 6 months after their first discharge for CHF.

Etiology

No matter what the etiology of the CHF, age-related changes in the cardiovascular system contribute to the development of CHF (see Box 11-6). Not only do older persons experience an age-related decrease in LV diastolic relaxation and early LV diastolic filling, they are more likely to have LV diastolic dysfunction because they have an increased prevalence of hypertension, myocardial ischemia attributable to CAD, LVH from hypertension, valvular aortic stenosis, and hypertrophic cardiomyopathy (Cobbs et al, 2002). In addition to these aging changes, cardiac conditions in the patient can lead to CHF acutely or gradually. Three-fourths of all CHF is associated with either hypertension or CAD. Causes of acute CHF are listed in Box 11-7.

More gradual development of CHF can occur in chronic hypertension, chronic ischemic heart disease, valvular disease such as aortic stenosis, hypertrophic cardiomyopathy, diabetic cardiomyopathy, restrictive cardiomyopathy such as infiltrative myocardial disease from amyloid, constrictive pericardial disease, and drugs such as nonsteroidal antiinflammatory drugs (NSAIDs) and corticosteroids, which may cause increased sodium and water. Because of the improvement in the therapy of hypertension, CAD and ischemia are now the main causes of chronic CHF. Ischemia with or without actual myocardial infarct leads to ventricular remodeling with scar and fibrosis, which ultimately affect both systolic and diastolic function.

Pulmonary hypertension causes right heart failure. Some other conditions that cause or mimic right heart failure are pulmonic stenosis, right ventricular infarction, right atrial myxoma, and intracardiac shunts. Some conditions mimic left-sided heart failure, such as LV outflow obstruction, left atrial abnormality, and acute or chronic volume overload. Any of these conditions over time could cause such an increased strain on the heart as to contribute to the development of true LV heart failure, or CHF. If the right side of the heart is continuously contracting against increased pulmonary vascular bed pressures, there is decreased venous return and eventually decreased filling of

---

Box 11-6
Age-related Changes Contributing to Congestive Heart Failure

- Increased peripheral vascular resistance because of arterial noncompliance
- Decreased left ventricular compliance
- Decreased maximum cardiac output
- Decreased maximum oxygen consumption
- Decreased peak heart rate with exercise
- Decreased glomerular flow rate

> **Box 11-7**
>
> *Causes of Acute Congestive Heart Failure*
>
> - Acute hypertensive episodes
> - Ischemic episodes or acute MI
> - Acute onset of arrhythmias
> - Volume overload as in intravenous fluid therapy
> - Pulmonary embolism
> - Tamponade from pericardial effusion
>
> - Acute decompensation (e.g., anemia or hyperthyroidism)
> - Acute illnesses such as pneumonia or other infection
> - Drugs (e.g., beta blockers and some calcium channel blockers)

the LV. This decreased filling increases demand on the LV, requiring increased rate or increased ejection fraction and stroke volume to deliver the same cardiac output.

Over time, the LV might be expected to hypertrophy; but even without hypertrophy, there would be increased oxygen demand. In the presence of CAD, this could result in relative ischemia of the LV myocardium and eventual failure of the pump function and CHF. Conditions that mimic LV failure do so because there is obstruction to systolic outflow, resulting in the same kind of demand on the LV to keep the cardiac output stable and eventually the same physiologic pattern.

Many comorbid states contribute to the development of CHF. Any condition that results in decreased coronary blood flow, decreased heart muscle function, decreased ventricular filling, and decreased ventricular contraction, along with increased heart rate and increased oxygen demand, contributes to the development of CHF. Therefore any acute infection or other acute physiologic stress such as surgery can contribute to the development of CHF. Box 11-8 lists the common cardiac etiologies of heart failure.

Systolic Versus Diastolic Congestive Heart Failure

Congestive heart failure can be the failure of contraction, systolic failure, or the failure of filling, diastolic failure. In CHF associated with LV systolic dysfunction, the LV ejection fraction is below 50%. The amount of myocardial fiber shortening is reduced, the stroke volume is decreased, the LV is dilated, and the patient is symptomatic. In CHF associated with LV diastolic dysfunction with normal LV systolic function, the LV ejection fraction is normal (50% or greater). The prevalence of a normal LV ejection fraction associated with CHF increases with age and is higher in older women

> **Box 11-8**
>
> *Cardiac Etiologies of Heart Failure*
>
> Ventricular overload
>   Pressure—aortic and pulmonary stenosis, systemic and pulmonary hypertension
>   Volume—valvular incompetence, shunt defects, hyperthyroidism
> Coronary artery disease
>   Myocardial infarction
>   Myocardial ischemia
>
> Cardiac muscle disease
>   Infiltrative cardiomyopathy–amyloid, sarcoid
>   Hypertrophic cardiomyopathy
>   Restrictive cardiomyopathy
>   Congestive cardiomyopathy
> Mechanical diastolic restrictive disorder
>   Mitral valvular stenosis
>   Constrictive pericarditis
>
> From Tresch D: The clinical diagnosis of heart failure in older patients, *J Am Geriatr Soc* 45:1128-1133, 1997.

than in older men. In one study, the prevalence of a normal LV ejection fraction associated with CHF in older persons was found to be 44% in black American men, 58% in black American women, 46% in Hispanic American men, 56% in Hispanic American women, 35% in white American men, and 57% in white American women (Cobbs et al, 2002).

It is important for therapeutic decisions to differentiate between diastolic dysfunction and systolic dysfunction as the type of CHF. Systolic dysfunction is very familiar. The LV loses its strength of contraction. The ventricle may be thinned and dilated, the musculature "floppy." Thus contractions are weak and ineffective in delivering the stroke volume. When ejection fraction falls below 20%, it is considered end-stage CHF with poor prognosis. Contraction is impaired at rest and worsens with any increase in demand. The causal factor in chronic, irreversible systolic dysfunction is most often CAD with previous myocardial damage from infarction, clinical or subclinical, resulting in hypokinesis of segments of the ventricular wall. Some dilated cardiomyopathies, as opposed to hypertrophic cardiomyopathies, have other causes, such as alcoholic cardiomyopathy (which shows components of both dilation and hypertrophy on autopsy) or viral cardiomyopathies. In older patients, however, the cause of dilated cardiomyopathy is overwhelmingly ischemic disease with prior MI.

Diastolic dysfunction results in poor filling of the ventricle, usually during the early rapid filling phase or diastole but can affect filling throughout the entire diastolic period. Systemic hypertension leading to LV and underlying ischemic heart disease are the most common causes of diastolic heart failure. In the first case the hypertrophied ventricle is stiff and thickened because of increased connective tissue matrix. With increased exercise this stiff ventricle cannot stretch to accommodate a larger filling volume; so no increased stroke volume and no increased cardiac output can occur.

In the second case, both transient and sustained ischemia can lead to profound alteration in LV diastolic function. As mentioned earlier, chronic ischemia causes remodeling of the LV, with scarring and fibrosing; however, acute transient ischemia can cause sudden compromise of the hypertrophied, scarred ventricle. In acute stress the ventricle has impaired relaxation and decreased compliance, and extremely high pressures are necessary to fill the ventricle during diastole. Thus acute stresses such as demand ischemia, tachycardia, and tachyarrhythmias can result in decompensation and acute CHF, even with normal systolic function. In fact, acute reversible CHF associated with an acute stress is often diastolic dysfunction alone. Diastolic dysfunction can occur alone, whereas systolic dysfunction never occurs without concomitant diastolic dysfunction.

The phenomenon, known as *flash pulmonary edema,* is usually due to acute ischemia in patients with severe CAD, hypertension, and LVH. It can happen with normal systolic function, meaning that flash pulmonary edema may be diastolic dysfunction alone. In fact, abrupt-onset CHF, prominent jugular venous distention (JVD), and prominent crackles or rales in the lungs, with little or no edema, in a setting of an acute stress, are characteristic of diastolic CHF. In treating this acute CHF, presume that myocardial ischemia is part of the picture and treat for it.

In some older people with diastolic dysfunction, the hypertrophied LV may resemble the hypertrophic cardiomyopathy patient. There may be asymmetric basal and septal hypertrophy. The LV, if studied by echocardiography, appears small, hypertrophied, and hyperdynamic; even LV outflow tract obstruction may occur during systole; and left atrial enlargement may develop. Yet these changes are the result of long-standing hypertension and not idiopathic changes such as the asymmetric hypertrophic cardiomyopathy of younger patients. In obese or diabetic patients, a type of cardiomyopathy that leads to diastolic dysfunction can develop even in the absence of hypertensive history. Box 11-9 lists the cardiovascular changes that occur with aging that affect diastolic dysfunction. Box 11-10 is a summary of the disorders known to be associated with the development of diastolic dysfunction.

Assessment

Clinical findings to look for in CHF include JVD, rales or crackles in the lungs, an S3 gallop on heart auscultation, displacement of the point of maximal impulse (PMI) compatible with cardiomegaly,

---

Box 11-9

Normal Aging Changes Affecting Diastolic Function

Increase in systolic blood pressure
Increase in ventricular wall thickness
Decrease in left ventricular cavity size
Decrease in rate of ventricular filling

Increase in myocardial interstitial fibrosis
Ventricular relaxation prolonged
Increase in left atrial size

From Tresch D: The clinical diagnosis of heart failure in older patients, *J Am Geriatr Soc* 45:1128-1133, 1997.

---

possibly hepatojugular reflux, and peripheral edema. Other data helpful to diagnosis include chest x-ray examination, ECG, and echocardiography. Clues to etiology may be obtained from a CBC, thyroid function tests, and chemistries.

In older patients looking for JVD may have lower yield because an uncoiled aorta may impair venous outflow from the neck and cause a false-positive JVD. Then, flattened neck veins obliterated by fibrosis can cause a false-negative JVD. Likewise, in the elderly, the sign of leg edema is less useful because of the high incidence of venous insufficiency. Cardiac enlargement on chest x-ray film and LVH by voltage on an ECG are both independently associated with increased risk for CHF. In hypertensive older patients LVH on echocardiography is also an independent risk factor for CHF. The ECG may also show ST and T wave changes compatible with ischemia to lend weight to the likelihood that CHF is present. The chest x-ray film may also show increased pulmonary vasculature, pulmonary vascular congestion, and the presence or absence of other pulmonary disease.

An echocardiogram can confirm the diagnosis of systolic or diastolic LV dysfunction and provide clues to the etiology. Chamber size and configuration and ejection fraction on echocardiography help to differentiate between systolic and diastolic dysfunction. Echocardiography can differentiate between a hypertrophied LV and a dilated one. Dimensions of the ventricle can be obtained. Echocardiography can estimate the ejection fraction, which is a measure of systolic contractile function. A normal ejection fraction is 45% to 50%. With Doppler flow studies and echocardiography, diastolic filling can be evaluated. Impaired relaxation can be seen, which affects the early phase of diastolic filling, or impaired distensibility can be detected, which affects late-phase ventricular diastolic filling. An LV that is normal in size and contractility or that is hypertrophied but not dilated, along with an ejection fraction that is normal but LV relaxation and distensibility that are abnormal, indicates that the patient's symptoms of CHF are due to diastolic dysfunction. The typical patient with diastolic dysfunction has these echocardiography findings and, in addition, is

---

Box 11-10

Disorders Associated with Diastolic Function

Systemic hypertension
Coronary artery disease
Hypertrophic cardiomyopathy
Diabetes
Chronic renal disease

Infiltrative cardiomyopathy
Idiopathic restrictive cardiomyopathy
Aortic stenosis
Atrial fibrillation

From Tresch D: The clinical diagnosis of heart failure in older patients, *J Am Geriatr Soc* 45:1128-1133, 1997.

likely to have a history of hypertension, CAD, or valvular disease; to be of advanced age; to be female; to have diabetes; and to have chest x-ray film findings compatible with CHF.

A dilated LV on echocardiography with a less than normal ejection fraction indicates systolic dysfunction. This patient probably has left atrial enlargement and regional wall motion abnormalities on echocardiography as well.

Additional information about valvular disease and even ischemic disease can be obtained from an echocardiogram. Valve orifice diameter and pressure gradients across the valves can be estimated with Doppler flow echocardiography. Also, the direction of flow can be determined; so valvular regurgitation can be seen. If valvular disease is shown on echocardiography, heart catheterization may be necessary later to evaluate further the degree of valvular disease. An echocardiogram can also give information about the presence or absence of prior ischemic muscle injury. Wall motion abnormalities suggest areas of prior infarct. Stress echocardiography with Doppler can give even more information about areas of wall motion abnormality, such as whether these abnormalities change with exercise. Such data might suggest still viable myocardium that is jeopardized during exercise. Similar data can be obtained from radionucleotide ventriculography, multigated angiogram (MUGA) testing, and stress thallium testing, but these tests have the disadvantage of not providing the information about the heart valves that echocardiography can.

An echocardiogram can also diagnose hypertrophic cardiomyopathy and identify LV outflow obstruction and subvalvular obstruction. Other conditions can mimic CHF when there is neither systolic nor diastolic dysfunction. Any condition that causes increased left atrial pressures can result in pulmonary vascular congestion without LV dysfunction. Valvular disease such as mitral stenosis and aortic stenosis can do this. Chronic renal failure, with accompanying volume overload and high-output states such as thyrotoxicosis and anemia, can also do this. Pericardial disease and restrictive heart disease can mimic CHF as well. Fortunately, echocardiography with Doppler is able to detect these conditions and thus is an excellent tool for diagnosis.

In diagnosing CHF, noncardiogenic causes of pulmonary edema must be ruled out. Adult respiratory distress syndrome results in pulmonary edema because the abnormal permeability of pulmonary capillaries causes leakage of fluid from the blood vessels into the extravascular space. Direct pulmonary injury such as inhalation injury, chemical pneumonitis, aspiration, or trauma can cause pulmonary vascular congestion secondary to the inflammatory process. Sepsis, pancreatitis, high altitude, narcotic overdose, and disseminated intravascular coagulation are all associated with pulmonary edema. One factor that differentiates these conditions from CHF is that in these conditions, if the pulmonary capillary wedge pressure (PCWP) is measured, it is normal. Actually, the definitive diagnosis of diastolic CHF requires findings of elevated PCWP, elevated LV end diastolic pressures, normal systolic function, and normal ejection fraction. To take these measurements, cardiac catheterization is necessary. Short of that invasive test, diagnosis of CHF, diastolic and systolic, can be made with a high level of reliability by using history, physical examination, ECG, chest x-ray examination, and echocardiography with Doppler flow studies. The Mayo Clinic Proceedings (Senni and Redfield, 1997) published a handy algorithm for the diagnosis of diastolic heart failure in its review of CHF in older patients (Figure 11-2).

Presentation

Before an older person becomes symptomatic from CHF, signs may be seen that are a manifestation of deteriorating myocardial function. An enlarged heart may be detectable by a displaced PMI on physical examination. An enlarged cardiac silhouette may be seen on chest x-ray film. The patient may have a rapid resting heart rate. Hematocrit may be elevated, reflecting erythrocytosis that is compensatory for decreased cardiac output. Exercise tolerance may be decreased. As the patient develops either increased pulmonary venous pressure or increased systemic venous pressure because of CHF, other signs and symptoms appear.

Increased pulmonary capillary wedge pressure causes pulmonary congestion, resulting in dyspnea. Dyspnea may progress from exertional dyspnea to orthopnea, to paroxysmal nocturnal dyspnea, to

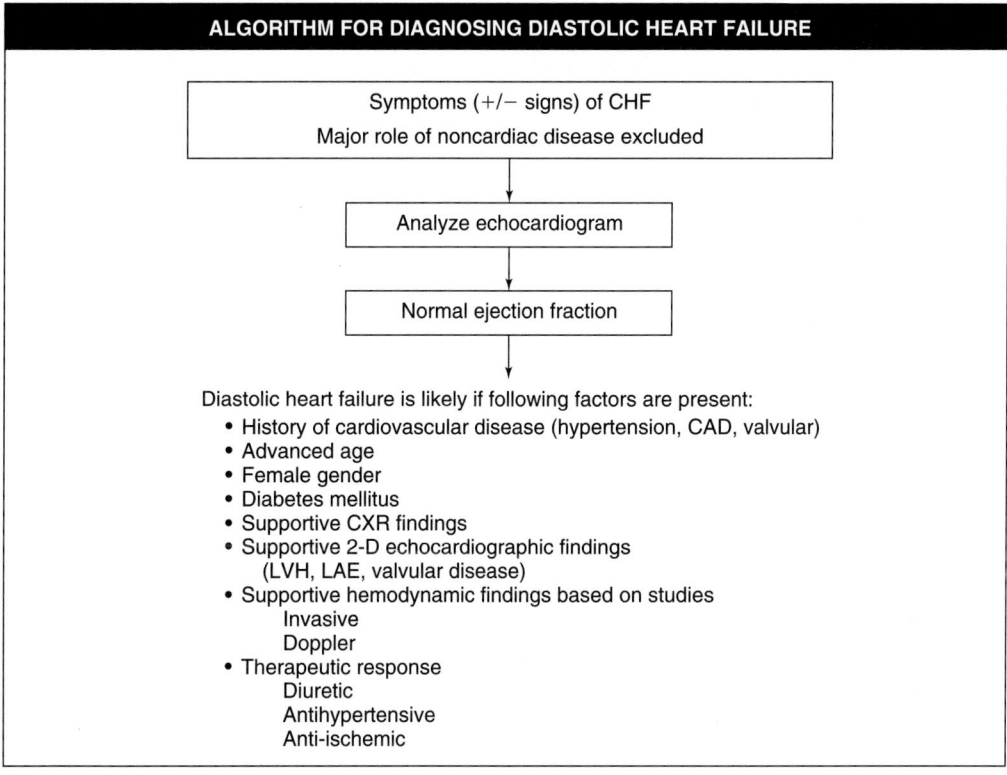

ALGORITHM FOR DIAGNOSING DIASTOLIC HEART FAILURE

Symptoms (+/− signs) of CHF
Major role of noncardiac disease excluded

Analyze echocardiogram

Normal ejection fraction

Diastolic heart failure is likely if following factors are present:
- History of cardiovascular disease (hypertension, CAD, valvular)
- Advanced age
- Female gender
- Diabetes mellitus
- Supportive CXR findings
- Supportive 2-D echocardiographic findings
   (LVH, LAE, valvular disease)
- Supportive hemodynamic findings based on studies
   Invasive
   Doppler
- Therapeutic response
   Diuretic
   Antihypertensive
   Anti-ischemic

Figure 11-2 Algorithm for diagnosing diastolic heart failure. (From Senni M, Redfield M: Concise review of primary care physicians: congestive heart failure in elderly patients, *Mayo Clin Proc* 72:453-460, 1997.)

dyspnea at rest, and to the development of acute pulmonary edema. Pulmonary congestion may cause coughing and wheezing. Wheezing as a manifestation of pulmonary vascular congestion and the presence of fluid in the pulmonary alveoli are sometimes called *cardiac asthma*. Decreased cardiac output may cause weakness, a feeling of heaviness in the limbs, nocturia, oliguria, confusion, insomnia, headache, anxiety, memory impairment, nightmares, and rarely, psychotic manifestations. Congestive hepatomegaly may cause epigastric or right upper quadrant heaviness or a dull ache, a sense of fullness after eating, anorexia, nausea, and vomiting (Cobbs et al, 2002). Liver function tests may be abnormal (e.g., elevated transaminases, elevated alkaline phosphatase, and elevated total bilirubin), and coagulation functions also may be abnormal, associated with congestion of the liver due to CHF.

Whether the CHF is primarily systolic or diastolic, pulmonary vascular congestion usually develops first; then, because of back pressure and back flow, eventually systemic venous congestion develops. In other words, the most common cause of right-sided heart failure is left-sided heart failure. The exception is the case of primary right-sided heart failure. In right-sided heart failure, as in primary and secondary lung diseases, there is increased resistance in the pulmonary vascular bed without any congestion. For instance, in primary pulmonary hypertension, acute pulmonary embolus, or COPD, increased pulmonary vascular pressure develops before and independent of any cardiac dysfunction. In such cases the right ventricle may fail. Failure of either pump or filling function of just the right ventricle presents first with the signs of systemic venous congestion. Lower-extremity edema develops first, progressing to abdominal wall and visceral edema. Because the circulation is circular, with the heart in the middle as the pump, any right-sided heart failure eventually leads to left-sided heart failure, and the reverse is also true.

It is also true that with CHF, as with other disorders, older adults may present atypically. With some older patients, the signs and symptoms of decreased cardiac output from CHF may be subtle. There may be only somnolence, fatigue, weakness, and motor retardation. Often there is confusion or increased confusion, and it may be the only major presenting symptom. Older patients are also likely to be diagnosed at a more advanced stage of their CHF. At earlier stages, when older adults experience increased fatigue, increased dyspnea on exertion, and decreased physical stamina, they may simply decrease their activities and become more sedentary. As a result, their average cardiac demand falls, and their CHF continues to go unnoticed and undiagnosed. These vague complaints are the predominant presentation of CHF in the very old. Thus CHF must be on the differential diagnosis list for an older patient who becomes confused rather acutely, stops eating, or stops being active on account of being "too tired." Their worsening air exchange while recumbent may lead to nocturnal anxiety, and poor sleep and nightmares are common. Nocturia with daytime oliguria is a frequent early complaint in older patients. It occurs because in the recumbent position venous return is no longer in an against-gravity direction and therefore increases. Increased venous return, with decreased cardiac demand from lack of muscular activity, results in increased renal perfusion and output at night. These vague complaints may be the first clue, before any dyspnea, rales, cough, wheezes, edema, or similar signs and symptoms appear, or they may be the only clue. As dyspnea in older patients is often the predominant symptom with CAD, dyspnea in a setting of new ECG changes or in the absence of any other signs and symptoms of CHF should be considered a possible anginal equivalent. Anorexia and a resultant weight loss *(cardiac cachexia)* can be a striking sign in CHF in older patients. This hepatic and gut congestion is a frequent cause of weight loss in older adults. Cough and wheezing in the older patient with CHF are often mistakenly attributed to COPD; however, when a patient has COPD and is experiencing frequent exacerbations or repeated pulmonary infections, the possibility of concomitant CHF should be strongly considered. Echocardiogram findings, and perhaps pulmonary function tests in addition, can help differentiate between the possible etiologies. In some cases stress testing, if necessary, with the several nonexercise nuclear stress tests that are available, can also be helpful.

Other comorbidities can confuse evaluation of the symptoms of CHF in older patients. The patient with dyspnea on exertion may simply be deconditioned or have orthopedic limitations, obesity, or the pulmonary fibrosis with restriction that can be a physiologic aging change in the lungs. The patient with edema may have venous insufficiency, renal disease, or fluid retention in response to medications such as some of the calcium channel blockers, NSAIDs, or hormones. Patients may simply be obese and inactive. Again, echocardiography is a simple, accessible, usually fast, noninvasive way to evaluate heart function.

Diastolic CHF may not be distinguishable from systolic CHF clinically. There are no ECG distinguishing factors. The chest x-ray film might show an enlarged heart, but this can be a finding with systolic or diastolic CHF. It is usually not possible to distinguish between cardiomegaly attributable to hypertrophy versus that attributable to dilation on chest x-ray film. A hugely enlarged heart on x-ray may be a dilated heart or may represent pericardial effusion. A history of hypertension or CAD in patients with CHF may be a useful clue but does not distinguish between diastolic and systolic CHF with any certainty. In fact, the history of hypertension, the history of CAD, a third heart sound, and a fourth heart sound are all findings that occur with equal frequency in diastolic and systolic CHF. The pattern of presentation can be helpful. Diastolic CHF is likely to be the cause when CHF develops abruptly with acute stresses such as pneumonia, surgery, or acute arrhythmias, in the absence of acute MI. Again, the most useful tool for determining the difference is an echocardiogram. The echocardiogram with Doppler flow studies is necessary to assess diastolic function.

Treatment

In general, treatment consists of inotropic support where needed, fluid mobilization accomplished by preload reduction, afterload reduction, and relief of ischemia. In terms of drug therapy, this translates into digoxin, diuretics, vasodilators such as hydralazine and nitrates, and ACE inhibitors. In older patients the effective doses of each are usually lower. A multidisciplinary case-management approach to patients with heart failure decreases the frequency of unplanned and repeat hospitalizations, increases functional status, and increases quality of life. Patient instruction in self-monitoring of daily weight and blood pressure, combined with frequent telephone follow-up from a nurse, has been proven to reduce readmissions and hospitalization days (McConaghy and Smith, 2002).

Digoxin is given in systolic dysfunction to increase inotropism, or the strength of ventricular contraction. Because of the decrease in renal function that occurs with normal aging, older patients are at greater risk for digoxin toxicity. Therefore it is prudent to use lower maintenance doses of digoxin in treating the geriatric patient. The goal of digoxin therapy is control of heart rate and symptoms. It is not necessary to achieve a therapeutic laboratory level of digoxin if these goals are achieved; however, it is still important to monitor the digoxin level at least every 6 months once the condition is stabilized to monitor for toxicity.

This same decreased renal function can make older patients rather resistant to the effect of diuretics. Often it is necessary to use loop diuretics to achieve effective diuresis. Yet, when using these loop diuretics, the minimum dose necessary should be used. If adequate diuresis is still not achieved, it often helps to add metolazone (Zaroxolyn), a thiazide diuretic, to the loop diuretic. Giving metolazone 30 to 60 minutes before the loop diuretic results in a synergism that can be quite effective. Because this regimen can result in severe hypokalemia, adequate potassium supplementation must be supplied. Any diuretics used in older patients can quickly deplete the intravascular volume faster than fluid in the interstitial spaces of the tissues (edema) and can be mobilized and resorbed, resulting in intravascular dehydration, decreased renal perfusion, prerenal azotemia, and hypotension. If there is hypotension, perfusion simply becomes worse. The balance between too "wet" and too dry can be a delicate one in older patients. To achieve this delicate balance, one should start with low doses of medications and increase or decrease minimally while observing the effects on urinary output, BUN and creatinine levels, and BP. The addition of spironolactone can help patients with severe heart failure. In NYHA class III and IV patients, spironolactone at doses ranging from 25 mg every other day to 50 mg every day reduced mortality rates and hospitalization (McConaghy and Smith, 2002). Patients must be monitored for hyperkalemia as well as breast pain and gynecomastia in men. The combination of hydralazine and isosorbide reduces mortality rates from heart failure, but tolerability is an issue (McConaghy and Smith, 2002).

Older patients likewise may be more sensitive to the effect of decreased volume from the decreased sodium and fluid retention ACE inhibitors cause. Renal function on ACE inhibitors must be monitored closely as well. They reduce the preload by reducing volume, and they also reduce afterload because of their vasodilating effect. Current clinical pathways developed by various medical communities for the treatment of CHF consider the use of ACE inhibitors for the treatment of CHF to be the standard of practice. Studies have demonstrated that mortality rates were lower in patients taking an ACE inhibitor, and there is a reduction in the combined endpoints of death and hospitalization. Most of the benefits occurred in the first 90 days of therapy, but benefits lasted for 4 to 5 years and were more pronounced in patients categorized in more severe NYHA heart failure classes (class I: no limitation of activities; class II: slight limitation of activity; class III: marked limitation of activity and comfortable only at rest; class IV: symptoms at rest) (McConaghy and Smith, 2002). If decreased renal function or development of cough or angioedema precludes the use of ACE inhibitors, hydralazine and nitrates can be used for their vasodilating effect. Angiotensin receptor blockers (ARBs) are an alternative for blocking sodium and fluid retention, although they, too, might cause the same side effects as ACE inhibitors (dizziness, altered taste, hypotension, hyperkalemia, and cough). Although the worsening renal function with ACE inhibitors and ARBs might be dose related, cough seems to be an idiosyncratic reaction. Therefore it is entirely possible that a patient who develops a cough with ACE inhibitors might not do so with ARBs. Table 11-10 lists the suggested dosage ranges for vasodilator therapy in older patients.

TABLE 11-10	Suggested Dosages of Vasodilators in the Treatment of Systolic Congestive Heart Failure		

| | **Dosages** | |
Vasodilator	**Initial**	**Goal**
Captopril	6.25 mg t.i.d.	50 mg t.i.d.
Enalapril	2.5 mg b.i.d.	10 mg b.i.d.
Lisinopril	5 mg/day	20 mg/day
Hydralazine/isosorbide dinitrate	10/5 mg t.i.d.	75/40 mg t.i.d.

From Senni M, Redfield M: Concise review of primary care physicians, congestive heart failure in elderly patients, Mayo Clin Proc 72:453-460, 1997.
b.i.d., Twice a day; *t.i.d.*, three times a day.

Calcium channel blockers may be indicated in the treatment of CHF if coronary artery insufficiency coexists. The chief contraindication to their use in CHF has been the depressive effect on strength of contraction or inotropy that some have. Verapamil, diltiazem, and nifedipine all have some negative inotropic effect. There are newer alternatives, however. Amlodipine (Norvasc) has not been demonstrated to have any negative inotropic effect. When CAD coexists, beta-blockers, which reduce mortality in CAD patients in part because they decrease myocardial oxygen demand, would be a desirable part of the treatment regimen; however, their known negative inotropic effect has caused them to be considered contraindicated in patients with CHF. Some recent studies, nevertheless, have shown that more than 95% of CHF patients are able to tolerate at least small doses of beta-blockers. Several small studies even suggest that besides decreasing mortality from CAD, they improve symptoms, and in some they may even result in improved systolic function. Their potential for benefit is even more understandable in treatment of CHF from diastolic dysfunction.

Other measures important in the treatment of CHF include elevating edematous legs; wearing compression (or thromboembolic disease, or TED) stockings; avoiding complete bed rest; and, if hospitalized, using subcutaneous heparin to reduce risk of deep vein thrombosis. In patients with chronic severe CHF, dilated cardiomyopathy, echocardiographic visualization of an LV thrombus, or concomitant atrial fibrillation, long-term anticoagulation with warfarin may be indicated (McConaghy and Smith, 2002). Oxygen supplementation may be important to relieve symptoms.

Moderate exercise training (60% of maximum exercise capacity) improves quality of life and decreases mortality in patients with stable chronic heart failure. Figure 11-3 provides an algorithm for the treatment of adults with heart failure.

Diastolic Dysfunction

Diastolic dysfunction requires adjustments in the therapeutic approach. In the patient with normal systolic function but CHF from diastolic dysfunction, small changes in intravascular volume can result in large changes in filling pressures. Therefore reducing the preload, which reduces the volume that reaches the LV, can actually further reduce filling pressures and cardiac output. Thus diuretic therapy, although perhaps necessary initially to control symptoms, can actually worsen the failure. As in hypertrophic cardiomyopathy, the stiff, noncompliant ventricle that does not relax and accommodate adequate filling volumes may need more volume to overcome that stiffness, "stretch" the ventricle, and fill adequately. As in aortic stenosis, there is already decreased stroke volume; so further decreasing preload can further compromise stroke volume and cardiac output. Therefore diuretics must be used with extreme caution.

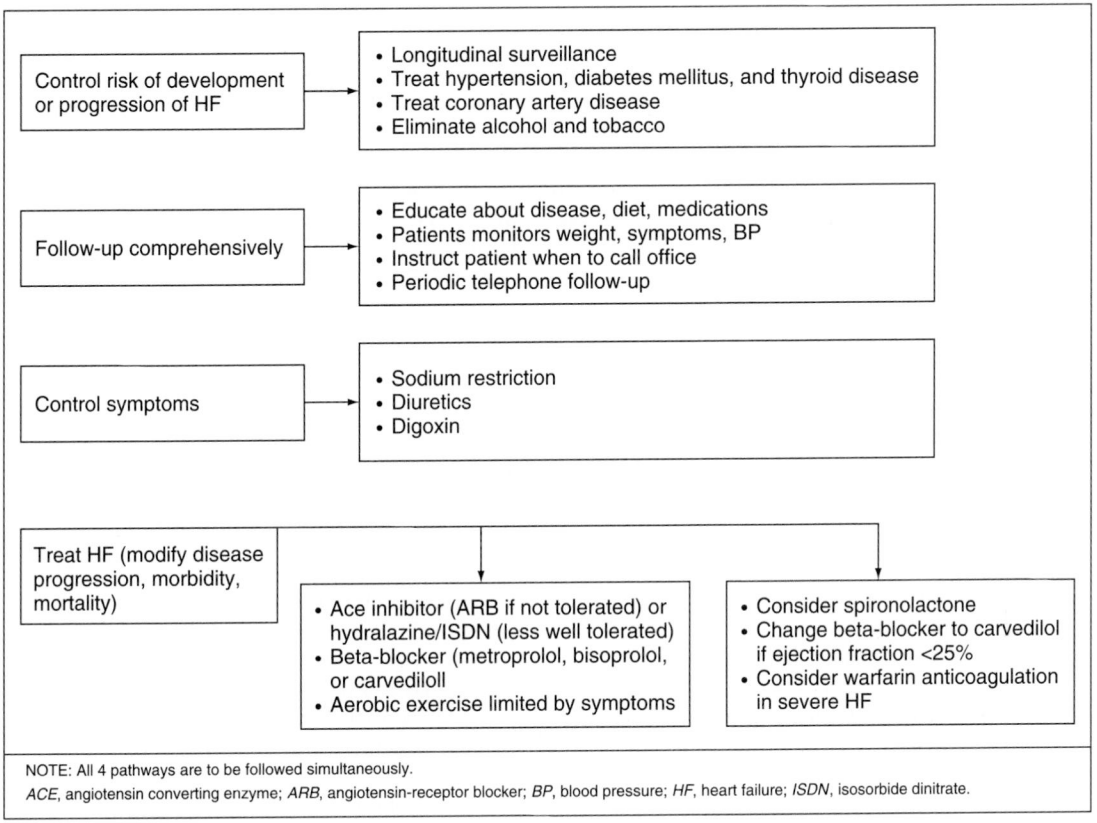

Figure 11-3 Management of adults with heart failure. (From McConaghy JR, Smith SR: Outpatient treatment of heart failure, *J Fam Pract* 51(6):519-525, 2002.)

Digoxin should be avoided. The stiff, noncompliant ventricle has a problem relaxing and stretching to fill. Increasing the strength of contraction is not necessary and may be counterproductive. The need is to improve relaxation. Again, a parallel can be seen in hypertrophic cardiomyopathy, in which digoxin is contraindicated.

The mainstay of therapy for diastolic dysfunction should be ACE inhibitors. Because they dilate both the venous and arterial tree, ACE inhibitors reduce preload, but they also reduce afterload, with a resultant increase in cardiac output. There is evidence that over time ACE inhibitors actually induce regression of LVH. They may accomplish this result by lessening the accumulation of myocardial collagen over time. Both the symptoms of CHF in the short term and survival in the long term may be increased by the use of ACE inhibitors in diastolic heart failure. The usual precautions in older patients hold, such as starting with the smallest effective dose and watching for renal insufficiency. The initial dose can cause marked drops in BP within the first 3 hours after it is given. This drop in BP is even more dramatic in patients who already are on diuretics. It may be wise to stop diuretic therapy while initiating ACE inhibitor therapy in the older patient, or at least to decrease the diuretic dose. For treatment of CHF with ACE inhibitors, the therapeutic goal is the maximum tolerated dose. The ACE inhibitor should be stopped only for symptomatic hypotension rather than holding it for arbitrary BP limits.

In diastolic heart failure calcium channel blockers and beta-blockers may have an even greater role. The negative inotropic effect of a particular calcium channel blocker may make it more desirable therapy. Reduced contractility may result in greater relaxation and therefore greater filling. At least one calcium channel blocker contraindicated in systolic dysfunction because of its suppression of ventricular contraction may have benefit in diastolic dysfunction. Verapamil not only has significant negative inotropism but also causes the regression of LVH; however, this benefit may not last with long-term use. Beta-blockers would be useful for the same reason: negative inotropic effect. Yet it is useful to remember that one of the physiologic changes in normal aging is decreased responsiveness to beta-adrenergic stimuli; so beta-blockers may not be as effective in older patients.

As in systolic dysfunction, it is important to treat and control coexisting disorders. If a patient is in atrial fibrillation, restoring normal sinus rhythm and thereby restoring the older person's "atrial kick," the final and active phase of diastolic filling may be the most effective therapy of all. Hypertension must be controlled. Angina needs to be treated.

For any patient with CHF of either modality, diet should be low in sodium, the exercise level should be maintained or increased if possible, and calorie supplementation may be necessary for "cardiac cachexia." If the patient's CHF is primarily systolic and the patient is severely compromised functionally or has an ejection fraction of less than 20%, fluid intake may need to be restricted as well.

Sequelae

The incidence of CHF increases with age. Therefore as the population of older adults increases, more and more patients will require treatment for CHF. Despite the increased longevity in Western developed nations and increased survival from CAD over recent decades, the overall prognosis of heart failure has improved little. Mortality data derived from several different sources, the largest being the Framingham Heart Study, have shown that heart failure remains highly lethal, with a 5-year survival rate of 25% in men and 38% in women with NYHA II-IV heart failure with the average 1-year mortality has been as high as 18%. Another study demonstrated survival rates of only 62% at 12 months and 57% at 18 months (McConaghy and Smith, 2002). Hospitalization increases and, perhaps with more impact, functional decline increases because of CHF. Diabetic patients with CHF and ischemia do worse than others. Those with CHF with LVH have an increased incidence of sudden death phenomena. Patients with ejection fractions less than or equal to 20%, even if they are already receiving maximum medical therapy with ACE inhibitors, diuretics, and vasodilators, have increased early mortality. The mortality rates for these patients increase even more in the presence of supraventricular tachyarrhythmias; ventricular arrhythmias; or a history of syncope, stroke, or previous cardiac arrest and cardiopulmonary resuscitation. The incidence of stroke in CHF increases fourfold. The incidence of ischemic events increases 2.5 to 5 times. The functional disability that results from heart failure may be the most important factor for older patients. They lose function in mobility and independence in activities of daily living. In addition, these losses are often associated with additional financial burdens. Currently, studies of cardiovascular physiology that seek to refine preventive therapy for CHF focus on measures to reduce cardiac muscle stress, lower cardiac oxygen demand, and suppress norepinephrine.

Despite dismal population-based data regarding mortality rates, predicting the likelihood of survival in persons with heart failure is largely unreliable. Estimating individual prognosis is only somewhat useful in making end-of-life care and hospice decisions for patients with advanced heart failure (McConaghy and Smith, 2002). It is important to facilitate patient and family education regarding the disease and its progression and to discuss the goals of care on an ongoing basis. Table 11-11 lists factors that affect prognosis for patients with heart failure.

Summary

Cardiovascular disease is the most common cause of disease and disability in the older adult. The practitioner must understand cardiovascular physiology and pathophysiology. Initial symptoms can be vague or misleading, and the possible causes can be numerous. The practitioner must be skillful in history taking and physical examination to differentiate the possibilities, initiate the appropriate diagnostic evaluation, and refer when appropriate. Treatments for various conditions are often influ-

TABLE 11-11	Factors that Affect Prognosis in Patients with Heart Failure (HF)

Factor	Result	Comment
Age	Increasing age and age older than 55 years decreases survival	Framingham data: survival rates of older women are twice as long as those of older men despite significant age difference (women: 72 years; men: 68 years).
Sex	Mortality higher in men	Women are underrepresented in HF trials and frequently have HF associated with diastolic dysfunction. Women rate their quality of inpatient care lower than men do.
Race	African Americans have higher mortality rates and higher rates of recurrent hospitalization	HF affects approximately 3% of all African Americans. They develop symptoms at an earlier age. The disease progresses more rapidly than in whites. African Americans are underrepresented in HF trials.
Attending physician specialty	No difference in 6-month cardiac and all-cause mortality between family physician or generalist and cardiologist care	Family physician or generalist: Twofold increased risk of readmission in 6 months; tend to overestimate risks of ACE inhibitors and therefore underprescribe them. Cardiologist (as attending or consultant): Increased testing, hospital lengths of stay, and hospital charges, but better patient-perceived quality of life.

From McConaghy: JR, Smith SR: Outpatient treatment of heart failure, *J Fam Pract*, 51(6):519-525, 2002.

enced by comorbidities, and it may take much consideration to determine the appropriate intervention. Education for the patient, family, and caregiver is critical to ensure the best possible outcome.

Resources

American Heart Association
7320 Greenville Avenue
Dallas, TX 75231
(214) 373-6300
www.americanheart.org

National Heart, Lung, and Blood Information
P.O. Box 30105
Bethesda, MD 20824-0105
(301) 251-1222

References

Brignole M: Sick sinus syndrome, *Clin Geriatr Med* 18(2):211-227, 2002.
Cobbs EL, Duthie EH, Murphy JB, editors: *Geriatrics review syllabus: a core curriculum in geriatric medicine,* ed 5, Malden, Mass, 2002, Blackwell Publishing for the American Geriatrics Society.

Duncan A, Vittone JM: Cardiovascular disease in elderly patients, *Mayo Clin Proc* 71:184-196, 1996.

Ehsani AA: Exercise in patients with hypertension, *Am J Geriatr Cardiol* 10(5):253-259, 2001.

Fleg JL: Stress testing in the elderly, *Am J Geriatr Cardiol* 10(6):308-313, 2001.

Gage BF, Fihn SD, White RH: Warfarin therapy for an octogenarian who has atrial fibrillation, *Ann Intern Med* 134(6):465-474, 2001.

Gladdish S, Rajkumar C: Prevention of cardiac disease in the elderly, *J Cardiovasc Risk* 8(5):271-277, 2001.

Go AS et al: Prevalence of diagnosed atrial fibrillation in adults: national implications for rhythm management and stroke prevention: the Anticoagulation and Risk Factors in Atrial Fibrillation (ATRIA) Study, *JAMA* 285(18):2370-2375, 2001.

Gregorato G: Clinical manifestations of acute myocardial infarction in older patients, *Am J Geriatr Cardiol* 10(6):345-347, 2001.

Hicks GL, Massey HT: Update on indications for surgery in aortic insufficiency, *Curr Opin Cardiol* 17(2):172-178, 2002

Jairath N: Implications of gender differences on coronary artery disease risk reduction in women, *AACN Clinical Issues* 12(1):17-28, 2001.

McConaghy JR, Smith SR: Outpatient treatment of heart failure, *J Fam Pract* 51(6):519-525, 2002.

National Institutes of Health: *The sixth report of the Joint National Committee on Prevention, Detection, Evaluation, and Treatment of High Blood Pressure*, Bethesda, Md, 1997, International Medical.

National Institutes of Health: *The seventh report of the Joint National Committee on Prevention, Detection, Evaluation, and Treatment of High Blood Pressure*, NIH Publication No. 03-5233, Bethesda, Md, May 2003.

Senni M, Redfield M: Concise review of primary care physicians: congestive heart failure in elderly patients, *Mayo Clin Proc* 72:453-460, 1997.

Tresch DD, Alla HR: Diagnosis and management of myocardial ischemia (angina) in the elderly patient, *Am J Geriatr Cardiol* 10(6):337-344, 2001.

Waldo AL: Long-term pharmacologic management of atrial fibrillation in the elderly, *Am J Geriatr Cardiol* 11(4):233-244, 2002.

12

Gastrointestinal: Common Conditions

Gastrointestinal (GI) problems in older people cause a great amount of anxiety, morbidity, and mortality. The management of GI problems is more difficult because in an older age group, functional changes can present in the same way as organic diseases. In addition, primary care practitioners may not have the same immediate access to diagnostic investigations as specialists (Newton, 2001). It is important for primary care practitioners to recognize and treat appropriately GI problems in older patients and to know when referral is appropriate and necessary.

Age-related Changes

The structure and function of the GI tract are affected both by physiologic changes of aging and by the effects of accumulating disorders involving many body systems. In association with advancing age, changes in connective tissue that limit elasticity of the gut and alterations in the nerves and muscles that impair mobility can occur. Accumulating disorders and diseases are often associated with increased use of medications by older persons, many of which have direct effects on intestinal mucosa and motility. Some disease states can adversely influence GI function and can lead to symptoms and complications. GI problems can quickly compromise the older person's ability to maintain adequate nutrition and can lead to fatigue and weight loss (Cobbs, Duthie, and Murphy, 2002). Age-related changes in the GI system include decreased saliva flow and in the stomach a decrease in the production of acid and an increase in gastrin production. In the small intestine transit time is increased with an accompanying increase in motility, but the absorption of vitamin D and B_{12}, folate, calcium, and iron are decreased; for fat-soluble vitamins the absorption rate is increased. In the colon the mucosa, musculature, and transit time are all decreased. The size of the liver decreases along with hepatic blood flow. The changes in the GI system, along with the progressive age-related decrease in creatinine clearance, increase the possibility of adverse drug reactions in the older adult.

GASTROESOPHAGEAL REFLUX DISEASE

Gastroesophageal reflux disease (GERD) is defined as chronic symptoms or mucosal damage produced by abnormal reflux of gastric contents into the esophagus. Highly specific symptoms for

GERD include heartburn, regurgitation, or both, which occur often after meals and are aggravated by recumbency and relieved by antacids. Among persons 65 years of age and older, symptoms of heartburn or acid regurgitation occur at least weekly in 20% of the population and at least monthly in 59% of the population, rates similar to those observed in young adults (Cobbs, Duthie, and Murphy, 2002).

The lower esophageal sphincter is a physiologic barrier to the transfer of gastric acid secretions from the stomach to the esophagus. In more than 80% of patients, GERD is caused by transient inappropriate lower esophageal sphincter relaxations that lead to acid reflux into the esophagus. Some patients have reduced lower esophageal sphincter tone, which permits reflux when intraabdominal pressure rises. Sliding hiatal hernia occurs in about 30% of patients 50 years of age or older and may contribute to acid reflux and regurgitation. Poor esophageal peristalsis leads to delayed clearance of the reflux and increased acid exposure time. In patients receiving anticholinergic drugs, reduced salivary secretion decreases the buffering capacity of the esophagus against refluxed acid and may aggravate mucosal injury (Cobbs, Duthie, and Murphy, 2002).

History

Heartburn is the most common manifestation of reflux esophagitis. Neither its severity nor its frequency predicts the degree of severity of the tissue damage seen on endoscopy. The presence of anemia, dysphagia, GI bleeding, recurrent vomiting, and weight loss suggests complicated GERD (Cobbs, Duthie, and Murphy, 2002).

Reflux esophagitis occurs more frequently in older patients and is more severe than in younger patients. Although the degree of symptom manifestation is similar between older and younger patients with high-grade esophagitis, older patients with mild reflux esophagitis tend to be less symptomatic than younger patients.

Differential Diagnosis

Reflux can also present with nonesophageal symptoms, such as noncardiac chest pain, chronic sinusitis, globus hystericus, hoarseness, wheezing, asthma, aspiration pneumonia, and poor dentition.

Treatment

Treatment should be conservative at first, starting with lifestyle modifications that include elevating the head of the bed at least 6 inches and avoiding late-night snacks, alcohol, smoking, caffeine derivatives, and any food that makes the patient symptomatic, including citrus juices or carbonated beverages. Weight reduction, along with reduction of dietary fat and meal size, may be beneficial.

When lifestyle modifications fail, drug therapy is recommended. Patients with uncomplicated heartburn or regurgitation should be treated empirically with acid-suppressing drugs. Proton-pump inhibitors are the treatment of choice for patients with GERD, but they are expensive. Use of these drugs heals esophagitis in 85% of cases and eradicates heartburn and regurgitation in 80%. In comparison, H_2 antagonists ameliorate symptoms and heal esophagitis in only 60% of cases. Regardless, therapy should be maintained for at least 8 weeks (Cobbs, Duthie, and Murphy, 2002).

Cost, adverse effects, and drug interactions have become important considerations in the treatment of reflux, especially in vulnerable older patients. Important drug interactions with antacids include the prevention of the absorption of antibacterials such as tetracycline, azithromycin, and quinolones. H_2 antagonists, proton-pump inhibitors, and prokinetic agents undergo metabolism by the cytochrome P450 system present in the liver and gastrointestinal tract. Cimetidine may cause significant interactions with certain drugs and is generally not recommended for use in older patients. Interactions with prokinetic agents carry significant potential for harm. Metoclopramide is a dopamine antagonist that may cause extrapyramidal effects when administered alone at high concentrations or when coadministered with antipsychotic agents such as haloperidol or phenothiazines (Flockhart, Desta, and Mahal, 2000). Cisapride, a prokinetic, has been withdrawn from the market in many countries because some patients experienced dangerous cardiac arrhythmias, especially when cisapride was administered with potent inhibitors of cytochrome P450 3A4 (Asante, 2001). It is important to ask patients whether they are continuing to take this medication from a previous prescription.

If empiric treatment with acid-suppressing drugs is unsuccessful, or if symptoms suggest complicated disease, an upper endoscopy should be performed. This is the procedure of choice to evaluate mucosal integrity and confirm the diagnosis of dysplasia or cancer in cases of Barrett's esophagus (Cobbs, Duthie, and Murphy, 2002). Gastrointestinal endoscopy is extremely safe and well tolerated even in very old patients. Age alone should not influence decisions relating to its use (Clarke et al, 2001).

The 24-hour continuous intraesophageal pH monitoring provides the ability to correlate symptoms with episodes of acid reflux, especially in the presence of atypical symptoms. This noninvasive test is also useful for patients with noncardiac chest pain or reflux-associated pulmonary and upper respiratory symptoms or to monitor esophageal acid exposure in patients with refractory symptoms.

Recurrence of symptoms is common after therapy is stopped, and lifelong therapy is commonly needed. Intermittent therapy with an H_2 antagonist or proton-pump inhibitor may be successful in some patients with mild to moderate symptoms without severe esophagitis. Recurrent symptoms in less than 3 months suggest that the disease will be best managed with continuous therapy (Cobbs, Duthie, and Murphy, 2002). Concerns regarding the long-term safety of proton-pump inhibitors necessitate ongoing monitoring and information seeking by practitioners.

When medical management fails or if lifelong medical treatment is not preferred, antireflux surgery is indicated. This can be performed laparascopically; success rates have been greater than 90%. Laparoscopic antireflux surgery (LARS) can be a safe, effective procedure that significantly improves quality of life in the older patient suffering from GERD. Age should not be a contraindication to LARS (Kamolz et al, 2001). Esophageal manometry is used to document the presence of effective esophageal peristalsis in patients for whom antireflux surgery is being considered (Cobbs, Duthie, and Murphy, 2002).

PEPTIC ULCER DISEASE

Risk Factors

In the United States, *Helicobacter pylori* infection is responsible for about 80% of duodenal ulcers and about 60% of gastric ulcers (Cobbs, Duthie, and Murphy, 2002). It has been suggested that cigarette smoking increases the incidence of peptic ulcer disease.

History

Most older persons with ulcers complain of dyspepsia, although bleeding, anemia, and acute abdominal pain may occur. The most common presenting symptom is burning epigastric pain that is nocturnal or postprandial and nonradiating. Pain that awakens the patient from sleep is highly suggestive of duodenal ulcer but can also be seen in nonulcer dyspepsia and gastric ulcers. About 10% of patients with peptic ulcer disease present with complications (i.e., GI bleed and perforation) without any history of epigastric pain.

Differential Diagnosis

The differential diagnosis of epigastric pain is vast and should include pain of esophageal, biliary, pancreatic, cardiac, and intestinal origin. Osteoarthritis is more common in older persons, and the use of nonsteroidal antiinflammatory drugs (NSAIDs) is particularly toxic in older patients. If NSAIDs are required, propionic acid derivatives such as naproxen are better tolerated. COX-2 (cyclooxygenase-2) inhibitors such as Celebrex and Vioxx are available; although they are preferred for patients who are at high risk for GI complications such as perforation or bleeding, some risk still exists. Contrary to popular thought, the greatest value of these agents may be in patients without risk factors because in this unconfounded group these drugs' ability to free patients of ulcer risk appears to be delivered in full (Hawkey, 2001).

Typically, the diagnosis of peptic ulcer is made by upper GI radiography or endoscopy. Endoscopy is more sensitive and specific than double-contrast barium study. To differentiate benign gastric ulcers from gastric cancer, mutiple endoscopic biopsies must be obtained, especially in patients who present with early satiety, weight loss, occult GI bleeding, or otherwise unexplained anemia (Cobbs, Duthie, and Murphy, 2002). The diagnosis of *H. pylori* can be made histologically by Giemsa stain and a Clotest or by the breath test and determining the *H. pylori* antibody titers in the serum.

Treatment

In treating peptic ulcer disease, one should eliminate the offending factors such as NSAIDs and smoking and also eradicate *H. pylori* infection. Such eradication helps decrease the relapse rate and prevent the possible transformation to mucosa-associated lymphoid tissue lymphoma seen in the stomach. Several therapy regimens have been highly effective in eradicating *H. pylori*, all of which should include an antisecretory agent with either one antibiotic plus bismuth or two antibiotics. One such plan consists of a 14-day regimen (taken before eating) of the following:
- One Prevacid (lansoprazole) 30-mg capsule administered orally twice a day
- Two amoxicillin 500-mg capsules taken orally twice a day
- One Biaxin (clarithromycin) 500-mg tablets taken orally twice a day

Lansoprasole 30 mg combined with amoxicillin 1g, clarithromycin 250 or 500 mg, or metronidazole 400 mg twice daily was associated with eradication rates ranging from 71% to 94%, and ulcer healing rates were generally greater than 80% in some studies (Matheson and Jarvis, 2001). Follow-up upper endoscopy may be indicated in cases in which healing needs to be documented.

DIVERTICULAR DISEASE

Risk Factors

Diverticula are herniations through the colonic wall and are therefore likely to be due to a weakness within the wall, an alteration in intracolonic pressures, or a combination of these factors (Simpson, Scholefield, and Spiller, 2002). The presence of diverticular disease is age dependent, increasing to 30% by 60 years of age and to 65% by 85 years of age. Although most patients remain asymptomatic, 20% develop diverticulitis, and 10% may develop diverticular bleeding (Cobbs, Duthie, and Murphy, 2002). A high-fiber diet appears to be associated with a reduced risk of the development of diverticular disease and may reduce the risk of subsequent complications.

Differential Diagnosis

Uncomplicated diverticulosis is often an incidental finding on screening sigmoidoscopy, colonoscopy, or barium enema. Some patients complain of nonspecific abdominal cramping, bloating, flatulence, and irregular bowel habits. Diverticular bleeding is usually painless and self-limited.

When microperforation of the diverticulae occurs, it starts an inflammatory process in the peridiverticulum area and causes diverticulitis. This inflammation may extend further and cause abscess formation that may in turn encase the colonic lumen and cause obstruction. One should differentiate this from acute appendicitis, inflammatory bowel disease, Crohn's colitis, infectious colitis, ischemic colitis, or any other process causing pericolonic abscess. The physical examination usually reveals left lower-quadrant tenderness, a tender mass, and abdominal distention.

Generalized tenderness suggests perforation and peritonitis. Low-grade fever and leukocytosis are common, but their absence in older adults does not exclude the diagnosis. Diverticulitis usually manifests with left lower-quadrant pain, although nausea, vomiting, constipation, diarrhea, dysuria, or frequency may occur. Complications may include obstruction and abscess formation (Cobbs, Duthie, and Murphy, 2002).

Diagnosis may be made by barium enema, which shows outpouching of the colonic wall. This also helps to rule out an obstructing lesion. Computed tomography scanning is the optimal imaging method in acute diverticulitis. In about 10% of patients, however, diverticulitis cannot be distinguished from colon cancer because both may show focal thickening of the bowel wall. In such cases, on resolution of the acute inflammation, a colonoscopy is indicated (Cobbs, Duthie, and Murphy, 2002).

Small bowel diverticula are usually asymptomatic and rare, but they may carry the risk of serious complication such as infection, rupture, obstruction, and bleeding (Kouraklis et al, 2002).

Treatment

Uncomplicated diverticulosis is usually treated with a high-fiber diet. Antispasmodic agents may be tried in patients with chronic, intermittent, nonspecific abdominal pain.

Most patients (85%) with simple diverticulitis respond to medical therapy, which includes fluid replacement, bowel rest (clear liquids), and oral antibiotics such as ciprofloxacin 500 mg twice a day or metronidazole 500 mg three times a day or both. Treatment of simple diverticulitis may be completed on an outpatient basis. For those with moderate to severe symptoms, treatment is with bowel rest, fluids, and intravenous antibiotics and possibly nasogastric suction if mechanical or functional obstruction is present.

Surgical resection is necessary in about 20% of patients with diverticulitis. Indications are peritonitis, perforation, colonic obstruction, poor response to conservative management, recurrent diverticulitis, or an abscess that cannot be drained percutaneously (Cobbs, Duthie, and Murphy, 2002).

The management of diverticular bleeding should be directed first toward volume replacement and resuscitation, followed by a colonoscopy. Angiography may be necessary if bleeding recurs or continues with the failure to identify the bleeding site by colonoscopy. Angiography should be the first step if the patient develops major persistent bleeding. Localizing the bleeding site and colonic involvement with diverticular disease helps the surgeon to direct the treatment plan to segmental colectomy versus total abdominal colectomy. In cases in which the bleeding ceases spontaneously, as occurs in most cases, surgery is not needed and the prognosis is good.

After successful medical therapy of the first episode of diverticulitis, one third of persons will remain asymptomatic, another third will have episodic abdominal cramps, and the remaining will proceed to a second attack of diverticulitis. Therefore, elective surgery is not necessary for all patients with diverticulitis who respond to medical therapy. If surgery is performed, progression of diverticulitis in the remaining colon occurs in only 15%, and the need for further surgery is reduced to less than 10% (Cobbs, Duthie, and Murphy, 2002).

COLORECTAL CANCER

Risk Factors

Colorectal cancer is the fourth most common cancer and second leading cause of cancer deaths in the United States. About 135,000 new cases were diagnosed in 2001, resulting in about 56,000 deaths.

Screening efforts have become considerably important in identifying early, curable colorectal cancer (Swaroop and Larson, 2002). Table 12-1 outlines the guidelines for screening for colorectal cancer by various agencies.

The long exposure to environmental carcinogens results in an increased incidence exponentially. Factors such as alcohol use, particularly beer; tobacco smoking; and dietary habits such as a high-fat, low-fiber or a red meat-rich diet have been implicated in adenoma or adenocarcinoma of the colon. Other factors, including the *p53* genes and the *APC* gene, have also been implicated in the adenoma to carcinoma sequence. Inflammatory bowel diseases, colonic adenomas, and prior exposure to radiation increase the risk for colorectal cancer.

Occult GI bleeding is generally the only manifestation of early colon cancer. Bright red blood per rectum may be seen with more distal lesions. In advanced cases, colonic obstruction, abdominal pain, and symptoms of local and distant invasion may be found. Wasting syndrome has been described even with small early tumors.

A family history of colorectal polyps increases the risk of cancer by about the same amount as a family history of colorectal cancer. Polyps are usually asymptomatic, but they may bleed. Colonic

TABLE 12-1	Guidelines for Screening for Colorectal Cancer in Average-Risk Individuals				
Organization	**FOBT**	**FS**	**FOBT and FS**	**BE**	**CS**
USPSTF	Annually	Yes, frequency unspecified	Yes, frequency unspecified	NR	NR
AHCPR	Annually	Every 5 yr	Annual FOBT and FS every 5 yr	DCBE every 5-10 yr	Every 10 yr
AGA (multi-disciplinary panel)	Annually	Every 5 yr	Annual FOBT and FS every 5 yr	Every 5 yr	Every 10 yr
ACG	Annually	Every 5 yr	Annual FOBT and FS every 5 yr	DCBE every 5-10 yr	Every 10 yr
ACS	Annually	Every 5 yr	Annual FOBT and FS every 5 yr	Every 5 yr	Every 10 yr
WHO	NR	NR	Annual FOBT and FS every 3-5 y	NR	NR
ACP	Yes (if patient refuses other options)	Every 10 yr	NR	Every 10 yr	Every 10 yr
CTFPHE	NR	NR	NR	NR	NR

From Swaroop VS, Larson MV: Colonoscopy as a screening test for colorectal cancer in average-risk individuals, *Mayo Clin Proc* 77(9):951-956, 2002.

ACG, American College of Gastroenterology; *ACP*, American College of Physicians; *ACS*, American Cancer Society; *AGA*, American Gastroenterological Association; *AHCPR*, Agency for Healthcare Policy and Research; *BE*, barium enema; *CS*, colonoscopy; *CTFPHE*, Canadian Task Force on the Periodic Health Examination; *DCBE*, double-contrast barium enema; *FOBT*, fecal occult blood test; *FS*, flexible sigmoidoscopy; *NR*, not recommended; *USPSTF*, U.S. Preventive Services Task Force; *WHO*, World Health Organization.

polyps are usually classified as neoplastic (adenomas) and nonneoplastic (hyperplastic). About 40% of the U.S. population 50 years of age or older have one or more adenomas. Detection and removal of adenomas significantly decrease the morbidity and mortality rates associated with colorectal cancer (Cobbs, Duthie, and Murphy, 2002). Older age, villous histology, and size are independent risk factors for malignancy within an adenoma. About 70% of polyps removed at colonoscopy are adenomas (Bond, 2000).

Screening

Five different screening strategies for colorectal cancer have been recommended by the Agency for Healthcare Policy and Research, now known as the Agency for Healthcare Research and Quality, for average-risk patients. These strategies include annual fecal occult blood test (FOBT), flexible sigmoidoscopy (FS) every 5 years, annual FOBT with FS every 5 years, double-contrast barium enema every 5 to 10 years, and colonoscopy every 10 years (Swaroop and Larson, 2002). There is much disagreement regarding the benefit of annual FOBT. If the stool is positive for occult blood, a colonoscopy versus a flexible sigmoidoscopy with air-contrast barium enema is indicated. Because adenomas typically do not bleed, FOBT is an insensitive screening method.

The adenoma carcinoma sequence takes an average of 15 years to occur. Therefore, screening asymptomatic patients is a crucial first step in diagnosing adenocarcinoma in the colon. The most sensitive and specific test available, especially in patients with small polyps or early cancers, is colonoscopy, which also provides the opportunity to obtain tissue biopsies. Barium enema is helpful in more advanced cases.

Treatment

Adenomatous polyps are treated with polypectomy or polyp fulguration based on the polyp size. Some large polyps may require segmental resection. Surgery is the mainstay treatment for adenocarcinoma. Adjuvant chemotherapy increases survival for patients with advanced disease. Self-expanding colonic metallic stent placement is a minimally invasive and cost-effective palliative approach. Older patients with comorbidities who have colon perforation and obstruction from colon cancer and require emergency surgical intervention may benefit from conservative surgery followed by staged resection. The same may be said for patients with intraoperatively established greater spread of tumor. This procedure permits delayed radical resection at the lowest rate of clinical mortality and is especially suitable for frail older patients in poor condition.

Age should not be the only parameter considered when addressing the treatment of a gastrointestinal malignancy. Management decisions for older patients should follow the same principles as those in younger patients. A thorough medical evaluation of older patients is necessary to evaluate the patient's risk and to optimize surgical, chemotherapeutic, and palliative outcomes (Sial and Catalano, 2001).

ACUTE ABDOMEN

Especially in older patients, the GI and hepatobiliary systems are responsible for a wide range of pathologies resulting in an acute abdomen. These include appendicitis, diverticulitis, perforated peptic ulcer disease, intestinal ischemia, obstruction and perforation, acute pancreatitis, acute cholangitis, acute cholecystitis, hepatic abscess, and ruptured hepatic neoplasm.

Because early diagnosis is essential in directing treatment, one should start first with a thorough history and physical examination that should provide clues to the diagnosis in most cases. One should pay attention to the pain characteristics and the presence of peritoneal irritation signs, masses, or GI bleeding.

Acute Appendicitis

Acute appendicitis has increased in incidence in the last decades, in part because of the increased longevity in the general population. Appendicitis is prevalent in the older population, accounting for up to 14% of all cases of acute abdomen. Mortality is reported to be higher in the older patient because of the nonclassic presentation, delayed diagnosis, and higher rate of complication in a patient with multiple preexisting diseases. The primary care provider needs to practice increased vigilance and have a high index of suspicion.

History

Typically the pain starts in the periumbilical area and is associated with nausea and possibly vomiting. This is thought to be due to the obstruction of the appendiceal lumen by a fecalith, a foreign body, or lymphatic hyperplasia. If the obstruction continues, the inflammation becomes transmural, resulting in serosal inflammation and then pain localization in the right lower quadrant.

Differential Diagnosis

The diagnosis of appendicitis is often made on clinical examination. It can be supported by leukocytosis, small bowel ileus, the presence of the appendicolith on the abdominal flat plate, the presence of pneumoperitoneum indicating a perforation, or the presence of a dilated appendix with a thickened wall on ultrasound. The accuracy of ultrasonography in nonperforated appendix is 93%, with a negative predicted value of 97%. In older patients, the diagnosis is often made late, with 40% to 80% of cases already perforated. The reasons for delayed hospitalization include atypical course, reduction in sensitivity to pain in old age, and inadequate ability to communicate.

Treatment

The treatment for acute appendicitis is emergent appendectomy. Delayed diagnosis or presentation may lead to increased mortality as a result of appendiceal perforation. The overall mortality rate increases with age, reaching up to 16% for patients above 70 years of age. Postoperative complications occur much more frequently in older patients, resulting in an increased morbidity and prolonged hospital stay.

Mesenteric Ischemia

The diagnosis of mesenteric ischemia requires a high degree of suspicion in the patient with abdominal pain. It is associated with a high mortality rate. It can result from an occlusive or a nonocclusive process and can be arterial or venous in origin. Acute occlusive arterial ischemia is a result of an embolic phenomenon most commonly caused by a mural thrombus from an underlying cardiac disease or an aortic embolus.

Presentation and Differential Diagnosis

Patients present with acute sudden onset of severe midabdominal pain that may be associated with peritoneal irritation and occult GI bleeding. The diagnosis is made clinically, but the presence of leukocytosis, hemoconcentration, and metabolic acidosis with an increase in serum lactate levels, which usually indicates a late presentation, is helpful. Once the diagnosis is suspected, emergent angiography is indicated. Once the embolus is identified, intraarterial injection of urokinase and systemic intravenous heparin may spare the patient an emergent surgery, which includes embolectomy and resection of necrotic bowels.

In cases of the low-flow state, nonocclusive mesenteric ischemia is due to vasoconstriction as a result of decreased cardiac output, hypovolemia, or medications such as digoxin. Angiography shows mesenteric vasoconstriction with a pruned appearance. Treatment is directed toward fluid and volume resuscitation. Surgery is reserved for necrotic bowel resection.

Mesenteric Thrombosis

Mesenteric thrombosis can manifest with acute abdominal pain, but more commonly it manifests as a chronic postprandial abdominal pain, resulting in decreased food intake and weight loss. Diagnosis is made angiographically, and treatment can be achieved by intraarterial stenting or surgical bypass. Patients older than 75 years of age with mesenteric ischemia have a higher overall mortality after exploratory laparotomy.

HEPATOBILIARY PANCREATIC DISEASES

Isolated abnormalities of liver enzymes have been noted occasionally in older patients. Isolated elevation of alkaline phosphatase is related to osteomalacia in 50% of patients and to liver disease in 25% and is idiopathic in 25%. An isolated elevation of serum bilirubin may reflect congestive hepatopathy seen with the congestive heart. Hepatocellular dysfunction and cholestatic damage are also seen in older patients and may reflect conditions such as hepatitis, drug toxicity, and hepatocellular carcinoma.

CHOLELITHIASIS AND CHOLEDOCHOLITHIASIS

Gallstones form primarily in the gallbladder and may obstruct the cystic or common bile duct, causing biliary pain, cholecystitis, and cholangitis. When stones obstruct the ampulla, pancreatitis may occur. The prevalence of cholelithiasis increases with age, with up to 30% of the geriatric population having this condition.

Presentation

Biliary colic is characterized by an epigastric or right upper-quadrant abdominal pain that gradually worsens before reaching a plateau of constant severe pain that may last for several hours. Spontaneous resolution of biliary colic reflects the dislodgment of the impacted stone from the cystic duct. The pain is most commonly postprandial, especially after a fatty meal, and is associated with nausea and vomiting.

Cholecystitis occurs as a result of the continued obstruction of the cystic duct, leading to gallbladder wall inflammation. When the inflammation reaches the serosal surface of the gallbladder, peritoneal irritation signs occur, leading to localization of the pain in the right upper quadrant. Murphy's sign is described as the inhibition of deep inspiration secondary to pain produced by the movement of an inflamed gallbladder against the parietal peritoneum. Fever, leukocytosis, and elevation of liver enzymes, including bilirubin, alkaline phosphatase, and transaminases, may be seen. Ultrasonographic findings may include gallstones, biliary obstruction and dilation, thickened gallbladder wall, or pericholecystic fluid. Isolated alkaline phosphatase elevation without jaundice may be a presenting manifestation of biliary obstruction in older patients and should always be evaluated (Cobbs, Duthie, and Murphy, 2002).

Differential Diagnosis

In the proper clinical setting and in the presence of gallstones, a positive sonographic Murphy's sign predicts acute cholecystitis in 90% of cases. When acalculus cholecystitis is suspected, cholescintigraphy can help in the diagnosis. Computed abdominal tomography scanning may be used if common bile duct stones or ductal obstruction are suspected. Magnetic resonance cholangiography and endoscopic ultrasonongraphy are two very accurate imaging modalities to detect common bile duct pathology, including gallstones. For patients with obstructive jaundice, cholangitis, or suspected biliary pancreatitis, however, where the probability of common bile duct stones is high, therapeutic endoscopic retrograde cholangiopancreatography (ERCP) is preferred (Cobbs, Duthie, and Murphy, 2002).

Treatment

Management includes fluid resuscitation, intravenous antibiotics, and cholecystectomy, which is the most effective management. Laparoscopic cholecystectomy is the procedure of choice. When patients are poor surgical candidates, percutaneous cholecystostomy is a safe, effective treatment for acute cholecystitis. For acalculus cholecystitis, cholecystostomy can be followed by elective surgery. Biliary obstruction may be complicated by acute pancreatitis, termed *biliary pancreatitis.*. If acute pancreatitis is severe, the abdominal pain may be periumbilical or midabdominal, radiating to the back; some relief may be obtained by adopting the fetal position. Acute pancreatitis is usually associated with amylase and lipase elevation. When biliary pancreatitis and continued biliary obstruction are suspected, ERCP with sphincterotomy and stone removal is indicated. This results in substantial improvement in the outcome of acute biliary pancreatitis.

In the rare older patient who is unable to undergo surgery, treatment with ursodeoxycholic acid or lithotripsy or both may be attempted. In patients with common bile duct obstruction from gallstones, endoscopic sphincterotomy and bile ductal drainage are adequate in preventing recurrent cholangitis, and the gallbladder may be left in place. In any older person with gallstones, the possibility of gallbladder cancer should be entertained (Cobbs, Duthie, and Murphy, 2002).

LIVER DISEASE

Viral Hepatitis

With the advances in novel technologies, eight distinct types of hepatitis virus have been described: A, B, C, D, E, G, TT, and SEN viruses. Hepatitis A and E viruses are transmitted by the fecal-oral route and do not induce a chronic carrier state. As a result of major changes in the epidemiology of hepatitis A virus, their significance is more pronounced in areas of intermediate endemicity. Because the available hepatitis A vaccine is rather expensive, cost-benefit studies should be performed with emphasis on the area under consideration or specialized vulnerable groups. Parenterally transmitted hepatitis B and C viruses are major causes of chronic liver disease, including cirrhosis, hepatocellular carcinoma, and end-stage liver failure. Hepatitis D virus is unable to replicate on its own; it requires an established hepatitis B virus infection to be able to replicate. Since its introduction, hepatitis B vaccine has been widely used, leading to a significant decrease in hepatitis B virus infection in countries with universal vaccination. Hepatitis G and TT viruses have been characterized within the latter part of the past decade, but their significance as to the causation of human liver disease has yet to be elucidated. Likewise, the precise impact of the most recently described SEN virus isolated from patients with posttransfusion hepatitis awaits further studies (Poovorawan, Chatchatee, and Chongsrisawat, 2002).

The contribution of hepatitis C to chronic liver disease is predicted to rise in the future. Vaccines can prevent hepatitis A and B. Interferon alpha is effective treatment in 25% to 30% of patients with chronic hepatitis B or C. The prospects for treating chronic hepatitis B have been improved by the introduction of reverse transcriptase inhibitors. Lamivudine is the first drug of this class to be licensed. The optimal use of these new drugs is currently being studied. The success rate for treating chronic hepatitis C can be raised to about 40% with combination therapy of interferon alpha and ribavirin. A large research effort to discover new antiviral agents against hepatitis C is already giving the prospect of more effective therapies in the next few years (Summerfield, 2000).

Hepatitis B virus is usually transmitted by inoculation of infected blood or blood products. The incubation period of hepatitis B is 6 weeks to 6 months (average 12 to 14 weeks) but may be prolonged by the administration of hepatitis B immune globulin. See Table 12-2 for recommended postexposure prophylaxis for exposure to hepatitis B virus. Table 12-3 outlines the interpretation of the hepatitis B panel to determine the patient's immune or infection status.

Hepatitis C virus is a ribonucleic acid virus that was first identified in 1989 and currently affects about 2% of the American population and 4.1% of patients 60 years of age and older. In the subgroup of geriatric patients, risk factors for acquiring hepatitis C are blood transfusion, surgical intervention,

TABLE 12-2 Recommended Postexposure Prophylaxis for Percutaneous or Permucosal Exposure to Hepatitis B Virus, United States		
	Treatment When Source Is	
Vaccination and Antibody Response Status of Exposed Person	**HBsAg* Positive**	**HBsAg Negative**	**Not Tested or Status Unknown**
Unvaccinated	HBIG† × 1; initiate HB vaccine series‡	Initiate HB vaccine series	Initiate HB vaccine series
Previously vaccinated:			
Known responder§	No treatment	No treatment	No treatment
Known non-responder	HBIG × 2 or HBIG × 1 and initiate revaccination	No treatment	If known high-risk source, treat as if source were HBsAg positive
Antibody response unknown	Test exposed person for anti-HBs‖ 1. If adequate,§ no treatment 2. If inadequate,§ HBIG × 1 and vaccine booster	No treatment	Test exposed person for anti-HBs 1. If adequate,§ no treatment 2. If inadequate, initiate revaccination

From Centers for Disease Control and Prevention: Immunization of health-care workers, *MMWR* 46(RR-18):1-42, 1997.
*Hepatitis B surface antigen.
†Hepatitis B immune globulin; dose 0.06 ml/kg intramuscularly.
‡Hepatitis B vaccine.
§Responder is defined as a person with adequate levels of serum antibody to hepatitis B surface antigen (i.e., anti-HBs ≥10 mIU/ml); inadequate response to vaccination defined as serum anti-HBs < 10 mIU/ml.
‖Antibody to hepatitis B surface antigen.

TABLE 12-3	Interpreting the Hepatitis B Panel

Interpretation of the Hepatitis B Panel

Tests	Results	Interpretation
HBsAg	Negative	Susceptible
anti-HBc	Negative	
anti-HBs	Negative	
HBsAg	Negative	Immune due to vaccination
anti-HBc	Negative	
anti-HBs	Positive with ≥10mIU/mL*	
HBsAg	Negative	Immune due to natural infection
anti-HBc	Positive	
anti-HBs	Positive	
HBsAg	Positive	Acutely infected
anti-HBc	Positive	
IgM anti-HBc	Positive	
anti-HBs	Negative	
HBsAg	Positive	Chronically infected
anti-HBc	Positive	
IgM anti-HBc	Negative	
anti-HBs	Negative	
HBsAg	Negative	Four interpretations possible†
anti-HBc	Positive	
anti-HBs	Negative	

From Immunization Action Coalition, 2002, 1573 Selby Avenue, St. Paul MN 55104. E-mail: admin@immunize.org, web: http://www.immunize.org/.

*Postvaccination testing, when it is recommended, should be performed 1-2 months following dose #3.

†1. May be recovering from acute HBV infection.
  2. May be distantly immune and the test is not sensitive enough to detect a very low level of anti-HBs in serum.
  3. May be susceptible with a false positive anti-HBc.
  4. May be chronically infected and have an undetectable level of HBsAg present in the serum.

and the use of nondisposable syringes. The most prevalent route of transmission is through parenteral transmission; in the older population it is most commonly from a blood transfusion before 1990. After exposure to hepatitis C, more than 80% of patients develop chronic hepatitis C, which has an insidious course and is usually discovered when abnormal liver enzymes are found and further investigated or when the patient with the chronic hepatitis C decompensates with cirrhosis.

Symptoms are usually mild, most commonly fatigue and malaise. Change of sleep pattern, easy bruisability, altered mental status resulting from hepatic encephalopathy, and GI bleeding are seen in the late stages when cirrhosis is present.

Diagnosis is made clinically and by laboratory values. Liver biopsy may be needed if treatment is planned or to assess the severity and stage of the liver involvement. Patients over 60 years of age were found to have mild histologic changes, which were thought to be related to the higher prevalence of genotype IIA found in most of these patients.

It is generally accepted that 10% to 20% of patients with chronic hepatitis C will develop cirrhosis within 10 years of first infection. The recommended treatment for naïve patients is interferon in subcutaneous injections for 12 to 18 months. Patients older than 65 years of age have been found to have a 30% virologic/complete response. Some studies have recommended postponing treatment in asymptomatic patients if liver biopsy specimens show no more than grade I necroinflammatory activity or stage I fibrosis. Therefore, one could argue that in a geriatric patient who fits the preceding description, clinical monitoring is a reasonable course of action.

Although it has been suggested in many studies that hepatitis C virus (or G or both) may play an etiologic role in non-Hodgkin lymphoma and other myeloproliferative diseases, this has not been confirmed (Kaya et al, 2002).

In patients with decompensated cirrhosis, the only treatment that would improve the 5-year survival rate is liver transplantation, which is less frequently done in the geriatric population because of the comorbid conditions that would make such a major intervention futile. Therefore, conservative management with diuretics for fluid retention in ascites and lactulose for portosystemic encephalopathy is indicated.

With the increased incidence of hepatocellular carcinoma in cirrhotic patients who do not tolerate surgical resection because of advanced cirrhosis, new modalities of treatment have recently been described that include thoracoscopic microwave coagulation therapy for tumor ablation and percutaneous ethanol injection, both of which have resulted in partial or complete resolution of liver lesions.

Summary

Several GI disorders are very common in the older population. It is important to be able to perform the appropriate evaluation to distinguish among them, especially the acute or malignant conditions. Numerous special considerations for diagnosing and treating GI conditions must be kept in mind, such as the presence of *H. pylori* in ulcer disease or the risk of hepatitis. Several laboratory and diagnostic examinations are available. The ability to determine the appropriate one (and to know when to refer) can save much discomfort and expense. In addition, the practitioner must be able to prescribe the appropriate treatment or intervention and provide adequate teaching to the patient or caregiver.

Resources

American College of Gastroenterology
www.acg.gi.org

American Institute for Cancer Research
www.aicr.org

GERD Information Resource Center
www.gerd.com
Hepatitis B Immunization Action Coalition
1573 Selby Avenue
St. Paul, MN 55104
(651) 647-9009
www.immunize.org

Immunization Action Coalition
www.immunize.org

National Cancer Institute
www.nci.nih.gov

References

Asante MA: Optimal management of patients with non-ulcer dyspepsia: considerations for the treatment of the elderly, *Drugs Aging* 10(11):819-826, 2001.

Bond JH: Polyp Guideline diagnosis, treatment and surveillance for patients with colorectal polyps, *Am J Clinical Gastroenterol* Pract Guideline 95(11):3053-3063, 2000.

Clarke GA et al: The indications, utilization and safety of gastrointestinal endoscopy in an extremely elderly patient cohort, *Endoscopy* 33(7):580-584, 2001.

Cobbs EL, Duthie EH, Murphy JB, editors: *Geriatrics review syllabus: a core curriculum in geriatric medicine,* ed 5, Malden, Mass, 2002, Blackwell Publishing for the American Geriatrics Society.

Flockhart DA, Desta Z, Mahal SK: Selection of drugs to treat gastro-oesophageal reflux disease: the role of drug interactions, *Clin Pharmacokinet* 39(4):295-309, 2000.

Hawkey CJ: Gastrointestinal safety of COX-2 specific inhibitors, *Gastroenterol Clin North Am* 30(4):921-936, 2001.

Kamolz T et al: Quality of life and surgical outcome after laparoscopic antireflux surgery in the elderly gastroesophageal reflux disease patient, *Scand J Gastroenterol* 36(2):116-120, 2001.

Kaya H et al: Prevalence of hepatitis C virus and hepatitis G virus in patients with non-Hodgkin's lymphoma, *Clin Lab Haematol* 24(2):107-110, 2002.

Kouraklis G et al: Clinical implications of small bowel diverticula, *Isr Med Assoc J* 4(6):431-433, 2002.

Matheson AJ, Jarvis B: Lansoprazole: an update of its place in the management of acid-related disorders, *Drugs* 61(12):1801-1833, 2001.

Newton JL: Care of the elderly with gastrointestinal problems in family practice, *Best Pract Res Clin Gastroenterol* 15(6):1013-1025, 2001.

Poovorawan Y, Chatchatee P, Chongsrisawat V: Epidemiology and prophylaxis of viral hepatitis: a global perspective, *J Gastroenterol Hepatol* 19(suppl S1):55-66, 2002.

Sial SH, Catalano MF: Gastrointestinal tract cancer in the elderly, *Gastroenterol Clin North Am* 30(2):565-590, 2001.

Simpson J, Scholefield JH, Spiller RC: Pathogenesis of colonic diverticula, *Br J Surg* 89(5):546-554, 2002.

Summerfield JA: Virus hepatitis update, *J R Coll Physicians Lond* 34(4):381-385, 2000.

Swaroop VS, Larson MV: Colonoscopy as a screening test for colorectal cancer in average-risk individuals, *Mayo Clin Proc* 77(9):951-956, 2002.

13

Gastrointestinal: Constipation and Diarrhea

CONSTIPATION

Constipation is a frequently cited problem in the older population, with more than 2.5 million annual visits to physicians for this complaint. This figure does not include the millions of self-treated people who use laxatives either routinely or during an acute occurrence. Chronic constipation affects about 30% of adults 65 years of age or older, more commonly women (Cobbs, Duthie, and Murphy, 2002).

The definition of constipation is misunderstood and misinterpreted, however, by both health care providers and patients. Although constipation in medical terms has been defined as a frequency of fewer than three bowel movements a week, a patient may define constipation as one or more of the following: straining at stool, painful bowel movements, perceived infrequent bowel movements, feelings of incomplete bowel movements, or loss of ability to recognize the urge to defecate. What is a normal pattern of bowel elimination for one person may constitute constipation for another.

Age-related Changes

Many age-related changes and other causes contribute to reports of constipation in older adults. Although no consistent changes of colonic or anorectal motility have been shown in older people, some studies have found a prolonged colonic transit time in immobile, frail older patients (Ron et al, 2002). Although aging per se affects function throughout the gut, particularly after 70 years of age, the observed changes are relatively modest and often asymptomatic. The proximal esophagus, anus, and pelvic floor are possible exceptions to this generalization, and the combination of aging and factors such as neurologic changes or obstetrical damage often results in dysphagia, constipation, or fecal incontinence (Bharucha and Camilleri, 2001).

Constipation frequently occurs as a side effect of drugs, a reduced amount of dietary fiber because of poor chewing ability, or a manifestation of metabolic or neurologic disease (Cobbs, Duthie, and Murphy, 2002; Muller-Lissner, 2002). Decreased motility of the colon, which leads to chronic slowing of transit time, may contribute to constipation. Being bedridden and having weak straining ability (Muller-Lissner, 2002) as well as decreased motility result in diminished capacity of the muscles controlling bowel elimination to coordinate properly, which leads to pain, incomplete evacuation,

319

> ## Box 13-1
> *Causes of Constipation*
>
> **Acute-onset Constipation**
>
> Bowel obstruction
> Colonic cancer
> Cancers of gastrointestinal tract
> Diverticulitis
>
> **Chronic Constipation**
>
> *Age-related Changes*
>
> Slowed transit time
> Decreased agility and mobility
> Loss of muscle tone
>
> *Response to Diseases*
>
> Stroke
> Parkinson's disease
> Thyroid conditions
> Irritable bowel syndrome
>
> **Chronic Constipation—cont'd**
>
> *Response to Mental Health Conditions*
>
> Depression
> Obsessive behaviors
>
> *Response to Medications*
>
> Laxative habituation
>
> *Environmental Factors*
>
> Institutional living
> Lack of privacy
> Lifestyle factors
> Diet and hydration
> Lack of exercise

and failure to defecate despite effort and urge. Other causes are diseases that affect motility such as hypothyroidism, neurologic disorders such as Parkinson disease or stroke, drugs, laxative habituation, psychologic disorders, and colorectal conditions (Box 13-1). Drug-induced constipation is particularly likely with anti-parkinsonism drugs (either anticholinergic or dopaminergic) and also with tricyclic antidepressants, opiates, iron, anticonvulsants, and aluminum or calcium-containing antacids (Muller-Lissner, 2002). Lumbosacral spinal disease may lead to colonic hypomotility and dilatation, decreased rectal tone and sensation, and impaired defecation.

Constipation and lower urinary tract symptoms frequently occur together in older adults, and several reports have suggested that dysfunction in either of these systems may affect the other. Medical relief of constipation can significantly improve lower urinary tract symptoms, which in turn improves the patient's mood, sexual activity, and quality of life (Charach et al, 2001). Figure 13-1 illustrates the anatomy of the anal canal and rectum showing the physiologic mechanisms important to continence and defecation (Whitehead, Wald, and Norton, 2001).

HISTORY

It is important to clarify what the patient is defining as constipation. Patients should be guided to include all dimensions of their constipation. A complete medical history, with particular emphasis on rectal bleeding and abdominal pain, must be carefully obtained from the patient during the review of systems. If the presentation is acute onset of constipation in a healthy older person, the practitioner should suspect a colonic obstruction. A review of all the patient's current medications, including all laxatives and over-the-counter (OTC) drugs, is an important consideration because many drugs can cause or contribute to constipation (Box 13-2). Lifestyle factors, including diet, functional ability, cognitive status, exercise patterns, bowel hygiene, and living conditions, need to be assessed (Figure 13-2).

Physical Examination and Diagnostic Testing

A focused examination centers on detecting a localized abdominal mass and local anorectal lesions such as internal or external hemorrhoids, an anal fistula, or a tumor. Confirmation of bowel sounds

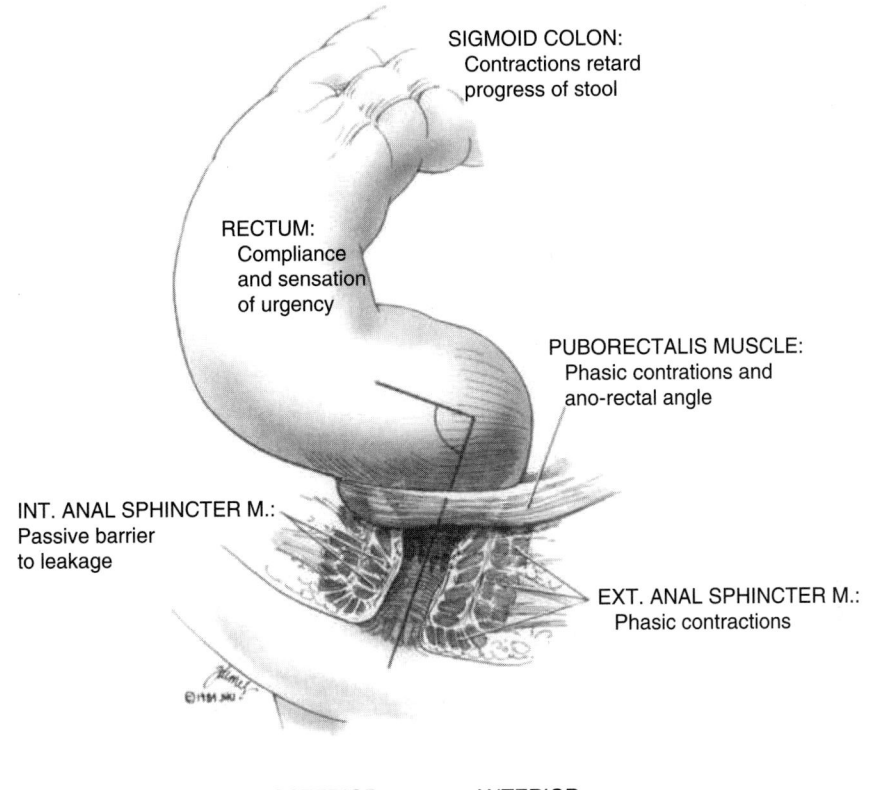

SIGMOID COLON:
Contractions retard
progress of stool

RECTUM:
Compliance
and sensation
of urgency

PUBORECTALIS MUSCLE:
Phasic contrations and
ano-rectal angle

INT. ANAL SPHINCTER M.:
Passive barrier
to leakage

EXT. ANAL SPHINCTER M.:
Phasic contractions

POSTERIOR ⟷ ANTERIOR

Figure 13-1 Anatomy of the anal canal and rectum showing the physiologic mechanisms important to continence and defecation. (From Whitehead WE, Schuster MM: *Gastrointestinal disorders: behavioral and physiological basis for treatment*, Orlando, Fla, 1985, Academic Press.)

by auscultation is essential. Digital examination of the rectum and anal canal assesses the tone and strength of the internal and external sphincter and the puborectalis muscles. A patient with a fecal impaction often complains of diarrhea. In these cases the digital examination finds hard, dry, rocklike stool in the rectal vault.

Flexible sigmoidoscopy may be appropriate for newly diagnosed patients, even if there is no report of rectal bleeding or pain. Stool testing for occult blood (guaiac) should be part of the rectal examination despite the many false-positive results that occur.

Box 13-2
Drugs that Contribute to Constipation

Antacids
   Aluminum hydroxide
   Calcium carbonate
Anticholinergics
Antidepressants (tricyclic)
Antihistamines

Barium
Iron preparations
Narcotics
Verapamil
Pseudoephedrine

Lifestyle Assessment Tool

DIET

1. What high-fiber foods do you eat on a daily basis?

2. How many glasses of water do you drink during a normal day?

3. What fluids and how many glasses or cups of each do you drink in a normal day (e.g., 2 cups of coffee and 1 small glass of juice)?

4. What did you eat yesterday? Please list all meals and anything between meals.

5. Are you now or have you been in the last 6 months on any type of a diet?

EXERCISE

1. On a scale of 1 to 10, with 10 being the highest, how active do you consider yourself?

2. What physical activities do you participate in?

3. How often do you participate?

4. What hinders your participation in physical activities?

BOWEL HYGIENE

1. How long have you had problems moving your bowels?

2. Do you have a particular time that you usually move your bowels?

3. What do you do when you feel constipated?

4. Have you taken any laxatives or enemas during the past 7 days?

5. Do you take or use laxatives or enemas on most days?

6. What helps the most when you are constipated?

Figure 13-2   Lifestyle assessment tool. (Patient should complete before appointment.)

Lifestyle Assessment Tool – cont'd

LIVING CONDITIONS

1. Do you live alone?

2. If not, with whom do you live?

3. Do you have free access to a bathroom?

4. Do you have enough privacy and time in the bathroom?

5. Are the conditions in the bathroom comfortable and pleasant?

FUNCTIONAL STATUS

1. Do you have any problems getting to the bathroom when you feel the urge to move your bowels?

2. Do you always realize you have the urge to move your bowels?

3. Do your bowels ever move when you are not expecting it?

Figure 13-2,   cont'd.

In chronic constipation, abdominal radiographs can determine the extent of a fecal impaction. Transit-time studies can provide information regarding bowel function. Additional studies include defecography, a technique in which thick barium simulating stool is introduced into the rectum and evacuation is monitored by fluoroscopy while the patient sits on a commode. Assessment of the anorectal structure and function is then made at rest and during barium expulsion. Anorectal manometry evaluates rectal sensation and compliance, reflex relaxation of the internal anal sphincter, and the competence of the anal sphincters (Cobbs, Duthie, and Murphy, 2002).

Acute onset of constipation may suggest colonic obstruction, and abdominal radiographs are sufficient to determine the level and, at times, the cause of the obstruction. To rule out more serious conditions, constipated patients with occult or gross rectal bleeding, patients with complaints of a change in bowel habits, and patients who complain of abdominal pain should be referred for barium enemas and colonoscopy.

Conditions to Consider

- Fecal impaction
- Diverticulitis
- Irritable bowel syndrome
- Anal stricture
- Hemorrhoids
- Bowel obstruction
- Colon cancer

Treatment

1. If causal, treat the underlying disease such as hypothyroidism.
2. If medication is suspected, change or stop medication.
3. For nonpathologic constipation, first try a lifestyle modification (step 1):
   Diet and fluid (fruits such as prunes and kiwi fruit may be beneficial [Rush et al, 2002])

Exercise
Fiber supplements (e.g., Metamucil)
Relaxed, unhurried toilet time after breakfast or dinner
4. If the first attempt at lifestyle changes fails or does not produce improvement, try step 2: add Milk of Magnesia at bedtime, which is to be used *only* during the beginning phase of the modification program. The goal is to continue the education and support needed to assist in the lifestyle change.
5. If the patient is found to have an impaction, the following treatments are appropriate:
Digital disimpaction
Suppositories
  Glycerin
Enemas
  Oil retention
6. Education, support, and follow-up

Laxatives

Unless the constipation complaint is acute and of fairly sudden onset, the patient most likely has been self-medicating for a significant period. In a nonthreatening and nonaccusatory manner, an accurate history is taken that includes all alternative treatments. It is usually safe to start with the premise that most patients whose complaint is constipation are already using laxatives. Trying to get the patient to stop or change to a less harmful laxative is actually more common than prescribing a laxative. It is essential to respect the patient's self-care practices by providing information that assists in decision making.

For most patients with constipation and normal colonic transit time, fluids, dietary fiber, and bulk laxatives, such as psyllium seed or calcium polycarbophil, are effective in increasing the frequency and softening the consistency of stool with a minimum of adverse effects. Patients who respond poorly or who do not tolerate fiber may require laxatives (Cobbs, Duthie, and Murphy, 2002).

Five types of laxatives are now available to the general public in OTC medications. Bulk-forming products (bran and psyllium mucilloid [Metamucil]) are the first choice for treatment of constipation. They tend to increase stool mass and soften its consistency. The dose needs to be adjusted to 15 g of fiber, and each dose has to be taken with 8 oz of fluids. The side effects of bulk laxatives include flatus, cramping, bloating, and, in extreme cases, obstruction related to inadequate fluid intake. The normal American diet is deficient in fiber, and foods high in fiber should be stressed, such as bran cereal, beans (baked, kidney, lima, and navy), fruits (prunes and prune juice), and vegetables.

Emollients or stool softeners are usually considered the second step in treatment to relieve idiopathic constipation. Docusate or dioctyl sodium sulfosuccinate (Colace) works by lowering surface tension and allowing water to enter the stool. These preparations are safe, well tolerated, and quite useful for even bed-bound older patients. By contrast, mineral oil is not safe and is not generally recommended; it may impede the absorption of fat-soluble vitamins and increase the risk of pneumonia by aspiration, especially in the older impaired population.

Saline and electrolyte laxatives and enemas are OTC treatments and are used by the public as Milk of Magnesia and Fleet Enema. These preparations are contraindicated for people with impaired renal function.

Stimulant laxatives are common and habituating. Senna (Senokot) and bisacodyl (Dulcolax) are effective but carry the risk of electrolyte imbalance and long-term toxicity. Bisacodyl has less toxicity than other stimulant laxatives. GoLYTELY and Colyte are lavage laxatives; these preparations are used mainly as bowel preparation before procedures.

DIARRHEA

Diarrhea is a common problem in older adults and a leading cause of mortality worldwide. In the developed world, 85% of its mortality affects older adults (Hoffmann and Zeitz, 2002). Symptoms include an increase in stool volume and bulk, usually with an increase in stool frequency and water content. Dehydration and cardiovascular collapse can result from acute or chronic diarrhea, with secondary complications of hypernatremia, hyponatremia, hypokalemia, renal failure, or syncope (Yoshikawa, Cobbs, and Brummel-Smith, 1998). Older patients may not admit to having chronic diarrhea, particularly if they are also incontinent.

Causes include intestinal malabsorption (even though diarrhea is a less common manifestation of malabsorption in older than in younger patients), drugs, pathogens, fecal impaction, enteral feeding, food additives, caffeine, alcohol, lactose intolerance, and inflammatory bowel disease (Holt, 2001; Yoshikawa, Cobbs, and Brummel-Smith, 1998). Box 13-3 lists drugs that commonly cause diarrhea. If diarrhea is of short duration, an infectious cause is at least as frequent as in young adults. Institutionalized older patients are particularly susceptible to gastrointestinal infections, but the manifestations may not be overt. When an intestinal infection and potential medication-induced gastrointestinal disturbances have been excluded, the differential diagnosis of diarrhea in older persons is the same as in younger persons. Although the causes of malabsorption are similar in older and younger patients, chronic pancreatic insufficiency or unknown cause and intestinal bacterial overgrowth without an anatomic abnormality of the small intestine are syndromes that are specific to older persons (Holt, 2001).

Diarrhea is common in diabetic patients and may have various causes, including autonomic neuropathy, exocrine insufficiency of the pancreas, celiac sprue, intestinal bacterial overgrowth, and colonic dysmotility in associated with impaction and overflow diarrhea (Yoshikawa, Cobbs, and Brummel-Smith, 1998).

Infectious diarrhea is a common complaint in clinical practice and an important disease in older adults. Infectious diarrhea is most often associated with group settings (e.g., nursing homes and skilled nursing facilities) or antibiotic use. Infectious diarrhea may be associated with abnormal immune function and certain bacterial infections such as *Clostridium difficile, Escherichia coli*, and *Salmonella* organisms (Slotwiner-Nie and Brandt, 2001). Routine empirical use of antibiotics for infectious diarrhea should be avoided because of the self-limited nature of most cases, the cost of antibiotics, and the potential to worsen the already significant problem of antibiotic resistance of enteric pathogens. For patients with severe invasive or prolonged diarrhea or who are at high risk of complications, such as older patients, diabetic patients, and immunocompromised patients, empirical treatment with a quinolone antibiotic for 3 to 5 days can be considered (Oldfield and Wallace, 2001). The institution of appropriate isolation and infection control measures is crucial in group settings (Slotwiner-Nie and Brandt, 2001).

Ischemic colitis is one of the most often seen disorders of the large intestine in older adults. Common predisposing factors are atherosclerosis, shock, and congestive heart failure, but often

---

Box 13-3

Drugs that Commonly Cause Diarrhea

Quinidine	Colchicine
Antibiotics	Theophylline
Magnesium-containing antacids	Nonsteroidal antiinflammatory agents
Misoprostol	Lactulose and sorbitol
Levodopa	Acarbose

older patients have no obvious predisposing or precipitating factors. The typical clinical presentation is acute sudden abdominal pain and distention with bloody diarrhea. Common early radiographic signs are bowel-wall thickening with thumb printing; later ulceration and strictures may be found. Patients should be referred for evaluation, including endoscopy. Within 48 hours, most patients show favorable response to conservative measures consisting of intravenous hydration, bowel rest, antibiotics therapy, and correction of precipitating processes. Surgical intervention may include resection of the ischemic segment (Alapati and Mihas, 1999).

Diagnosis

Most cases of acute diarrhea are self-limited and can be managed supportively for 1 to 2 days without pursuing a diagnostic evaluation if the patient is not seriously ill or dehydrated. The physical examination should focus on the general appearance, the presence or absence of fever, pallor, tachycardia, orthostatic blood pressure change, mucous membrane appearance, and skin turgor. Examination of the abdomen should include evaluation of the presence of tenderness, distention, and palpable stool in the colon. Rectal examination should be performed to determine the presence of masses, tenderness, or stool in the rectal vault; however, the absence of stool does not exclude a high impaction (Yoshikawa, Cobbs, and Brummel-Smith, 1998).

Further testing may include a plain abdominal radiograph and stool specimen for fecal leukocytes, *C. difficile* toxin, and culture and examination for ova and parasites. Patients should be referred for sigmoidoscopy and biopsy if they are acutely ill and diagnosis cannot be made by less invasive testing.

Treatment

In cases of diarrhea that are self-limited, treatment is primarily supportive with aggressive oral hydration. If diarrhea persists for more than 24 hours, intravenous fluids should be considered to prevent hypotension and organ failure in the frail older patient who often has multiple morbidities (Hoffmann and Zietz, 2002). For the patient who is seriously ill or has a protracted course of diarrhea, specific therapy should be instituted. Loperamide and diphenoxylate hydrochloride with atropine are useful in suppressing diarrhea but should be reserved until an infectious cause is excluded. For diabetic patients in whom bacterial overgrowth is suspected, a 2-week course of broad-spectrum antibiotics may be beneficial (Yoshikawa, Cobbs, and Brummel-Smith, 1998).

If diarrhea occurs as a result of enteral feeding, the formula should be diluted, and the patient receiving bolus feedings should be changed to continuous feedings. Consultation with a dietician is helpful and important in caring for patients receiving enteral feedings.

Clostridium difficile

Clostridium difficile, a spore-forming toxigenic bacterium, is one of the most common causes of infectious diarrhea and colitis in the United States (Moyenuddin, Williamson, and Ohl, 2002). The incidence of infection with this organism is increasing in hospitals worldwide, consequent to the widespread use of broad-spectrum antibiotics. Pathogenic strains of *C. difficile* produce two protein exotoxins, toxin A and toxin B, that cause colonic mucosal injury and inflammation (Kyne, Farrell, and Kelly, 2001). Most patients with *C. difficile* infection recently received antimicrobial therapy, usually clindamycin, cephalosporins, or the extended-spectrum penicillins. Clinical presentation varies from asymptomatic colonization to mild diarrhea to severe colitis. The mainstay of diagnosis is detection of *C. difficile* toxin A, toxin B, or both with a cytotoxin test or enzyme immunoassay of the stool of patients who have received antibiotic therapy and have features of *C. difficile*-associated diarrhea. If the first assay is negative and *C. difficile*-associated diarrhea is strongly suspected, a second assay should be performed. Ten days of oral metronidazole is the preferred therapy for most initial infections. Vancomycin is considered second-line therapy because of its cost and potential to select for vancomycin resistance. About 20%

to 25% of patients experience reinfection or relapse after initial therapy and require retreatment. The disease can best be prevented by limiting the use of broad-spectrum antibiotics and adhering to infection control techniques (Moyenuddin, Williamson, and Ohl, 2002).

In older patients, *C. difficile*-associated diarrhea is almost always acquired in institutions and may not be obvious among patients' other problems (Brandt et al, 1999). It has been suggested that severe cases of *C. difficile* or *C. difficile*-associated sepsis are probably not rare and that routine testing of fecal specimens for the presence of *C. difficile* toxins should be considered not only in nosocomial gastrointestinal infections but also in community-acquired gastrointestinal infections of older adults (Siemann, Koch-Dorfler, and Rabenhorst, 2000).

It should be remembered that not all antibiotic-associated diarrhea is due to *C. difficile;* antibiotics may also cause diarrhea by altering gut motility (e.g., erythromycin) or gastrointestinal flora (Yoshikawa, Cobbs, and Brummel-Smith, 1998).

FECAL INCONTINENCE

Fecal incontinence, defined as the recurrent uncontrolled passage of fecal material for at least 1 month (Whitehead et al, 2001), is a disturbing disability because it greatly affects the quality of life and may lead to social isolation. Fecal incontinence may be minor, with inadvertent passage of flatus or soiling of underwear with liquid stool, or it may be major with involuntary leakage of feces. Fecal incontinence affects 2% to 7% of adults, mostly older persons in poor general health (Cobbs, Duthie, and Murphy, 2002); however, the symptoms deserve the same thoughtful evaluation and management in older patients as in younger patients (Schiller, 2001). The 1995 National Nursing Home Survey identified fecal incontinence in 45% of nursing home residents. Long-lasting or permanent fecal incontinence has been associated with increased mortality, suggesting that this symptom is a marker of poor health in older adults (Chassagne et al, 1999). Reluctance to disclose incontinence is recognized to be an impediment to obtaining accurate estimates of the prevalence of fecal incontinence; only one-third of patients with fecal incontinence have discussed the problem with a health care provider (Whitehead et al, 2001).

Fecal continence depends on many factors, such as mental function, stool consistency, colonic transit, rectal compliance, internal and external anal sphincter function, as well anorectal sensation and reflexes. Continence is influenced by the volume and consistency of the stool delivered to the rectum, which is determined in part by motility, secretion, and absorption in the small and large intestines. The compliance of the rectum determines the ability to store stool while delaying defecation (Whitehead, Wald, and Norton, 2001). Normal defecation is a complex sequential process that starts with the entry of stool into the rectum, leading to reflex relaxation of the internal anal sphincter. If defecation is desired, the anorectal angle is voluntarily straightened, and abdominal pressure is increased by straining. This results in descent of the pelvic floor, contraction of the rectum, and inhibition of the external anal sphincter, which causes evacuation of the rectal contents (Cobbs, Duthie, and Murphy, 2002).

Table 13-1 describes common causes for fecal incontinence (Whitehead, Wald, and Norton, 2001). Decreased anal sphincter tone can result from trauma (e.g., anal surgery) or neurologic disorders (e.g., spinal cord injury or a secondary effect of diabetes mellitus). Fecal impaction is a common cause of incontinence in older persons because it inhibits the internal anal sphincter tone, permitting leakage of liquid stool.

Vaginal delivery associated with anal sphincter tears or trauma to the pudendal nerve may result in fecal incontinence immediately or after many years. Acquired laxity of the pelvic floor muscles that contribute to the external sphincter of the rectum can occur in middle-aged and older women, contributing to problems with fecal incontinence (Cobbs, Duthie, and Murphy, 2002).

Older patients with megacolon or megarectum have chronic fecal retention, increased rectal compliance and elasticity, and blunted rectal sensation, all leading to fecal impaction and soiling. Decreased rectal compliance resulting from radiation proctitis leads to increased fecal frequency and urgency.

TABLE 13-1	Common Causes for Fecal Incontinence	

Category	Mechanism	Common Causes
Functional		
	Fecal impaction: dilated internal anal sphincter	Pelvic floor dyssynergia (difficulty relaxing sphincter when defecating), drug side-effect, idiopathic, spinal cord injury
	Diarrhea: rapid transit or large volume	Irritable bowel syndrome, infectious and metabolic causes of diarrhea
	Cognitive/psychological: social indifference	Dementia, psychosis, willful soiling
Sphincter weakness		
	Sphincter muscle injury	Obstetrical trauma, motor vehicle accident, foreign body trauma
	Pudendal nerve injury	Obstetrical trauma, diabetic peripheral neuropathy, multiple sclerosis, idiopathic
	CNS injury	Spina bifida, traumatic spinal cord injury, cerebrovascular accident, multiple sclerosis
Sensory loss		
	Afferent nerve injury: unable to detect rectal filling	Diabetic neuropathy, spinal cord injury, multiple sclerosis

From Whitehead WE, Wald A, Norton NJ: Treatment options for fecal incontinence, *Dis Colon Rectum* 44(1): 131-144, 2001.
CNS, Central nervous system.

The history and physical examination often provide the clues to the cause of fecal incontinence. The most common causes of fecal incontinence, diarrhea and constipation, can often be identified by a careful history and physical examination, and empirical treatment can be initiated without further testing. A plain abdominal radiograph is a useful adjunct to physical examination in detecting fecal impaction as a contributing cause (Whitehead, Wald, and Norton, 2001). A flexible sigmoidoscopy may be considered to exclude inflammation or tumor. Anorectal manometry measures resting anal sphincter tone, the squeeze pressure, the rectoanal inhibitory reflex, rectal sensation, and rectal compliance. Abnormalities may be further evaluated using endorectal or transvaginal ultrasound (Cobbs, Duthie, and Murphy, 2002).

Most patients with fecal incontinence can be diagnosed and treatment initiated in the primary care setting. Only patients who fail to respond within a reasonable time (4 to 8 weeks) need to be referred for further evaluation (Whitehead, Wald, and Norton, 2001). The goal of therapy is to reduce stool frequency (such as with antidiarrheal drugs such as loperamide) and improving stool consistency (such as with bulking agents such as methylcellulose) with attention to quality-of-life issues. Biofeedback therapy may be effective in retraining the pelvic floor and the abdominal wall musculature. Surgery may involve sphincter repair or implantation of an artificial sphincter. Colostomy may be needed for patients with intractable symptoms in whom other treatments have failed. A synthetic sphincter device, consisting of an inflatable cuff that maintains continence, is a valve that allows the cuff to deflate for defecation (Cobbs, Duthie, and Murphy, 2002).

IRRITABLE BOWEL SYNDROME

Irritable bowel syndrome (IBS) is a functional gut disorder. Diagnosis is based on clinical symptoms including constipation, which alternates with periods of diarrhea or normal bowel evacuation. Such patients have normal colonic transit times. As the population ages, especially with the population of patients 75 years of age and older expanding greatly over the next 10 years, IBS is becoming one of the most common diseases of older adults (Dunphy and Verne, 2001). Whether advancing age impacts IBS is largely unknown, and how the disorder manifests in older persons remains unclear (Bennett and Talley, 2002).

Most patients will show improvement with simple attention to diet, stress management, and fiber intake; however, antidiarrheals and antispasmodics may play a role in the symptomatic treatment of IBS. With the evolution of IBS as a disorder of visceral hypersensitivity, new drugs have been developed to target the enteric nervous system. Tricyclic antidepressants target the enteric neurons and play a role in pain modulation but are reserved for severe cases of IBS pain. Also now approved for use in IBS are the serotonin (5-HT) antagonists, especially for the control of symptoms in female patients (Dunphy and Verne, 2001).

Summary

Gastrointestinal complaints, especially constipation and diarrhea, are extremely common in the older population and should be evaluated carefully. Although most cases are not of great concern, much potential exists for complications and comorbid illness. Many conditions can be successfully treated in the primary care setting; however, more complicated courses or patients who are extremely frail may require consultation with a specialist.

Resources

American Gastroenterological Association
www.gastro.org

Henry Ford Health System
Patient Information website
www.henryfordhealth.org/cancer/constipation.htm

References

Alapati SV, Mihas AA: When to suspect ischemic colitis: why is this condition so often missed or misdiagnosed? *Postgrad Med* 105(4):177-180, 183-184, 187, 1999.

Bennett G, Talley NJ: Irritable bowel syndrome in the elderly, *Best Pract Res Clin Gastroenterol* 16(1):63-76, 2002.

Bharucha AE, Camilleri M: Functional abdominal pain in the elderly, *Gastroenterol Clin North Am* 30(2):517-529, 2001.

Brandt LJ et al: Clostridium difficile-associated diarrhea in the elderly, *Am J Gastroenterol* 94(11):3263-3266, 1999.

Charach G et al: Alleviating constipation in the elderly improves lower urinary tract symptoms, *Gerontology* 47(2): 72-76, 2001.

Chassagne P et al: Fecal incontinence in the institutionalized elderly: incidence, risk factors and prognosis, *Am J Med* 106(2):185-190, 1999.

Cobbs EL, Duthie EH, Murphy JB, editors. *Geriatrics review syllabus: a core curriculum in geriatric medicine*, ed 5, Malden, Mass, 2002, Blackwell Publishing for the American Geriatrics Society.

Dunphy RC, Verne GN: Drug treatment options for irritable bowel syndrome: managing for success, *Drugs Aging* 18(3):201-211, 2001.

Hoffmann JC, Zeitz M: Small bowel disease in the elderly: diarrhea and malabsorption, *Best Pract Res Clin Gastroenterol* 16(1):17-36, 2002.

Holt PR: Diarrhea and malabsorption in the elderly, *Gastroenterol Clin North Am* 30(2):427-444, 2001.

Kyne L, Farrell RJ, Kelly CP: *Clostridium difficile, Gastroenterol Clin North Am* 30(3):753-777, ix-x, 2001.

Moyenuddin M, Williamson JC, Ohl CA: *Clostridium difficile*-associated diarrhea: current strategies for diagnosis and therapy, *Curr Gastroenterol Rep* 4(4):279-286, 2002.

Muller-Lissner S: General geriatrics and gastroenterology: constipation and faecal incontinence, *Best Pract Res Clin Gastroenterol* 16(1):115-133, 2002.

Newton JL: Care of the elderly with gastrointestinal problems in family practice, *Best Practices Res Clin Gastroenterol* 15(6):1013-1025, 2001.

Oldfield EC, Wallace MR: The role of antibiotics in the treatment of infectious diarrhea, *Gastroenterol Clin North Am* 30(3):817-836, 2001.

Ron Y et al: Colonic transit time in diabetic and non-diabetic long-term care patients, *Gerontology* 48(4):250-253, 2002.

Rush EC et al: Kiwifruit promotes laxation in the elderly, *Asia Pacific J Clin Nutr* 11(2):164-168, 2002.

Schiller LR: Constipation and fecal incontinence in the elderly, *Gastroenterol Clin North Am* 30(2):497-515, 2001.

Siemann M, Koch-Dorfler M, Rabenhorst G: *Clostridium difficile*-associated diseases: the clinical courses of 18 fatal cases, *Intens Care Med* 26(4):416-421, 2000.

Slotwiner-Nie PK, Brandt LJ: Infectious diarrhea in the elderly, *Gastroenterol Clin North Am* 30(3):625-635, 2001.

Whitehead WE, Wald A, Norton NJ: Treatment options for fecal incontinence, *Dis Colon Rectum* 44(1):131-144, 2001.

Yoshikawa TT, Cobbs EL, Brummel-Smith K: *Practical ambulatory geriatrics,* St Louis, 1998, Mosby.

14

Endocrine Conditions

This chapter discusses the care of older adults who have significant but common disturbances within their endocrine system. The focus of this chapter is on the assessment, diagnosis, and treatment of three conditions of the endocrine system. The condition that occurs most frequently is diabetes mellitus, followed by thyroid conditions, which are frequent but at times undiagnosed, and, third, conditions of the parathyroid gland, which are uncommon but often misdiagnosed.

DIABETES MELLITUS

Diabetes mellitus is a heterogeneous group of metabolic disorders characterized by hyperglycemia secondary to defects in insulin secretion, insulin action, or both. In the United States, an estimated 16 million persons have diabetes, although many are undiagnosed. Among the 7.9 million persons 18 to 75 years of age diagnosed with diabetes, many receive less than optimal care for the disease (Kulkarni, 2002). At diagnosis, about half of patients with type 2 diabetes are already experiencing diabetes-related complications, indicating that the disease is often present long before the patient receives a diagnosis.

Prediabetes is a condition that occurs when blood glucose levels are higher than normal but not high enough for a diagnosis of type 2 diabetes. An estimated 16 million Americans have prediabetes (American Diabetes Association, 2002).

Clinical Features

Diabetes in older adults is characterized by a variety of nonspecific clinical manifestations (see Box 14-1 for common symptoms of diabetes in older persons). It is widely known that advancing age is associated with impaired glucose handling. Hypotheses explaining the relationship between aging and insulin resistance include the following: (1) anthropometric changes (relative and absolute increases in body fat combined with a decline in fat-free mass), which could explain the reduction in active metabolic tissue; (2) environmental causes, mainly diet and physical activity; (3) neurohormonal variations; and (4) the rise in oxidative stress (Barbieri et al, 2001).

Box 14-1

Common Symptoms of Diabetes in the Older Person

General

Unexplained weight loss
Fatigue
Slow wound healing
Mental status changes
Recurrent bacterial or fungal infections

Eyes

Cataracts
Retinal detachment, hemorrhages
Microaneurysms
Macular disease

Gastrointestinal

Gastroparesis

Neuromuscular

Paresthesias
Cranial nerve palsies
Pain
Muscle weakness

Cardiovascular

Angina
Silent cardiac ischemia
Myocardial infarction
Transient cerebral ischemia
Stroke
Diabetic foot ulcers

Renal

Proteinuria
Glomerulopathy
Uremia

The classic polyuria, polydipsia, and polyphagia are uncommon in the older population. Long-term complications involve the vasculature, including vision, renal, and neural function (Zielinski et al, 2002).

Classifications of Diabetes

TYPE 1 DIABETES

Type 1 diabetes, which is said to account for about 10% of cases in the United States, generally has its onset in childhood; however, this type of diabetes can also develop in adulthood. Its essential characteristic is that insulin dependence is eventually absolute; at this stage, without replacement insulin therapy, ketosis-acidosis ensues within hours. Type 1 diabetes is now considered a chronic autoimmune disease characterized by the destruction of beta cells in pancreatic islets and eventual failure to synthesize sufficient insulin. Various autoantibodies have been identified early in the course of the illness. There is clearly a genetic susceptibility to this process, and environmental influences also play a role, but the precise pathogenesis of type 1 disease has not been established (Barker, Burton, and Zieve, 2003).

TYPE 2 DIABETES

Type 2 diabetes is the most common form of diabetes mellitus and accounts for about 80% of patients with an overt abnormality of glucose metabolism. More than 10 million people in the United States are affected. Patients with type 2 disease are ordinarily neither absolutely dependent on treatment with insulin nor ketosis prone.

Type 2 diabetes is often only one component of a complex of abnormalities variously termed metabolic syndrome, syndrome X, the metabolic syndrome X, or the insulin-resistance syndrome. Hyperinsulinemia with or without obvious hyperglycemia is present and denotes the presence of insulin resistance. Other components of the syndrome are obesity (central type), hypertension, fasting and postprandial hyperlipidemia, abnormal concentrations of blood coagulation factors, and premature cardiovascular atherosclerosis. Its pathogenesis remains unclear (Barker, Burton, and Zieve, 2003).

OTHER TYPES OF DIABETES

Diabetes may exist from other causes such as genetic defects in B-cell function, genetic defects in insulin action, diseases of the exocrine pancreas, and drugs or other chemicals (American Diabetes Association, 2002).

Diagnosis

Diabetes is diagnosed by a fasting plasma glucose level of 126 mg/dL or higher or a casual plasma level exceeding 200 mg/dL on more than one occasion, with *casual* defined as anytime, without regard to time since last meal.

Prediabetes is indicated by impaired glucose tolerance or impaired fasting glucose (i.e., between 110 and 126 mg/dL) or a 2-hour post-load glucose reading between 140 and 200 mg/dL (Kulkarni, 2002).

Chronic Complications

MICROANGIOPATHY

Microvascular complications of type 2 diabetes cause significant morbidity, including renal failure, blindness, and lower-extremity amputations. Older persons with diabetes have a high incidence of renal disease, retinopathy, and neuropathy, usually as a result of a long duration of untreated disease before detection.

DIABETIC NEPHROPATHY

Diabetes is the most common single cause of end-stage renal disease (ESRD) in the United States, accounting for close to a third of all cases. About 20% to 30% of patients with diabetes develop evidence of nephropathy; more than half who begin dialysis have type 2 disease (O'Connor, Spann, and Woolf, 1998). Persistent albuminuria of 30 to 300 mg/24 hours has been shown to be the earliest stage of diabetic nephropathy (American Diabetes Association, 1998).

Hypertension can hasten the progression of renal disease. Intensive diabetes control and maintaining blood pressure below 130/85 will decrease the rate of progression of diabetic nephropathy. Current consensus-based clinical guidelines recommend screening for microalbuminuria on a yearly basis to detect early diabetic nephropathy. Screening is recommended to begin 5 years after diagnosis for type 1 patients and immediately on diagnosis for patients with type 2 disease (O'Connor, Spann, and Woolf, 1998).

Angiotensin-converting enzyme (ACE) inhibitors are recommended for all type 1 patients with microalbuminuria with or without hypertension and for hypertensive type 2 patients with microalbuminuria. Protein restriction to 0.8 g/kg daily should be instituted with onset of overt nephropathy.

DIABETIC RETINOPATHY

Retinopathy is a common microvascular complication and is estimated to be the most frequent cause of new blindness among Americans 20 to 74 years of age. The prevalence and severity of diabetic retinopathy depend on the duration of diabetes and on the individual patient's control of glycosylated hemoglobin (Hgb A1c) (O'Connor, Spann, and Woolf, 1998). More than 60% of persons with type 2 diabetes show some degree of retinopathy. Optimal screening intervals have not yet been determined; however, most consensus-based guidelines call for yearly, dilated, comprehensive examinations by ophthalmologists or optometrists, beginning 3 to 5 years after diagnosis with type

1 diabetes and beginning immediately on diagnosis for patients with type 2 diabetes (O'Connor, Spann, and Woolf, 1998).

DIABETIC NEUROPATHY

Diabetic neuropathy can affect almost any part of the nervous system except the brain. It manifests as peripheral polyneuropathy, mononeuropathy, radiculopathy, autonomic neuropathy, and amyotrophy. Peripheral polyneuropathy is the most common form, with sensory involvement more common than motor. Peripheral neuropathy, combined with peripheral vascular disease, increases the risk of diabetic foot ulcers and amputations. About 50% of lower-extremity amputations (i.e., almost 55,000 amputations per year) in the United States are related to diabetes. Patients who undergo an amputation are at greater risk for a second amputation on either the same leg or on the other leg. The risk for amputation is 15 times that of persons without diabetes. Yet it has been estimated that half of the amputations in patients with diabetes are preventable (O'Connor, Spann, and Woolf, 1998).

MACROANGIOPATHY

Macroangiopathy manifests as silent myocardial ischemia, angina, myocardial infarction, cerebrovascular accidents, and peripheral vascular disease with foot ulcers. Diabetes doubles the risk for cardiovascular disease in the older person and is more pronounced in women with diabetes than in men. Cardiovascular mortality is higher in older persons with diabetes compared with those without diabetes. More than 70% of adults with type 2 diabetes die of heart attacks or strokes (O'Connor, Spann, and Woolf, 1998). Hypertension and hyperlipidemia increase the risk of the patient with diabetes for cardiovascular disease complications. Hyperinsulinemia, insulin resistance, and hereditary factors all increase the risk of atherosclerosis.

Assessment

HISTORY

A comprehensive history is important and should include presenting symptoms, family history, other medical conditions, surgical history, medications, allergies, and tobacco and alcohol use. Information should be obtained regarding any previous treatments for diabetes and success of glycemic control, cardiovascular risk factors, and presence of diabetic complications. Functional abilities, including vision and fine motor skills, and the ability to manage medications will determine the patient's ability to self-manage his or her diabetes control via blood glucose monitoring and insulin administration, if necessary. A social history will help to ascertain who might be available to help the patient manage his or her diabetes treatments. Information regarding insurance coverage is helpful in ensuring the patient's ability to afford medications, diagnostics, and services that might be needed.

PHYSICAL EXAMINATION

The physical examination should include blood pressure determination with orthostatic measurements, ophthalmoscopic examination, cardiac examination, abdominal examination, evaluation of pulses, and foot examination. Current consensus-based guidelines recommend that comprehensive foot evaluations, including vascular, neurologic, musculoskeletal, and skin and soft tissue assessments, be performed at least annually. These guidelines recommend that once a high-risk abnormality is identified, the patient should have a foot examination at each visit (i.e., several times a year).

The vascular examination should involve palpation of lower-extremity pulses and inspection of the legs and feet for ischemic changes. The neurologic examination should include a sensorimotor test to ascertain whether protective sensation has been lost. A 10-g Semmes-Weinstein monofilament is recommended. This inexpensive but valuable tool is simple to use. It can be obtained from Sensory Testing Systems and Curative Health Services (see Resources). Patients identified as having a loss of sensation should participate in a comprehensive, ongoing program of patient education concerning self-care and podiatric care and always wear appropriate footwear.

Laboratory Testing

The initial laboratory evaluation should include fasting plasma glucose, glycosylated hemoglobin level (HgbA1c), fasting lipid profile, serum creatinine, urinalysis, test for microalbuminuria, and electrocardiogram. Hgb A1c levels should be drawn every 3 to 6 months for ongoing monitoring.

Screening

Testing for diabetes should be considered in all persons 45 years of age and older and, if normal, it should be repeated at 3-year intervals. The American Diabetes Association (2002) recommends targeted screening for high-risk populations such as those with a family history of diabetes, cardiovascular disease, obesity (body mass index [BMI] 25 kg/m^2 or higher), sedentary lifestyle, and certain ethnicities (African Americans, Hispanic Americans, Native Americans, Asian Americans, Pacific Islanders), persons with prediabetes, hypertension (blood pressure 140/90 or higher), elevated triglyceride levels (250 mg/dl or higher), or low levels of high-density lipoprotein (35 mg/dl or lower), a history of gestational diabetes, delivery of an infant weighing more than 9lb, polycystic ovary syndrome, or acanthosis nigricans (Kulkarni, 2002). At-risk persons should undergo fasting blood glucose screening that is confirmed by a plasma glucose laboratory test.

Treatment

The optimal strategy for a particular patient depends not only on research evidence but also on other concerns, including timing of the intervention and its appropriateness to the patient's circumstances, other existing patient problems, medications the patient is taking, patient preference, and the anticipated adherence of the patient to the contemplated course of action. The management of diabetes requires a multidisciplinary approach, including the primary care provider, nurses, dietitians, and possibly mental health professionals (American Diabetes Association, 2002). Any plan should recognize diabetes self-management education as an integral component of care. In developing the plan, consideration should be given to the patient's age, work schedule and conditions (if applicable), physical activity, eating patterns, social situation and personality, cultural factors, and the presence of complications of diabetes or other medical conditions (American Diabetes Association, 2002).

The American Diabetes Association has recommended the following goals for glycemic control for all patients with diabetes:
- Preprandial glucose of 80 to 120 mg/dl
- Bedtime glucose of 100 to 140 mg/dl
- Hgb A1c levels of less than 7%

Treatment regimens that reduce average Hgb A1c levels to 7% have been associated with fewer long-term, microvascular complications; however, intense control increases the risk of hypoglycemia and weight gain. An average Hgb A1c level greater than 8% is associated with a greater risk of complications, at least in patients with reasonably long life expectancies (American Diabetes Association, 2002).

Treatment goals should take into consideration the patient's ability to understand and carry out the management regimen, risk factors for severe hypoglycemia, patient factors that may increase risk or decrease the benefit of tight glycemic control (such as advanced age, ESRD, or advanced cardiac or cerebrovascular disease), or other conditions that may shorten life expectancy. It may be preferable to allow slightly higher glucose levels to minimize the risk of hypoglycemia.

Diet

The American Diabetes Association has long recognized that the concept of a specific diabetic diet should be abandoned and that the dietary recommendations for patients must be individualized. The American Diabetes Association recommends a diet that contains 55% carbohydrates, 20% proteins, and less than 30% fat. Weight loss should be a goal for patients with diabetes who are overweight. A nutritionist or dietitian is an important member of the interdisciplinary team.

Exercise

Physical activity improves insulin sensitivity and enhances cardiovascular fitness. Although older persons with diabetes may find certain forms of exercise (such as brisk walking or swimming) difficult because of other comorbid conditions, it is important to encourage some sort of aerobic activity lasting at least 20 minutes three times per week. This may be as simple as wading in a pool, performing chair exercises, or walking at the mall.

Smoking Cessation

Smoking cessation should be strongly recommended to reduce the risk of cardiovascular events, peripheral vascular disease and foot ulcers, retinopathy, and nephropathy.

Oral Hypoglycemic Agents

Medical nutrition therapy and regular exercise are the mainstay of management for type 2 diabetes, but nearly all patients require oral medication to stimulate insulin production or to exert other important metabolic mechanisms (Kulkarni, 2002). Currently five classes of oral hypoglycemic agents with different modes of action are available: the sulfonylureas, metformin, acarbose, troglitazone, and meglitinides. Table 14-1 provides information about these five classes of agents (Kulkarni, 2002). Figure 14-1 provides an algorithm for medical management of type 2 diabetes (Kulkarni, 2002).

Insulin

As beta-cell function declines, more than half of patients with type 2 diabetes will eventually need insulin therapy, as do all patients with type 1 diabetes. In addition, patients may proceed to taking a combination of oral medication with insulin (Kilkarni, 2002). Insulin preparations consist of either animal or human insulin. The short-acting insulins are regular, Lispro, and Semilente. When given intravenously, they exert their effects within 10 to 15 minutes. When given subcutaneously, the regular and Semilente insulins reach peak effect in 2 to 3 hours, whereas the Lispro reaches peak effect in 0.5 to 1.5 hours. The intermediate-acting insulins are NPH and Lente. Their peak effect is reached in 6 to 9 hours. Therapy is initiated with a dose of 5 to 10 U daily, to be increased by 2 to 3 U every 4 days until the fasting plasma glucose goal is reached. Insulin is relatively inexpensive. The major risk of insulin therapy is hypoglycemia. Table 14-2 provides information about the actions of different types of insulin (Kulkarni, 2002).

Insulin regimens can range from a single dose of long-acting insulin (with a goal of preventing symptomatic hyperglycemia) to multiple doses of short- and long-acting insulin (with a goal of achieving normal levels of glycemia).

Rapid-acting insulin doses are determined by preprandial and 2-hour postprandial blood glucose levels because they reflect the amount of insulin needed to metabolize the usual intake of carbohydrates at a meal. If rapid-acting insulin is initiated, the background insulin may have to be adjusted. For example, when a patient is changed from preprandial regular (short-acting) insulin to a rapid-acting insulin, the background insulin dose may have to be adjusted upward by 10% to 15% and the rapid-acting

| TABLE 14-1 | Oral Medications Prescribed for Patients with Type 2 Diabetes |

Class (Generic Names)	Mechanism of Action	Advantages	Adverse Effects	Precautions
Sulfonylureas (glyburide, glipizide, glimepiride)	Stimulate the pancreas to secrete insulin in response to meals	Economy	Hypoglycemia, possible weight gain	Not to be used during pregnancy or lactation; requires caution in patients who are elderly or have hepatic dysfunction
α-Glucosidase inhibitors (acarbose, miglitol)	Block enzymes that metabolize starches in the intestine	Cannot cause hypoglycemia if used alone	Abdominal discomfort, flatulence, diarrhea	Must be taken with first bite of food
Meglitinides (repaglinide, nateglinide)	Stimulate insulin release from the pancreas when glucose is present in the bloodstream	Low risk of between-meal and nighttime hypoglycemia	Hypoglycemia (if taken without a meal)	Must be taken only before meals or large snacks containing carbohydrates; dosage must be adjusted for added or skipped meals; contraindicated by liver problems; not recommended during pregnancy or lactation
Biguanides (metformin, metformin-extended release)	Reduce hepatic glucose production; slow glucose uptake in the intestine; increase insulin sensitivity in the muscles	Lower lipid levels, decrease appetite, cannot cause hypoglycemia if used alone	Cramping, gas, diarrhea; rarely, lactic acidosis	Should be taken with first bite of food; contraindicated in those with renal or hepatic disease, respiratory insufficiency, alcohol abuse, heart failure; not recommended during pregnancy or lactation
TZDs (rosiglitazone, pioglitazone)	Reduce insulin resistance, decrease hepatic glucose output, facilitate peripheral glucose uptake	Cannot cause hypoglycemia if used alone	Weight gain, edema	Liver disease or heart failure, contrain-dications; liver function must be monitored

Source: Kulkarni K: Managing type 2 diabetes: the struggle to maintaining control, *Clin Rev* 12(9):62-67, 2002. Data extracted from American Diabetes Association: *Medications for the treatment of diabetes,* Alexandria, Va, 2000, American Diabetes Association; and American Diabetes Association: *Medical management of type 2 diabetes,* ed 4, Alexandria, Va, 1998, American Diabetes Association.
TZDs, Thiazolidinediones.

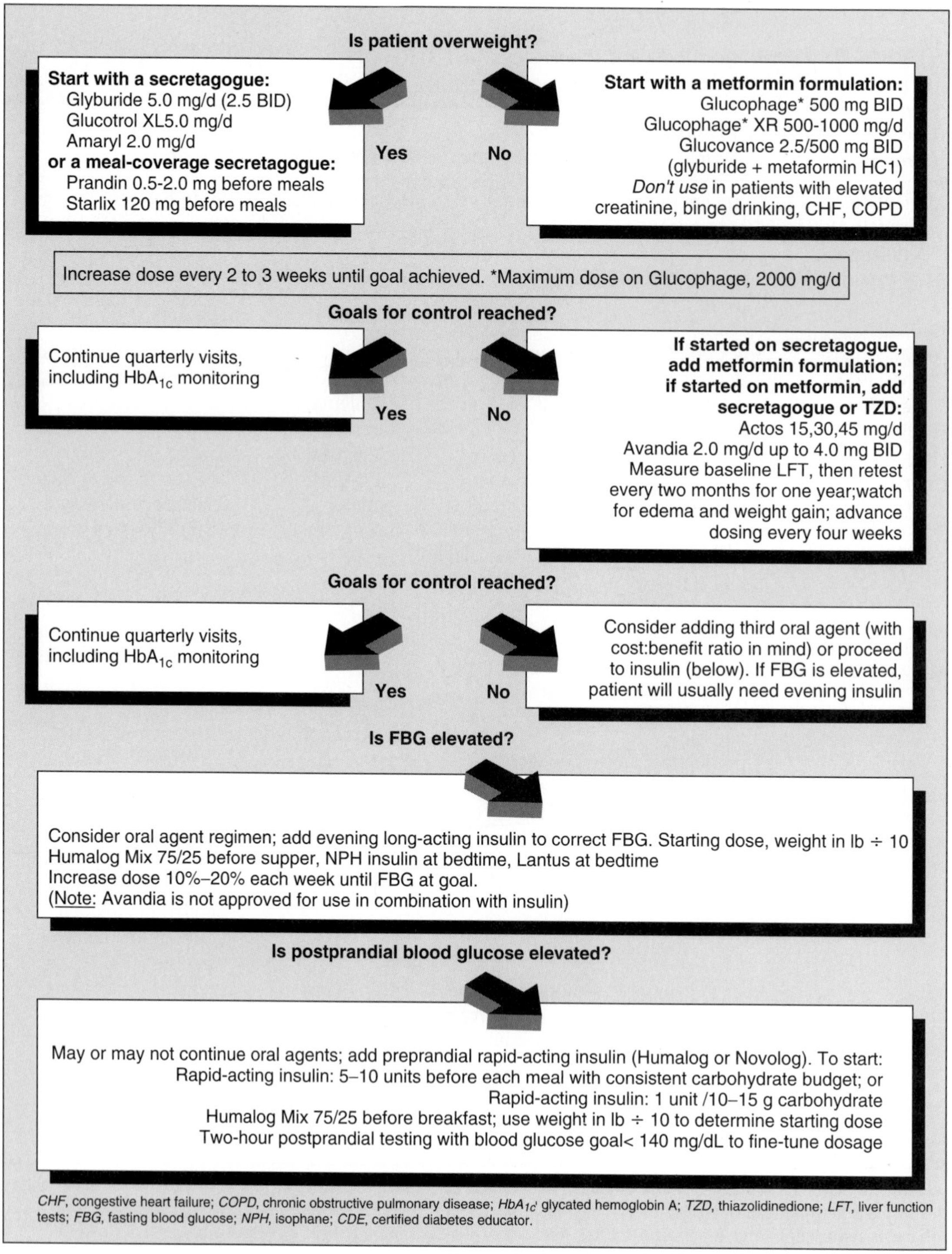

Is patient overweight?

Start with a secretagogue:
  Glyburide 5.0 mg/d (2.5 BID)
  Glucotrol XL5.0 mg/d
  Amaryl 2.0 mg/d
or a meal-coverage secretagogue:
  Prandin 0.5-2.0 mg before meals
  Starlix 120 mg before meals

Yes   No

Start with a metformin formulation:
  Glucophage* 500 mg BID
  Glucophage* XR 500-1000 mg/d
  Glucovance 2.5/500 mg BID
  (glyburide + metformin HC1)
  Don't use in patients with elevated
  creatinine, binge drinking, CHF, COPD

Increase dose every 2 to 3 weeks until goal achieved. *Maximum dose on Glucophage, 2000 mg/d

Goals for control reached?

Continue quarterly visits,
including HbA$_{1c}$ monitoring

Yes   No

**If started on secretagogue,
add metformin formulation;
if started on metformin, add
secretagogue or TZD:**
  Actos 15,30,45 mg/d
  Avandia 2.0 mg/d up to 4.0 mg BID
  Measure baseline LFT, then retest
  every two months for one year;watch
  for edema and weight gain; advance
  dosing every four weeks

Goals for control reached?

Continue quarterly visits,
including HbA$_{1c}$ monitoring

Yes   No

Consider adding third oral agent (with
cost:benefit ratio in mind) or proceed
to insulin (below). If FBG is elevated,
patient will usually need evening insulin

Is FBG elevated?

Consider oral agent regimen; add evening long-acting insulin to correct FBG. Starting dose, weight in lb ÷ 10
Humalog Mix 75/25 before supper, NPH insulin at bedtime, Lantus at bedtime
Increase dose 10%–20% each week until FBG at goal.
(Note: Avandia is not approved for use in combination with insulin)

Is postprandial blood glucose elevated?

May or may not continue oral agents; add preprandial rapid-acting insulin (Humalog or Novolog). To start:
Rapid-acting insulin: 5–10 units before each meal with consistent carbohydrate budget; or
Rapid-acting insulin: 1 unit /10–15 g carbohydrate
Humalog Mix 75/25 before breakfast; use weight in lb ÷ 10 to determine starting dose
Two-hour postprandial testing with blood glucose goal< 140 mg/dL to fine-tune dosage

CHF, congestive heart failure; *COPD*, chronic obstructive pulmonary disease; *HbA$_{1c}$* glycated hemoglobin A; *TZD*, thiazolidinedione; *LFT*, liver function tests; *FBG*, fasting blood glucose; *NPH*, isophane; *CDE*, certified diabetes educator.

Figure 14-1   Algorithm for medical management of type 2 diabetes. (Adapted from Valentine V: *Algorithm for control: algorithm for medication management—type 2 diabetes*, 2002, Diabetes Network.)

TABLE 14-2	Actions of Different Types of Insulin		
Insulin Type	**Starts**	**Peaks**	**Ends**
Rapid-acting (mealtime) insulin			
Insulin lispro	10 min	60 min	3–4 h
Insulin aspart	10 min	60 min	3–4 h
Short-acting (mealtime) insulin			
Regular insulin	30–60 min	2–4 h	6–8 h
Intermediate-acting (background) insulin			
NPH insulin	1.5 h	4–12 h	10–16 h
Insulin lente	2.5 h	7–15 h	10–16 h
Long-acting (background) insulin			
Insulin ultralente	4 h	8–16 h	18–20 h
Insulin glargine	4–6 h	None	24 h
Insulin mixtures*			
70/30, 50/50	0.5–1.0 h	Dual (NPH/R)	12–20 h
75/25	10 min	Dual (NPH/L)	12–20 h

Source: Kulkarni K: Managing type 2 diabetes: the struggle to maintain control, *Clin Rev* 12(9):62-67, 2002. Data extracted from American Diabetes Association: *Medical management of type 1 diabetes*, ed 3, Alexandria, Va, 1998, American Diabetes Association; and American Diabetes Association: Insulin administration, *Diabetes Care* 25(Suppl 1):S112-S115, 2002.
NPH, Isophane; NPH/R, intermediate-acting/rapid-acting; NPH/L, intermediate-acting/long-acting.

insulin dose decreased from that of the regular insulin by 10% to 15%. This is because regular insulin overlaps with the background insulin, whereas rapid-acting insulin does not (Kulkarni, 2002).

Initial treatment may be started by instituting a sliding-scale administration of regular insulin based on fingersticks before each meal and at bedtime. For example:

Blood Sugar	Insulin Dose (U)
< 200	0
201 to 249	2
250 to 299	4
300 to 349	6
350 to 399	8
> 400	Call medical provider

Total amount of insulin administered within 24 hours is then added, and an initial dose of long-acting insulin is thereby determined. Patients receiving a bedtime insulin dose must be instructed to eat a bedtime snack, such as a piece of fruit or a half sandwich.

INSULIN PUMPS

Insulin pumps, which have been available for two decades, are now becoming a more widely available technology for insulin delivery. Compared with syringe-injected insulin and pen-injected insulin, continuous subcutaneous insulin infusion (CSII) via an insulin pump is being marketed as the most sophisticated and flexible method of providing insulin therapy. It has been suggested that CSII can help achieve enhanced glycemic control with a reduced risk of hypoglycemic events. Data in favor of the use of insulin pumps are most substantial in relation to patient acceptance, flexibility of injection regimen, and reduction in omissions of scheduled doses. No clear evidence exists that CSII enhances glycemic control compared with other forms of insulin therapy, although evidence does suggest that CSII reduces the risk of hypoglycemia for the same level of control (Kanakis, Watts, and Leichter, 2002).

Cost can be a formidable obstacle to CSII therapy. The most popular insulin pumps and initial supplies, including tubing, syringes, cartridges, and dressings, cost more than $5000. The infusion set and catheters must be purchased regularly for as long as CSII; annual cost is about $1500. Most insurance companies, including Medicare and Medicaid, cover the cost of CSII after prospective approval; however, patients whose plans cover 80% of the total cost may still face substantial initial and recurrent out-of-pocket expenses (Kanakis, Watts, and Leichter, 2002). CSII therapy poses financial issues for providers as well. Initiating this type of treatment requires a substantial investment of time and effort to assess patient suitability and to teach proper pump use.

Management of Subsequent Health Risks

Attention must also be given to other health issues, such as hyperlipidemia, coronary artery disease (CAD), renal disease, and stroke risk. These problems may exist independently or as a result of the diabetes. Recommendations include the following:

- Hyperlipidemia
  Lowering low-density lipoprotein (LDL) cholesterol below 100 mg/dl regardless of the presence of CAD
  Lower high triglyceride levels (> 1000 mg/dl) to below 400 mg/dl.
- Blood pressure
  Maintain blood pressure at < 130/85 mm Hg.
- Renal disease
  Nephrology consult is necessary when glomerular filtration rate drops below 60 ml per minute, serum creatinine rises to 2 mg/dl, or when difficulties occur in management of hypertension or hyperkalemia.
- Risk of CAD and stroke
  Daily aspirin administration has been shown to reduce adverse clinical outcomes, especially subsequent major cerebrovascular events (O'Connor, Spann, and Woolf, 1998).

Table 14-3 Provides the standards of care for the patient with type 2 diabetes (Kulkarni, 2002).

Management

The management plan should include short- and long-term goals, medications, nutritional recommendations, home blood-glucose monitoring, annual comprehensive dilated eye examinations, Pneumovax and yearly influenza vaccine administration, and follow-up plans. Patients starting oral antidiabetic agents need to be in contact with their provider weekly until reasonable glucose control is achieved. Patients starting insulin therapy or having a major change in their regimen need to be in contact with their provider daily until glucose control is achieved. Patients are seen at least every 3 months until their treatment goals are achieved and then every 6 months (American Diabetes Association, 1998).

During follow-up visits an interim history is obtained that includes questioning about hypoglycemic episodes, results of self-monitoring blood glucose, current medications, and other medical illnesses. The health provider should examine the feet and measure weight and blood pressure. Hgb

A1c should be measured every 3 months; lipid profile, urinalysis, and microalbuminuria should be checked every year.

Managing Diabetes During Glucocorticoid Therapy

Although glucocorticoid therapy carries a risk of promoting or exacerbating hyperglycemia, currently no medical guidelines have been examined for detecting or managing diabetes in patients starting such therapy. The importance of having a strategy to detect, monitor, and, if necessary, aggressively treat diabetes during glucocorticoid therapy is underscored, however, by the potential seriousness of diabetic metabolic emergencies (Braithwaite et al, 1998). Glucocorticoid therapy makes patients insulin resistant. Therefore patients who have used insulin before moderate- or high-dose glucocorticoid therapy often must increase insulin doses 1.5 to 2 times the previously established doses. Other medications and agents that alter glucose control are listed in Table 14-4.

Management of Hypoglycemia

Patients, caregivers, and family members must be educated about the signs and symptoms of hypoglycemia as well as how to manage this problem. Table 14-5 describes the levels of hypoglycemia and the treatment of each.

Education

Patients should be given as much verbal and written information as they can manage to encourage self-care and prevention of complications. Education should include issues discussed previously, such as diet, exercise, medication management, and glucose monitoring. The patient or caregiver must be able to administer the correct medication or insulin dosage, monitor blood sugar at home, and recognize the symptoms of hypoglycemia and their management. Referral to a local home nursing agency can provide the patient and caregivers with at-home initial instruction and observation of blood glucose monitoring, medication or insulin administration, nutrition counseling, and monitoring of complications. Patients must first purchase their own glucose monitoring machine and test

TABLE 14-4	Medications or Agents that Alter Glucose Control

Drugs that Increase Blood Glucose	Drugs that Decrease Blood Glucose
Corticosteroids	Insulin
Thiazides	Oral hypoglycemic agents (sulfonylureas; acetohexamide,
Thyroid preparations	chlorpropamide, glipizide, glyburide, tolazamide, and
Phenytoin	tolbutamide)
Epinephrine	Alcohol
Sugary preparations (many over the	Salicylates (high doses)
counter cold medications)	Reserpine
Estrogens	Clonidine
Glucagon	Phenylbutazone
Acetazolamide	Probenecid
Caffeine	Allopurinol
Cyclophosphamide	Pentamidine
Ethacrynic acid	Chloroquine
Nicotine	Dicumarol
Calcium-channel blockers	Beta-blockers
Nonsteroidal anti-inflammatory drugs	Clofibrate
Phenobarbitol	Monoamine oxidase inhibitors
Chloramphenicol	Anabolic steroids
	Potassium salts

Modified from Steil D: Prescription drugs and diabetes, *Diabetes Spectrum* 3(2):119-122, 1990.

strips (available from most pharmacies). The monitor, supplies, and nursing services are usually covered by Medicare.

Another important issue is foot care and prevention of foot ulcers. Teaching should include proper footwear, avoidance of walking barefoot, and soaking the feet. Daily assessment of skin integrity of the feet should be performed by the patient by using a mirror and flashlight to see all surfaces of the foot, if necessary. If the patient is unable to do this, a caregiver should be taught to do it. Feet should be washed daily in water that is not too hot and lubrication applied to avoid skin cracks that can lead to infection. Regular evaluations by a podiatrist may be beneficial.

THYROID CONDITIONS

Thyroid disease is the second most frequent endocrine problem for older people. Many of the signs and symptoms of both hypothyroidism and hyperthyroidism in older persons are blunted in their presentation, the presentation is atypical, or the presentation may be dismissed as a normal reaction to aging. Although laboratory tests are remarkably improved in reliability, they still can pose difficulties in reaching a firm diagnosis. Patients with thyroid disease need to be initially diagnosed and managed by a team of health professionals with expertise in this area. If the health care team does not include specialists, consultation with an endocrinologist is essential in managing patients with hyperthyroidism and selected cases of hypothyroidism.

TABLE 14-5	Levels of Hypoglycemia and Treatment	
Hypoglycemia Level	**Symptoms**	**Treatment**
Mild	Hunger, diaphoresis, nervousness, shakiness, tachycardia, and pale skin	15 g of carbohydrate (4 oz. of juice, no sugar added)
Moderate	Headache, irritability, fatigue, blurred vision, and mood changes	15 g of carbohydrate; may repeat Glucagon, intravenous glucose
Severe	Unresponsiveness, confusion, coma, or convulsions	

Hypothyroidism

Epidemiology

Hypothyroidism is a clinical syndrome resulting from a deficiency of thyroid hormone. This disorder can range from subclinical hypothyroidism with no obvious symptoms to severe hypothyroidism, which is myxedema coma. The prevalence of hypothyroidism varies depending on ethnicity, the iodine content of the diet, and the criteria used to define the diagnosis. The prevalence of hypothyroidism ranges from 0.5% to 6% and 14% to 18%, depending on the study population. It is more frequent in hospitalized patients, whites, and older women (Li, 2002). Autoimmune thyroiditis and postoperative hypothyroidism are the main causes of thyroid hypofunction in patients older than 55 years (Diez, 2002).

Physiology

The production of thyroid hormones is regulated by the hypothalamic-pituitary-thyroid axis. Thyrotropin-releasing hormone (TRH) is synthesized in the hypothalamus and stimulates the release of thyroid-stimulating hormone (TSH) from the anterior pituitary. TSH is regulated by the negative feedback of the thyroid hormones thyroxine (T4) and triiodothyronine (T3) acting on the pituitary gland and probably the hypothalamus. In response to TSH activity, T4 and T3 stored in thyroid follicles are hydrolyzed from thyroglobulin and released into the circulation, where they bind to albumin, thyroid-binding prealbumin (TBPA), and thyroid-binding globulin (TBG). Fewer than 0.1% of the hormones circulate in the free form. The small proportion of T4 and T3 in the free state (FT4 and FT3) are the biologically active forms of the hormones. The primary thyroid hormone acting on peripheral tissue and responsible from the broad range of thyroid actions in T3 (Li, 2002).

Causes

Hypothyroidism has several causes and generally develops as a primary thyroid gland disorder. The most common cause of primary hypothyroidism is Hashimoto thyroiditis, an autoimmune disorder with chronic lymphocytic infiltration of the thyroid gland leading to tissue fibrosis, and decline of hormone production. Other causes include prior treatment of hyperthyroidism, especially Graves disease; prior radiotherapy of Hodgkin's disease; previous thyroidectomy; and medications, especially lithium, amiodarone, and iodine. Fifteen percent of patients treated with external radiotherapy or surgery for cancers of the head and neck have developed hypothyroidism (Li, 2002). Iodide and iodine-containing drugs can result in inhibition of thyroid-hormone synthesis, causing hypothyroidism, which is usually reversible once the external iodine sources are removed. Common sources of external iodine ingestion are amiodarone and iodinated radiographic contrast agents. Lithium, interferon-alpha, and interleukin-2 have been claimed by many researchers to cause hypothyroidism (Li, 2002).

Central hypothyroidism is a term used to describe secondary and tertiary hypothyroidism. Impaired production or release of TSH from the anterior pituitary or impaired production or release of TRH from the hypothalamus leads to secondary and tertiary hypothyroidism, respectively. These alterations can be the consequences of pituitary or hypothalamic tumors, surgical or traumatic injury, radiotherapy, or infiltrative diseases, such as human immunodeficiency (HIV) infection (Li, 2002).

Features

The signs and symptoms of hypothyroidism often develop insidiously. Common symptoms include dry skin, hair loss, cold intolerance, paresthesias, confusion, unsteadiness, constipation, fatigue, lethargy, hoarseness, slowed speech, depression, and muscle cramps. Table 14-6 describes the classic presentation of hypothyroidism (Li, 2002). Physical findings of hypothyroidism include delayed deep-tendon reflexes, bradycardia, diastolic hypertension, hypoventilation, hypothermia, ataxia, carpal tunnel syndrome, cool pale skin, and puffy face and hands. Symptoms of peripheral neuropathy such as mild to severe burning and knife-like pain in the extremities may be the only symptoms in an older patient. Hypothyroidism is a cause of reversible dementia, and even subclinical hypothyroidism may be associated with cognitive dysfunction, mood disturbance, and diminished response to standard psychiatric treatments. Anemia may be the only manifestation in some cases. Clinicians need to be aware that many older people and family members may mistake the signs of hypothyroidism and believe that these are "only signs of aging."

Diagnosis

A comprehensive medical history and physical examination can uncover signs and symptoms that may help confirm the diagnosis of hypothyroidism. Patients should be asked about weakness, fatigue, sleepiness, cold intolerance, hoarseness, constipation, joint pains, muscle cramps, and depression. Cardiovascular, neurologic, musculoskeletal, skin, gastrointestinal, and respiratory systems should be included in the physical examination.

TABLE 14-6	Classic Presentation of Hypothyroidism
System	**Symptoms**
Cardiovascular	Cardiomyopathy, peripheral edema, bradycardia, hypertension
Gastrointestinal	Constipation, anorexia
General	Fatigue, lethargy, hoarseness, slurred speech
Metabolic	Cold intolerance, hypothermia, weight gain
Neuromuscular	Impaired memory, depression, delay of deep tendon reflex, physical slowing, weakness
Respiratory	Sleep apnea
Skin	Dry skin, diminished sweating, yellowing skin

Li TM: Hypothyroidism in elderly people, *Geriatr Nurs* 23(2): 88-93, 2002.

The best test for diagnosis of primary hypothyroidism is the serum TSH concentration (Li, 2002). The circulating TSH concentration is regulated by the circulating free T4 concentration in a negative-feedback manner and is elevated in primary hypothyroidism. When serum thyroid hormone concentrations decrease below an individual patient's threshold for thyroid hormone sufficiency, serum TSH concentration increases. Serum TSH levels will be elevated in subclinical and overt hypothyroidism. Free T4 should be measured when TSH level is high. If free T4 level is normal, TSH levels should be repeated in 4 to 6 weeks because they may be transiently elevated during the recovery phase of nonthyroid illness. Serum T3 levels should not be used as a major test of thyroid function because low-serum T3 is often seen in ill older persons. Other tests, including reverse T3, radioactive iodine uptake, thyroid antibodies, and serum TRH, may be useful in the differential diagnosis. Table 14-7 outlines various tests of thyroid function (Li, 2002).

Disorders often confused with hypothyroidism are nonthyroidal illness (NTI) and low T3 and low T4 syndromes. Malnutrition, infections, septic illness, major surgery, poorly controlled diabetes, hepatic disease, renal failure, cerebrovascular disease, heart failure, respiratory failure, malignancy, trauma, burns, coma, and medications (e.g., salicylates, phenytoin, carbamazepine) may alter thyroid function test results (Li, 2002). Table 14-8 lists factors that influence thyroid status.

The American Thyroid Association recommends the measurement of both TSH and free T4 as initial tests in patients with suspected hypothyroidism. The American College of Physicians recommends a total T4, free thyroxine index (T4I), or sensitive TSH as the best initial test in patients with suspected hypothyroidism. Isolated elevated TSH levels should be repeated in 4 to 6 weeks. The

TABLE 14-7	**Tests of Thyroid Function**
Thyroid-stimulating hormone:	An extremely sensitive indicator of thyroid function. Normal test results rule out hyperthyroidism or hypothyroidism, except in central thyroid dysfunction.
Free T4 (FT4):	FT4 level is not influenced by the level of binding protein, and this test provides a more accurate assessment of thyroid function than total T4.
Total T4 (TT4):	Affected by alternation in the binding protein level in plasma and by drugs that affect protein binding. It is not a reliable indicator of thyroid function.
Thyroid scan:	Useful to evaluate functional status of nodular thyroid disease and structural abnormalities
Ultrasonography:	Ninety percent accuracy in discriminating between cystic and solid nodules thyroid disease
Antithyroid antibody:	High titers in hypothyroidism patients suggest Hashimoto's or lymphocytic thyroiditis. High titers in hyperthyroidism patients suggest Graves' disease.
Radioactive iodine uptake (RAIU):	Difficult to distinguish low values from low normal value when dietary iodine is high; less diagnostic usefulness in establishing a diagnosis of hypothyroidism
Total T3 (TT3):	Affected by alteration of binding protein level (although less than T4) and by drugs that affect binding. Total T3 is easily affected by nonthyroidal illness.
Free T3 (FT3):	Levels remain constant over the age span; decreased level should be considered consequence of illness.
Thyrotropin-releasing hormone test:	May be useful in distinguishing pituitary hypothyroidism from hypothalamic hypothyroidism

From Li TM: Hypothyroidism in elderly people, *Geriatr Nurs* 23(22):88-93, 2002.

TABLE 14-8	Factors that Influence Thyroid Status

Factors Increasing T_4	Factors Decreasing T_4
Laboratory error	Severe illness (e.g., chronic renal failure, major surgery,
Autoimmunity	caloric deprivation)
Acute illness (e.g., viral hepatitis, chronic	Acute psychiatric problems
active hepatitis, primary biliary	Cirrhosis
cirrhosis, acute intermittent	Nephrotic syndrome
porphyria, AIDS)	Hereditary TBG deficiency
High-estrogen states (may also increase T_3)	Drugs
Oral estrogen-containing contraceptives	Phenobarbital
Pregnancy	Phenytoin (T_4 may be as low as 2 μg/dL)
Estrogen replacement therapy	Carbamazepine
Neonatal period	T_3 therapy
Acute psychiatric problems	Androgens
Hyperemesis gravidarum and morning	Fluorouracil
sickness (may also increase T_3)	Halofenate (lowers triglycerides and uric
Familial thyroid hormone binding abnormalities	acid; not marketed in USA)
Generalized resistance to thyroid hormone	Mitotane
Drugs	Phenylbutazone
Amiodarone	Fenclofenac (nonsteroidal antiinflammatory agent;
Amphetamines	not marketed in USA)
Clofibrate	Salicylates (large doses)
Heparin (dialysis method)	Chloral hydrate
Heroin	Asparaginase
Levothyroxine (T_4) replacement therapy	
Methadone (may also increase T_3)	
Perphenazine	

From Fitzgerald P: Endocrinology. In Tierney LM et al: *Current medical diagnoses and treatment*, ed 36, Stamford, Conn, 1997, Appleton & Lange.
AIDS, Acquired immunodeficiency syndrome; T_3, triiodothyronine; T_4, thyroxine; *TBG*, thyroxine-binding globuline.

findings of concentrated low serum FT4 and elevated serum TSH clearly establish a diagnosis of primary hypothyroidism. Table 14-9 presents a simplified guide to diagnosis (Li, 2002).

Treatment

Thyroid hormone replacement therapy is the treatment of overt hypothyroidism. The goal should be full physiologic replacement. The preferred agent is levothyroxine (Synthroid) because of its long half-life and its conversion to T3. Brand-name products have been preferred over generic ones because they vary less in bioavailability from batch to batch; however, generic preparations are significantly less expensive. It is important to maintain consistency of brand and not to switch between generic and brand name prescriptions to avoid fluctuations in response and TSH levels.

Levothyroxine therapy for hypothyroid older patients with or without overt heart disease should start at 25 μg per day. The dose is increased in increments of 25 μg at 8-week intervals until the serum TSH level returns to normal. The TSH should also be checked after 8 to 12 weeks in patients

TABLE 14-9	Diagnosis of Diseases

Primary hypothyroidism: Decreased free T4, increased TSH
Central hypothyroidism: Decreased free T4, decreased or normal TSH
Subclinical hypothyroidism: Normal free T4, increased TSH, absence of clinical symptoms

From Li TM: Hypothyroidism in elderly people, *Geriatr Nurs* 23(2): 88-93, 2002.

who had their dosage, type, or brand changed. Once the TSH has been normalized, the patient should be monitored with a TSH level annually.

Precautions

Side effects associated with treatment include accelerating osteoporosis, increased risk of fracture, anginal pain, myocardial infarction, congestive heart failure, arrhythmia, and left ventricular hypertrophy (Li, 2002).

Thyroxine treatment with patients who have known CAD need to be treated initially with caution. T4 increases cardiac muscle demand and can precipitate angina or a myocardial infarction in patients with CAD. If cardiac symptoms develop or worsen, therapy should be stopped pending evaluation of the cardiac disease. To protect women from bone loss, the dosage of levothyroxine should not suppress the TSH below normal even if T4 levels are normal.

Subclinical Hypothyroidism

Of people with subclinical hypothyroidism, 20% to 50% develop overt hypothyroidism within 4 to 8 years. Overt hypothyroidism develops within 4 years in 80% of patients over the age of 65 with subclinical hypothyroidism and elevated antithyroid antibodies (Wallace and Hoffman, 1998). Treatment of subclinical hypothyroidism must be individualized and considered a strong possibility in the presence of antithyroid antibodies (Wallace and Hoffman, 1998). Patients with subclinical hypothyroidism may notice increased energy, decreased skin dryness, and constipation after treatment with T4. Once a decision is made to treat the person with subclinical hypothyroidism, the same treatment plan as for overt hypothyroidism is followed.

Myxedema Coma

Myxedema coma occurs almost exclusively in older adults with long-standing primary hypothyroidism and usually is precipitated by a concomitant medical illness. Clinial presentation includes rapid development of stupor, seizures, or coma, often associated with infection, stress, exposure to cold, or after administration of sedatives, tranquilizers, or narcotics. Respiratory depression with hypoxia and carbon dioxide retention is common and may require mechanical ventilatory assistance. Blood pressure may be low, along with bradycardia and features of shock. Localized neurologic signs, hypothermia, hyponatremia, and hypoglycemia are the hallmarks of myxedema coma.

Treatment is with intravenous L-thyroxine and corticosteroids until evidence of clinical improvement and stabilization has occurred or central hypothyroidism can be ruled out (Li, 2002).

Hyperthyroidism

Prevalence

Hyperthyroidism is a metabolic disorder that results when tissues are exposed to excess thyroid hormone. The prevalence of hyperthyroidism in older persons (55 years of age and older) has been reported to be 0.5% to 2.3%, depending on the population studied and the criteria used for diagnosis. About 15% of all patients with hyperthyroidism are 60 years of age and older.

Causes

Graves disease is the most common cause of hyperthyroidism in older patients. Clinicians need to be aware that radiographic examinations that use iodine-containing contrast materials (gallbladder and others) may contribute to an increased risk of an older person developing iodine-induced thyrotoxicosis such as that caused by amiodarone.

Clinical Manifestations

Older patients with hyperthyroidism have fewer signs and symptoms than their younger counterparts. Weight loss and nonspecific failure to thrive are the most common manifestations of hyperthyroidism in older persons. The common signs and symptoms of hyperthyroidism are weight loss (44%), palpitations (36%), weakness (32%), heat intolerance (4%), constipation or diarrhea, anorexia, depression and apathy, tachycardia (28%), atrial fibrillation (32%), lid lag (12%), fine skin (40%), and tremor (36%). Atrial fibrillation may be the only manifestation of hyperthyroidism in older patients.

Diagnosis

The preferred test for hyperthyroidism is TSH measurement using one of the newer, sensitive TSH assays. The American Thyroid Association recommends free T4 and a sensitive thyrotropin assay for hyperthyroidism measurement. The American College of Physicians recommends the free T4 index as the best initial test; however, free T4 index is not a good test for hyperthyroidism in chronically ill, institutionalized older patients. Patients with hyperthyroidism will have TSH levels below the detection limit of the assay. If TSH levels are low, free T4I should be measured and, if it is normal, T3 should be measured. If free T4 and T3 levels are normal, the TSH measurement should be repeated in 4 to 6 weeks. Radioactive iodine uptake will help to identify the cause of hyperthyroidism (see Table 14-10 for screening using thyroid tests).

Treatment

Radioactive iodine therapy is the preferred treatment of hyperthyroidism in older adults. It carries the risk of a transient worsening of the hyperthyroidism. Some recommend achieving a euthyroid state using antithyroid drugs before the iodine radiotherapy. After completing radioactive iodine treatment, 80% of the patients will be euthyroid, 10% will be hypothyroid, and 10% will remain hyperthyroid. Propylthiouracil and methimazole are the most widely used antithyroid drugs in the United States. Their major side effects include skin rash, fever, agranulocytosis, arthritis, and hepatitis. The major concern when treating older patients with hyperthyroidism is to eliminate the hyperthyroidism before any complications arise. Patients must be followed up closely during therapy.

| **TABLE 14-10** | Thyroid Testing | |

Purpose	Test	Comment
Screening	Serum TSH (sensitive assay)	Most sensitive test for primary hypothyroidism and hyperthyroidism
	Free T_4	Excellent test
	T_4 (RIA)	Varies directly with TBG
	T_3 resin uptake (T_3 RU)	Varies inversely with TBG
	Free thyroxine index	Useful combination of T_4 and T_3U
For hypothyroidism	Serum TSH	High in primary and low in secondary hypothyroidism.
	Antithyroglobulin and antithyroperoxidase antibodies	Elevated in Hashimoto's thyroiditis
For hyperthyroidism	Serum TSH (sensitive assay)	Suppressed except in TSH-secreting pituitary tumor or hyperplasia (rare)
	T_3 (RIA)	Elevated
	^{123}I uptake and scan	Increased diffuse vs. "hot" areas
	Antithyroglobulin and antimicrosomal antibodies	Elevated in Graves' disease
	TSH receptor antibody (TSH-R Ab [stim])	Usually positive in Graves' disease
For nodules	FNA	Best diagnostic method for thyroid cancer
	^{123}I uptake and scan	Cancer is usually "cold"; less reliable than FNA
	^{99m}Tc scan	Vascular versus avascular
	Ultrasonography	Solid versus cystic; pure cysts are usually not malignant

From Fitzgerald P: Endocrinology. In Tierney LM et al: *Current medical diagnoses and treatment*, ed 36, Stamford, Conn, 1997, Appleton & Lange.
FNA, Fine-needle aspiration; *RIA*, radioimmunoassay; T_3, triiodothyronine; T_4, thyroxine; *TSH*, thyroid-stimulating hormone; *TBG*, thyroxine-binding globulin.

Euthyroid Multinodular Goiter

Euthyroid multinodular goiter is caused by excessive replication of thyroid epithelial cells as a result of various stimuli. With time, size and nodularity increase. The clinical manifestations arise solely from thyroid enlargement. Treatment of euthyroid multinodular goiter is indicated only when thyroid enlargement causes symptoms of obstruction, such as dysphagia and dyspnea. Treatment options are radioiodine (iodine-131), surgery, and TSH suppression therapy (Manders and Corstens, 2002).

Primary Hyperparathyroidism

Hyperparathyroidism is a metabolic disorder of calcium, phosphorus, and bone metabolism caused by increased circulating levels of parathyroid hormone (PTH).

Epidemiology

Hyperparathyroidism occurs with increasing frequency in older people and is the most common cause of hypercalcemia in healthy outpatients. The estimated incidence is 1 case per 1000 men and 2 to 3 cases per 1000 women. Improvements in testing since the 1970s have led to an increase in recognized cases, and the severe complications of hyperparathyroidism (osteitis fibrosa cystica and nephrocalcinosis) are rarely seen today. Distinguishing primary hyperparathyroidism from malignancy, the next common cause of hypercalcemia, is generally not difficult based on clinical grounds alone (Kearns and Thompson, 2002).

Causes

Hyperparathyroidism is considered *primary* when there is autonomous excessive secretion of PTH and consequent hypercalcemia. Single adenomas cause 80% to 85% of cases of primary hyperparathyroidism. Hypertrophy of all four parathyroid glands causes hyperparathyroidism in 15% of patients. A small number of cases of hyperthyroidism result from parathyroid carcinomas and multiple adenomas (Allerheiligen, 1998). No etiologic agent is identified in most cases; however, previous neck exposure to radiation and lithium intake has been associated with hyperparathyroidism. Multiple endocrine neoplasia syndromes (I and II) and familial hyperparathyroidism cause a few number of cases of hyperparathyroidism.

Clinical Features

The presenting signs and symptoms of patients with hyperparathyroidism vary from a lack of symptoms to the rare hypercalcemic crisis. Most patients have no symptoms until their calcium level exceeds 12 mg/dL, but nearly all patients with a calcium level higher than 14 mg/dL are symptomatic (Kearns and Thompson, 2002). Currently hyperparathyroidism manifests as an unexpected elevation in calcium found incidentally on a serum chemistry profile in an asymptomatic person. Most of the specific signs and symptoms involve the skeleton or the kidneys.

Hyperparathyroidism causes an increased bone remodeling that leads to the rare pathologic diagnosis of osteitis fibrosa cystica. It causes osteopenia or osteosclerosis, which has the "salt and pepper" appearance on a skull X-ray; however, there has been no increased incidence of vertebral fractures with primary hyperparathyroidism. The effects of hyperparathyroidism include nephrolithiasis, proximal renal tubular acidosis, nephrocalcinosis, and nephrogenic diabetes insipidus.

Most of the other signs and symptoms associated with hyperparathyroidism can be attributed to the resultant hypercalcemia, and several organ systems are involved. Symptoms associated with central nervous system involvement range from inability to concentrate to confusion to altered levels of consciousness, depending on the severity of the hypercalcemia. Gastrointestinal symptoms include constipation, anorexia, nausea, vomiting, and abdominal pain. Pancreatitis and peptic ulcer disease are also associated with hypercalcemia. Polyuria, polydipsia, and kidney stones are common urologic symptoms. Hypercalcemia induces a mild nephrogenic diabetes insipidus-like picture with altered urine-concentrating ability. Cardiac manifestations include prolongation of the QT interval and occasionally bradycardia or other arrhythmias. Some patients with longstanding primary hyperparathyroidism may develop bone pain because of brown tumors in the skeleton. Brown tumors represent a severe form of osteitis fibrosa cystica, with brownish fibrous tissue connections in cystic spaces in the skeleton, which gradually heal over time once the primary hyperparathyroidism is cured. Less specific manifestations of hypercalcemia include fatigue, depression, arthralgias, myalgias, and chondrocalcinosis (Kearns and Thompson, 2002).

Diagnosis

Hypercalcemia in the presence of elevated PTH measured by double immunoradiometric assay confirms the diagnosis of primary hyperparathyroidism (Allerheiligen, 1998). The scattergram plot of PTH versus calcium provided by the laboratory helps to interpret the result. The differential diagnosis should include all causes of hypercalcemia. Common causes of hypercalcemia are primary hyperparathyroidism, humoral hypercalcemia of malignancy, renal failure, malignancy via direct bone destruction, and thiazide diuretics. Uncommon causes of hypercalcemia are immobilization, lithium use, hyperthyroidism, vitamin D toxicity, granulomatous diseases, and familial hypocalciuric hypercalcemia.

Treatment

Treatment of hyperparathyroidism depends on the presenting signs and symptoms and on a clear diagnosis based on biochemical confirmation. Serum calcium can be lowered by hydration and by a variety of pharmacologic agents; however, none of these agents is effective in the long-term management of primary hyperparathyroidism (Udelsman, 2001). Because most of the cases are asymptomatic, no immediate treatment is needed.

Nonsurgical Management

Patients who are not surgical candidates for parathyroidectomy appear to do well when they are managed conservatively. On average, these patients remain stable, with little progression to the more serious manifestations of hyperparathyroidism over 10 years. It would seem, therefore, that the overall population of older patients with mild asymptomatic primary hyperparathyroidism can be safely monitored without intervention. Because certain proportion of cases do progress, however, surveillance is necessary. Individual patients can have worsening hypercalcemia or hypercalciuria, and in a small percentage of patients, bone density can decrease over time. In most patients, deferral of surgery is not a one-time decision but rather one that is reviewed and reconsidered in conjunction with meticulous monitoring (Boonen et al, 2001).

At this time no effective medical therapy for primary hyperparathyroidism is available; the current acceptable treatment is surgery. Asymptomatic patients with calcium levels below 11 mg/dl and no evidence of disease can be monitored safely with serum calcium, serum creatinine, creatinine clearance, urinary calcium, bone density, and kidney-ureter-bladder x-ray. Although there is still no agreement on how often these tests should be done, some have recommended doing them on an annual basis. There is no evidence that surgery will improve symptoms or neuropsychiatric disturbances in patients with serum calcium below 11 mg/dl. During medical management, avoidance of dehydration and immobilization, maintenance of a modest dietary calcium intake, treatment of hypertension, cautious use of diuretics, and estrogen replacement in postmenopausal women are advised.

Management of hypercalcemic crisis should take precedence over diagnostic workup. This involves intravenous hydration; diuresis with fluids and furosemide; and administration of pamidronate, calcitonin, glucocorticoids, and mithramycin.

Surgical Management

The extraordinarily high success rate of surgery, combined with its low morbidity and the ever-increasing acceptance of minimally invasive techniques, makes surgical resection the recommended treatment for virtually all patients (Udelsman, 2001). Computed tomographic scan, magnetic resonance imaging, ultrasonography, and radionuclide scans have been used to locate adenomas before surgery. Preoperative localization can decrease the time and lower the incidence of complications;

however, preoperative localization in patients without a previous neck operation has not proven cost effective. Indications for surgical treatment of hyperparathyroidism include (1) typical parathyroid-related symptoms, (2) markedly elevated serum calcium level (1 to 1.6 mg/dl above accepted normal range), (3) history of an episode of life-threatening hypercalcemia, (4) reduced creatinine clearance (30% less than expected), markedly elevated urinary calcium excretion (greater than 400 mg/day), (5) substantially reduced bone mass, (6) significant neuromuscular or psychological symptoms, (7) a patient who requests surgery, (8) consistent follow-up is unlikely, (9) coexistent illness complicates management, or (10) the patient is young (< 50 years of age).

When a patient requires surgical repair of a pathologic fracture because of hyperparathyroidism, the procedures can be safely performed simultaneously. This corrects the underlying endocrinopathy, thereby improving the outcome of the orthopedic surgery (Singhal, Johnson, and Udelsman, 2001).

Parathyroid surgery has the following complications: (1) damage to the recurrent laryngeal nerve, (2) transient hypocalcemia in the immediate postoperative period, and (3) recurrence of symptoms. Recurrence of hyperparathyroidism is less likely after a solitary adenoma than after multiglandular disease (Allerheiligen, 1998).

Summary

Endocrine disorders such as thyroid disease and diabetes are common in the older population; however, they may manifest in a somewhat vague fashion, making them more difficult to diagnose. It is important to be adept in obtaining history that will lead the practitioner to the appropriate diagnostic evaluation. Several medications have been added to the available options for managing diabetes. Although many of these are promising, most have special considerations for use in the older population. Hypothyroidism is often well managed in the primary care setting, whereas hyperthyroidism requires evaluation and treatment by a specialist. Referral to an endocrinologist or other specialist may be necessary to ensure the best outcome for the patient's health. Management, monitoring, and education of endocrine disorders require ongoing care; these disorders are often ideally managed by a multidisciplinary team.

Resources

American Diabetes Association
National Office
1660 Duke Street
Alexandria, VA 22314
www.diabetes.org
(800)-DIABETES

Curative Health Services
150 Motor Pkwy.
Hauppague, NY 11788
(800) 966-5656, ext. 7078

Diabetes-Related Sites on the Internet
www.diabetes.org/internetresources.asp

Sensory Testing Systems
1815 Dallas Dr., Suite 11A
Baton Rouge, LA 70806-1454
(888) 289-9293

References

Allerheiligen DA et al: Hyperparathyroidism, *Am Fam Physician* 57(8):1795-1802, 1998.

American Diabetes Association: Clinical practice recommendations, *Diabetes Care* 21:S5-S31, 1998.

American Diabetes Association: www.diabetes.org. Accessed October 2002.

Barbieri M et al: Age-related insulin resistance: is it an obligatory finding? The lesson from healthy centenarians, *Diabetes/Metabolism Research Reviews* 17(1):19-26, 2001.

Barker LR, Burton JR, Zieve PD: *Principles of ambulatory medicine,* ed 6, Philadelphia, 2003, Lippincott Williams & Wilkins.

Boonen S et al: Primary hyperparathyroidism: pathophysiology, diagnosis and indications for surgery, *Acta Otorhinolaryngol Belg* 55(2):119-127, 2001.

Braithwaite SS et al: Managing diabetes during glucocorticoid therapy, *Postgrad Med* 104(5):163-176, 1998.

Diez JJ: Hypothyroidism in patients older than 55 years: an analysis of the etiology and assessment of the effectiveness of therapy, *J Gerontol A Biol Sci Med Sci* 57(5): M315-M320, 2002.

Kanakis SJ, Watts C, Leichter SB: The business of insulin pumps in diabetes care: clinical and economic considerations, *Clin Diabetes* 20:214-216, 2002.

Kearns AE, Thompson GB: Medical and surgical management of hyperparathyroidism, *Mayo Clin Proc* 77(1): 87-91, 2002.

Kulkarni K: Managing Type 2 Diabetes: the struggle to maintain control, *Clin Rev* 12(9):62-67, 2002.

Li TM: Hypothyroidism in elderly people, *Geriatr Nurs* 23(2):88-93, 2002.

Manders JM, Corstens FH: Radioiodine therapy of euthyroid multinodular goiters, *Eur J Nucl Med Mol Imaging* 29(suppl 2):S466-S470, 2002.

O'Connor PJ, Spann SJ, Woolf SH. Care of adults with type 2 diabetes mellitus: a review of the evidence, *J Fam Pract* 47 (5)(suppl):S13-S22, 1998.

Singhal S, Johnson CA, Udelsman R: Primary hyperparathyroidism, *Orthopedics* 24(10):1003-1009, 2001.

Udelsman R: Primary hyperparathyroidism, *Curr Treat Options Oncol* 2(4):365-372, 2001.

Wallace K, Hoffman MT: Thyroid dysfunction: how to manage overt and subclinical disease in older patients, *Geriatrics* 53:32-34, 1998.

Zielinski MB et al: Oral health in the elderly with non-insulin dependent diabetes mellitus, *Special Care Dentistry* 22(3):94-98, 2002.

15

Musculoskeletal: Osteoporosis

About 10 million people living in the United States have osteoporosis (Ankrom and Blackman, 2003). Both men and women may develop osteoporosis, but women are disproportionately affected because of lower peak bone mass and the influence of menopause on bone mass. Annually 1.5 million fractures related to osteoporosis occur, the most frequent being fractures of the vertebrae (Fitzgerald, 2002). The annual cost of osteoporosis-related fractures in the United States is estimated at $8 billion. Of white women 50 to 59 years of age, 14% have osteoporosis, 22% of those 60 to 69, 39% of those age 70 to 79, and 70% of women age 80 years of age and older (Bellantoni, 2003).

The World Health Organization (WHO) has proposed a definition of osteoporosis as a deficit in bone-mineral density (BMD) of 2.5 standard deviations on or below peak bone-mineral density (BMD). This definition is based on study populations of white postmenopausal women that found a fracture prevalence of 50% in women with bone mass at this level (Bellantoni, 2003; Henry et al, 2002). There is a need to develop guidelines for more diverse populations, such as men and women of other races.

Age-related Changes

The process of osteoporosis involves increased bone resorption over bone formation. Physiologically, bone is continuously turning over, with the bony skeleton acting as a reservoir for calcium. The increase in bone resorption that causes osteoporosis is mediated primarily by the osteoclast and normally initiates bone remodeling. Increased bone formation, which is mediated primarily by the osteoblast, follows 40 to 60 days afterward. The process of osteoporosis may be primary or secondary. *Primary osteoporosis* is usually senile or postmenopausal and is mediated by estrogen. Estrogen receptors have been found in osteoclastic-like cells. Estrogen decreases bone resorption by decreasing the responsiveness of the osteoclast. *Secondary osteoporosis* may be mediated by one of several factors: vitamin D metabolites (osteomalacia), calcitonin (Paget's disease), parathyroid hormone (hyperparathyroidism or malignant tumors), thyroxine (hyperthyroidism), cortisol (Cushing's disease or exogenous cortisol excess), and other biomarkers.

Risk Factors

A slow loss of bone mass begins as a natural aspect of aging in about the 35th to 40th year of life. The amount of bone mass that a person acquires during a lifetime is influenced by genetics, nutrition, exercise, drug exposures, and health status. Bone loss is influenced by intake of beverages high in phosphates (carbonated sodas), which in turn influences excessive urinary excretion of calcium. Caffeine, alcohol, and smoking are directly harmful to bone metabolism; the use of systemic glucocorticoids has a significant negative impact on bone formation. Up to 50% of patients taking chronic corticosteroids sustain osteoporotic fractures (Lucasey, 2001).

Bone loss related to menopause can reach 4% a year for a period of 10 years, but it is important to remember that great individual variations within these ranges are found. Other risk factors include age, female gender, inadequate intake of calcium and vitamin D, lack of weight-bearing exercise, lack of sufficient body fat, weight of less than 127 pounds, and white race (Cummings and Melton, 2002; Messinger-Rapport and Thacker, 2002).

Screening and Assessment

Counseling women for lifestyle modification should be the first aspect of any program dealing with osteoporosis. These modifications include smoking cessation, weight-bearing exercise, and calcium intake. The positive benefits of certain exercise activities are reported in a study of 2914 women and 2296 men 45 to 74 years of age. Findings of the study show that bone density increases significantly only among those reporting more than 2 hours a week of high-impact physical activity (e.g., jogging). Among women, bone density was significantly increased among those reporting stair climbing or any high-impact activity. Swimming, bicycling, and walking had no detectable effect on bone density (Jakes et al, 2001).

Controversy continues about the cost-effectiveness of universal screening of postmenopausal women. The Medicare guidelines were effective as of 1998 (Box 15-1). Medicare will cover bone mass measurement once every 2 years for beneficiaries, and more frequent screening may be covered if it is considered medically necessary. Medicare reimbursement for central bone densitometry is about $140, and ultrasound studies and peripheral densitometry are reimbursed at $50 (Health Care Financing Administration, 1998).

The three current methods used for osteoporosis screening include heel ultrasound (HUS), dual-energy x-ray absorptiometry (DEXA), and quantitative computed tomography (QCT) (Moyad, 2002). DEXA is the current standard for assessing bone mass. Bone mass of the lumbar spine and hip are used for diagnostic evaluation and monitoring treatment. Inconsistencies occur within an individual's bone loss sites. For example, heel bone mass may be normal, but the same person can have clinically significant loss of the bone mass of the spine. Furthermore, vertebral compression fractures may also result in falsely elevated bone-density measurements (Bellantoni, 2003).

Box 15-1

Medicare Guidelines for Bone Densitometry

- Estrogen-deficit women at risk for osteoporosis (may include estrogen users)
- Individuals with vertebral abnormalities
- Individuals receiving chronic glucocorticoid therapy defined as prednisone 7.5 mg or greater daily for 3 months or longer
- Individuals with primary hyperparathyroidism
- Individuals being monitored in an osteoporosis drug therapy approved by the FDA

From Health Care Financing Administration Medicare Program: Medicare coverage and payment for bone mass measurements, *Federal Register* 63(121):34320, 1998.
FDA, Food and Drug Administration.

Manufacturers of the bone density machines are not standardized in their method of calibration; so bone-density readings can vary by up to 12% in some cases (Bellantoni, 2003). The same bone densitometer must be used over time to ensure correct understanding of the results of the screening. A bone-density study provides current bone mass but does not assess the rate of loss or predict the future loss level; but older women with low BMD have a risk of hip fracture more than twice the average risk of women the same age (Dargent-Molina et al, 2002).

LABORATORY STUDIES

Laboratory studies, recommended at initial diagnosis, should include serum calcium and alkaline phosphatase; if history is pertinent, serum thyroxine (T4), thyroid-stimulating hormone (TSH), and serum hydroxyvitamin D measurements should be done.

SIGNS AND SYMPTOMS

Signs and symptoms in early disease are completely absent. Signs and symptoms of advanced osteoporosis include loss of height, chronic pain secondary to muscle spasm, kyphosis with abdominal protuberance, constipation (as a result of spine curvature), pulmonary insufficiency secondary to thoracic cage deformity, painful rubbing of the ribs on the iliac crest with severe disease, and pain secondary to vertebral or hip fracture. Nursing home residents are at high risk because of the lack of sunlight, which converts the inactive form of vitamin D to the active form involved in calcium absorption from the gut.

Secondary osteoporosis should be a consideration in the patient, male or female, with a pathologic fracture (one not associated with significant trauma or incidental findings of advanced osteoporosis noted when the patient is evaluated by radiology for other medical reasons). Other indications include chronic smokers; patients with diabetes; patients who use steroids chronically; patients with hyperparathyroidism or hyperthyroidism; those taking oral thyroxine; patients with Paget's disease, multiple myeloma, hypercalcemic states, or malabsorption syndromes; and immobilized patients.

Treatment

Initial treatment of osteoporosis should be modification of risk factors such as cessation of smoking and moderation of alcohol consumption, regular (weight resistance) exercise, and adequate dietary calcium intake (1500 mg daily for the postmenopausal and 1000 mg daily for the premenopausal female), and 400 IU of vitamin D. Secondary causes of osteoporosis should be managed by treating the underlying disease process.

Studies indicate that the process of primary osteoporosis can be slowed and to some extent prevented through regular exercise, regular calcium and vitamin D intake, and weight-bearing exercise. Immobilization and lack of exercise can hasten its onset. Prevention of osteoporosis is obviously less expensive and associated with better quality of life than treatment of hip and vertebral fractures with their associated morbidity and mortality.

PHARMACOLOGIC THERAPY

Early menopausal estrogen replacement therapy (ERT) results in maximum benefits regarding the prevention of significant bone loss. Questions arise concerning long-term use of ERT. A more detailed discussion of ERT is available in Chapter 21. The use of estrogen does carry risks and may be relatively or absolutely contraindicated in some women. Recent advances have made alternatives available for women who are unable to or choose not to take ERT.

Selective estrogen receptor modulators (SERMs) are a relatively new class of drugs that have both estrogen receptor agonist and antagonist effects. Raloxifene (Evista), the only SERM approved by the U.S. Food and Drug Administration (FDA) for treatment and prevention of osteoporosis, offers a choice for women who are unable to or choose not to take estrogen.

The FDA approval in 1998 of raloxifene offers clinical advantages over estrogen. Raloxifene significantly increased BMD of the hip, spine, and total body at 24 months' follow-up in 601 postmenopausal women but to a lesser extent than estrogen when used in doses of 30, 60, and 150 mg per day compared with placebo. No difference in the frequency of hot flashes, vaginal bleeding, or thickness of the endometrium was found in women taking raloxifene compared with placebo. The drug also had a positive effect on the lipid profile that was similar to that of estrogen (except with no increase in the high-density lipoprotein [HDL] fractions) (Delmas et al, 1997). In a study involving 390 healthy postmenopausal women involved in a double-blind, randomized, parallel trial, raloxifene did not increase the triglyceride level and significantly decreased fibrinogen levels by 12% to 14% at 3 and 6 months' follow-up, respectively. No difference was found in the incidence of the side effects of hot flashes or vaginal bleeding compared with placebo at 24 months' follow-up. Raloxifene has a profile like estrogen regarding relative contraindications, including deep venous thrombosis or history of the disease and previous pulmonary embolus (Walsh, 1998).

The effects of raloxifene on bone are comparable to ERT with a reduced risk for adverse effects on breast or endometrium, although raloxifene use has a risk of thromboembolic disease as great as or greater than estrogen. Among 5129 postmenopausal women taking raloxifene compared with 2576 women taking placebo, the incidence of breast cancer was reduced by 76% in the raloxifene group during a 40-month follow-up. The incidence of venous thromboembolic disorders was increased threefold, however (Cummings et al, 1999). Another aspect of raloxifene is that the cost of the drug is significantly higher than the traditional estrogen regimen.

The bisphosphonates constitute a class of drugs that has been shown to prevent accelerated bone loss in newly postmenopausal women. In 3-year clinical trials, alendronate (Fosamax) 10 mg daily or risedronate (Actonel) 5 mg daily reduced the risk of new vertebral and hip fractures by 50% (Harris et al, 1999). Alternative dosing of once a week of 70 mg of alendronate is an available alternative to daily therapy. The efficacy of this class of drugs is not confirmed for more than 2 years of the therapy.

Common gastrointestinial side effects include nausea, acid reflux symptoms, and constipation. Gastric and duodenal ulcers have been reported after approval of these drugs and after the original clinical trials. Significant erosion of the gastric antrum and esophagus was reported after just 7 to 14 days of treatment with alendronate (Graham et al, 1999). The combined use of bisphosphonates and nonsteroidal antiinflammatory drugs (NSAIIDs) increases the incidence of gastrointestinal bleeding and side effects. Esophageal adverse effects are significant, and any patient with a history of esophagus problems should be treated with great caution. The drug must be taken on an empty stomach with water only, and the patient must wait standing or sitting erect for 30 to 60 minutes before eating or drinking. Also, to realize the drug's potential, adequate calcium and vitamin D must be part of the daily therapy. Any patient who is unable to conform to the strict protocol for taking the drug needs daily supervision (*Physicians' Desk Reference*, 2001).

Calcitonin is considered a second-line treatment for those who cannot tolerate bisphosphonate therapy. The risk of vertebral fractures has been shown to be reduced, but the effects on the hips is not significant. Calcitonin is administered by nasal spray with one metered puff daily in alternating nostrils. Side effects include nasal irritation and rare sinusitis, epistaxis, or rhinitis. Calcitonin increases spinal bone in postmenopausal women with established osteoporosis but not in women in early menopause. Calcitonin should be used in conjunction with calcium and vitamin D (*Physicians' Desk Reference*, 2001).

Summary

Just as the cardiovascular era raised interest in cholesterol, the period of transition during which the public will become increasingly aware of media coverage of the benefits of prevention and the deleterious effects of untreated osteoporosis has been evident since the first edition of this book.

Recent events that have revolutionized the awareness and treatment of osteoporosis include published guidelines for the evaluation and management of osteoporosis, Medicare reimbursement of densitometry, and advent of the bisphosphonates and estrogen designer drugs.

Health care professionals are being bombarded by medical journals and the pharmaceutical industry regarding new therapies for osteoporosis promoting pharmacologic agents with better side effect profiles, more efficacy, lower cost, and better compliance. It is the responsibility of all primary care providers to be ever vigilant concerning new therapies and to be knowledgeable about the risks and benefits of all therapies, old and new.

Resources

Doctor's Guide to Osteoporosis: Information and Resources
www.pslgroup.com/osteoporosis.html

National Institutes of Health
Osteoporosis and Related Bone Diseases

National Resource Center
www.osteo.org

References

Ankrom MA, Blackman MR: Metabolic bone disease. In Barker LR et al: *Principles of ambulatory medicine,* ed 6, Philadelphia, 2003, Lippincott Williams & Wilkins.

Bellantoni M: Osteoporosis. In Barker LR et al: *Principles of ambulatory medicine,* ed 6, Philadelphia, 2003, Lippincott Williams & Wilkins.

Cummings SR, Melton LJ: Epidemiology and outcomes of osteoporotic fractures, *Lancet* 359(9319):1714, 2002.

Cummings SR et al: the effect of raloxifene on the risk of breast cancer in postmenopausal women: the results from the MORE randomized trial: multiple outcomes of raloxifene evaluation, *JAMA* 281:2189, 1999.

Dargent-Molina P et al: Use of clinical risk factors in elderly women with low bone mineral density to identify women at higher risk of hip fracture: the EPIDOS prospective study, *Osteoporosis Int* 13(7):593-599, 2002.

Delmas PD et al: Effects of raloxifene on bone mineral density, serum cholesterol concentrations and uterine endometrium in postmenopausal women, *N Engl J Med* 337:164-1647, 1997.

Fitzgerald P: Metabolic bone disease. In Lawerence T et al: *Current medical diagnosis and treatment: adult ambulatory and inpatient management,* ed 41, New York, 2002, Lange Medical Books—McGraw-Hill.

Graham DY et al: Alendronate gastric ulcers, *Aliment Pharmacol Ther* 13:515, 1999.

Harris ST et al: Effects of risedronate treatment on vertebral and nonvertebral fractures in women with postmenopausal osteoporosis: a randomized controlled trial. Vertebral Efficacy with Risedronate Therapy (VERT) Study Group, *JAMA* 282(14):1344-1352, 1999.

Health Care Financing Administration Medicare Program: Medicare coverage and payment for bone mass measurements, *Federal Register* 63(121):34320, 1998.

Henry MJ et al: Fracture thresholds revisited, Geelong Osteoporosis Study, *J Clin Epidemiol* 55(7):642-646, 2002.

Jakes RW et al: Patterns of physical activity and ultrasound attenuation by heel bone among Norfolk cohort of European Prospective Investigation of Cancer (EPIC Norfolk): population based study, *BMJ* 322:140, 2001.

Lucasey B: Corticosteroid–induced osteoporosis. *Nurs Clin North Am* 36(3):455-466, 2001.

Messinger-Rapport BJ, Thacker HL: Prevention for the older woman: a practical guide to prevention and treatment of osteoporosis. *Geriatrics* 57(4):16-18, 21-24, 27, 2002.

Moyad MA: Osteoporosis—Part I: Risk factors and screening. *Urol Nurs* 22(4):276-279, 2002.

Physicians' Desk Reference, ed 56, Montvale, NJ, 2001, Medical Economics.

Walsh BW et al: Effects of raloxifene on serum lipids and coagulation factors in healthy postmenopausal women, *JAMA* 279(18):1445-1451, 1998.

16

Musculoskeletal: Common Injuries

Age-related Changes

Musculoskeletal problems are among older adults' most common complaints. They affect quality rather than quantity of life and often lead to disabilities that are costly to manage. Muscular changes include a decrease in the strength and speed of contraction of the muscles in the extremities, although overall muscle endurance is minimally affected. Bone mass decreases significantly after 35 years of age, with declines of 0.5% to 1% per year. Women suffer increased bone loss, especially during the first 5 years after menopause. In the United States, of the 10 million people who have osteoporosis, two million are men (Ankrom and Blackman, 2002).

Degenerative arthritis is a disorder of movable joints resulting from cartilage degeneration. It is associated with mild, inflammatory degeneration in the synovium and with faulty bone and cartilage regeneration. Between one third and half of the adult population have radiographic evidence of osteoarthritis, with a striking rise in prevalence that parallels advancing age. Men and women are affected with equal frequency, but the findings are more advanced and generalized in women. Musculoskeletal disease is not an inevitable consequence of aging and thus should be regarded as a specific disease process, not just the result of normal aging.

Social Changes

With increased emphasis on maintaining physical fitness throughout the life span, participation of older people in all types of recreational activities and exercise training activities has increased. As a result more older people with minor injuries seek professional advice for treatment that will restore their ability to continue their participation. Because a lack of fitness increases the likelihood of risk of injury, the primary care provider needs to assess the older person's baseline fitness (Byank et al, 2002). The following questions should be asked of patients who have minor injuries related to activities:

1. Describe the activity.
2. How long has it been since first recognition of this injury?
3. What have you done to improve your condition?
4. Describe the frequency and intensity of the physical activity.

5. Has there been a recent increase in the level of the activity?
6. Is there repetitive activity?
7. Has there been a similar injury in the past?

Neck Pain

Neck pain is a common problem. Nearly 50% of adults 50 years of age and older experience neck pain at some time. Because of the multiple sources of referred pain, as well as the many structures in the neck that may cause pain when diseased, patients who complain of new or persistent neck pain should be systematically evaluated.

The cervical spine consists of seven vertebral bodies connected by an anterior and posterior longitudinal ligament. These ligaments provide stability when the neck is flexed and extended. The vertebral bodies are joined by intervertebral disks composed of a gel-like material (the nucleus pulposus) that absorbs increased pressure applied to the spine. The nucleus pulposus is contained within an annulus fibrosus, a fibrous structure ringing the outer margin of the disk. During the fourth decade of life, both the nucleus pulposus and the annulus fibrosus undergo progressive degeneration, which is seen microscopically as a loss of the fibrous pattern and the collagen alignment. As a result, the ability of the disk to absorb shocks is reduced.

Facet joints are located between vertebral elements posteriorly, one on each side of the spine; they are apophyseal (projecting) joints with a synovium-lined capsule. Osteoarthritis (a breakdown of the articular cartilage within the joints) can occur within these small joints in the posterior spine. The intervertebral neural foramina, located laterally on either side of the vertebral bodies, are the canals through which the individual nerve roots emerge from the spinal canal. Eight pairs of nerve roots arise from the cervical spinal cord. Each nerve exits above the vertebra of the same number. Thus the sixth nerve root exits at the C5-6 disk space. Except for the first two pairs, each nerve leaves the spinal column by passing through an intervertebral foramen (Figures 16-1 and 16-2). The spinal canal and the foramina can be encroached by a bulging intervertebral disk or an osseous proliferation (bony spur) originating in a vertebral body, by a facet joint, or from the bony margin of a neural foramen. When the encroachment involves a nerve root, pain in the distribution of that root (radicular pain) can occur. The facet joint capsules and the intervertebral disk are innervated by fine nerves with simple nerve endings. When these nerve endings are stimulated by degenerative disease

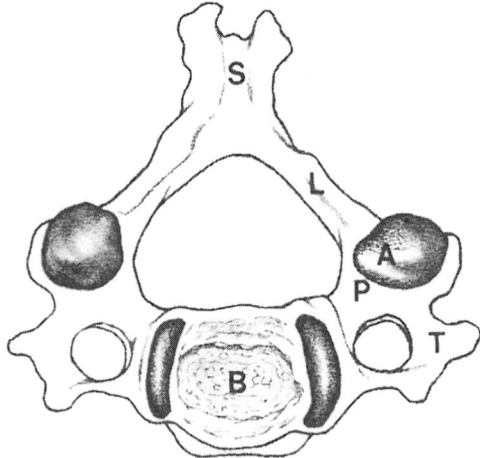

Figure 16-1   A typical cervical vertebra. *S*, Spinous process; *L*, lamina; *A*, articular facet; *P*, pedicle; *T*, transverse process; *B*, body. (From Mercier LR: *Practical orthopedics*, ed 5, St Louis, 2000, Mosby.)

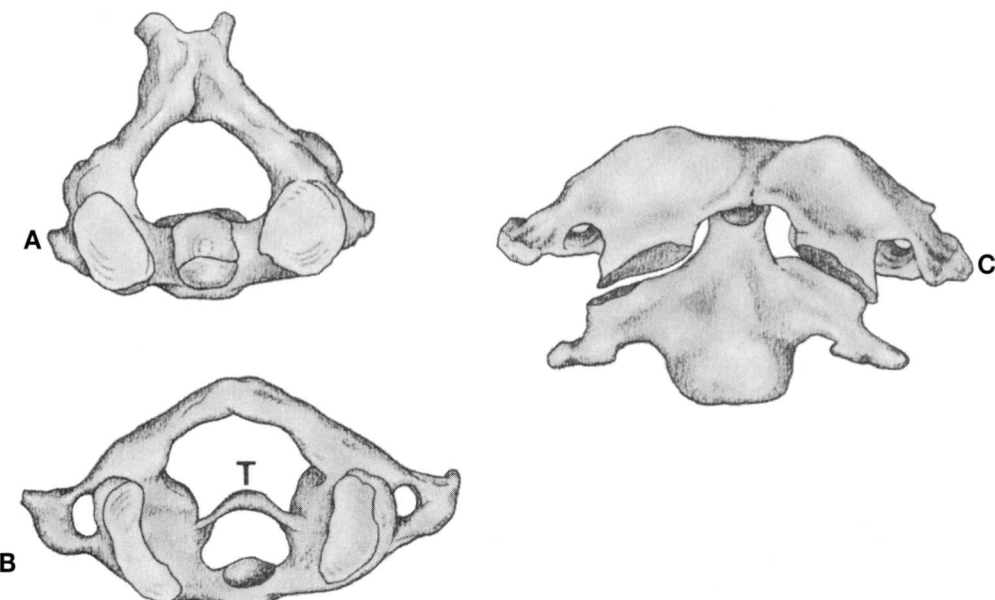

Figure 16-2   A, The axis. **B,** The atlas and transverse ligament *(T)*. **C,** Articulation of the atlas and the axis.
(From Mercier LR: *Practical orthopedics*, ed 5, St Louis, 2000, Mosby.)

within the disk or joint capsules, the patient may experience pain that is referred to the posterior aspect of the neck at any level. The pain felt in the neck may not be at the cervical level from which the nerve is arising. In addition, stimulation of the nerves can cause pain to be referred to the interscapular area, superiorly and laterally over the shoulders. Spasm of any of the many muscles of the neck region is also a common source of pain (Lenz, 2002).

Neck Ache or Strain

Neck ache or neck strain involves nonradiating discomfort or pain around the neck area and is associated with loss of motion or stiffness. It may manifest as a headache, but most often the pain is located in the middle or lower portion of the back of the neck. The source of the pain is often the ligaments of the cervical spine or surrounding muscles. Patients involved in rear-end automobile accidents, in which a relaxed person in the stationary car is struck from behind and the torso moves forward as the neck is hyperextended, may suffer acute hyperextension injuries to the neck, commonly called *whiplash.* Recoil forward flexion occurs, and the chin strikes the chest. Individuals often feel little discomfort at the scene but develop neck stiffness 12 to 14 hours after the accident.

HISTORY

- Area of maximal tenderness
- Radiation of pain
- Presence of numbness or weakness in the extremities
- Precipitating events (e.g., car accident or prolonged hyperextension, such as painting the ceiling)
- History of similar problems
- Headache or migraine
- Dizziness with lateral rotation
- Meningeal irritation signs (e.g., photophobia, fever)
- Gradual or sudden onset

- Constant or intermittent pain
- Alleviating or exacerbating activities: rest, motion
- Proper or improper neck positions at home or at work
- Bruxism (grinding or clenching the teeth) at night or jaw complaints after sleep
- Sensory impairment (vision, hearing) that causes unconscious head tilting
- Previous trauma
- Occupation
- Hobbies
- Changes in daily activity patterns

SYMPTOMS

- Headache
- Dull, aching pain exacerbated by neck motion
- Pain abated by rest or immobilization
- Pain that may be referred to other structures: scapula, posterior shoulder, occiput, or anterior chest wall
- Dysphagia (may result from an esophageal tear with hyperextension)
- Hoarseness (may result from a laryngeal tear)
- Pain in the temporomandibular joint
- Neck ache
- Neck stiffness

FOCUSED PHYSICAL EXAMINATION

- If a fracture is suspected, do not test range of motion (ROM).
- Assess for localized tender area of neck lateral to the spine.
- Assess for loss of cervical motion.
- Pain on neck motion may be variable.
- The presence of true spasm is rare, except in severe cases where the head may be tilted to one side (torticollis).
- Perform a neurologic examination (usually normal).
- Horner syndrome, nausea, and dizziness may result from longus colli muscle tears.
- Assess the strength of contraction of trapezius and sternocleidomastoid muscles.
- Inspect for laceration, swelling, or bruising.
- Palpate lymph nodes for enlargement and tenderness.

DIFFERENTIAL DIAGNOSES

- Muscle strain
- Muscle spasm
- Cervical spondylosis
- Cervical root compression
- Lymphadenopathy
- Thyroiditis
- Angina pectoris
- Meningitis
- Trigger points
- Tumor
- Infection

DIAGNOSTIC TESTS

Plain x-ray films are usually not warranted at the first visit unless the patient has a history of trauma or neurologic findings. If pain continues for longer than 2 weeks or the patient develops other physical findings, x-ray films should be obtained to rule out other conditions, such as neoplasia or instability.

It is essential to visualize the cervical spine radiologically down to C7-T1. If plain x-ray films are normal, flexion-extension x-ray films should be obtained. Any patient with neurologic findings in these circumstances should be immobilized in a collar and seen immediately by a neurosurgeon or orthopedic surgeon before flexion extension x-ray films are taken.

A complete blood count (CBC) with differential is useful when infection or inflammatory arthritis is suspected.

TREATMENT

Therapeutics

- Immobilization in a cervical collar for no more than 2 to 4 weeks is done to prevent atrophy of nonworking muscles.
- Analgesics such as acetaminophen or nonsteroidal antiinflammatory drugs (NSAIDs) are administered.
- Heat, either moist or dry, may provide symptomatic relief but does not speed healing.
- Activity is restricted based on the severity of symptoms. "Let pain be your guide."
- Narcotics may be administered for the first 2 weeks if necessary but should be avoided.

Education

- Encourage the patient to perform work and daily activities as much as possible. When the pain subsides and the patient has full ROM without muscle spasm, the cervical collar can be gradually discontinued. Initially decrease the length of time the collar is worn during the day; however, instruct the patient to continue using the collar at night, when the neck is unprotected and subjected to awkward movements. Once the patient is pain free, use of the cervical collar can be discontinued.
- When patients are pain free, they should begin a program of isometric strengthening exercises. Using the hand for resistance, the muscles controlling flexion, extension, rotation, and lateral bend should be strengthened.
- If the patient has severe pain and muscle spasm at initial injury, the clinical course will probably last 4 to 6 weeks.
- If headaches persist, consider head computed tomography (CT) studies.
- If arm or shoulder pain persists, consider a neck and thoracic CT to rule out conditions such as mass or brachial plexus injury.
- If tests are negative for organic causes of pain, consider emotional overlay.
- Although medications such as NSAIDs may be adjuncts to pain relief, they do not alter the natural history of the disorder.
- The patient should avoid driving during the acute phase, when neck mobility is limited.
- Teach the patient proper body mechanics for sitting, standing, lifting, and so on.

Follow-up

Because this condition is usually self-limited, follow-up or referral to a specialist is dictated by either worsening symptoms or the persistence of symptoms after 4 to 6 weeks (Figure 16-3).

Cervical Spondylosis

Degenerative disease of the disk and facet joints is included under this heading because it occurs simultaneously and may be difficult to distinguish clinically. This condition is commonly encountered in people over 45 years of age.

Cervical spondylosis is thought to result from chronic cervical disk degeneration with herniation of disc material, secondary calcification, and associated osteophytic outgrowths (Aminoff, 2001). Cervical nerve roots may be compressed, stretched, or angular. Myelopathy may also develop related to compression, vacular insufficiency, or recurrent minor trauma to the spinal cord.

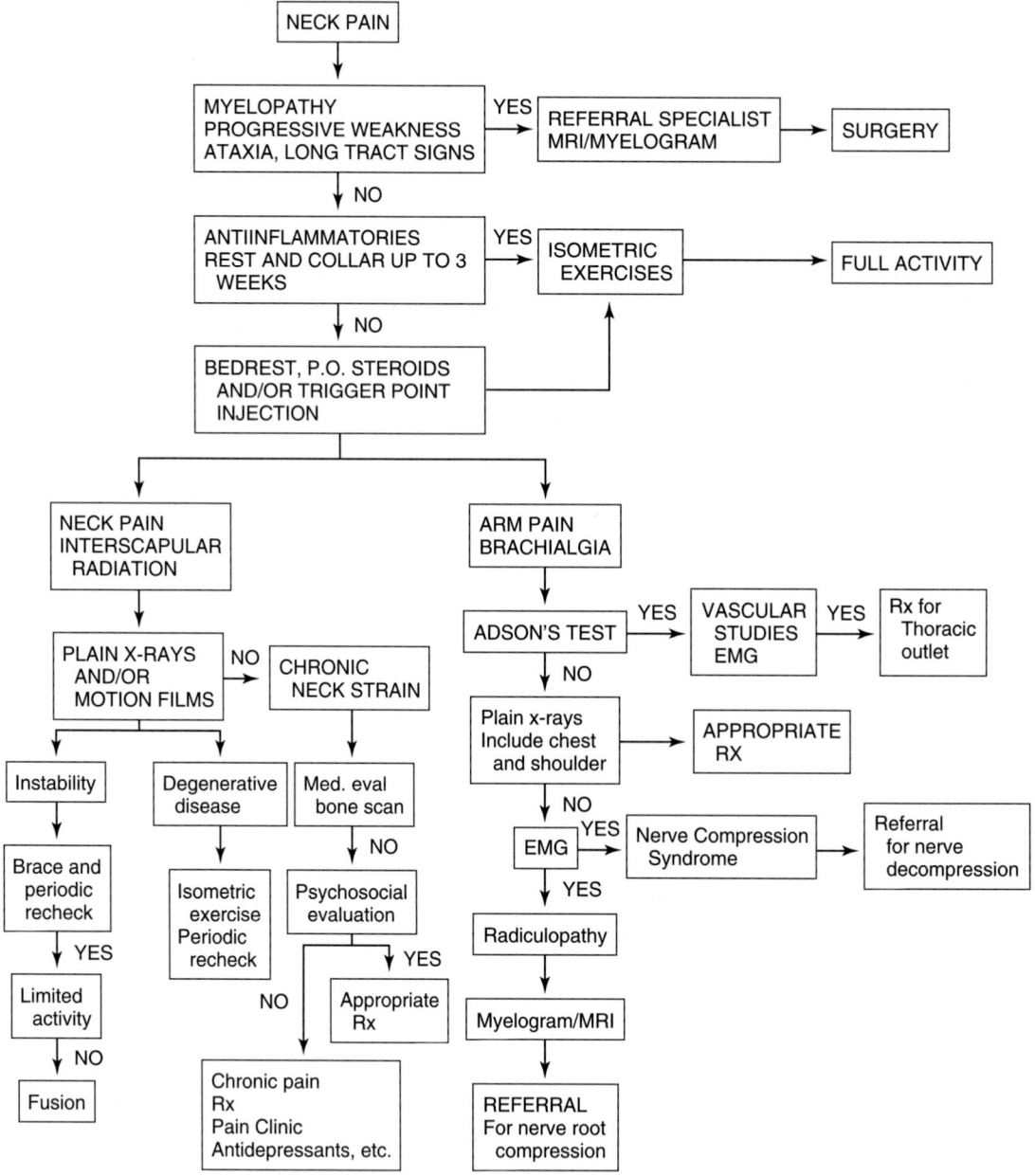

Figure 16-3 Cervical spine algorithm.

HISTORY

- Past neck pain
- Onset of symptoms that is usually insidious but may be acute, with exacerbations and remissions
- Acute exacerbations that may be brought on by excessive activity, such as reading (especially with bifocals) or painting a ceiling with the neck in extension
- Pain that is aggravated by movements and may be worse after activities

- Compression fracture
- Pain that is relieved by lying down and avoiding certain activities
- Symptoms that improve when the patient is at rest or asleep
- Proper or improper neck positions at home or at work
- Bruxism (grinding or clenching the teeth) at night or jaw complaints after sleep
- Sensory impairment (vision, hearing) that causes unconscious head tilting
- Previous trauma
- Motor vehicle accident
- Occupation
- Hobbies
- Changes in daily activity patterns

SYMPTOMS

- Occipital headache
- Neck pain with referred pain patterns
- Restricted head movement
- Pain in the shoulder or arm with possible radiation to one side
- Sensory disturbances in arms with weakness of arms or legs
- Tendon reflexes of affected nerve root are depressed
- Most commonly affected nerve roots are C5 and C6 (Aminoff, 2001)

FOCUSED PHYSICAL EXAMINATION

- Inspection: Patient avoids all movements of the neck and holds it still and straight.
- Normal lordosis of the cervical spine is lost.
- Paraspinal muscles may be tender and firm because of muscle spasms.
- Coexisting localized trigger points are present.
- Compression test: **This test should not be performed if instability of the cervical spine is suspected.** While the patient is in a sitting position, downward pressure is exerted with the palms of the examiner's hands placed on the patient's head. This test may reproduce pain if narrowing of the intervertebral foramen and pressure on the nerve root are present. If there is no pain, the patient is asked to bend the neck to the affected side, and similar pressure is exerted.
- A neurologic examination is performed.

DIFFERENTIAL DIAGNOSES

- Trigger points of the paraspinal muscles
- Carpal tunnel syndrome
- Peripheral neuropathy
- Prolapsed intervertebral disk
- Tumor
- Infection

DIAGNOSTIC TESTS

Anteroposterior (AP), lateral, and oblique radiographs of the cervical spine in cervical spondylosis show varying degrees of changes: disk space narrowing, osteophytosis, foraminal narrowing, degenerative changes of the facets, and instability. These findings, however, do not necessarily correlate with symptoms. In large part, the radiographs serve to rule out more serious causes of neck and referred pain, such as tumors. Further diagnostic testing is usually not warranted.

TREATMENT

Therapeutics

- Rest
- Immobilization in a cervical collar

- Analgesics: aspirin, acetaminophen, or NSAIDs must often be administered on a chronic basis or at least intermittently.
- Triggerpoint injections with local anesthetics (lidocaine) and corticosteroids (triamcinolone)
- Isometric exercises for neck strengthening: using the hand for resistance, strengthening of the muscles controlling flexion, extension, rotation, and lateral bend
- Restricted activity based on severity of symptoms

Education

- Educate the patient regarding proper sleep positions (e.g., side-lying versus prone) and proper body mechanics for sitting, standing, lifting, and so on.
- When the patient's pain subsides, the cervical collar can be gradually discontinued. Initially decrease the length of time the collar is worn during the day; however, instruct the patient to continue using the collar at night, when the neck is unprotected and subjected to awkward movements. Once the patient is pain free, use of the collar can be discontinued.
- Although medications such as NSAIDs may be adjuncts to pain relief, they do not alter the natural history of the disorder.

Follow-up

Follow-up or referral to a specialist is dictated by either worsening or persistence of symptoms.

Cervical Spondylosis with Radiculopathy

Aching or burning pain that follows a radicular distribution (dermatome) is cervical spondylosis with radiculopathy. Most often the C5-6 and C6-7 interspaces are involved, with compromise of the sixth and seventh cervical roots, respectively.

HISTORY

- Aching or burning pain that follows a radicular or dermatomal distribution
- Symptoms that are worse at rest or during sleep than at other times
- Proper or improper neck positions at home or at work
- Bruxism (grinding or clenching the teeth) at night or jaw complaints after sleep
- History of migraine
- Sensory impairment (vision, hearing) causing unconscious head tilting
- Previous trauma
- Motor vehicle accident
- Occupation
- Hobbies
- Changes in daily activity patterns

SYMPTOMS

- Pain in neck, shoulder, medial border of scapula, lateral arm, and dorsal forearm, with sensory changes in the thumb and index finger, indicate compromise of C6 nerve root.
- Pain plus sensory changes in the index and middle finger suggests a C7 lesion.

FOCUSED PHYSICAL EXAMINATION

Neurologic examination: Motor and reflex changes involving the biceps indicate C6 compromise versus triceps changes indicate C7 compromise (Table 16-1).

DIFFERENTIAL DIAGNOSES

- Trigger points of the paraspinal muscles
- Cervical spondylosis

TABLE 16-1		Symptoms and Findings in Cervical Radiculopathy

Disk Level	Nerve Root	Symptoms and Findings
C2-3	C3	**Pain:** Back of neck, mastoid process, pinna of ear **Sensory change:** Back of neck, mastoid process, pinna of ear **Motor deficit:** None readily detectable except by EMG **Reflex change:** None
C3-4	C4	**Pain:** Back of neck, levator scapula, anterior chest **Sensory change:** Back of neck, levator scapula, anterior chest **Motor deficit:** None readily detectable except by EMG **Reflex change:** None
C4-5	C5	**Pain:** Neck, tip of shoulder, anterior arm **Sensory change:** Deltoid area **Motor deficit:** Deltoid, biceps **Reflex change:** Biceps
C5-6	C6	**Pain:** Neck, shoulder, medial border of scapula, lateral arm, dorsal forearm **Sensory change:** Thumb and index finger **Motor deficit:** Biceps **Reflex change:** Biceps
C6-7	C7	**Pain:** Neck, shoulder, medial border of scapula, lateral arm, dorsal forearm **Sensory change:** Index and middle finger **Motor deficit:** Triceps **Reflex change:** Triceps
C7-T1	C8	**Pain:** Neck, medial border of scapula, medial aspect of arm and forearm **Sensory change:** Ring and little finger **Motor deficit:** Intrinsic muscles of hand **Reflex change:** None

Adapted from Wiesel SW, Delahay JN: *Essentials of orthopaedic surgery,* ed 2, Philadelphia, 1997, Saunders.

- Carpal tunnel syndrome
- Peripheral neuropathy
- Prolapsed intervertebral disk
- Radiculopathy
- Tumor
- Infection

DIAGNOSTIC TESTS

Lateral, AP, and oblique radiographs of the cervical spine show varying degrees of changes with cervical spondylosis: disk space narrowing, osteophytosis, foraminal narrowing, degenerative changes of the facets, and instability. These findings, however, do not necessarily correlate with symptoms. In large part, radiographs serve to rule out more serious causes of neck and referred pain, such as tumors.

TREATMENT

Therapeutics

- Rest: Restricted activity based on severity of symptoms
- Immobilization in a cervical collar

- Analgesics: acetaminophen or NSAIDs
- Triggerpoint injections with local anesthetics (lidocaine) and corticosteroids (triamcinolone)
- Isometric exercises for neck strengthening: using the hand for resistance, strengthening of the muscles controlling flexion, extension, rotation, and lateral bend
- Possible use of cervical traction, in slight flexion, of 5 to 10 pounds
- Heat, either moist or dry, which may provide symptomatic relief

Education

- Educate patient regarding proper sleep positions (e.g., side-lying versus prone) and proper body mechanics for sitting, standing, lifting, and so on. Chiropractic manipulation is contraindicated.
- For 75% to 80% of persons with radiculopathy, nonsurgical interventions are successful in relieving pain.
- When the patient's pain subsides, the cervical collar can be gradually discontinued. Initially decrease the length of time the collar is worn during the day; however, instruct the patient to continue using the collar at night, when the neck is unprotected and subjected to awkward movements.
- Although medications such as NSAIDs can be used as adjuncts to pain relief, they do not alter the natural history of the disorder.

Follow-up

If these therapeutic measures fail, referral to a neurosurgeon or orthopedist for intervention may be appropriate.

Cervical Myelopathy

When the secondary bony changes of cervical spondylosis encroach on the spinal cord, a pathologic process called *myelopathy* develops. If this process involves both the spinal cord and nerve roots, it is called *myeloradiculopathy*. Regardless of its etiology, radiculopathy causes shoulder or arm pain (Wiesel and Boden, 1997).

Myelopathy is the most serious sequela of cervical spondylosis and is the most difficult to treat effectively. Fewer than 5% of patients with cervical spondylosis develop myelopathy, and they are usually between 40 and 60 years of age. The changes of myelopathy are most often gradual and are associated with posterior osteophyte formation (spondylitic bone or hard disk) and spinal canal narrowing (spinal stenosis). Acute myelopathy is most often the result of a central soft disk herniation that produces a high-grade block that may be visualized on myelogram.

HISTORY

- Cervical spondylosis

SYMPTOMS

- Patients gradually notice a peculiar sensation in the hands that is associated with clumsiness and weakness.
- Lower-extremity symptoms may include difficulty in walking, peculiar sensations, leg weakness, and spasticity. These symptoms may antedate the upper extremity findings.
- Neck pain is not a prominent feature of myelopathy.
- Abnormal urination indicates more severe disease.

FOCUSED PHYSICAL EXAMINATION

- Stooped posture; gait that is wide stance
- Possible hyperreflexia or clonus
- Upper-extremity weakness
- Loss of vibration and position sense that is more common in feet than in hands and may be unilateral
- Possible electric sensation down the spine when neck is flexed (Lhermitte's sign)

- Signs of cord compression: increased reflexes in the upper and lower extremities with a positive Babinski's sign

DIFFERENTIAL DIAGNOSES

- Cervical spondylosis
- Myelopathy
- Herniated nucleus pulposus
- Peripheral neuropathy
- Multiple sclerosis
- Localized compression of vascular structures
- Peripheral nerve entrapment
- Spinal stenosis
- Tumor
- Infection

DIAGNOSTIC TESTS

- X-ray films of the cervical spine often reveal advanced degenerative disease, including spinal canal narrowing by prominent posterior osteophytosis, variable foraminal narrowing, disk space narrowing, facet joint arthrosis, and instability.
- Congenital stenosis of the cervical canal is often seen; this condition predisposes the patient to the development of myelopathy.
- Consider a myelogram.
- Consider magnetic resonance imaging (MRI).

TREATMENT

Therapeutics

Conservative therapy that consists of immobilization and rest with a soft cervical collar and cervical pillow offers a viable option to the patient with myelopathy who is not a good operative risk. Surgery is clearly indicated if the myelopathy is progressive despite a trial of conservative treatment. Surgical decompression yields satisfactory results in 75% to 80% of cases.

- Local heat
- Gentle ROM exercises
- Analgesics: acetaminophen or NSAIDs, which may help to relieve pain
- Injection of triggerpoints with local anesthetic agents (xylocaine), which provides immediate relief of pain
- Physical therapy

Education

- Educate the patient regarding proper sleep positions (e.g., side-lying versus prone) and proper body mechanics for sitting, standing, lifting, and so on.
- Chiropractic manipulation is contraindicated.
- Although medications such as NSAIDs may be adjuncts to pain relief, they do not alter the natural history of the disorder.

Follow-up

Referral to an orthopedist or neurosurgeon should be considered if symptoms persist despite conservative measures.

Cervical Herniated Nucleus Pulposus

Protrusion of the nucleus pulposus through the fibers of the annulus fibrosus produces cervical herniated nucleus pulposus. Most acute disk herniations occur posterolaterally around the fourth decade of life, when the nucleus is still gelatinous. The most common areas of disk herniation are C5-6 and C6-7. Unlike the lumbar herniated disk, the cervical herniated disk may cause both myelopathy and radiculopathy because of the presence of the spinal cord in the cervical region (Wiesel and Delahay, 1997).

Disk herniation usually affects the root numbered lowest for the given disk level (e.g., the C5-6 disk affects the sixth cervical root, and the C6-7 disk affects the seventh cervical root).

Not every herniated disk is symptomatic. The presence of symptoms depends on the spinal reserve capacity, the presence of inflammation, the size of the herniation, and the presence of concomitant disease, such as osteophyte formation.

HISTORY

- Symptoms that are worse when at rest or asleep than at other times
- Proper or improper neck positions at home or at work
- Bruxism (grinding or clenching the teeth) at night or jaw complaints after sleep
- History of migraine
- Sensory impairment (vision, hearing) that causes unconscious head tilting
- Previous trauma
- Motor-vehicle accident
- Occupation
- Hobbies
- Changes in daily activity patterns

SYMPTOMS

The major complaint is arm pain, not neck pain. The pain is often perceived as starting in the neck area, but it radiates from this point down the shoulder, forearm, and usually into the hand, commonly in a dermatomal distribution.

The onset of radicular pain is often gradual, although there can be a sudden onset associated with a tearing or snapping sensation.

As time passes, the magnitude of the arm pain clearly exceeds that of the neck or shoulder pain. The arm pain can vary in intensity from severe enough to precluding any use of the arm without severe pain to a dull cramping ache in the arm muscles with use of the arm. The pain is usually severe enough to awaken the patient at night.

FOCUSED PHYSICAL EXAMINATION

There is motion limitation in the neck. Occasionally, the patient may tilt head in a "cocked robin" toward the side of the herniated disk.

Extension of the spine often exacerbates the pain because it further narrows the intervertebral foramina. Axial compression, the Valsalva maneuver, and coughing may also recreate or exacerbate the pain pattern.

Palpate the posterior neck muscles for spasm and symmetry. Determine whether shoulder ROM elicits pain within the shoulder itself.

The presence of a positive neurologic finding is the most helpful aspect of the diagnostic workup, although the neurologic examination may remain normal despite a chronic radicular pattern. To be significant, the neurologic examination must show objective signs of reflex diminution, motor weakness, or atrophy. An objective sensory deficit is one that conforms to a dermatomal distribution.

DIFFERENTIAL DIAGNOSES

- Herniated nucleus pulposus
- Cervical myelopathy
- Cervical radiculopathy

- Shoulder impingement
- Carpal tunnel syndrome
- Infection
- Tumor

DIAGNOSTIC TESTS

Plain x-ray films are usually not diagnostic; however, disk space narrowing may be visualized in the AP view. The value of an x-ray examination is to exclude other causes of neck and arm pain. Tests such as an electromyogram (EMG) or MRI are confirmatory examinations and should not be used as screening tests because misinformation may ensue.

TREATMENT

Therapeutics

- Immobilization in a soft cervical collar and rest
- Decreased activity for at least 2 weeks
- Analgesics: acetaminophen or NSAIDs
- Avoid narcotics, which can be administered for the first 2 weeks if necessary

Education

- A well-informed patient who is willing to follow through on suggestions will have improved outcomes.
- Educate the patient regarding proper body mechanics, such as sitting, standing, and lifting.
- Educate the patient regarding the proper use of the cervical collar: Wear it 24 hours per day for the first 2 weeks.
- When the pain subsides and the patient has full ROM without muscle spasm or radicular pain, the cervical collar can be gradually discontinued. Initially decrease the length of time the collar is worn during the day; however, instruct the patient to continue using the collar at night, when the neck is unprotected and subjected to awkward movements. Once the patient is pain free, use of the cervical collar can be discontinued.
- Although medications such as NSAIDs may be adjuncts to pain relief, they do not alter the natural history of the disorder.

Follow-up

Most patients respond to a 4- to 6-week course of conservative treatment. Follow-up or referral to a specialist is dictated by either worsening or persistence of symptoms.

SHOULDER PAIN

Shoulder pain is a frequently encountered complaint in adult primary care practice. Prevalence ranges from 8% to more than 20% in the population 30 years of age and older, and it is most prevalent in the older population (Kerr, 2002). A proper diagnosis requires (1) a sound understanding of the anatomy of the shoulder region, (2) a realistic differential diagnosis, and (3) a focused history and physical examination.

Pain originating in the shoulder region, as opposed to referred pain, is typically exacerbated by activities requiring ROM. The shoulder is best described as a region (Figures 16-4 to 16-6) of three large bones (the scapula, clavicle, and humerus) and four joints (the glenohumeral, sternoclavicular, acromioclavicular [AC], and scapulothoracic). Most of the shoulder's stability depends on muscular and ligamentous attachments. The acromion projects from the scapula to form the roof of the shoulder. Together with the coracoid and attaching ligaments, it forms a socket called the *glenoid fossa*. The ball-like head of the humerus is cradled here, forming the glenohumeral joint, or shoulder joint.

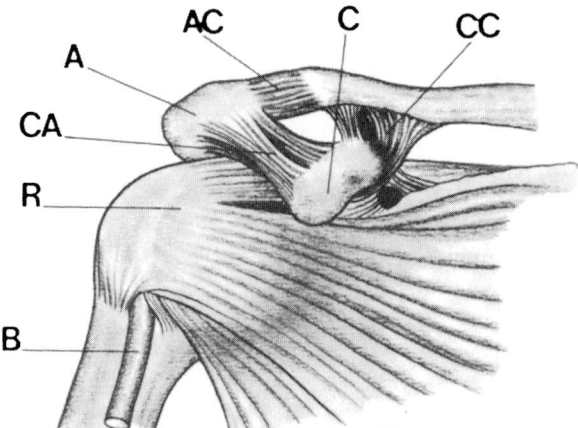

Figure 16-4   Bones and ligaments of the shoulder. *R,* rotator cuff; *B,* long head of the biceps; *AC,* acromio-clavicular joint capsule; *CC,* coracoclavicular ligaments; *A,* acromion; *C,* coracoid process; *CA,* coracoacromial ligaments. (From Mercier LR: *Practical orthopedics,* ed 5, St Louis, 2000, Mosby.)

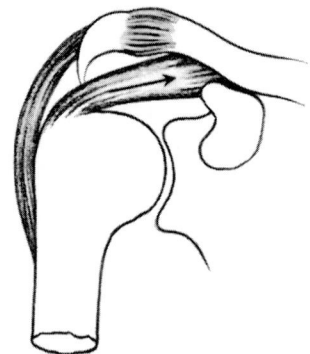

Figure 16-5   Abduction of the shoulder. By stabilizing the humeral head in the glenoid *(arrow),* the superior portion of the rotator cuff prevents it from being forced into the acromion by the deltoid muscle. (From Mercier LR: *Practical orthopedics,* ed 5, St Louis, 2000, Mosby.)

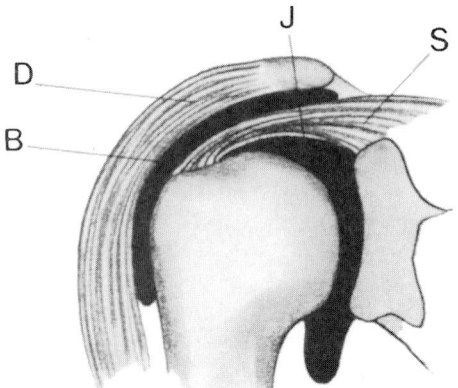

Figure 16-6   The subacromial bursa *(B)* is shown between the deltoid *(D)* and supraspinatus *(S)* muscles. Deep to the rotator cuff is the glenohumeral joint cavity *(J).* (From Mercier LR: *Practical orthopedics,* ed 5, St Louis, 2000, Mosby.)

The shallow glenohumeral joint, the lax ligamentous capsule, and the interplay of the other regional joints allow maximum mobility.

This mobility comes at a price, however. The shoulder's dependence on soft tissue articulation makes it vulnerable to injury and accounts for the relatively high prevalence of problems in this region. The most significant shoulder stabilizers are the four scapulohumeral muscles collectively known as the *rotator cuff.* These supraspinatus, infraspinatus, subscapularis, and teres minor muscles function in countertraction to abduction by the deltoid muscle. The tendons of these muscles converge under the acromion and coracoid processes and attach to the capsular ligaments. The tendon of the long head of the biceps runs through the joint capsule and along the bicipital groove of the humerus. Between the acromion and the rotator cuff lies a bursa that cushions the tendon from the bone. This small sac is a common trouble spot. The shoulder anatomy is unique in that surrounding bursae communicate with the joint, thus providing a pathway for extraarticular infection to invade the joint (Sykes, 1997).

Dermatomes represented in the shoulder area are those originating from C4, C5, and T1-4. In addition, the sensory branch of the axillary nerve (C5) supplies the area over the deltoid.

A rotator cuff tear should be considered in all patients over 40 years of age, even though they may not complain of severe pain or limitations in activity. For individuals under age 70, the prevalence is 30%. For persons 71 to 80 years of age the prevalence is nearly 60%, and for those over 80, nearly 70%. Older patients who have mild chronic impingement symptoms but sustain an episode of trauma may experience tears of the rotator cuff. The most common differential diagnosis in patients who experience shoulder pain with exertion of the joint is rotator cuff tear. Another key point to keep in mind during the evaluation of shoulder pain is that disorders can coexist (Millstein, 1997).

With the anatomy of the shoulder region in mind, the practitioner can arrive at a differential diagnosis by examining the pathophysiology and clinical epidemiology of shoulder pain in the adult patient population. Despite advances in sophisticated imaging studies, the history and physical examination remain the benchmark of diagnostic success.

HISTORY

The most common complaints are pain, stiffness, instability, and weakness. In reviewing the history, consider the following points:

- Whether the pain has a sudden or insidious onset
- Whether it is a burning pain or a dull ache over the shoulder
- Cervical spine symptoms: neck pain, neck stiffness, paresthesias (Figure 16-7)
- Pain that occurs during a specific activity or with a particular position
- Nocturnal awakening
- Pain at rest
- Stiffness
- Weakness (the least common complaint)
- Activities the patient is unable to perform: lift arm over the head, wash under opposite axilla
- History of trauma: whether or not the patient has experienced a snapping, popping, or tearing sensation
- Gastrointestinal, pulmonary, or cardiovascular symptoms
- Arm dominance
- Current medications
- Allergies
- Occupation
- Hobbies
- Alleviating factors

FOCUSED PHYSICAL EXAMINATION

The five components to the physical examination are inspection, palpation, ROM, strength, and neurovascular examination:

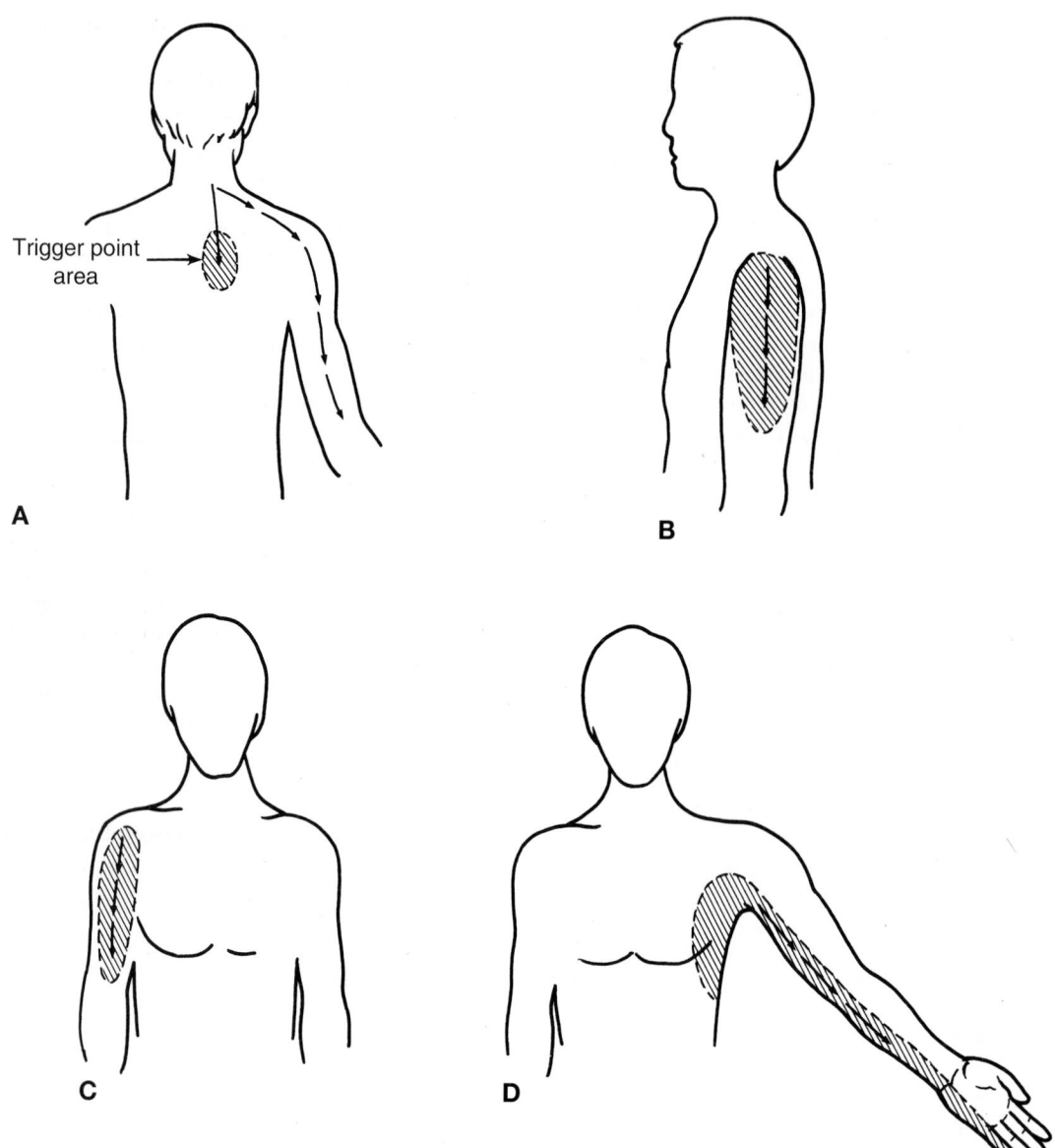

Trigger point area

A

B

C

D

Figure 16-7 General pain distribution of common neck and arm disorders. **A,** Cervical disk syndrome; **B,** Rotator cuff syndrome; **C,** Bicipital tendinitis; **D,** Disorders involving the lower portion of the brachial plexus (Pancoast tumor, thoracic outlet syndrome). When the shoulder pain has a visceral origin, the patient sometimes recognizes it as "deep" and perhaps not arising in the exact region where it is felt. (From Mercier LR: *Practical orthopedics,* ed 5, St Louis, 2000, Mosby.)

Inspection

- Check for shoulder symmetry, masses, swelling, erythema, ecchymosis, and muscular atrophy.
- With an AC joint separation, a stepoff at the AC joint is present.
- With an anterior shoulder dislocation, anterior fullness and lateral flatness occur.

- With a posterior shoulder dislocation, flattening of the anterior aspect of the shoulder occurs, best seen from above as the patient sits on a stool.
- With a tear of the long head of the biceps, the biceps muscle has a globular appearance.
- Note the position of the scapula in relation to the thorax and spine (Figure 16-8).
- Observe spinal curvature.

Palpation

Palpation is done to look for tenderness, masses, warmth, and crepitus. Beginning at the sternoclavicular joint, palpation follows along the clavicle to the AC joint, the coracoid, the acromion, and the scapular spine. Palpation also includes the trapezius and deltoid muscles, noting any focal tenderness over the sternoclavicular or AC joints, which indicates joint strain. Palpation then is done to look for triggerpoints along the superior border of the trapezius, paraspinal, supraspinatus, and infraspinatus muscles and the axillae for enlarged or tender lymph nodes.

Range of Motion

Never perform ROM in a traumatized, obviously fractured, or dislocated shoulder until x-ray films have been obtained. ROM of the shoulder is measured from the neutral position with the arm by the side of the body. Evaluation of forward elevation can be done by asking the patient to lift the arm overhead, and evaluation of external rotation can be done by having the patient stand with the elbows at the side and rotating the arms out as far as possible. The internal rotation is evaluated by asking the patient to put a hand behind the body and touching that hand as high as possible with the thumb on the spinal column. At this time, it is important to note the level of the spinal column reached. (The tip of the scapula is T7.) If a discrepancy is noted in comparing either side, the patient should lie supine and perform passive ROM, which disallows spine or trunk compensation. Mild restriction is common after immobilization, trauma, arthritis, or rotator cuff pathology.

Strength

Strength can be tested by asking the patient to perform a wall pushup and to shrug shoulders to assess strength of the scapular rotators. Two tests are used to assess the rotator cuff muscles. To evaluate the supraspinatus, the patient elevates both arms to 90 degrees, points the thumbs down,

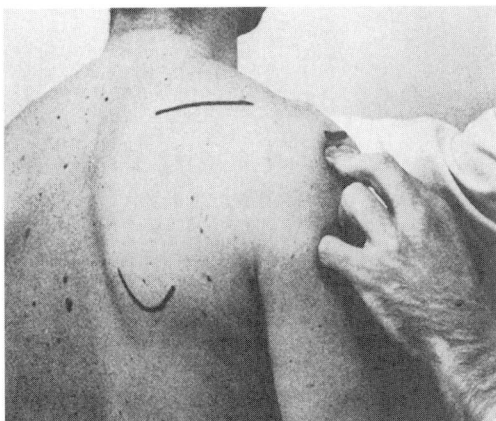

Figure 16-8   Superficial landmarks of the shoulder. The spine of the scapula lies at the level of the third dorsal vertebra. The inferior angle lies at the level of the seventh rib and eighth dorsal vertebra. The rotator cuff is palpated just distal to the acromion process. (From Mercier LR: *Practical orthopedics*, ed 5, St Louis, 2000, Mosby.)

and holds the arms at 90 degrees against resistance. If the patient exhibits weakness or an arm drops, it is considered cuff pathology. To evaluate the infraspinatus and teres minor, the patient is asked to put elbows at the side, with forearms parallel to the floor, and externally rotate against resistance.

Neurovascular Examination

- Perform thorough reflex and sensory testing. The biceps tendon correlates with the C5 nerve, the brachioradialis correlates with C6, and the triceps correlates with C7.
- Sensory: Evaluate light touch over the thumb web space (radial nerve), the radial aspect of the index finger (median nerve), and the ulnar aspect of the little finger (ulnar nerve).

DIFFERENTIAL DIAGNOSES

- Rotator cuff tendinitis or tear
- Subdeltoid or subacromial bursitis
- Adhesive capsulitis (also known as *frozen shoulder*)
- AC arthritis or strain
- Biceps tendinitis
- Cardiac sources (referred pain)
- Carpal tunnel syndrome (referred pain)
- Cerebral vascular accident with hemiparesis (referred pain)
- Cervical and neck disorders (referred pain)
- Neoplasm (local or referred pain)
- Fracture
- Dislocation
- Arthritis
- Infection
- Polymyalgia rheumatica
- Reflex sympathetic dystrophy
- Nerve entrapment
- Visceral sources (referred pain)

Most commonly, shoulder pathology falls in one of three areas: trauma (dislocations, fractures, sprains, strains), inflammation (acute rotator cuff tear or tendinitis, bursitis, adhesive capsulitis), and infection.

Trauma

Dislocation

Dislocation most commonly occurs after an outstretched hand with forceful abduction, extension, and external rotation of the shoulder. Anterior dislocation accounts for 95% of shoulder dislocations; posterior dislocations account for 5%, are less obvious, and are more likely to be overlooked on examination and on x-ray films. Posterior dislocations result from direct or indirect trauma that forces the humeral head posteriorly out of the glenoid fossa and may follow an electrical shock or convulsion.

FOCUSED PHYSICAL EXAMINATION

Anterior Dislocation

The finding of a sulcus or hollow in the skin beneath the acromion, together with fixed external rotation of the arm, should be easily diagnosed. In addition, displacement of the humeral head is seen and felt inferior to the clavicle.

The patient may have a positive apprehension test. With this test, the arm is abducted and externally rotated. Just before the joint is about to dislocate, an expression of anxiety appears on the patient's face because the patient knows the joint is about to dislocate.

Posterior Dislocation

The arm is adducted and fixed in internal rotation. Anteriorly, the shoulder contour is flattened and the coracoid process is prominent. Posteriorly, more prominence and rounding of the shoulder than normal is present, and markedly limited external rotation and elevation of the arm are seen.

DIFFERENTIAL DIAGNOSIS

- Shoulder dislocation

DIAGNOSTIC TESTS

The findings on standard AP x-ray films are subtle. An additional axillary lateral view should also be ordered to assist in revealing posterior displacement of the humeral head.

If the diagnosis is still in question after an axillary view, a CT scan should be ordered.

Dislocations can be accompanied by rotator cuff injury, neurovascular compromise (commonly the axillary nerve in anterior dislocation), or fracture; therefore posttreatment x-ray films should be obtained to evaluate these complications and ensure the adequacy of the reduction.

TREATMENT

Therapeutics

Treatment of dislocations requires prompt reduction and referral to an orthopedist or emergency department.

Education

Postreduction immobilization in a sling allows capsular structures to tighten. This is followed by physical therapy to build strength. Passive exercises are started early to prevent stiffness. The range and intensity are increased as tolerated by the patient.

Follow-up

At completion of the course of physical therapy, the patient should be reevaluated. In the event of recurrent dislocation, a referral for possible surgical intervention should be considered.

Fractures

The constriction around the articular surface of the proximal end of the humerus is the anatomic neck of the humerus. The *surgical neck* is the region where the expanded proximal end meets the shaft of the humerus. Fractures commonly occur at the surgical neck (Figure 16-9). In older patients fractures usually occur after a fall, although they may accompany traumatic dislocation.

SYMPTOMS

Pain occurs in the shoulder region after a fall or dislocation. The severity of pain depends on the severity of trauma; in an older osteoporotic patient with an impacted fracture, much pain may not be present.

FOCUSED PHYSICAL EXAMINATION

The injured arm is supported by the other hand, and swelling is visible in the upper arm. Later, ecchymosis appears, which may track down to the elbow or forearm (within 1 to 2 days after fracture). Localized tenderness occurs at the fracture site. All active and passive movements are painful.

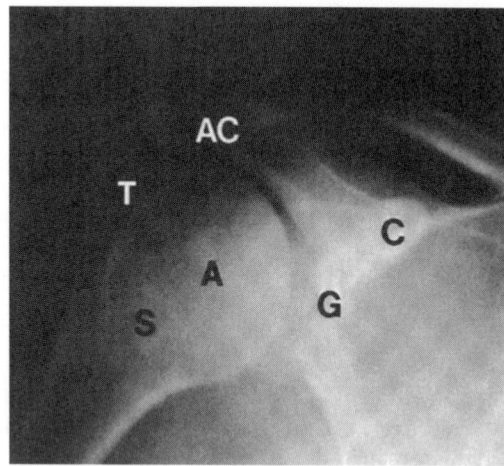

Figure 16-9   Roentgenographic anatomy of the shoulder. *S,* surgical neck of the humerus; *A,* anatomic neck of the humerus; *T,* greater tuberosity; *C,* coracoid process; *AC,* acromion process; *G,* glenoid fossa. (From Mercier LR: *Practical orthopedics,* ed 5, St Louis, 2000, Mosby.)

Evaluation by neurologic examination and radial and ulnar artery pulsations should be done to rule out axillary artery injury.

DIFFERENTIAL DIAGNOSIS

- Humeral fracture

DIAGNOSTIC TESTS

Plain x-ray film establishes the diagnosis.

TREATMENT

Therapeutics

- Referral to an orthopedist for definitive treatment
- Analgesics to control pain
- Support in a sling until evaluation by an orthopedist

Education

Gentle passive ROM exercises are started as soon as pain permits. Later, pendulum exercises and active exercises against gravity are started. Pendulum exercises may be performed with a weight (an iron works well). Patients are instructed to bend over and stabilize themselves by holding onto an object, such as a chair. They then move the arm back and forth, sideways, and in clockwise and counterclockwise circles.

Follow-up

Reevaluation of the patient should be done at completion of the course of physical therapy.

Strains and Sprains

The diagnosis of shoulder strain is reserved for a muscle injury, usually of the large deltoid muscle, and is a diagnosis of exclusion. When all other conditions have been ruled out and the shoulder is sore from an acute injury, look to the muscles as the cause, and look to rest, ice, and compression as the treatment (Sykes, 1997).

Inflammation

Rotator Cuff Tendinitis

Tendinitis is the most common cause of shoulder pain. The tendinous fibers of the rotator cuff muscles undergo degenerative changes with advancing age. The tendons, particularly the supraspinatus (which are the most superior), are thought to be worn down by repetitive excursion between the greater tuberosity of the humerus and the acromion and the AC ligament. Pain is caused by edema, hemorrhage, and inflammation associated with the repeated trauma. *Impingement syndrome* and *pericapsulitis* are less specific terms applied to these degenerative and inflammatory disorders of the tendons and bursae. Risk factors for tendinitis include repetitive overhead work or activities and increasing age.

SYMPTOMS

- Acute severe pain occurs in the shoulder.
- Radiation of pain depends on the severity of the lesion.
- Initially, all movements may be painful.
- Pain radiates laterally to the deltoid insertion.

FOCUSED PHYSICAL EXAMINATION

- Pain on resisted abduction

Painful Arc Sign

The patient should be asked to perform abduction from the resting position. At 45 degrees of abduction, pain can be felt as inflamed tissue is forced under the acromion. Pain persists until the 120-degree portion of the arc is reached. The tissue has now moved from under the acromion. No pain from 120 to 180 degrees is present. Passive ROM is normal or exceeds active ROM, which may or may not be limited by pain.

Drop Sign

The arm is passively abducted to 180 degrees, and the patient is asked to let it come down slowly to the neutral position. At about 90 degrees of abduction, the arm falls abruptly because of weakness. The smooth lowering of the arm is replaced by sudden drop.

DIFFERENTIAL DIAGNOSES

- Rotator cuff tendinitis
- Rotator cuff tear
- Subacromial bursitis
- Bicipital tendinitis

DIAGNOSTIC TESTS

Plain x-ray films are usually normal. Degenerative changes, such as sclerosis and cysts, appear on the undersurface of the acromion and over the greater tuberosity of the humerus. Consider MRI to evaluate rotator cuff tear.

TREATMENT

Therapeutics

- NSAIDs help reduce pain and inflammation.
- Local injection of steroids may be used to reduce inflammation and pain.
- Local ice or heat may be applied.
- Physical therapy: Start with passive exercises to increase ROM.

Education

Exercises must be continued. As pain decreases and ROM increases, active assisted exercises are integrated to strengthen various muscle groups. If pain worsens with exercise, the exercises can be withheld until pain decreases and then restarted.

Follow-up

Failure to resolve symptoms with conservative therapy warrants referral to an orthopedist.

Subacromial Bursitis

The subacromial bursa and rotator cuff are squeezed between the head of the humerus and the coricoacromial arch when the arm is abducted beyond 45 to 60 degrees. Normally, full abduction is achieved by external rotation of the humerus, which helps to ease the subacromial bursa under the coricoacromial arch. Abduction of the arm becomes painful if there is swelling or inflammation in the subacromial region because of increased pressure on the inflamed structures. Clinically, subacromial bursitis, rotator cuff tendinitis, painful arc syndrome, and other impingement syndromes may present with similar symptoms, and these conditions may be difficult to distinguish from one another. Management of all these conditions is conservative and similar, however.

SYMPTOMS

- A dull ache is felt in the shoulder region and may extend down to the middle of the arm or even the wrist, depending on the severity of the condition.
- Pain is worse at night and may interfere with sleep. Movements of the shoulder, especially abduction, aggravate the pain. Sometimes the pain is severe enough to compel the patient to go to an emergency room in the middle of the night.
- The patient may describe an inability to comb hair or hook bra.

FOCUSED PHYSICAL EXAMINATION

- Inspection: Wasting of the deltoid and supraspinatus muscles may develop as a result of disuse.
- Tenderness in the subacromial region over the lateral aspect of the shoulder may be present.
- Pain may occur with active abduction beyond 50 to 60 degrees.
- Active abduction of the arm against resistance produces pain.
- A painful arc is demonstrated.

DIFFERENTIAL DIAGNOSES

- Subacromial bursitis
- Calcific tendinitis
- Fracture of greater tuberosity
- Bicipital tendinitis
- Degenerative joint disease of AC joint
- Cervical radiculopathy

DIAGNOSTIC TESTS

Plain x-ray films are usually normal. Degenerative changes, such as sclerosis and cysts, appear on the undersurface of the acromion and over the greater tuberosity of the humerus. MRI should be done to evaluate rotator cuff tear.

TREATMENT

Therapeutics

- NSAIDs to help reduce pain and inflammation
- Local injection of steroids to reduce inflammation and pain

- Local ice or heat
- Physical therapy, with passive exercises to increase ROM

Education

Continuing with exercises is important. As pain decreases and ROM increases, active assisted exercises can be done to strengthen various muscle groups. If pain worsens with exercise, the exercises can be withheld until pain decreases and then restarted.

Follow-up

Failure to resolve symptoms with conservative therapy warrants referral to an orthopedist.

Bicipital Tendinitis

With aging, the biceps tendon, like the rotator cuff tendon, is subject to inflammation, erosion, and rupture. Because the biceps tendon runs through the joint space and next to the rotator cuff and subacromial bursa, bicipital tendinitis may coexist with inflammation of these structures.

SYMPTOMS

- Pain

FOCUSED PHYSICAL EXAMINATION

Palpation elicits tenderness over the biceps tendon in the bicipital groove. The elbow is flexed to 90 degrees with the shoulder in a neutral rotation, and the palpating finger moves over the anterior aspect of the shoulder. The forearm is moved gently to rotate the humerus into a position of external and internal rotation. The long head of the biceps will slip under the palpating fingers and give rise to pain if bicipital tendinitis is present.

Tenderness over the lateral aspect of the shoulder may also be felt if coexisting rotator cuff pathology or subacromial bursitis is present. Evaluation is done by having the patient flex the elbow to 90 degrees and supinate the forearm against resistance. Then the patient flexes the shoulder forward against resistance to elicit reproducible pain over the anterior shoulder.

DIFFERENTIAL DIAGNOSES

- Bicipital tendinitis
- Rotator cuff pathology
- Degenerative arthritis of the AC joint

DIAGNOSTIC TESTS

- None: Diagnosis is mainly clinical.

TREATMENT

Therapeutics

- NSAIDs or local injection of long-acting steroid

Education

- Rest: Discontinue activities that precipitate tendinitis.
- Heat
- Gentle, passive ROM exercises; active exercises as tolerated by the patient

Follow-up

Persistence or worsening of symptoms warrants further evaluation or referral.

Adhesive Capsulitis

Adhesive capsulitis, or frozen shoulder, is of uncertain etiology but may be a sequela of shoulder pain of diverse causes, such as diabetic neuropathy, reflex sympathetic dystrophy, or previous shoulder trauma. Progressive restriction of motion occurs with this condition, usually after prolonged immobility. The glenohumeral capsule thickens, and adhesions to the humeral head form. Older patients are at especially high risk of developing adhesive capsulitis. This disorder is somewhat more common in women than in men and generally occurs in the fifth decade or later (Sykes, 1997).

SYMPTOMS

Insidious onset of diffuse pain and limitation of motion in the shoulder occur. The patient notes difficulty with reaching the arm overhead, reaching the hip pocket, or hooking the bra. Pain subsides in late stages, but stiffness persists.

FOCUSED PHYSICAL EXAMINATION

- The normal swing of the arm during walking may be limited on the affected side. Later, when the shoulder has lost all movements, wasting of the deltoid and other muscles may develop because of disuse atrophy. The arm is kept adducted and close to the body in a neutral or internally rotated position.
- Tenderness in the shoulder area occurs with palpation; however, tenderness and pain subside when inflammation is controlled.
- Initially, active ROM is affected more than passive ROM. External rotation and abduction are restricted to a greater extent than other movements.
- During the stage of inflammation, movements are restricted and painful. When inflammation subsides and fibrosis sets in, all movements are restricted and there may be little pain.

DIFFERENTIAL DIAGNOSIS

- Subacromial bursitis
- Adhesive capsulitis

DIAGNOSTIC TESTS

Plain x-ray films are not helpful because there are no abnormal findings.

TREATMENT

Therapeutics

- NSAIDs
- Injection of an anesthetic agent into the glenohumeral joint may result in improved pain control but does not result in improved ROM. Intraarticular and periarticular corticosteroid injections, weekly for several weeks, may assist in pain control and patient progress in mobility.
- Physical therapy: During the acute painful stage, very gentle exercises are prescribed. Exercises are stepped up as the patient is able to tolerate increased activity.

Education

In mostly uncontrolled trials, a combination of corticosteroid injections and progressive exercise has been associated with recovery periods of 4 to 8 weeks. In contrast, treatment with analgesics yields a recovery rate only within 2 to 3 years. Therefore the value of passive and active exercise, either with or without the guidance of a physical therapist, must be stressed as an important tool in recovery.

Follow-up

In the past, referral to an orthopedist for free capsular adhesions by manipulation of the shoulder under anesthesia was commonly recommended for patients who did not improve with conservative management. The efficacy of this treatment has not been studied in a controlled fashion, however; thus it is generally not recommended and should be considered only in recalcitrant cases.

Infection

Infection is uncommon, but any patient with immune system depression should be considered at risk. This category includes all patients with rheumatoid disease, diabetes, vascular disease, and human immunodeficiency virus. The shoulder anatomy is unique in that surrounding bursae communicate with the joint, thus providing a pathway for extraarticular infection to invade the joint. The devastating effects of irreversible cartilage damage in a septic joint make early diagnosis and treatment mandatory (Sykes, 1997).

SYMPTOMS

- Pain
- Loss of motion
- Effusion
- Increased temperature in the joint
- Arm that is usually adducted
- Sudden onset of systemic symptoms

FOCUSED PHYSICAL EXAMINATION

- X-ray films that show a widened glenohumeral joint space
- Erythematous, warm, swollen shoulder joint
- Intense pain on palpation or any attempt at ROM
- Constitutional symptoms such as fever and chills

DIFFERENTIAL DIAGNOSES

- Septic joint
- Gout
- Rotator cuff tear
- Shoulder dislocation

DIAGNOSTIC TESTS

- CBC with differential is used to rule out systemic infection.
- Blood cultures are obtained.
- Joint fluid aspiration with smear, culture, and sensitivity is used.
- Indium scan is probably the best indicator of sepsis. If the scan is negative, infection is unlikely.
- Consider a CT scan, which is helpful in identifying small lytic lesions often missed by plain films.

TREATMENT

Therapeutics

- Consult with a specialist regarding the course and treatment plan. The initial antibiotic of choice is a broad-spectrum cephalosporin followed by the appropriate antibiotic as determined by sensitivity studies. The antibiotic regimen should be altered if the patient does not respond.
- Rest the affected joint until the acute episode subsides. To avoid the development of adhesive capsulitis, introduce gentle, passive ROM exercises until the patient can tolerate more active ROM without pain.
- For an analgesic, consider narcotics.

Education
- Instruct in the appropriate use of antibiotics.
- Instruct in ROM exercises to prevent loss of motion.
- Stress the importance of follow-up.

Follow-up
- Daily phone follow-up
- Office visit in 3 days
- Follow-up with referring practitioner as necessary

Low Back Pain

Low back pain is second only to the common cold as a cause for primary care office visits. More than 75% of people 75 years of age have one or more episodes of low back pain secondary to disorders of the intervertebral disks; these episodes vary in intensity and frequency. Low back pain can be medically and economically devastating. Between 70 and 80% of the total population experience back pain at some point during their lifetime, and as many as 30% do not seek medical assistance (Borenstein, 2002).

Acute low back problems are defined as activity intolerance because of lower back or back-related leg symptoms of less than 3 months' duration. Back pain may be due to a variety of disorders, including gynecologic, genitourinary, and gastrointestinal diseases, but the most common causes are disorders of the lumbar disk. Many nonspinal conditions can masquerade as low back pain or create symptoms analogous to those commonly originating from the lumbar spine:

1. Sacroiliac joint pain: Pain is referred into the gluteal area, similar to facet joint pain.
2. Piriformis syndrome: Pain is referred in the distribution of the sciatic nerve, particularly an S1 distribution.
3. Myofascial pain: Pain referral can be radicular in quality and mimic a lumbar radiculopathy.
4. Peroneal nerve-root entrapment at the fibular head: Pain referral in the peroneal nerve distribution may mimic an L5 radiculopathy.

An additional life-threatening cause of low back pain may be a leaking abdominal aortic aneurysm, and careful evaluation of patients, especially older men with a history of hypertension, is important to exclude this diagnosis.

The structure of the lumbosacral spine is complex. The lumbar spine is composed of five vertebrae with interposed intervertebral disks that consist of a gelatinous nucleus pulposus and a surrounding annulus fibrosus (Figure 16-10). The vertebrae and disks are supported by strong ligamentous structures and paraspinous muscles. The posterior aspects of the vertebrae surround the spinal canal, form the neural foramina, and interlock to form apophyseal (facet) joints, whose main purpose is motion. The sacrum is the part of the spine that interdigitates with the iliac bones to form part of the pelvis.

An understanding of the nerve supply to the lumbosacral spine is essential in recognizing the patterns of pain associated with disease processes that affect individual anatomic components of the back. The sinuvertebral nerve is the major sensory nerve supplying structures in the lumbar spine.

Several organs are situated in the retroperitoneum, anterior to the lumbar spine. The kidneys, ureters, aorta, inferior vena cava, pancreas, and periaortic lymph nodes are retroperitoneal organs. Diseases that affect these organs may result in referred pain that is localized to the lumbar spine.

The lumbar vertebrae are exposed to tremendous forces, principally because of the magnification of stresses that result from the lever effect of the arm in lifting and the vertical forces associated with the human upright position. Because each intervertebral disk is a fluid system, hydraulic pres-

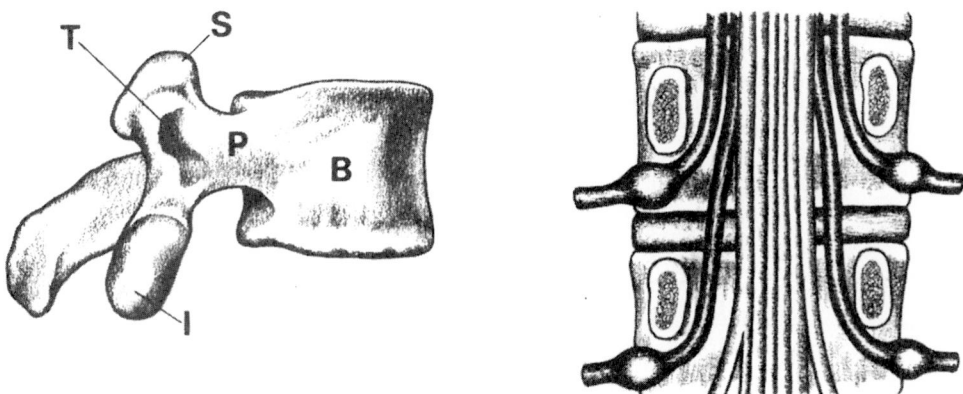

Figure 16-10   *Left:* A typical lumbar vertebra: *S,* superior articular facet; *I,* inferior articular facet; *P,* pedicle; *T,* transverse process; *B,* body. *Right:* Relationship of nerve roots to disks in the lumbar spine. (From Mercier LR: *Practical orthopedics,* ed 5, St Louis, 2000, Mosby.)

sure is created whenever a load is placed on the axial skeleton. This hydraulic pressure magnifies three to five times the force that occurs on the annulus fibrosus. This force is akin to the hoop stress that occurs in a barrel when pressure is applied to its liquid content. The ability of the annulus fibrosus to withstand stress decreases significantly with age; by 60 years of age, many persons have only 50% of the strength in these fibers that they had at 30 years of age (Borenstein, 2002).

The lumbar spine is not just an isolated structure. Much support is obtained from the muscles and ligaments of the spine and by the muscles of the thoracic and abdominal cavities. The natural history of low back pain is reported to be self-limited and to have a favorable prognosis. About 90% of patients with acute low back problems spontaneously recover activity tolerance within 1 month. In primary care, the task is to distinguish accurately between the 90% of low back complaints that are the result of simple strain or overuse and the 10% that may be caused by serious pathology (Hellmann, 2001).

As a general guideline, the patient's age can yield the first clue to diagnosis. Diseases of middle age that can cause back pain include osteomyelitis, Paget's disease, and hemangioma. The older person with back pain is most likely to have underlying neuropathy, degenerative disease, metabolic disorder, or malignancy; however, disorders can develop in any age group. A general medical review, especially in the older patient, is imperative. Metabolic, infectious, and malignant disorders may initially present as low back pain (Figure 16-11, Box 16-1).

HISTORY

The history is the most powerful diagnostic tool. A thorough history allows an accurate working diagnosis to be made in 90% of patients with low back pain. The history helps to determine the patient's current emotional state and the effect of pain on the patient's life. In reviewing the history, consider the following:

- Past medical history: diabetes, hypertension, cardiac disease, cancer, infections, rheumatologic disease, gastrointestinal disorders (tolerance for NSAIDs)
- Smoking
- Surgical history
- Present medications
- Allergies
- Operations, injuries, and previous hospitalizations
- Onset of pain: when it began

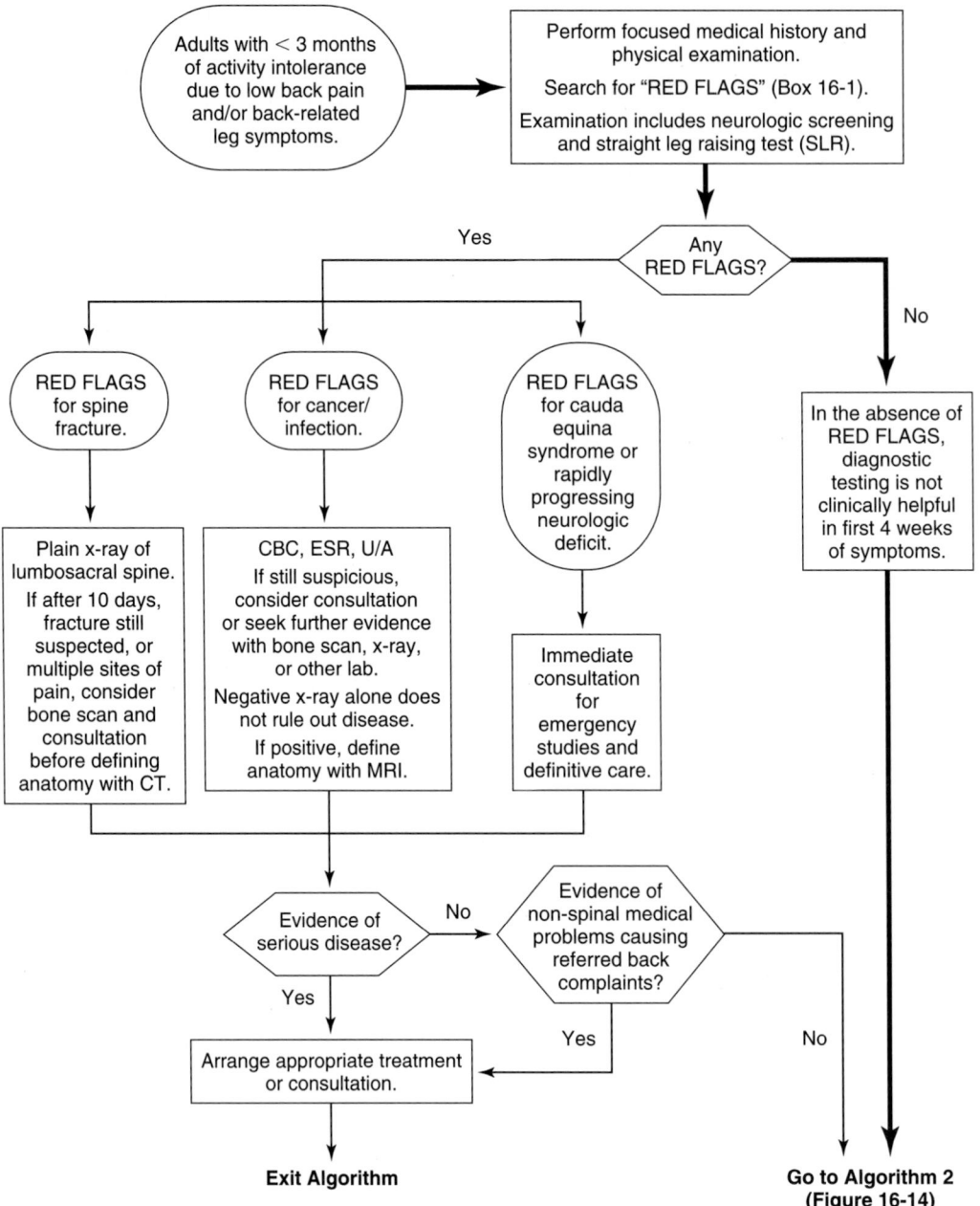

Figure 16-11   Algorithm 1. Initial evaluation of acute low back problem. (Modified from Bigos S et al: *Acute low back problems in adults: clinical guideline, quick reference guide,* AHCPR No. 95-0643, Rockville, Md, 1994, US Department of Health and Human Services.)

- How pain began: spontaneously with sudden or gradual onset or traumatically via a motor-vehicle accident or other mechanism (e.g., flexion, extension, twist, lift, fall, sneeze, cough, strain)
- Work-related injury: details of specific injury, pending litigation, compensation for time off work
- Sports-related injury

Box 16-1

Red Flags in Initial Evaluation of Acute Low Back Problem

Spinal Fractures

Significant trauma
Motor vehicle accident
Fall from height
Minor fall
Heavy lifting

Cancer/Infection

Unexplained weight loss
Immunosuppression
Intravenous drug use
Pain increased by rest
Presence of fever

Cauda Equina Syndrome

Bladder dysfunction
Saddle anesthesia
Major limb motor weakness

Modified from Bigos S et al: *Acute low back problems in adults: clinical practice guidelines, quick reference guide*, AHCPR No. 95-0642, Rockville, Md, 1994, US Department of Health and Human Services.

- Intensity of pain: Have patient assign a numeric or percent value to pain.
- Location: A pain diagram is helpful. If the patient describes primarily back pain, think of annular tear, facet syndrome, local muscular pathology, bony lesion. If the patient describes primarily distal lower-extremity pain, think of extruded or lateral herniated nucleus pulposus (HNP), stenosis, nerve lesion.
- Whether or not the location has changed over time and in response to specific treatments
- Relationship of pain to daily routine: positions that increase pain. If the answer is "prone," think of facet pain, lateral HNP, systemic process. If the answer is "sitting," think of annular tear, paramedian HNP. If the answer is "standing," think of central stenosis, facet syndrome, lateral HNP.
- Whether or not there is pain on arising from a seat, which is typical of discogenic pain
- Relationship of walking and pain: Consider distance walked, posture with walking, and whether walking up or down hills aggravates or alleviates the pain. If pain is less while walking uphill, think of stenosis because the lumbar spine is flexed, which increases the foraminal and central canal space. If pain is less when walking downhill, think of discogenic symptoms because the lumbar spine is extended and disks are unloaded. If pain is less with spinal flexion, think of stenosis.
- Time of day: If pain awakens patient from sleep, think of systemic process; if morning stiffness of a duration of 20 to 30 minutes, think of discogenic source; if it lasts 2 hours, think of rheumatic process. Does pain increase or decrease as the day progresses?
- Whether or not pain is intensified by coughing, sneezing, laughing, or Valsalva maneuver; think of discogenic source
- Reproduction of distal pain strongly supports a discogenic source
- Activities patient is unable to perform
- Positions or maneuvers that relieve the pain
- Associated neurologic symptoms: location of anesthesia, hypoesthesia, hyperesthesia, and paresthesias; regional, dermatomal, sclerotomal, or nonphysiologic
- Weakness: Differentiate inability to perform a task because of pain versus weakness.
- Bladder, bowel, or sexual dysfunction: Think of cauda equina syndrome.
- Review of systems: Include questions to investigate a differential diagnosis of organic problems such as aortic aneurysm, duodenal ulcer, abdominal tumor, fibroids, pelvic inflammatory disease, and prostate tumor.
- Emotional issues should always be considered a potential factor that could add to the patient's anxiety. It is wise to ask a few questions concerning activities of a normal day and the extent of relationships with family members or friends.

FOCUSED PHYSICAL EXAMINATION

General Observation

How the patient walks into the office, the gait, how the patient sits, any facial expressions, and, if possible, how the patient undresses should be noted. The patient's back shows the alignment of the spine. While observing from the sides, normal cervical and lumbar lordosis and dorsal kyphosis can be noted. From the front, the head and neck, level of shoulders, anterior-superior iliac spines, and the relation of the trunk to the lower extremities can be noted.

Palpation

The spinous processes, supraspinous ligaments, paraspinous muscles, sacroiliac joints, coccyx, and greater trochanters should be palpated, noting generalized or point tenderness, muscle spasm, and spinous process alignment. An infection, tumor, or fracture can cause localized soft tissue tenderness.

Evaluation of Range of Motion

The quality and the symmetry of movement are more important than the actual range. Flexion, extension, lateral bending, and rotation should be noted. Focus should be especially on the L5-S1 and L4-5 levels, where most movement occurs.

Testing for Muscle Strength with Neurologic Evaluation

- Ability to toe walk: calf muscles, mostly S1 nerve root
- Ability to heel walk: ankle and toe dorsiflexion muscles, L5 and some L4 nerve roots
- Single squat and rise: quadriceps muscles and mostly L4 nerve root
- Dorsiflexor muscles of the ankle and great toe: L5 and some L4 nerve root
- Hamstring and ankle evertors: L5-S1
- Toe flexors: S1

Reflexes

The reliability of reflex testing can be diminished in the presence of joint or muscle problems:
- Ankle jerk: S1 nerve root
- Knee jerk: L4 nerve root

Upgoing toes in response to stroking the plantar footpad (Babinski's sign) may indicate upper motor neuron abnormalities (such as myelopathy or demyelinating disease) rather than a common low back problem (Cole and Herring, 1997).

Evaluate sensory examination via light touch and pressure: medial foot (L4), dorsal foot (L5), and lateral foot (S1) (Figure 16-12).

The straight leg-raising test (also known as a tension sign) is a maneuver that tightens the sciatic nerve and further compresses an inflamed nerve root against a herniated lumbar disk. It may be performed with the patient supine or seated at the edge of an examination table. The leg is then raised, in an extended position, by the heel. The test is positive if leg pain below the knee, not in the back and buttocks, is reproduced or intensified. Reliability is age dependent. Older patients who have desiccated disks have less disk volume to herniate and are therefore less likely to have a positive sign (Figure 16-13).

Patrick's or Faber's test to differentiate between hip problems and sacroiliac joint pain as the cause of low back pain involves maneuvers of flexion, abduction, and external rotation. Direct the supine patient to place heel on knee, and then place gentle downward pressure on the knee toward the table. The test is positive for hip pain if the patient complains of same-side hip pain. If the patient complains of pain in the ipsilateral pelvis, the sacroiliac joint may be the source of pain.

Measure bilateral limb length.

Rectal examination for an enlarged prostate gland or a rectal carcinoma may suggest a cause for back pain. Abdominal examination is also appropriate.

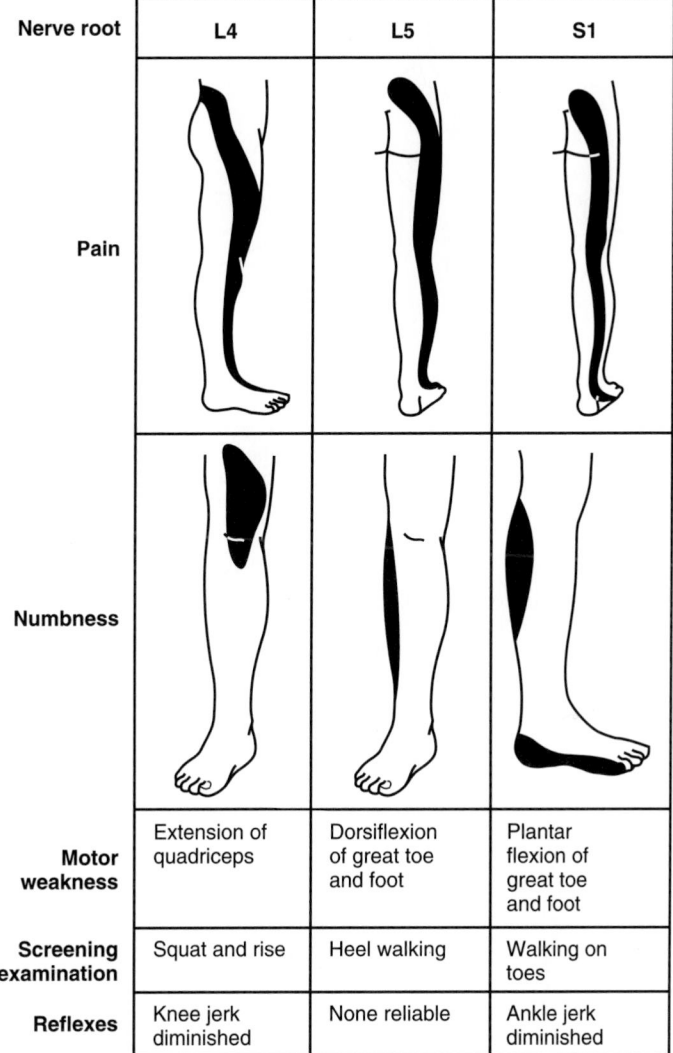

Nerve root	L4	L5	S1
Pain			
Numbness			
Motor weakness	Extension of quadriceps	Dorsiflexion of great toe and foot	Plantar flexion of great toe and foot
Screening examination	Squat and rise	Heel walking	Walking on toes
Reflexes	Knee jerk diminished	None reliable	Ankle jerk diminished

Figure 16-12 Sensory examination. (Adapted from Bigos S et al: *Acute low back problems in adults: clinical guideline, quick reference guide,* AHCPR No. 95-0643, Rockville, Md, 1994, US Department of Health and Human Services.)

DIFFERENTIAL DIAGNOSES

- Trauma: acute soft tissue strain, chronic strain
- Overuse syndromes
- Trigger points
- Generalized inflammatory joint disease such as ankylosing spondylitis
- Degenerative disk disease
- HNP
- Degenerative facet joint disease
- Spinal stenosis
- Osteoporosis
- Compression fracture

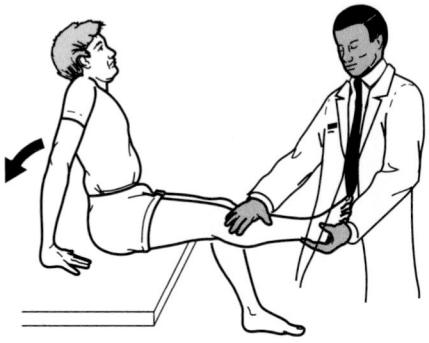

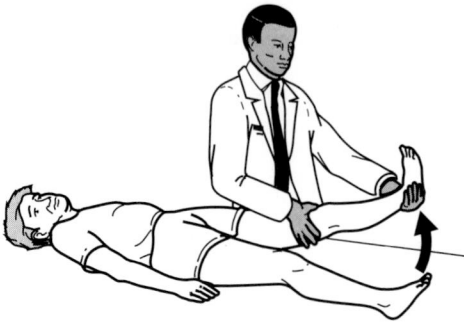

A   With the patient sitting on a table, both hip and knees flexed at 90 degrees, slowly extend the knee as if evaluating the patella or bottom of the foot. This maneuver stretches nerve roots as much as a moderate degree of supine SLR.

B   Ask the patient to lie as straight as possible on the table in the supine position. With one hand placed above the knee of the leg being examined, exert enough firm pressure to keep the knee fully extended. Ask the patient to relax.

C   With the other hand cupped under the heel, slowly raise the straight limb. Tell the patient, "If this bothers you, let me know, and I will stop."

D   Monitor for any movement of the pelvis before complaints are elicited. True sciatic tension should elicit complaints before the hamstrings are stretched enough to move the pelvis.

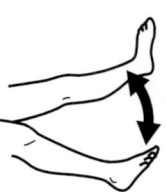

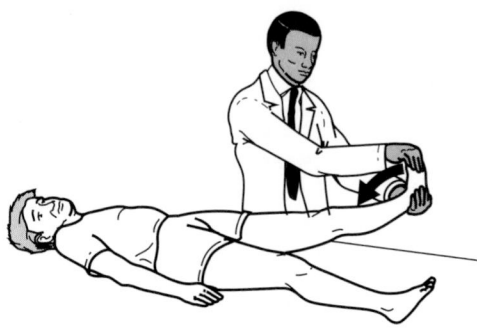

E   Estimate the degree of leg elevation that elicits complaint from the patient. Then determine the most distal area of discomfort: back, hip, thigh, knee, or below the knee.

F   While holding the leg at the limit of straight leg raising, dorsiflex the ankle. Note whether this aggravates the pain. Internal rotation of the limb can also increase the tension on the sciatic nerve roots.

Figure 16-13   Instructions for sitting knee extension test. (Adapted from Bigos S et al: *Acute low back problems in adults: clinical guideline, quick reference guide,* AHCPR No. 95-0643, Rockville, Md, 1994, US Department of Health and Human Services.)

- Infection
- Metastases, tumor
- Spondylolisthesis
- Viscerogenic source, such as abdominal aortic aneurysm, degenerative disease of the hip
- Sacroiliitis
- Cauda equina syndrome
- Herpes zoster radiculopathy
- Diabetic radiculopathy
- Arachnoiditis
- Sciatica
- Psychogenic or nonorganic source
- Vascular claudication

A number of conditions can present as low back pain in any given person. The following seven conditions are the most important of those typically evaluated in the primary care setting.

Back Strain

Back strain is ligamentous or muscular strain secondary to postural inadequacy, either continuously or with a single event. Pain may be limited to one spot or cover a larger area. Pain may radiate to the buttock or posterior thigh; however, pain referral does not necessarily indicate any mechanical compression of the neural element. The etiology is not always clear but may be related to muscular, ligamentous, or fascial strain. Attacks vary in intensity. Findings may include muscle spasm.

SYMPTOMS

- Pain that may be severe in the back, buttock, or one or both thighs
- Recent increase in physical activity for the patient
- Pain that begins 12 to 36 hours after an event
- Muscular stiffness
- Pain accentuated by standing and bending
- Pain alleviated by rest and lying down

FOCUSED PHYSICAL EXAMINATION

- Tenderness over the involved area
- Muscle spasm
- No evidence of nerve root impingement
- Posture may be tilted forward or to side, with difficulty in ambulating

DIFFERENTIAL DIAGNOSIS

- Lumbosacral strain syndrome

DIAGNOSTIC TESTS

Routine lumbosacral spine films are generally not indicated at the first visit; however, if a patient fails to respond after 2 weeks of conservative therapy, consider lumbosacral x-ray films. Plain x-ray films do show the changes of degenerative disk and facet joint disease, but these conditions are so common after the fifth decade of life that x-ray films are not useful in confirming the structure that is causing pain in a patient.

TREATMENT

Therapeutics

- Limited physical activity, particularly bending, stooping, heavy lifting, twisting
- Heat or ice

- Analgesics: acetaminophen, or NSAIDs on a regular rather than on an as-needed basis
  See Box 16-2 for guidelines for management of acute low back pain.

Education

Patients with uncomplicated low back pain can be managed conservatively and directed toward exercise programs that provide acute treatment and long-term prevention of future injury. Patients should return to normal activity as soon as possible and advised against activities such as vacuuming, which increase the force applied to the lower spine (Box 16-2, Figure 16-14).

Follow-up

If therapy fails to effect a response or pain recurs, the patient should be reexamined 3 to 4 weeks later to investigate the possibility of a medical (systemic) cause of back pain.

Degenerative Disk Disease

The disk begins to degenerate early in life. The intervertebral disk allows spinal mobility while retaining axial stability. Proteoglycan content decreases with age, leading to lower imbibition pressure, reduced water content, and associated fibrous replacement of the nucleus pulposus. Changes in the blood supply to the disk occur such that repair cannot keep pace with degeneration.

Degenerated disks have the following characteristics: decreased disk height, increased lateral bulging, reduced imbibition pressure, and increased mobility. Degenerative disk disease is a syndrome initiated by degenerative changes in the disk that secondarily involve other spinal elements that contribute to the symptom complex. Degenerative disk disease and prolapsed intervertebral disks are common causes of low back pain. Lumbar disk disease is most common at the L4-5 and L5-S1 levels and is less common between other vertebral bodies. Not all low back pains are due to prolapsed disk, and not all prolapsed disks need to be removed by surgery. At least 30% of asymptomatic individuals have abnormal imaging studies. Therefore it is important to treat the patient, not the imaging study. Most patients with back pain due to prolapsed disks can be treated successfully by conservative means.

HISTORY

Pain is usually located in the low back or gluteal region on one or both sides. Radiation of pain into the buttock or thigh is likely to be radiated from adjacent spinal joints or muscles rather than from the nerve root. Radiation of pain into the lower leg or foot may be caused by disk pressure on the nerve root.

Box 16-2

Comfort Options for Patients with Acute Low Back Problems

Oral medications
  Acetaminophen
Gradual return to normal activity
  Bedrest not recommended

Exercise
  Low-stress aerobics
  Gradual increase to walking, biking, or swimming
  Shoe insoles or shoe lifts
  Ice or heat if patient finds comfort

Modified from Bigos S et al: *Acute low back problems in adults: clinical practice guidelines, quick reference guide,* AHCPR No. 95-0642, Rockville, Md, 1994, US Department of Health and Human Services

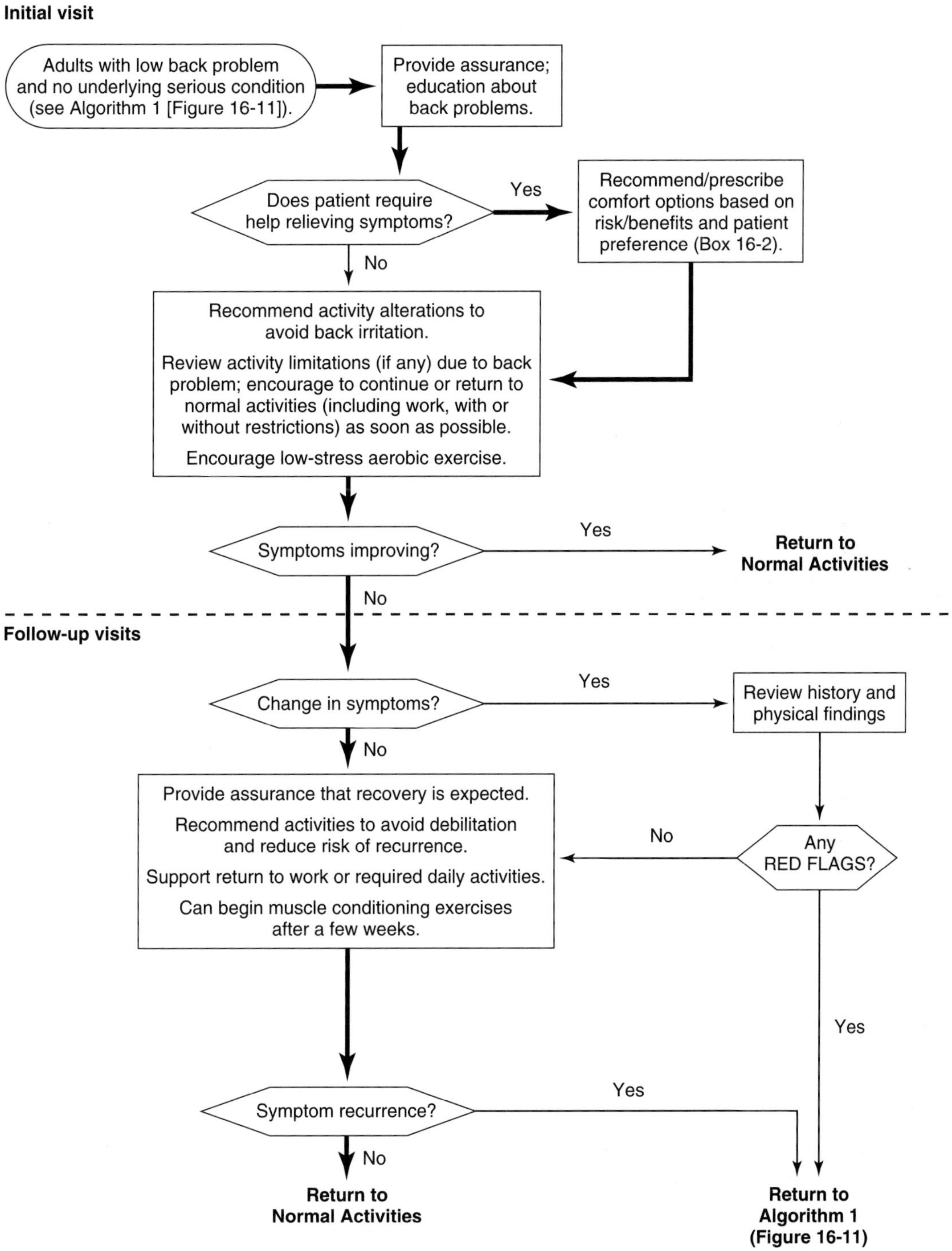

Initial visit

Adults with low back problem and no underlying serious condition (see Algorithm 1 [Figure 16-11]).

Provide assurance; education about back problems.

Does patient require help relieving symptoms?

Yes → Recommend/prescribe comfort options based on risk/benefits and patient preference (Box 16-2).

No

Recommend activity alterations to avoid back irritation.

Review activity limitations (if any) due to back problem; encourage to continue or return to normal activities (including work, with or without restrictions) as soon as possible.

Encourage low-stress aerobic exercise.

Symptoms improving? → Yes → **Return to Normal Activities**

No

- -

Follow-up visits

Change in symptoms? → Yes → Review history and physical findings

No

Any RED FLAGS?

No → Provide assurance that recovery is expected.

Recommend activities to avoid debilitation and reduce risk of recurrence.

Support return to work or required daily activities.

Can begin muscle conditioning exercises after a few weeks.

Yes → **Return to Algorithm 1 (Figure 16-11)**

Symptom recurrence? → Yes → **Return to Algorithm 1 (Figure 16-11)**

No → **Return to Normal Activities**

Figure 16-14 Algorithm 2. Treatment of acute low back problem on initial and follow-up visits. (Adapted from Bigos S et al: *Acute low back problems in adults: clinical guideline, quick reference guide,* AHCPR No. 95-0643, Rockville, Md, 1994, US Department of Health and Human Services.)

SYMPTOMS

- Symptoms are of variable duration.
- A traumatic event may precede pain. Coughing, sneezing, straining, lifting weight out in front of body, twisting, or bending at the waist may exacerbate the pain.
- Bed rest may provide some relief from the pain.
- Muscle stiffness is present.

FOCUSED PHYSICAL EXAMINATION

- Pain with back flexion
- Limited ROM
- Muscle spasms
- Possible neurologic signs with nerve root compression

DIFFERENTIAL DIAGNOSIS

- Degenerative disk disease

DIAGNOSTIC TESTS

- Lumbosacral spine films: Disk space is narrowed with horizontally directed osteophytes and reactive sclerosis of vertebral endplates. Vacuum phenomenon (description for a dark line seen in the intervertebral space) is considered a definite sign of disk degeneration. Degenerative changes of the facet joints occur with osteophyte encroachment on the intervertebral foramen.
- Consider MRI.

TREATMENT

Therapeutics

- Rest: Limit activities that contribute to pain.
- Analgesics: Consider NSAIDs.
- Use local heat.
- Consider local trigger point injections.

Education

- Exercises to increase mobility and strengthen muscles begin after the acute pain episode or spasm is over. Continue for maintenance of benefits.
- Avoid prone-lying activities, which accentuate lumbar lordosis. Consider lumbosacral support.

Follow-up

If the patient does not respond or pain recurs, the patient should be reexamined 3 to 4 weeks later to investigate the possibility of a medical (systemic) cause of back pain.

Herniated Nucleus Pulposus

Most disk ruptures occur during the third, fourth, and fifth decades of life. More than 80% of all lumbar disk herniations occur at L4-5 and L5-S1. Tears in the annulus fibrosus allow the contents of the nucleus pulposus to herniate beyond their normal confines. Tears in the annulus may be associated with transient episodes of low back pain. Herniation of the nucleus may result in sudden, severe pain if neural elements are compressed and inflamed by the nuclear contents. Sudden pressure placed on the lumbar spine that may occur with flexion (e.g., bending over to lift a heavy object or lifting with the arms extended) can precipitate the rupture; however, many patients who have a herniated disk do not give a history of injury or a sudden increase in pressure (Borenstein, 2002).

HISTORY

The major complaint is pain. Classic discogenic history factors that worsen the pain are sitting, standing, lying, arising from seated position, the first 20 to 30 minutes of the day, coughing, sneezing, straining, lifting weight out in front of body, twisting, and bending at the waist.

Features common to symptomatic presentations include prolonged sitting, twisting and rotation, occupations involving vibration such as truck drivers or operators of heavy machines, and chronic cough. The patient may have a prior history of low back pain.

SYMPTOMS

Onset is usually spontaneous. A sharp, lancinating pain may be insidious or sudden and is associated with a snapping or tearing sensation. Pain radiates from the back down the leg in the anatomic distribution of the affected nerve root. The patient may complain of thigh pain or calf pain with accompanying numbness and paresthesias. Leg pain is usually more pronounced than back pain when herniation has occurred.

FOCUSED PHYSICAL EXAMINATION

- Decreased ROM in flexion.
- Pain can be so severe that the patient resists examination and splints the back in lateral lumbar flexion and hip flexion.
- Patient tends to drift away from the involved side during bending.
- Antalgic gait: The patient holds the involved leg flexed to put as little weight as possible on the extremity.
- The neurologic examination may be undependable because the nerve may still function or the patient may have a deficit from a previous injury (Table 16-2).
- Reflex changes, weakness, atrophy, or sensory loss must conform to the rest of the clinical picture. The clinical picture varies depending on the level involved and the degree of herniation.
- The straight leg-raising test is positive (see Figure 16-13).

DIFFERENTIAL DIAGNOSIS

- Herniated lumbar nucleolus pulposus

DIAGNOSTIC TESTS

The initial diagnosis of a herniated disk is ordinarily made on the basis of the history and physical examination. Plain x-ray films of the lumbosacral spine rarely help the diagnosis but should be obtained to rule out other sources of pain, such as infection or tumor. Other tests, such as electromyelography, CT scan, or MRI are confirmatory by nature and can be misinformative when used as screening devices. CBC, sedimentation rate, and chemistries should be considered to evaluate systemic illness in patients for whom conservative therapy has failed.

TREATMENT

Therapeutics

- Controlled physical activity, sometimes bed rest
- Analgesics: NSAIDs
- Local heat

Education

- Increase activity as pain improves.
- Instruct patient in exercises for strengthening low back and abdominal musculature.
- Instruct patient not to bend, twist, stoop, stretch, lift, sit for prolonged periods, or carry anything heavier than the Sunday newspaper.

TABLE 16-2	Symptoms and Findings in Lumbar Disk Syndromes

Disk Level	Nerve Root	Symptoms and Findings
L3-4	L4	**Pain:** Low back, posterolateral aspect of the thigh, across patella, anteromedial aspect of leg **Sensory change:** Anterior aspect of knee, anteromedial aspect of leg **Motor deficit:** Quadriceps (knee extension) **Reflex change:** Knee jerk
L4-5	L5	**Pain:** Lateral, posterolateral aspect of thigh, leg **Sensory change:** Lateral aspect of leg, dorsum of foot, first webspace, great toe **Motor deficit:** Great toe extension, ankle dorsiflexion, heel walking difficult (footdrop may occur) **Reflex change:** Minor (posterior tibial jerk depressed)
L5-S1	S1	**Pain:** Posterolateral aspect of thigh, leg, heel **Sensory change:** Posterior aspect of calf, heel, lateral aspect of foot (3 toes) **Motor deficit:** Calf, plantarflexion of foot, great toe; toe walking weak **Reflex change:** Ankle jerk
Cauda equina syndrome	Massive midline protrusion	**Pain:** Low back, thigh, legs; often bilateral **Sensory change:** Thighs, legs, feet, perineum, often bilateral **Motor deficit:** Variable; may be bowel, bladder incontinence **Reflex change:** Ankle jerk (may be bilateral)

Adapted from Bigos S et al: *Acute low back problems in adults,* AHCPR No. 95-0642, Rockville, Md, 1994, US Department of Health and Human Services.

The long-term prognosis for patients with disk herniation is quite good. Between 85% and 90% of patients respond to conservative measures. Patience is a virtue. It may take up to 6 weeks before there is any appreciable decrease in pain.

Lumbar Spinal Stenosis

Spinal stenosis is a narrowing of the spinal canal that leads to mechanical pressure on structures within the canal. Activities involved in extension, which narrows the foramina and spinal canal, are associated with increased symptoms. The narrowing is usually slowly progressive and gradually advances over several years unless other conditions intervene. Back and radicular symptoms increase with walking variable distances and are relieved by lumbar flexion or sitting. Stenosis may occur as early as the fourth decade but is uncommon before age 55. A history of significant prior disk or facet joint degenerative disease is common. The intermittent nature of symptoms may be due to increased venous congestion within the confined space of the spinal canal. Many patients with spinal stenosis have symptoms mimicking those of peripheral vascular insufficiency or claudication. These patients develop lower-extremity pain while standing, walking, or hyperextending the spine in the absence of any evidence of peripheral vascular disease. Painful paresthesias are present in the feet or legs and may radiate to the hip girdle or lower trunk. Patients may experience lower-extremity numbness and weakness. These symptoms are relieved by rest or by flexion of the spine (the patient may report relief by bending forward as if to tie shoelaces) (Borenstein, 2002). With central canal stenosis, symptoms are generally noted bilaterally, fairly symmetrically, but in a nonspecific distribution. With lateral foraminal stenosis, symptoms are generally noted unilaterally in a fairly specific dermatomal distribution.

HISTORY

The history is the absolute key to diagnosis:
- Obtain a medical history. Onset of pain: Gradual progression of pain is usual; sudden changes in symptoms require an explanation other than stenosis, such as HNP or tumor.
- Symptoms: walking > standing > lying.
- While sitting, the patient is often asymptomatic, and sitting relieves symptoms.
- The patient may complain of weakness, pain, tingling, or numbness of one or both legs after walking.
- Legs feel "heavy" or rubbery.
- Valsalva maneuver should not affect symptoms in pure stenosis.
- While the patient is walking, relief is obtained with positions that increase lumbar flexion, such as squatting, stooping, going uphill, or leaning on a walker or cart.
- Late in the course of the disease, patients walk with a kyphotic posture and spend most of their time sitting. Patients report sitting in a flexed position while sleeping. Sitting is comfortable until late in the course of the disease.
- Bicycling and long car rides are well tolerated.

SYMPTOMS

- Back pain
- Buttock pain
- Radiating lower-extremity pain or dysesthesias, which are worse with standing and walking
- Main symptoms are sensory: vague dysesthesias, coldness, vague sense of weakness or "giving way," bizarre sensations such as water trickling down leg

FOCUSED PHYSICAL EXAMINATION

- Muscle atrophy and asymmetric reflex changes may appear late in the course of the disease. Neurologic changes occur only after the patient is stressed. The following stress test can be used in an outpatient clinic: After a neurologic examination, the patient is asked to walk up and down the corridor until the symptoms occur or the patient has walked 300 feet. A repeat examination is then performed; in many cases the second examination is positive for a focal neurologic deficit when the first was negative.
- ROM: Forward flexion is usually normal. At times, the patient is more supple and is able to touch the floor easily. Extension of the spine may be limited.
- Straight leg-raising test is negative in most patients.

DIFFERENTIAL DIAGNOSIS

- Lumbar spinal stenosis

DIAGNOSTIC TESTS

Plain x-ray films of the lumbosacral spine, with AP, lateral, and oblique views, are usually sufficient for diagnosis. CT or MRI may be ordered to support clinical findings or if surgery is considered.

TREATMENT

Therapeutics
- No treatment is necessary for asymptomatic patients.
- Analgesics or NSAIDs are given as needed when patients are symptomatic.
- A lumbosacral corset may be considered.
- Relative rest (supine with slight lumbar flexion) is used.

- Consider epidural steroid injections.
- Use an exercise program to increase flexibility and strengthen abdominal and back muscles.
- Stationary bicycles and walking either on level surfaces or uphill are generally well tolerated.

Education

- Poor posture is acceptable.
- Symptoms may be intermittent, and patients need encouragement to get through the episodes.
- Have patients use chairs that place them in a flexed position.
- Discuss potential surgery when conservative treatment fails to relieve symptoms and pain interferes with daily activities.

Follow-up

The patient should return to see the health care provider if symptoms persist or worsen. Refer for possible surgical intervention if symptoms persist despite aggressive conservative care.

Spondylolisthesis

Spondylolisthesis is a spinal condition in which all or part of a vertebra has slipped forward on another. There are several different types of spondylolisthesis, but in the most common type the lesion is in the isthmus or pars interarticularis. In this type, symptoms appear in late childhood and adolescence. Most commonly, L5-S1 is involved, and the location of the pain is in the L5-S1 dermatome. Some patients have radicular symptoms. This diagnosis should be considered for patients who have a history of involvement in sports with significant lumbar extension and rotation and that stress the pars interarticularis (e.g., gymnastics, dance, martial arts).

The next type of spondylolisthesis is degenerative and is the result of long-standing segmental instability with remodeling of articular processes. This type of spondylolisthesis presents in the fifth or sixth decade of life. Most commonly, L4-5 is involved, and pain is typically unilateral radicular, probably because of resultant foraminal stenosis. Bilateral calf pseudoclaudication is less common. The incidence increases with age; on rare occasions onset can be as early as age 40. The female-to-male ratio is 6:1. A slip of up to 10% (isthmic subtype) does not appear to increase the likelihood of back problems, but slippage beyond 25% increases the likelihood of low back symptoms, as does wedging of L5. In degenerative spondylolisthesis, slip rarely progresses past 33%. Footdrop may occur, but dural signs are rare. Most patients can be treated effectively with conservative measures (Figure 16-15).

HISTORY

Half of patients relate an acute episode of back and leg pain after a sudden twisting or lifting motion. Low back pain predominates initially, but over time leg pain develops and becomes the most annoying part of the problem. Pain is aggravated by activity and relieved by rest. The patient is seldom aware of any sensory or motor deficits. Occasionally, muscle spasm and local tenderness can be elicited.

SYMPTOMS

- Low back pain
- Leg pain
- Hamstring tightness
- Acute back and leg pain after a sudden twisting or lifting motion

FOCUSED PHYSICAL EXAMINATION

- Exaggeration of the lumbar lordosis with a palpable step-off and a dimple at the site of the abnormality

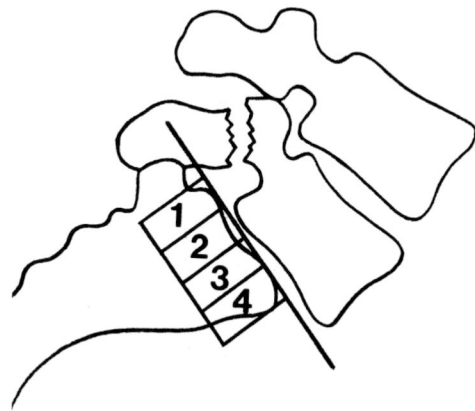

Figure 16-15   Meyerding's classification of spondylolisthesis. The amount of slippage is graded 1 to 4. Grade 1 represents 25% forward displacement; grade 2, 25% to 50%; grade 3, 50% to 75%; and grade 4, greater than 75%. (From Mercier LR: *Practical orthopedics*, ed 5, St Louis, 2000, Mosby.)

- Hamstring tightness
- Normal ROM
- Pain with back hyperextension
- No postural scoliosis in the absence of any radicular pain
- Morning stiffness
- Mild muscle spasm

DIFFERENTIAL DIAGNOSIS

- Spondylolisthesis, isthmic versus degenerative

DIAGNOSTIC TESTS

X-ray films, particularly the lateral views, confirm the diagnosis. Even the slightest amount of forward slipping of the body of the involved vertebra is readily discernible, and the oblique views disclose the actual defect in the pars.

TREATMENT

Therapeutics

- Relative rest should be provided during times of flares.
- Antiinflammatories or analgesics can be beneficial if leg pain is a significant problem.
- Exercises, usually a flexion exercise program, should be started when the patient is asymptomatic.

Education

- Educate the patient about proper body mechanics.
- Reinforce the need to continue exercise program to prevent further injury or exacerbation of symptoms.

Follow-up

Patient should return to the provider if symptoms persist or worsen. Refer for surgical intervention if symptoms persist despite aggressive conservative care.

Cauda Equina Syndrome

Cauda equina syndrome results from a mechanical compression of the neural elements, usually a result of an acute disk rupture at the L4-5 disk space. Only a small percentage of patients with low back pain have cauda equina, and it typically affects those in the third decade of life. The incidence is less than 1% of patients with lumbosacral pain. Because a missed diagnosis can have disastrous consequences, patients with suspected cauda equina syndrome require immediate referral to a specialist. This entity is the only one affecting the lumbosacral spine that requires emergent operative intervention.

HISTORY

- Pain as major complaint
- Saddle anesthesia
- Urinary retention
- Bowel incontinence
- Possible episode of trauma
- Classic discogenic factors that worsen the pain: sitting > standing > lying; arising from seated position; coughing, sneezing, straining; lifting weight out in front of body; twisting; or bending at the waist
- Possible history of low back pain

SYMPTOMS

- Severe low back pain
- Bilateral lower extremity weakness
- Bilateral sciatic pain
- Saddle anesthesia
- Bowel or bladder incontinence, with urinary retention the most common complaint
- Frank paraplegia

FOCUSED PHYSICAL EXAMINATION

- Confirmation of the previous signs plus major progressive motor weakness
- Neurologic abnormalities that are consistent with location of disk herniation

DIFFERENTIAL DIAGNOSIS

- Cauda equina compression syndrome

DIAGNOSTIC TESTS/THERAPEUTICS/EDUCATION/FOLLOW-UP

- Emergent advanced imaging (e.g., CT or MRI) and referral to a specialist for emergency decompression

Fractures of the Vertebrae

Vertebral fractures are common in the lower thoracic and upper lumbar regions. Most vertebral body fractures occur after some mechanical stress such as slipping on a stair, lifting, or jumping. Upper and middle thoracic regions are more stable and less prone to fractures because of the ribs, the shape of the articular processes, and the direction of the facets. Unique anatomic features of the thoracolumbar spine, T12-L1, predispose it to a high incidence of fracture. It is the junction between the relatively immobile thoracic spine (stabilized by the thoracic ribs) and the mobile lumbar spine (surrounded by soft tissue). It is also the junction between the kyphotic (forward curve) thoracic spine and the lordotic (reverse curve) lumbar spine. Change in facet orientation from the coronal plane (thoracic spine) to the sagittal plane (lumbar spine) predisposes the thoracolumbar junction to rotation and flexion strain.

Stable compression fractures of the vertebral bodies with intact spinal ligaments occur after a trauma such as a fall from a height and landing on the feet or buttocks. In addition, a downward blow to the shoulders may cause a fracture of the vertebral body. This force compresses the anterior part of the vertebra and leads to a compression fracture. Usually the force needed to compress the vertebral body in healthy bone is considerable. Sometimes the anterior and posterior surfaces of a vertebra are compressed to the same extent, especially in metastatic disease.

Vertebral compression fractures are common, especially among older adults, and usually are the result of a flexion injury when the spine is abruptly flexed. Compression fractures may occur after only a minimum of trauma in diseased bone, as in osteoporosis, multiple myeloma, metastatic cancer, or hyperparathyroidism. Also, they may occur with minimal stress, such as with sneezing, bending, or lifting a light object. In older patients one vertebral fracture is associated with a fivefold increase in the risk for subsequent vertebral fractures (Bellantoni, 2002). Back pain begins acutely and is sometimes associated with pain that radiates laterally and anteriorly. With multiple vertebral fractures, usually with anterior wedging, patients lose height and develop the characteristic dorsal kyphosis and cervical lordosis sometimes known as the "dowager's hump." At least one third of all vertebral compression fractures are asymptomatic. The overwhelming majority occur in people with osteoporosis.

HISTORY

- Mechanism of injury
- History of osteoporosis, multiple myeloma, metastatic cancer, hyperparathyroidism
- History of corticosteroid use
- Positions such as sitting or walking that exacerbate pain
- Cigarette smoking
- Family history
- Early or surgically induced menopause

SYMPTOMS

- In acute fracture, severe pain is localized over the affected vertebral body. Occasionally the pain radiates into the flanks, upper portion of the posterior thighs, or abdomen. Back motion, especially spinal flexion, aggravates the discomfort, as does prolonged sitting, standing, and the Valsalva maneuver.
- The most common locations of painful vertebrae are T10, T11, T12, and L1, with resultant lumbar pain. Lumbar fractures may result in lower extremity pain and, occasionally, neurologic symptoms. Neurologic or radicular symptoms distant from an area of fracture are unusual; if they are present, other pathologic conditions must be considered.
- Some patients are left with persistent, nagging, dull spinal pain after a vertebral body fracture secondary to osteoporosis, and this pain may persist even in the absence of new fractures on x-ray films. The source of this pain may be microfractures too small to be detected by x-ray films or biomechanical effects of the deformity on the lumbar spine below.
- Spasm of the paraspinous muscles contributes to the back pain.

FOCUSED PHYSICAL EXAMINATION

- Inspection: Abrasions and bruises indicate the direction and severity of forces involved. Visible deformity suggests a displaced, unstable fracture.
- Palpation: Tenderness over the spinous processes helps localize the fracture. The interspinous ligament normally feels firm on palpation. When this ligament is torn, the interspinous space feels softer. In addition, palpation of the paraspinous muscles reveals spasm.
- ROM: These tests are not performed when a fracture is suspected to avoid damaging the spinal cord or cauda equina.
- Special tests: A detailed neurologic examination is carried out and is often normal. On abdominal examination, patients with severe pain secondary to an acute fracture may demonstrate a loss of bowel sounds, ileus, or bladder distention secondary to acute urinary retention.

DIFFERENTIAL DIAGNOSES

- Vertebral compression fracture
- Back strain

- Tumor
- Multiple myeloma

DIAGNOSTIC TESTS

The AP view may appear nearly normal, whereas the lateral view shows wedging or compression of the normally square vertebra. A T12 fracture may be hidden by the liver and an underexposed lateral x-ray film. Compression of more than 20% should arouse suspicion that the fracture is an unstable burst fracture, and a CT scan should be obtained to check for fracture of the middle and posterior columns. The review of the CT scan is helpful in deciding on surgical intervention to relieve pressure on neurologic structures.

A bone scan is useful in demonstrating whether there are single or multiple fractures. A healing compression fracture may continue to be abnormal on bone scan for up to 2 years. The bone has healed before the bone scan becomes normal because of continued remodeling. More rapid resolution of an abnormal bone scan is usually seen in younger patients (Cole and Herring, 1997).

TREATMENT

Therapeutics

With lumbar or thoracic vertebral compression fractures, management includes rest, adequate analgesia, and gradual ambulation when the patient is free of severe pain. A lumbosacral support or, for the patient with thoracic vertebral fracture, a chairback or hyperextension brace may be helpful in alleviating pain. Bending and lifting activities should be restricted for 6 to 12 weeks.

Education

- Instruct in appropriate use of the support or brace.
- Inform the patient that pain from a vertebral fracture may persist for several months, although the incapacitating component is usually only 2 to 3 weeks in duration. Instruct the patient to contact the health care provider immediately if neurologic symptoms develop.
- Instruct the patient in proper body mechanics, including prevention of falls, if appropriate. Review the patient's home environment for safety issues.

Follow-up

Telephone follow-up is in 2 to 3 weeks. Further evaluation or referral should be done if symptoms persist or worsen.

Summary

Older persons are at high risk for musculoskeletal injury, which can lead to significant loss of function, pain, further morbidity, and even mortality. Age-related changes are significant, especially in bone mass and muscle strength. A history and physical examination are critical in localizing the area of injury and in determining whether the injury is muscular or skeletal in origin. The list of differential diagnoses can be significant. Diagnostic tests such as radiology studies, electromyelography, or MRI may be necessary to locate the source of pain and to determine appropriate therapy. Treatment often requires a multifaceted approach of medication, therapy, education, and surgery. The decision to pursue surgical intervention in a frail, older adult requires consideration of a number of issues, including comorbidities.

Resources

American Academy of Orthopedic Surgeons
www.aaos.org

National Institute of Aging health information
www.nia.nih.gov/health/

References

Aminoff M: Nervous system. In Tierney L et al: *Current medical diagnosis and treatment 2002*, ed 41, New York, 2001, Lange Medical Books—McGraw-Hill.

Ankrom M, Blackman M: Metabolic bone disorders. In Barker LR, Burton JR, Zieve PD, editors: *Ambulatory medicine*, ed 6, Baltimore, 2002, Lippincott Williams & Wilkins.

Bellantoni M: Osteoporosis. In Barker LR, Burton JR, Zieve PD, editors: *Ambulatory medicine*, ed 6, Baltimore, 2002, Lippincott Williams & Wilkins.

Borenstein D: Low back pain. In Barker LR, Burton JR, Zieve PD, editors: *Ambulatory medicine*, ed 6, Baltimore, 2002, Lippincott Williams & Wilkins.

Byank D et al: Approaches to musculoskeletal injuries. In Barker LR, Burton JR, Zieve PD, editors: *Ambulatory medicine*, ed 6, Baltimore, 2002, Lippincott Williams & Wilkins.

Cole AC, Herring SA: *The low back pain handbook: a practical guide for the primary care clinician*, St Louis, 1997, Mosby.

Hellmann D: Arthritis and musculoskeletal disease. In LM Tierney et al, editors: *Current medical diagnosis and treatment 2002*, ed 41, New York, 2001, Lange Medical Books—McGraw-Hill.

Kerr D: Shoulder and elbow pain. In Barker LR, Burton JR, Zieve PD, editors: *Ambulatory medicine*, ed 6, Baltimore, 2002, Lippincott Williams & Wilkins.

Lenz, F: Neck pain. In Barker LR, Burton JR, Zieve PD, editors: *Ambulatory medicine*, ed 6, Baltimore, 2002, Lippincott Williams & Wilkins.

Millstein JH: Three steps to diagnosing shoulder pain, *Intern Med* 18(11):14-30, 1997.

Sykes TF: A systematic approach to acute shoulder pain, *Patient Care* 11:34-51, 1997.

Wiesel SW, Boden SD: Low back pain: medical diagnosis and comprehensive management, ed 2, Philadelphia, 1997, Saunders.

17

Musculoskeletal: Common Disorders

Physiologic Age-related Changes

Along with aging comes a gradual loss of bone mass and an incremental process of bone resorption without successful formation of new bone mass. With age, bone mineral density decreases in people. Several factors appear to be predictive of bone mass: family and reproductive history, nutritional factors, medication use, and exercise. This loss of bone mass is combined with the diminished muscle strength that results from the age-related decrease in muscle fiber. Studies have shown, however, that regular exercise, especially resistance training, demonstrates a reduced rate of decline in muscle strength. Function, rather than the negative results of age-related change or pathology, is the major defining characteristic of musculoskeletal health in older adults.

This chapter discusses the following conditions: osteoarthritis (OA), rheumatoid arthritis (RA), polymyalgia rheumatica (PMR), giant cell arteritis (GCA), fibromyalgia, gout, and Dupuytren's contracture.

OSTEOARTHRITIS

Epidemiology

Osteoarthritis is the most common form of joint disease. The latest estimates of prevalence rates for arthritis reported by the Centers for Disease Control and Prevention (CDC) estimated that 33% of the adult population, or about 69.9 million U.S. adults, are afflicted with this condition (CDC, 2002). Major annual economic costs of OA are estimated at $15.5 billion (Townes, 2003). The significant prevalence of OA brings a high cost to society through loss of productivity and loss of self-care abilities, with a resulting drain on health care costs.

More than 90% of adults over 55 years of age have radiographic features of OA, and 90% of adults over 40 years of age have radiographic features of OA in weight-bearing joints (Hellmann, 2003). No relationship has been found, however, between radiographic features of OA and symptoms; only 10% to 30% of the older group report symptomatic pain and disability. Primary idiopathic OA is one of the leading causes of disability in both men and women by 65 years of age (Townes, 2002).

Osteoarthritis is a chronic disease that involves the entire joint. It is characterized by dynamic biochemical and biomechanical changes that cause the central loss of articular cartilage and active remodeling, especially on subchondral bone, which affects the joint structures. Inflammation is usually minimal. The radiographic features of OA are joint-space narrowing, osteophytes, subchondral sclerosis, and subchondral cysts. It affects weight-bearing joints (hip, knee, spine, hand, and feet) and is thought to result in part from mechanical wear and tear; however, the precise cause is unknown (Townes, 2003; Hellman and Stone, 2002).

Pathology

With OA, the articular cartilage becomes thinner, tears, and disrupts the joint capsule, resulting in bone remodeling and deformity. As the cartilage wears away, less protection and reduced cushioning cause ulceration (eburnation), spurs (osteophytes), synovitis, hypertrophy of the capsule, and periarticular muscle wasting. General disruption of collagen and the other elements necessary for joint integrity also occur. Joint inflammation is rare in OA, but soft tissue damage can result from osteophytes and bone remodeling.

Risk Factors

Although significant risk factors such as age and family history are not modifiable risks, obesity is also a significant risk for the development of OA in weight-bearing joints, especially in women (Sowers, 2001). The risk of OA of the knee is associated with high physical workload occupations, such as agriculture, forestry, and fishing, and in soccer players (Manninen et al, 2002). Recreational running does not increase the risk of OA, but participation in competitive contact sports does (Hellman and Stone, 2002). Primary care providers need to concentrate on the prevention of OA by addressing the association of obesity and OA with their obese patients. The protection of joints from joint trauma reduces the risk for OA, and this factor can be discussed with younger patients.

History

The frequent, classic clinical presentation of OA usually includes joint pain, swelling, decreased range of motion, and crepitus with movement. Pain and stiffness are the major complaints described by patients with OA. The practitioner gathers information about the dimensions of the pain and the description of affected joints and associated muscle spasms. An asymmetric joint pattern is typical. Duration of morning stiffness is an important aspect; most OA patients report less than 30 minutes of morning stiffness. Pain is usually relieved by rest, and pain at rest is often an indication of disease severity (Hellmann and Stone, 2002).

The practitioner needs to probe symptoms of fatigue, a vague general malaise, recent febrile illness, and general emotional state, with an awareness that some older patients may underreport by discounting symptoms. OA does not usually have any systemic manifestations. During history taking, the differential diagnosis becomes paramount (Table 17-1).

Focused Physical Examination

Palpation for joint tenderness is an essential part of the examination. A grimace by the patient when shaking hands certainly is an indication of tenderness. The practitioner must exert sufficient pressure to elicit a painful response from a tender joint. Pressing gently is of no value and can lead to considerable confusion. Certainly good sense would dictate that a red, swollen joint is painful, and therefore there is no need to confirm this observation. In a systematic method, each joint is assessed for tenderness, swelling, skin temperature, the presence of crepitus, and muscle strength. Both passive and active range of motion of all joints are essential aspects of the

TABLE 17-1	Differential Diagnosis of Arthritis

	Degenerative	*Inflammatory*	*Psychogenic*
Symptoms			
Stiffness (duration)	Few minutes; "gelling" after prolonged rest	Hours (often); most pronounced after rest	Little or no variation in intensity with rest or activity
Pain	Follows activity; relieved by rest	Even at rest; nocturnal pain may interfere with sleep	Little or no variation in intensity with rest or activity
Weakness	Present, usually localized and not severe	Often pronounced	Often a complaint; "neurasthenia"
Fatigue	Not usual	Often severe with onset in early afternoon	Often in A.M. on arising
Emotional depression and lability	Not usual	Common; coincides with fatigue; often disappears if disease remits	Often present
Signs			
Tenderness localized over afflicted joint	Usually present	Almost always; the most sensitive indication of inflammation	Tender "all over"; "touch-me-not attitude"; tendency to push away or to grasp the examining hand
Swelling	Effusion common; little synovial reaction	Effusion common; often synovial proliferation and thickening	None
Heat and erythema (skin)	Unusual but may occur	More common	None
Crepitus	Coarse to medium	Medium to fine	None, except with coexistent arthritis
Bony spurs	Common	Sometimes found, usually with antecedent osteoarthritis	None, except with coexistent osteoarthritis

From McCarty D: Differential diagnosis of arthritis: analysis of signs and symptoms. In Koopman WJ, editor: *Arthritis and allied conditions*, 13th ed, Baltimore, 1997, Williams & Wilkins.

focused physical examination. The characteristic distribution of involved joints is distal interphalangeal (Heberden's nodes), proximal interphalangeal (Bouchard's nodes), the thumb, carpal and metacarpal joints, the hallux metatarsophalangeal, and the hip, knee, and spine (Levy and Sethi, 1998) (Figure 17-1).

It is important to measure height accurately for baseline data. Observation of gait allows the practitioner to assess for limping or uneven gait, which is indicative of hip or knee involvement. Certain

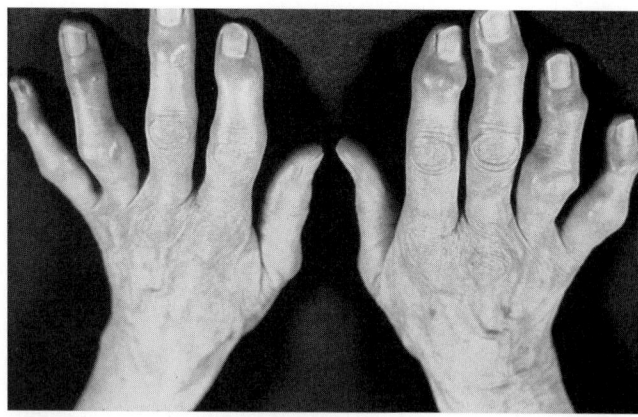

Figure 17-1   Degenerative joint disease; Heberden's nodes at the distal interphalangeal joints and Bouchard nodes at the proximal interphalangeal joints. (From Moskowitz RW et al: *Osteoarthritis,* ed 3, Philadelphia, 2001, Saunders.)

laboratory tests for OA can be performed on a routine basis (Table 17-2). For diagnostic tests for differential diagnosis, see Table 17-3.

Treatment
INTERVENTIONS

In the last few years realization of the multiple levels of treatment for patients with OA has increased. First and foremost, efforts need to reduce or modify risk factors, to encourage weight reduction, to establish a well-designed education program, and to enact an exercise regimen.

An important aspect of a treatment program is the prevention of further injury. If the patient is obese, the primary care provider has an obligation to impress on the patient the health risks inherent in obesity as well as the relationship of obesity to the development and, most likely, the progression of OA. There is a need for compassionate consideration in such a warning. It is not appropriate to "blame the victim" for the disease; instead, the provider must recognize the importance of building a relationship with the patient to increase compliance and self-care abilities.

TABLE 17-2	**Laboratory Investigations**
Test	***Results***
Erythrocyte sedimentation rate	Normal in osteoarthritis
	Elevated in polymyalgia rheumatica
	Elevated in rheumatoid arthritis
Rheumatoid factor	Negative in osteoarthritis
	Positive in rheumatoid arthritis
Antinuclear antibody	Negative in osteoarthritis
	20% of rheumatoid arthritis patients test positive
Uric acid	Elevated in gout
C-reactive protein	Elevated in rheumatoid arthritis

TABLE 17-3	Laboratory Investigations	
Class of Test	*Category*	*Example of Abnormality*
Hematology	Hemoglobin	Anemia in rheumatoid arthritis
	White cell count	Leukocytosis in septic arthritis
	Platelet count	Thrombocytopenia in systemic lupus
	ESR	erythematosus
		Elevated in polymylagia rheumatica
Biochemistry	Creatinine	High with involvement in systemic vasculitis
	Uric acid	Elevated in gout
	CPK	Elevated in polymyositis
Immunology	Rheumatoid factor	Positive in rheumatoid arthritis
	Antinuclear antibody	Positive in systemic lupus erythematosus
	C-reactive protein	Elevated in rheumatoid arthritis
	Immunoglobulins	Elevated in Sjögren syndrome
	Complements C_3 and C_4	Low in active systemic lupus erythematosus
Synovial fluid microscopy	Crystals	Present in gout and pyrophosphate crystal deposition disease
Culture	Bacteria in septic arthritis	

From Scott D: Authorities in the elderly. In Allis RCT, Fillit HM editors: *Brocklehurst's textbook of geriatric medicine and gerontology*, ed 6, London, 2003, Churchill Livingstone.
ESR, Erythrocyte sedimentation rate; *CPK*, creatine phosphokinase.

The goals of an exercise program for patients with OA are to increase function and reduce joint pain. After pain relief has been achieved, a graded exercise program can begin. Depending on the severity of the functional limitations attributed to the disease, some patients need formal physical therapy to develop their program; others need only minimal instruction. A joint-protection program that reduces sudden impact loads and optimizes the patient's muscular capacity can be considered both as a treatment and as a preventive measure (Box 17-1).

The primary care provider needs to dispel the old myth that any exercise will exacerbate the already painful joints and should also stress that a graded exercise program does not cause pain and does not advance quickly. Strength training improves function in patients with OA of the knee, reduces pain, prevents loss of bone mineral density, increases endurance performance, and reduces the risk of falls (Hurley and Roth, 2000). Studies of physical fitness exercise for older adults with joint disease demonstrate a positive effect on pain and or disability of OA (Baker and McAlindon, 2000; O'Grady et al, 2000). Figure 17-2 shows strengthening exercises.

Box 17-1
Joint Protection

1. Wear properly fitted shoes with well-cushioned soles.
2. Sit rather than stand for activities longer than 10 minutes.
3. Avoid low chairs, low beds, low toilet seats, bathtubs.
4. Do not kneel, squat, or sit cross-legged on the floor.
5. Do consider exercise by swimming or walking.

**Quadriceps Strengthening
Exercise**

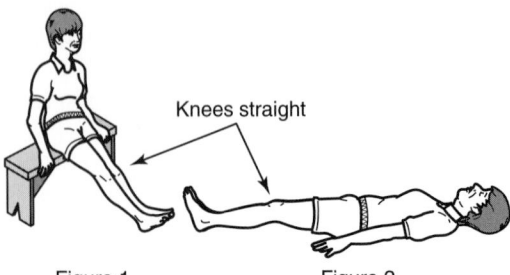

Knees straight

Figure 1   Figure 2

**Quadriceps Strengthening
Exercise Concentrating on the
Vastus Medialis Oblique Muscle**

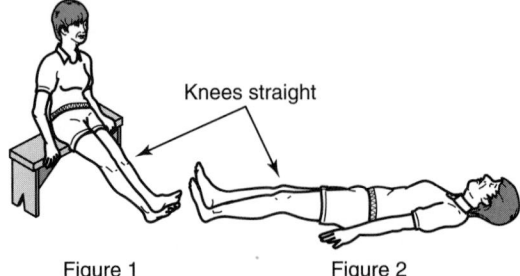

Knees straight

Figure 1   Figure 2

1. Sit on a firm surface (Figure 1) or lie flat in bed (Figure 2).

2. Perform this exercise in either of the following positions:
   a. Sit in a chair (Figure 1) with your legs straight, heels on the floor or on a footstool. Squeeze your thigh muscles, pushing your knees downward toward the floor.
   b. Lie in bed (Figure 2) with your legs straight and squeeze your thigh muscles, pushing the back of your knees into the bed.

3. Hold this position for a full 5 seconds. Use a clock or watch with a second hand, or count: one-one thousand, two-one thousand, three-one thousand, four-one thousand, five-one thousand.

4. Relax the muscles.

1. Sit on a firm surface (Figure 1) or lie flat in bed (Figure 2).

2. Cross your ankles with right leg above and left leg below. Legs should be stretched out straight.

3. With your heels on the floor or on the bed, push down with right leg, push up with left leg, squeezing your ankles together. (Pretend that you're crushing a walnut between your ankles.) There should be little actual movement except for the muscle tightening.

4. Hold this position for a full 5 seconds. Use a clock or a watch with a second hand, or count: one-one thousand, two-one thousand, three-one thousand, four-one thousand, five-one thousand.

5. Relax the muscles.

6. Reverse the position of the legs so that the leg that was on top is now on the bottom.

7. Repeat steps one, two and three.

Instructions

If your arthritis is causing knee pain, apply heat to your knees for 15 to 20 minutes prior to performing your exercises.

Begin your strengthening program with 10 repetitions, holding each contraction for a full 5 seconds. Perform this exercise 7 times daily and increase the number of repetitions you perform with each set by three to five daily during the first week.

Caution: In most patients, these knee exercises will not cause joint pain or increase the pain from your arthritis. If, however, you have significant pain lasting more than 20 minutes after you perform these exercises, decrease the number of repetitions by five per set. Maintain this number of repetitions until your knee discomfort subsides. Then, each day thereafter, increase the number of repetitions by three per set until you reach a maximum of 15 per set.

Figure 17-2   *Left,* Quadriceps-strengthening exercise. *Right,* Quadriceps strengthening exercise concentrating on the vastus medialis oblique muscle. (Modified from Brandt KD: *Diagnosis and nonsurgical management,* Indianapolis, 1996, Professional Communications.)

If pain is not relieved by these measures, the first drug of choice should be the analgesic acetaminophen at 4 g a day. It often provides sufficient pain relief, has a low cost, and has fewer side effects and adverse interactions with other drugs. Still, with acetaminophen there is an increased risk for hepatotoxicity in overdoses exceeding 10 g (2.5 times the normal dose). People with chronic high alcohol intake have been reported to be at risk for liver toxicity, and regular alcohol use increases the risk for induced liver damage.

Nonsteroidal antiinflammatory drugs (NSAIDs) have been more effective than acetominophen in relieving moderate to severe pain, reducing inflammation, and improving function (Pincus et al, 2001). Despite the favorable outcome, clinicians cannot overlook the increase in serious side effects of this class of drugs, especially in older adults.

The NSAIDs produce serious adverse side effects in the older population (gastric bleeding, renal insufficiency, and precipitation of confusion) and are known to have adverse interactions with multiple other drugs (Table 17-4). The availability of a new class of NSAIDs that inhibit cyclooxygenase-2 (COX-2) has somewhat reduced the risks of gastrointestinial bleeding (Bombardier et al, 2002). The effects of celecoxib (Celebrex) and rofecoxib (Vioxx) on the renal system and liver

---

TABLE 17-4	**Adverse Side Effects of Nonsteroidal Antiinflammatory Drugs**

	Approximate Incidence
Gastrointestinal	10%–20%
Epigastric pain, nausea	
Anorexia, dyspepsia, peptic ulceration	
Overt or occult bleeding	<1%
Hypersensitivity Reactions	1%–5%
Rashes, rarely Stevens–Johnson syndrome	
Very rarely, anaphylactoid reactions	
Aggravation of Allergic Rhinitis or Asthma	10% of sufferers
Renal Effects	>5%
Transient renal failure	
Water and salt retention	
Hypokalemia, inhibit diuretic action	
Interstitial nephritis, nephrotic syndrome	>1%
Hepatic Effects	5%–15%
Cholestatic hepatitis	
Central Nervous System	>5%
Tinnitus/deafness	Primary aspirin
Headache, vertigo, confusion	Higher with indomethacin
Others	
Diarrhea	10%–15% (mefenamic acid, other fenamates)
Aggravation of congestive heart failure, angina	>1%
Toxic amblyopia	<1% (ibuprofen)

From Matsumoto A: Rheumatrid arthritis. In Barker LR et al: *Principles of ambulatory medicine*, ed 6, Philadelphia, 2003, Lippincott Williams & Wilkins.

function are the same as other NSAIDs and should not be prescribed to patients with a compromised system. Celecoxib is contraindicated in patients with a history of allergic reaction to sulfonamide. Rofecoxib is contraindicated in patients taking rifampen, methrotrexate, and warfarin. Extreme caution should be taken when prescribing rofecoxib for a patient taking an ACE inhibitor or for one who has evidence of allergic asthma (Hay et al, 2001). See Table 17-5 for complete list of NSAIDs.

Topical agents can be used in conjunction with other medications. Capsaicin is a nonprescription drug available in two strengths. It can be used two to four times a day, but to remain effective it should not be used continuously.

The nutritional supplement glucosamine has low toxicity and may offer an alternative for older patients with mild or moderate pain who are unable or unwilling to take NSAIDS or other drugs

TABLE 17-5 | Nonsteroidal Antiinflammatory Drugs

Generic Names	*Trade Names*
Propionic Acid Derivatives	
Ibuprofen[a]	Motrin, Rufen, IBU Nuprin, Advil
Naproxen[a]	Naprosyn Anaprox, Aleve
Ketoprofen[a]	Orudis
Flurbiprofen[a]	Ansaid
Oxaprozin[a]	Daypro
Oxicams	
Piroxicam[a]	Feldene
Acetic Acids	
Indomethacin[a]	Indocin
Sulindac[a]	Clinoril
Tolmetin[a]	Tolectin
Diclofenac[a]	Voltaren
Etodolac[a]	Lodine
Nabumetone[a]	Relafen
Pyrazoles	
Ketorolac tromethamine	Toradol
Nonacetylated Salicylates	
Diflurisal	Dolobid
Magnesium choline salicylate[a]	Trilisate
Salsalate[a]	Disalcid
Cyclooxygenase-2 Inhibitors	
Celecoxib	Celebrex
Rofecoxib	Vioxx

From Matsumoto A: Rheumatoid arthritis. In Barker LR et al: *Principles of ambulatory medicine*, ed 6, Philadelphia, 2003, Lippincott Williams & Wilkins.
[a]Approved for use in rheumatoid arthritis.

(Reginstar et al, 2001). More long-term studies are needed to validate the claims surrounding glucosamine.

Intraarticular injection of depocorticosteroids is considered useful if there is evidence of inflammation. Synovial effusions should be removed before the injection is done. No conclusive evidence has been found to show that intraarticular injections of depocorticosteroids are of any benefit in OA. They should be limited to a maximum of four per year to an individual joint (Townes, 2003).

Surgical intervention, usually joint replacement, is an elective orthopedic procedure performed for either intractable pain or restoration of compromised function. For most patients, the results are good to excellent and have long-term benefits. Arthroscopic intervention with debridement is useful to patients with meniscal injury, loose cartilage, or large osteophytes (Townes, 2003).

RHEUMATOID ARTHRITIS

Epidemiology

Rheumatoid arthritis has a worldwide distribution, but different diagnostic criteria make accurate worldwide prevalence rates difficult to determine. The prevalence of RA among white populations is 1% to 2%; Native Americans have a high prevalence rate at 3.5% to 5.3%; and South African blacks and Japanese have a rate of 0.1%. Prevalence increases with age, approaching 5% of women over 55 years of age. In the United States the average annual incidence is about 70 per 100,000 and two to three times greater in women than men (Matsumoto, 2003).

Pathology and Definition

Rheumatoid arthritis is a chronic systemic inflammatory disorder of unknown origin that chiefly affects synovial membrane of multiple joints (Hellman and Stone, 2002). Susceptibility to RA is genetically determined (Matsumoto, 2003).

The pathologic hallmark of RA consists of infiltration of the subsynovia lining cells and blood vessels into a tumor-like structure called *pannus.* The pannus erodes cartilage, bone, ligaments, and tendons. In the acute stage, effusion and other manifestations of inflammation are common. In both the acute and chronic phases, inflammation of soft tissue around the joints may be prominent and is a significant factor in joint damage (Hellman and Stone, 2002).

In 1987 the American Rheumatism Association established criteria for RA (Table 17-6). RA can be considered a clinical syndrome with features that can vary from one patient to another and also can vary from time to time in the same patient.

History

The typical presentation of RA begins insidiously with a slow progression of signs and symptoms. Morning stiffness is accompanied by pain on movement and joint tenderness in three fourths of older people. Although in a few patients the onset is acute apparently following a stressful event such as infection, surgery, trauma, or emotional strain (Hellman and Stone, 2002).

If the patient presents with polyarticular inflammatory arthritis, especially of the hands or feet, the primary care provider begins to consider a diagnosis of RA. Patients with early disease usually report a general malaise with fatigue, severe morning stiffness that lasts more than an hour, and joint swelling and tenderness. The initial presentation of RA may lack the aspect of symmetric involvement, but the symmetry becomes evident as the disease progresses. A definitive diagnosis of RA requires a period of 6 weeks with symptoms.

TABLE 17-6	Revised Criteria for the Classification of Rheumatoid Arthritis

Criterion	Definition
Morning stiffness	Morning stiffness in and around the joints, lasting at least 1 hour before maximum improvement
Arthritis of 3 or more joint areas	At least 3 joint areas simultaneously with soft tissue swelling or joint fluid observed by a physician. The 14 possible areas are (right or left): PIP, MCP, wrist, elbow, knee, ankle, and MTP joints
Arthritis of hand joints	At least 1 area swollen in a wrist, MCP, or PIP joint
Symmetric arthritis	Simultaneous involvement of the same joint areas on both sides of the body (bilateral involvement of PIP, MCP, or MTP acceptable without perfect symmetry)
Rheumatoid nodules	Subcutaneous nodules over bony prominences or extensor surfaces, or in juxtaarticular regions, observed by a physician
Serum rheumatoid factor	Abnormal amount of serum rheumatoid factor by any method for which the result has been positive in < 5% of control subjects
Radiographic changes	Erosions or unequivocal bony decalcification localized in or most marked adjacent to the involved joints (osteoarthritis changes excluded), typical of rheumatoid arthritis on posteroanterior hand and wrist radiographs

From Arnett FC et al: The American Rheumatism Association 1987 revised criteria for the classification of rheumatoid arthritis, *Arthritis Rheum* 31:315-324, 1988.
For classification purposes, a patient is said to have rheumatoid arthritis if 4 of 7 criteria are satisfied. Criteria 1-4 must have been present for at least 6 weeks. Patients with 2 clinical diagnoses are not excluded.

A baseline for functional status should be completed on the first visit. A four-point scale that rates limitations in self-care and vocational and avocational activities was developed by the American College of Rheumatology for the classification of functional status in rheumatoid patients (Table 17-7).

Focused Physical Examination

Examination of affected joints for the signs of inflammation is important for early diagnosis because there are reversible aspects of inflammatory synovitis. RA criteria are to be considered only as guidelines for diagnosing RA. Essential for diagnosis is identification of inflammatory synovitis, which can be one of the following: synovial fluid leukocytosis (white blood cells > 2000/mm^3), histologic demonstration of chronic synovitis, or radiologic evidence of characteristic erosions (Weinblatt, 1997). The presence of deformity in non-weight-bearing joints (metacarpophalangeal, wrists) is highly indicative of RA unless there is a history of trauma.

Laboratory Tests

Aspiration of a joint with a palpable effusion is a first consideration. Rheumatoid factor (RF) is found in the serum of about 85% of people with RA, but it is of little prognostic value and may be present in other inflammatory processes. High titers of RF are more likely to be diagnostic of RA

TABLE 17-7	American College of Rheumatology Revised Criteria for Classification of Functional Status in Rheumatoid Arthritis
Class	**Functional Status**
Class I	Completely able to perform usual activities of daily living (self-care, vocational, and avocational)
Class II	Able to perform usual self-care and vocational activities but limited in avocational activities
Class III	Able to perform usual self-care activities but limited in vocational and avocational activities
Class IV	Limited in ability to perform usual self-care, vocational, and avocational activities

From Hochberg MC et al: The American College of Rheumatology 1991 revised criteria for the classification of global functional status in rheumatoid arthritis, *Arthritis Rheum* 25:498-502, 1992.
Usual self-care activities include dressing, feeding, bathing, grooming, and toileting. Avocational (recreational and/or leisure) and vocational (work, school, homemaking) activities are patient-desired and age- and sex-specific.

(Hellman and Stone, 2002). Some patients with early disease may be negative for RF but become positive as the disease progresses.

The erythrocyte sedimentation rate (ESR) and the gamma globulins (most commonly IgM and IgG) are typically elevated (Hellman and Stone, 2002). Joint fluid examination may be helpful, reflecting abnormalities associated with levels of inflammation.

Differential Diagnosis

- Osteoarthritis
- Polymyalgia rheumatica (Table 17-8)

Treatment

The goals of treatment are as follows:
- To provide pain relief
- To decrease joint inflammation
- To maintain or restore joint function
- To prevent bone and cartilage destruction

If at all feasible, patients should be monitored either by a specialist or in a specialty clinic. An interdisciplinary team needs to be responsible for care given by primary care providers, who may at times be in charge of follow-up after the diagnosis is confirmed.

Because the complexities surrounding the treatment of RA continue, it is imperative that the primary care provider consult the latest literature and investigate all information about new drug treatment. It is beyond the scope of this book to cover the extensive field of treatment options that exist. For information purposes, a summary will be presented that outlines options for treatment, but the primary care practitioner should be following the recommendations of the specialist for the follow-up care of the patient with RA, or the patient should be under the direct care of the specialist.

EDUCATION AND EMOTIONAL SUPPORT OF PATIENT AND FAMILY

After the diagnosis is confirmed, patients should be taught all aspects of the disease, the course of the disease, the causes of the pain, and expectations of treatment. Motivation to continue the daily

TABLE 17-8   Differential Diagnosis

	Pain Pattern	Common Systemic Symptoms	Onset and Course	Anatomy Affected	Laboratory Findings, X-Ray	Age at Onset
Rheumatoid arthritis	On arising, after prolonged inactivity	Fever, fatigue, weight loss, malaise, and organ-specific extraarticular symptoms such as shortness of breath	Acute or subacute onset, with chronic and variable course	Wrists, MCP joints, any synovial joints; symmetric; extraarticular (e.g., heart, lung, eye, integument)	Elevated ESR, +RA, +ANA; normochromic anemia; x-ray: joint changes and deformities; osteoporosis	Childhood to old age
Osteoarthritis	End of day or after heavy use of joints	Not prominent	Chronic, may emerge after injury	Weight-bearing joints, axial skeleton, distal hand joints; oligoarticular and asymmetric	Characteristic degenerative changes of joints on x-ray	>40 (unless posttraumatic)
PMR	On arising, after prolonged inactivity	Low-grade fevers, fatigue, general malaise, weight loss, depression, headache	Acute or subacute onset and chronic steady course	Proximal muscles, periarticular tissues of limb girdles	Elevated ESR, normochromic anemia	>55

Fibromyalgia	On arising and with active use	Insomnia, malaise, weakness, irritable bowel syndrome	Chronic but evanescent	Periarticular muscle insertion sites: "trigger points"	None	Middle age
Depression	Highly variable and changeable	Weakness, anxiety, malaise, insomnia, weight and appetite changes	Subacute to slow onset, with variable chronic course	Diffuse aches difficult to characterize; trigger points not prominent	No specific abnormalities	Childhood to old age
Chronic infection	Diffuse aching not clearly related to use	Spiking fevers, sweats, chills, malaise, anorexia, nausea, headache, weakness	Acute or subacute with variable course	Nonarticular diffuse aches and stiffness; varies with type of infection	Elevated ESR, elevated WBC; normochromic anemia; + skin test or serology; + cultures	Childhood to old age

Modified from Ham R, Sloane P: *Primary care geriatrics*, ed 4, St Louis, 2001, Mosby.
ESR, Erythrocyte sedimentation rate; *MCP*, metacarpophalangeal joints; *RA*, rheumatoid factor; *ANA*, antinuclear antigen; *EMG*, electromyography.

treatment prescription is essential to maintaining function and requires responsibility and sustained commitment by patients and their social support systems. Older patients with new-onset RA are often overwhelmed by the magnitude of the disease and need extra support from primary care providers.

LIFESTYLE CHANGES

The goal of reduction of joint stress is an underlying principle of the necessary changes that the individual patient can accomplish. The most essential goal is to provide for rest; the amount of rest is determined by the presence and severity of inflammation. Eight to 10 hours of sleep with a 2-hour rest period in the day is an accommodation that is appropriate for many persons to make. Achieving ideal body weight is another important goal.

PHYSICAL AND OCCUPATIONAL THERAPIES

The expertise of physical and occupational therapists is a necessary ingredient in any plan of care of RA patients of all ages. These health professionals are able to design a plan of care throughout the course of the disease that has the following goals:
- Preventing contractures and muscle atrophy by a progressive exercise program and use of splinting devices
- Nonpharmologic pain-controlled methods (i.e., hot showers and heat application and water therapy)
- Use of assistive devices for activities of daily living

DRUG TREATMENT

The NSAIDs are considered by some to be the first drug of choice, although it is widely recognized that these drugs do not retard the progress of the disease. Some rheumatologists move more aggressively to new and old drugs now described as disease-modifying antirheumatic drugs (DMARDs). These include hydroxychloroquine, sulfasalazine, methotrexate, and tumor necrosis factor (TNF) inhibitors. Low-dose corticosteroids (less than 10 mg a day) are also used as an adjunct therapy for some patients who are severely disabled (Hellman and Stone, 2002; Matsumoto, 2003). All drugs have side effects and contraindications, and the NSAIDs and DMARDs have significant problems, especially for older adults. Consultation with a rheumatologist, the patient, and family members is essential early in the drug treatment phase and throughout an aggressive treatment protocol. A list of NSAIDs and side effects of NSAIDs are listed in Tables 17-4 and 17-5.

All providers need to stay informed about the latest clinical trials and reports regarding adverse reactions to RA drugs. The medication regimens of older adults are indeed different from those for younger RA patients because of the higher risk of adverse drug reactions (Weinblatt, 1997).

ALTERNATIVE THERAPIES

Because RA and OA do not have a predictable disease course but rather an unpredictable pattern of flareups and remissions, patients may attribute remission to a variety of causes. Because health professionals are at a loss to explain the actual cause of either the positive or negative happenings, this chapter discusses a few of the alternative therapies that patients find and use in the informal health care system.

Use of alternative therapies is considered a universal phenomenon, especially in chronic conditions such as RA. In an Indian study of 114 RA patients, 43% had used alternative medicines. Ayurveda and homeopathy thereafter were the two most common modalities used. Most patients believed conventional medicine had no cure for RA, and adverse reactions are rare in alternative medicine modalities (Chandrashekra et al, 2002). Plant extractions are used in the Asian-Indian Ayurvedic medicinal system. A randomized double-blind trial of a standard plant formula that is considered safe and effective as a antiarthritic treatment was tested for efficacy. The study reported that the plant extract was not more effective than placebo, but the demonstrated safety of the plant extract was considered a benefit (Chopra et al, 2000). An Austrian study tested a plant extract and found relative safety of the plant extract but only modest benefit (Mur et al, 2002).

A randomized controlled study of 112 RA patients at a rheumatology clinic in a teaching hospital tested the efficacy of homeopathic medicine compared with placebo. The study results found no difference between groups in pain scores, joint tenderness, morning stiffness, and ESR (Fisher and Scott, 2001).

In a small study of the benefits of yoga training, researchers reported improved hand grip in both normal volunteers and RA patients (Dash and Telles, 2001). Spirituality and the power of prayer have also been studied as alternative therapies but have not produced significant improvement (le Gallez et al, 2000).

Copper bracelets were used by the ancient Greeks to relieve aches and pains, and many Americans wear copper bracelets for the same reason. Copper in the bracelets may be absorbed through the skin, but the effects of subjective well-being are considered a placebo effect. Copper salts have been used in the past, but severe adverse effects occurred (Sorenson, 1981; Sorenson and Hangarter, 1977).

Practitioners must note the unpredictable pattern of the disease and understand the difficulty that patients have in bringing a sense of order and causality to their experience. The important aspect for the primary care provider is to stay informed about the latest trends in alternative therapies, read the research, and talk to the patient about the risks and benefits of unregulated drugs and untested therapies. If the therapy is safe and works for the patient, the practitioner should document it and ask about its use and any effects at the next visit.

POLYMYALGIA RHEUMATICA AND GIANT CELL ARTERITIS

Epidemiology

Polymyalgia rheumatica (PMR) and giant cell (temporal) arteritis (GCA) are closely related syndromes that occur almost exclusively in people over 50 years of age; the average age of onset is 65 to 70 years of age. PMR is 10 times more common in people after 80 years of age. Prevalence estimates are higher in women, and it is much more common in whites than in other racial groups. The PMR prevalence rate in the United States is estimated to be 700 per 100,000, and the GCA rate is estimated to be 200 per 100,000 (Lawrence et al, 1998; Levy and Sethi, 1998).

Definition

The PMR syndrome is of unknown origin and includes joint and muscle pain, muscle stiffness, and systemic illness; it precedes or follows GCA in up to 20% of cases but also exists independently. Genetic factors appear to be important, and PMR has also been linked with RA (Bahlas, Ramos-Remus, and Davis, 1998).

Clinical Features of Polymyalgia Rheumatica

- Muscle pain in neck, shoulder girdle, or pelvic girdle (usually bilateral) for at least 4 weeks
- Stiffness after rest
- Elevated (> 50 mm/hour) ESR
- Frequent general malaise, fever, weight loss
- Clinical response to corticosteroid treatment (Labbe and Hardouin, 1998; Weyand and Goronzy, 1997)

Criteria for Classification of Giant Cell Arteritis

- Age at disease onset > 50 years of age
- Headache of new onset or new type

- Tenderness or decreased pulsation of temporal artery
- Elevated (> 50 mm/hour) ESR
- Positive temporal artery biopsy (Johnson, 2003)
- Histologic changes of arteritis (Weyland and Goronzy, 1997)

Treatment

Patients with PMR and GCA need to be followed up by a specialist or seen in a specialty clinic. An interdisciplinary team needs to be responsible for any care by primary care providers, who may at times be in charge of follow-up after the diagnosis is confirmed.

POLYMYALGIA RHEUMATICA

If diagnosed and treated promptly, PMR has an excellent prognosis. Corticosteroids are the treatment of choice. The goal is to control the pain, stiffness, and general constitutional symptoms with low doses; however, the schedule for the initial dose, the duration of treatment, and the optimal tapering are much debated (Labbe and Hardouin, 1998). One current recommendation is to initiate treatment with 15 to 20 mg of prednisone per day, with the expectation that relief is obtained within either hours or days. Tapering of the daily dose needs to be supervised by the interdisciplinary team, but the recommended trial is a 2.5-mg reduction of the daily dose every 2 weeks until a dose of 5 to 7.5 mg daily is reached. After that level is reached, a 1-mg incremental reduction every 4 weeks can begin. Some patients cannot tolerate this reduction system, and the problem is that to regain control of the disease, the dose of prednisone must be increased (Weyland and Goronzy, 1997). In a controlled 96-week study of 55 patients, side effects from oral prednisolone for the treatment of polymyalgia were weight gain, eight fractures, moon face, hypertension, cataracts, back pain, and depression; however, the numbers were small (Dasgupta et al., 1998).

Patients need to be followed up for 6 to 12 months after treatment with corticosteroids has been discontinued. Every patient with PMR needs to be considered at increased risk for the development of GCA. Nonsteroidal drugs are considered unsuitable for long-term treatment of PMR. Although long-term treatment with corticosteroids can lead to steroid side effects, they remain the mainstay of treatment (Labbe and Hardouin, 1998).

GIANT CELL ARTERITIS

High-dose corticosteroids in a range of 40 to 60 mg daily are the recommended treatment for GCA and need to be continued until reversible symptoms are in remission and laboratory values are normal. Tapering doses too rapidly may be harmful and has been associated with relapses. Treatment usually continues for 2 years, with clinical monitoring for an additional 6 to 12 years. Up to 50% of patients are unable to discontinue therapy in 2 years (Weyland and Goronzy, 1997). Again, the importance of a specialty or team approach to this type of patient must be noted.

FIBROMYALGIA

Fibromyalgia is a syndrome of unknown etiology, although it has been recognized for decades and has been described as nonarticular arthritis, psychogenic arteritis, and fibrositis. In 1990 the American College of Rheumatology established criteria that include pain over a wide area that persists for at least 3 months and specific point tenderness over at least 11 of 18 anatomic sites (Wolfe et al, 1990). The diagnosis is purely clinical because no laboratory tests are available to establish the diagnosis (Hellman, 2003).

Epidemiology

Prevalence rates are difficult to approximate because many uninsured people do not seek care for this non-life-threatening condition and because it is a difficult condition to diagnose. Available data, however, suggest that prevalence rates are lower in men (0.5%) than in women (3.4%). The prevalence of fibromyalgia increases with age, with an estimate at age 80 of 59 per 100,000 compared with a rate of 34 per 100,000 at 40 years of age (Lawrence et al, 1998).

Clinical Characteristics

- Widespread pain (Figure 17-3)
- Decreased pain threshold
- Sleep disturbance
- Fatigue
- Psychological distress

Laboratory Tests

The purpose of laboratory testing in fibromyalgia is to exclude other causes of the symptoms. This is important because the failure to diagnose accurately and treat this condition often leads to the patient having multiple consultations, needlessly expensive testing, and inappropriate treatment.

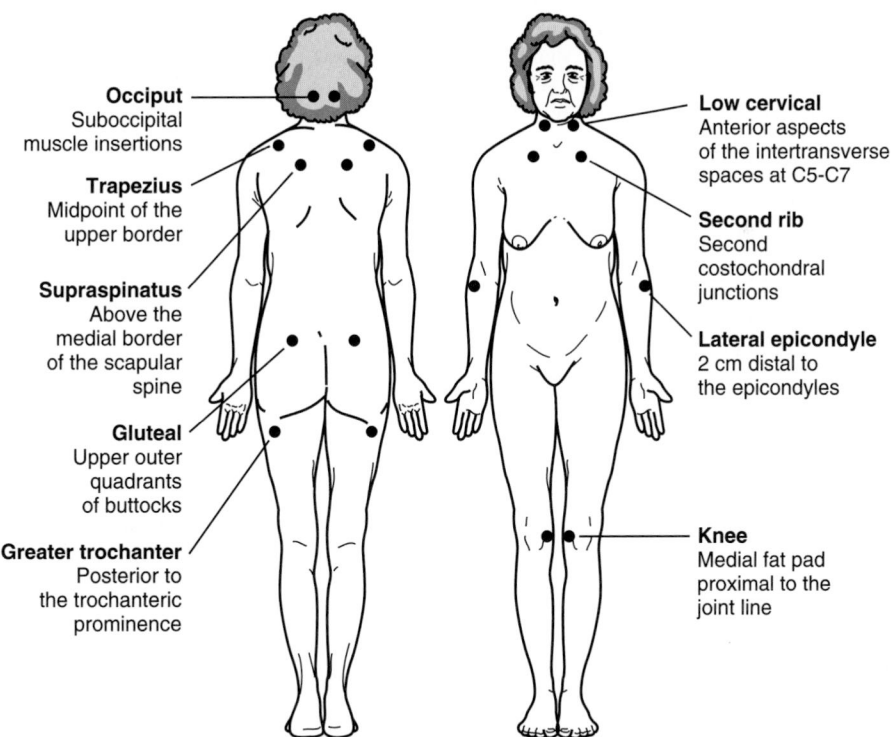

Occiput
Suboccipital muscle insertions

Trapezius
Midpoint of the upper border

Supraspinatus
Above the medial border of the scapular spine

Gluteal
Upper outer quadrants of buttocks

Greater trochanter
Posterior to the trochanteric prominence

Low cervical
Anterior aspects of the intertransverse spaces at C5-C7

Second rib
Second costochondral junctions

Lateral epicondyle
2 cm distal to the epicondyles

Knee
Medial fat pad proximal to the joint line

Figure 17-3 Location of tender points for diagnostic classification of fibromyalgia. (Redrawn from McCance KL, Huether SE: *Pathophysiology: the biologic basis for disease in adults and children*, ed 4, St Louis, 2001, Mosby.)

Conditions to rule out include all other causes of musculoskeletal problems; the most obvious will be polymyalgia and Parkinson's disease in older adults. Thyroid conditions, cancer, and chronic fatigue syndrome also must be ruled out. Basic laboratory tests should include complete blood cell count, sedimentation rate, thyroid function tests, and muscle enzyme levels. These tests will all be normal in patients with fibromyalgia (Hellman, 2003).

Treatment

In general, there is no accepted pathway for the treatment of patients with fibromyalgia. Education of the patient and reassurance that the disorder is not life threatening or associated with any type of joint deformity must be the first elements of treatment. Training in pain management and coping skills may be helpful to many patients. Physical therapy to include relaxation, heat massage, and a graded exercise program has been useful to some patients. Tricyclic antidepressants produce moderate improvement in up to one third of patients (Hillman, 2003).

GOUT

Clinical Characteristics

Gout affects both men and women in the United States. The prevalence rate has been estimated to be 8.4 per 1000 adults for a total of 2.1 million people. Men far outweigh women with this disease with a 3:1 ratio. Obesity and excessive weight gain are significant risk factors for men and increased age and the use of thiazide diuretics are significant risk factors for both women and men (Lawrence, 1998; Townes, 2003). Gout classically presents as an acute distal monoarthritis with extreme pain, swelling, redness, tenderness, and warmth over the involved joint. The course of the disease has wide variations even if left untreated; the attack abates after 1 to 2 weeks and may not return for weeks or years. If left untreated in some patients, the progression includes joint destruction, progressive renal impairment, and hypertension. Factors that can precipitate an attack are uricosuric agents, alcohol, diuretics, and stress.

Diagnosis

The definitive diagnosis of gout is made by the observation of urate crystals in the aspirated synovial fluid from an involved joint (Townes, 2003). Hyperuricemia, defined as a serum uric acid value above 7 mg/dl, has been thought to be responsible for the development of gout. An elevated uric acid level is not sufficient for a diagnosis, however.

Treatment

For the acute phase, treatment should include joint rest, cold compresses, and NSAIDs. Colchicine is effective for acute gout, but more than 80% of treated patients develop significant abdominal effects such as diarrhea or nausea. It is most effective when given in the first few hours of the onset of symptoms. The dose is 0.5 or 0.6 mg every hour until pain is relieved or side effects appear and not to exceed 8 mg (Hellman and Stone, 2002). Another recommendation for acute attack is administration of indomethacin 50 mg every 6 hours for six to eight doses; then the dosage is reduced to 25 mg every 6 to 8 hours for no more than 5 to 7 days (Townes, 2003). This drug has severe side effects and is not to be given to any patient with renal problems.

After the acute phase resolves, long-term treatment is intended to reduce acute occurrences and to minimize urate deposition in tissues, which causes chronic tophaceous arthritis. Diet low in purines, weight loss, diminished intake of alcohol, avoidance of beer, and avoidance of thiazade and loop diuretics are significant aspects of a prevention program. Avoidance of most aspirin but not single low-dose enteric tablets used for cardiac prophylaxis is also highly recommended (Harris et al, 2000). Lack of understanding of the disease and lack of compliance with therapy are major problems (Hellman and Stone, 2003; Townes, 2003).

Long-term drug therapy is generally a response to the uric acid level and the frequency of attacks. For persons who have mild hyperuricemia and occasional attacks of gouty arthritis, colchicine prophylaxis may be sufficient (Hellman and Stone, 2002). For patients not controlled by colchicine the intent is to lower the uric acid level below 6 mg/dl. The two classes of drugs effective in lowering uric acid levels are uricosuric drugs and allopurinol. A 24-hour urine collection to determine the uric acid level is needed; although many practitioners used the serum plasma level of uric acid as their measure, cost to the patient may be an issue. Patients with levels greater than 750 to 800 mg are considered overproducers and require allopurinol (Townes, 2003; Hellman and Stone, 2002), whereas others will be treated with uricosuric drug probenecid. Hydration to maintain a daily output of 2000 ml or more is an important consideration for patients taking these drugs. The toxicity of allopurinol is important because it can precipitate severe life-threatening reactions. Therefore the patient taking this drug needs to be monitored (Studenski and Laird, 1998).

DUPUYTREN'S CONTRACTURE

Dupuytren's contracture most commonly affects primarily middle-aged and older men. The palmar fascia for unknown causes undergoes nodular hypertrophis fibroplasia, resulting in the development of flexion contracture. The contracture is usually painless but may cause functional disability. Most frequently, digits 4 and 5 are affected. The contracture does not respond to passive extension, oral inflammatory drugs, or local cortisone injections. If there is disability the patient should be referred to an orthopedic surgeon (Hellman, 2003).

Summary

Most older adults are affected by OA. In addition, RA, PMR, GCA, fibromyalgia, gout, and Dupuytren's contracture cause severe pain, expense, and loss of function in a significant number of people in this population. Proper diagnosis requires knowledge of the risk factors and diagnostic criteria for each, a thorough history and physical examination, and use of the appropriate diagnostic tests. Treatment can involve both pharmacologic and nonpharmacologic interventions, including diet and alternative therapies. Proper use of assistive devices, exercise, and safety considerations can ease pain, prevent injury, and enhance function and independence.

Resources

Arthritis Foundation
1330 West Peachtree Street
Atlanta, GA 30309
(404) 872-7100
www.arthritis.org

Arthritis Net
www.arthritisnet.com

References

Bahlas S, Ramos-Remus C, Davis P: Clinical outcome of 149 patients with polymyalgia and giant cell arteritis, *J Rheumatol* 25(1):99-104, 1998.

Baker J, McAlindon T: Exercise in knee osteoarthritis, *Curr Opin Rheumatol* 12(5):456-463, 2000.

Bombardier C et al: An evidence-based evaluation of gastrointestinial safety of coxibs, *Am J Cardiol* 89(6A): 3D-9D, 2002.

Chandrashekara S et al: Complementary and alternative drug therapy in arthritis, *J Assoc Physicians India* 50:225-7, 2002.

Centers for Disease Control and Prevention (CDC): Prevalence of self-reported arthritis or chronic joint symptoms among adults—United States, 2001, *MMWR Morb Mortal Wkly Rep* 51(42):948-950, 2002.

Chopra A et al: Randomized double blind trial of ayurvedic plant derived formulation for treatment for rheumatoid arthritis, *J Rheumatol* 27(6):1332-1333, 2000.

Dash M, Telles S: Improvement in hand grip strength in normal volunteers and rheumatoid arthritis patients following yoga training, *Indian J Physiol Pharmacol* 45(3):355-360, 2001.

Dasgupta B et al: An initially double-blind controlled 96 week trial of depot methylprednisolone against oral prednisolone in the treatment of polymyalgia rheumatica, *Br J Rheumatol* 37(2):189-195, 1998.

Fisher P, Scott DL: A randomized controlled trial of homeopathy in rheumatoid arthritis, *Rheumatology (Oxford)* 40(9):1052-1055, 2001.

Harris M, Byrant LR, Danaker P et al: Effect of low dose daily aspirin on serum urate levels and urinary excretion in patients receiving probenecid for gouty arthritis, *J Rheumatol* 27:2873, 2000.

Hay E et al: Fatal hyperkalemia related to combined therapy with a Cox-2 inhibitor, ACE inhibitor and potassium rich diet, *J Emerg Med* 22(4):349-352, 2002.

Hellman D: Nonarticular rheumatic disorders. In Barker LR et al, editors: *Principles of ambulatory medicine*, ed 6, Philadelphia, 2003, Lippincott Williams & Wilkins.

Hellmann D, Stone J: Arthritis and musculoskeletal disorders. In Tierney LM, McPhee SJ, Papadakis MA, editors: *Current medical diagnosis and treatment*, ed 41, New York, 2002, Lange Medical Books—McGraw-Hill.

Hurley BF, Roth SM: Strength training in the elderly: effect on risk factors for age-related disease, *Sport Med* 30(4):249-268, 2000.

Johnson C: Headaches and facial pain. In Barker LR et al, editors: *Principles of ambulatory medicine*, ed 6, Philadelphia, 2003, Lippincott Williams & Wilkins.

Labbe P, Hardouin P: Epidemiology and optimal management of polymyalgia rheumatica, *Drugs Aging* 13(2):109-118, 1998.

Lawrence RC et al: Estimates of the prevalence of arthritis and selected musculoskeletal disorders in the United States, *Arthritis Rheum* 41(5):778-799, 1998.

Le Gallez P et al: Spiritual healing as adjunct therapy for rheumatoid arthritis, *Br J Nurs* 9(11):695-700, 2000.

Levy J, Sethi P: Joint pain in the elderly patient, *J Am Acad Orthopaed Surg* 2(1):66-73, 1998.

Manninen P et al: Physical workload and the risk of severe knee osteoarthritis, *Scand J Work Environ Health* 28(1):25-32, 2002.

Matsumoto AK: Rheumatoid arthritis. In Barker LR, et al, editor: *Principles of ambulatory medicine*, ed 6, Philadelphia, 2003, Lippincott Williams & Wilkins.

Mur E et al: Randomized double blind trial of extract from the pentacyclic alkaloid-chemotype of uncaria tomentosa for the treatment of rheumatoid arthritis, *J Rheumatol* 29(4):656-658, 2002.

Nishihara K, Furst D: Aspirin and other nonsteroid anti-inflammatory drugs. In Koopman WJ, editor: *Arthritis and allied conditions*, ed 13, Baltimore, 1997, Williams & Wilkins.

O'Grady M, Fletcher J, Ortiz S: Therapeutic and physical fitness exercise prescription for older adults with joint disease: an evidence based approach, *Rheum Dis Clin North Am* 26(3):617-648, 2000.

Pincus T et al: A randomized double-blind crossover clinical trial of diclofenac plus misoprostol versus acetaminophen in patients with osteoarthritis of the knee or hip. *Arthritis Rheum* 44:1587, 2001.

Rasker JJ et al: Lack of beneficial effect of zinc sulfate in rheumatoid arthritis, *Scand J Rheumatol* 11(3): 168-170, 1982.

Reginster JY et al: Long term effects of glucosamine sulfate on osteoarthritis: a randomized, placebo controlled clinical trial, *Lancet* 357:247, 2001.

Sorenson J: Development of copper complexes for potential therapeutic use, *Agents Actions Suppl* 8:305-325, 1981.

Sorenson J, Hangarter W: Treatment of rheumatoid and degenerative diseases with copper complexes, *Inflammation* 2:217-238, 1977.

Sowers M: Epidemiology of risk factors for osteoarthritis: systemic factors, *Curr Opin Rheumatol* 13(5): 447-451, 2001.

Townes A: Osteoarthritis. In Barker LR et al: *Principles of ambulatory medicine*, ed 6, Philadelphia, 2003, Lippincott Williams & Wilkins.

Weinblatt M: Rheumatoid arthritis: the clinical picture. In Koopman WJ, editor: *Arthritis and allied conditions*, ed 13, Baltimore, 1997, Williams & Wilkins.

Weyland C, Goronzy J: Polymyalgia rheumatica and giant cell arteritis. In Koopman WJ, editor: *Arthritis and allied conditions*, ed 13, Baltimore, 1997, Williams & Wilkins.

Wolfe F et al: The American College of Rheumatology 1990 criteria for the classification of fibromyalgia: report of the multi-center criteria committee, *Arthritis Rheum* 33:160-172, 1990.

18

Foot Problems

Foot problems in older adults are extremely common. About 75% to 80% of the older population exhibit pathologic conditions of the foot (Beiser and Shuman, 1998). Diminished opportunities for walking because of social factors and health conditions; increased foot neglect; and deterioration of vascular, neurologic, skeletal, and dermatologic structures all contribute to foot problems in older adults.

Walking is a low-impact, relatively safe form of aerobic exercise for the older adult and is essential to a person's overall health, including foot health. Walking with proper footwear tones and strengthens foot and leg muscles, maintains joint flexibility and motion, increases arterial blood flow, and helps evacuate venous blood flow (Figure 18-1). Unfortunately, many older adults become isolated, less active, and less ambulatory because of a variety of social and health conditions. Social factors that commonly affect the older person's desire to walk include a fear of falling, a loss of driving privileges, and a loss of friends and family. Health conditions such as vision deterioration, arthritic pain, chronic heart or lung disease, and foot and leg pain and weakness also limit an older person's ability to walk.

Foot neglect also contributes to problems in the older person. Visual impairment, an inability to reach the feet, unmanageable hypertrophic toenails, and transportation limitations to health care providers all contribute to foot neglect and the development of foot problems.

In addition, both natural and pathologic deterioration of vascular, neurologic, skeletal, and dermatologic structures contribute to foot problems. Peripheral vascular disease is often diagnosed in older patients and can be detrimental to ambulation capability and healing potential. Disease or neuropathy in lower-extremity nerves accompanies many systemic diseases and nervous system traumas (Lebowitz and Kern, 2003).

Neuropathic pain, weakness, and sensory loss can cause a variety of foot problems. Skeletal or orthopedic foot changes in the older patient are responsible for a great percentage of foot problems. Causes for the foot's mechanical and functional deterioration and its adaptive orthopedic changes include increased weight gain, decreased muscle strength, inadequate or ill-fitting shoes, decades of ambulation, limited exercise, and systemic diseases. Dermatologic changes such as dystrophic nails and painful corns and calluses are responsible for the majority of foot complaints in older adults.

Common Foot Problems and Treatments

Orthopedic, mechanically induced, and dermatologic changes are common reasons for foot complaints in the older patient. Understanding what causes these changes helps the primary care provider to recognize and treat current problems and also to foresee and prevent future problems.

429

Maintaining a normal gait requires the foot to accomplish four major functions: (1) to adapt to an uneven surface (ground topography adaptation), (2) to become a rigid lever for propulsion, (3) to translate rotary forces generated by the hip, and (4) to absorb shock (Beiser and Shuman, 1998). Shock absorption and ground topography adaptation are achieved with foot flexibility caused by subtalar joint pronation (foot abduction and eversion). Pushing off the ground requires foot rigidity and stability, which is achieved with subtalar joint supination (foot adduction and inversion). With age, the subtalar joint of the foot progresses to function in the pronated position and loses supination capacity. This adaptation causes excessive flexibility and instability during foot propulsion, which can lead to significant mechanically induced foot changes and problems.

Ambulation on a pronated, unstable foot can cause arch and heel pain, bunion deformities, hammertoe deformities, metatarsalgia, neuroma pain, tendinitis, arthritis, and an apropulsive gait. Reducing subtalar joint pronation via adequate shoe gear or generic or custom-molded orthotics is an important treatment consideration for these conditions. Running shoes and cross-training shoes provide the best foot support and usually help mild to moderate cases of tendinitis, heel pain, arch pain, neuroma pain, and metatarsalgia. Moderate to severe cases should be treated with some degree of arch support. Moderate cases can be treated with generic arch supports, which can be purchased in most pharmacies. Severely pronated feet should receive custom-molded arch supports made by a podiatrist.

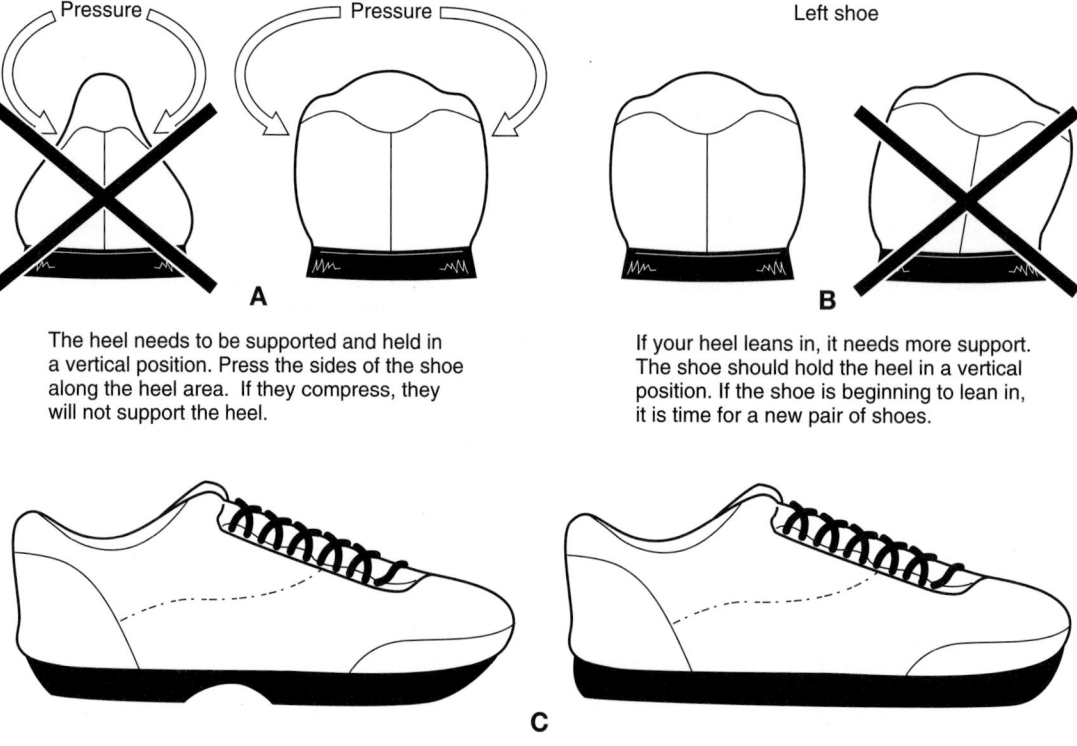

A The heel needs to be supported and held in a vertical position. Press the sides of the shoe along the heel area. If they compress, they will not support the heel.

B If your heel leans in, it needs more support. The shoe should hold the heel in a vertical position. If the shoe is beginning to lean in, it is time for a new pair of shoes.

C The midsole and outer-sole (in black) play an important role in absorbing shock. Unfortunately, this part of the shoe is the heaviest. However, since the foot only bears weight on the heel and forefoot, contouring the middle and ends of this area (left picture) results in a lighter shoe without disturbing the shock absorption under the heel and forefoot. It is a positive feature.

Figure 18-1   Choosing a proper walking shoe.

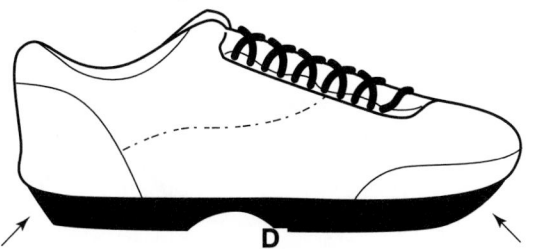

Contouring of the midsole and outer-sole on the ends of the shoe has an advantage in addition to making the shoe lighter. Look below.

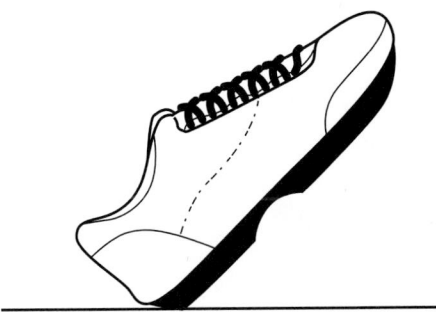

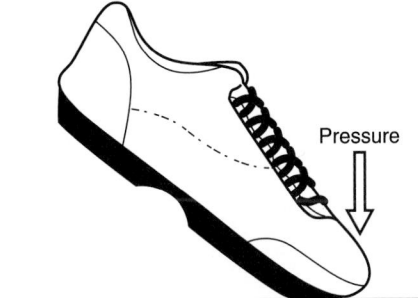

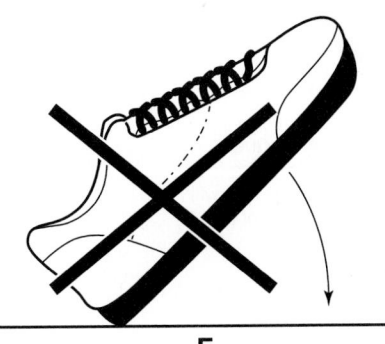

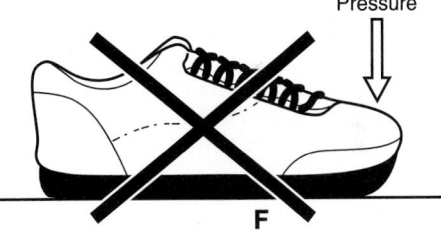

When a step is taken, the bevelled edge on the back (top picture) allows the foot to be balanced on the heel until it is ready to come down. A sharp angle (bottom picture) forces the foot down when the heel hits the ground, and this puts strain on the muscles in front of the lower leg.

The bevelled edge on the front of the midsole and outer-sole assists in elevating the heel when you lean forward. This reduces the strain on the muscles in back of the lower leg (top picture). These features make walking easier.

Figure 18-1, cont'd.

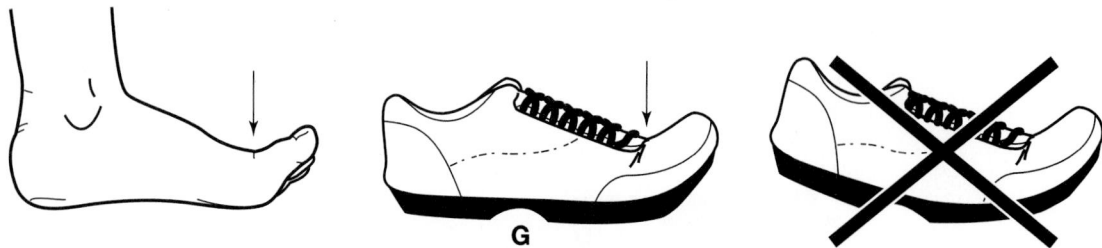

The foot only bends in one place (see arrow). Therefore the shoe should only bend in that one place. If the shoe bends in areas that the foot does not, the shoe will not support the foot well.

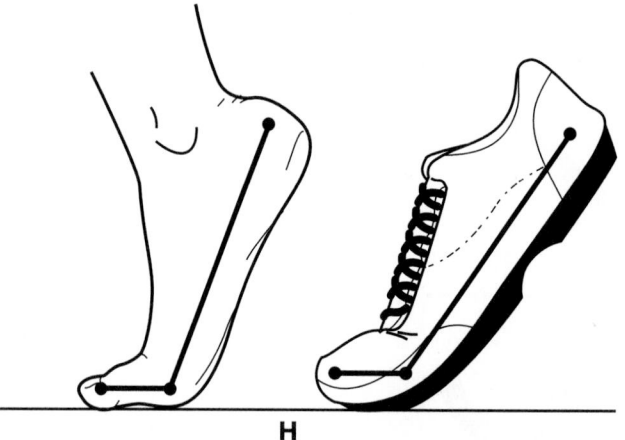

It is important that the shoe be as flexible as the foot in the area where the foot bends. If the shoe can not bend as much as the foot, the heel of your foot will pull out of the shoe when walking. This will result in excessive movement and rubbing between your heel and shoe and result in blistering, soreness, or infection.

Figure 18-1,   cont'd.

SUBTALAR JOINT PRONATION

Subtle increases in subtalar joint pronation are responsible for painful conditions but may be difficult to recognize. Recognition of the signs of pronation requires both a non-weight-bearing and a weight-bearing foot examination. While not bearing weight, the patient will exhibit excessive flexibility of the subtalar joint with passive range of motion, and some degree of bunion and hammertoe deformity will be present. While bearing weight, the patient will show a noticeable arch reduction, and the degree of bunion and hammertoe deformity will increase. The foot will be in some degree of abduction, and some degree of detectable rear foot valgus will be present. During walking, the heel may demonstrate an abductory twist as it elevates off the ground during propulsion.

The most applicable use of arch support and pronation reduction is for the treatment of heel pain and plantar fasciitis (Figure 18-2). Pronation reduction and arch elevation relax the plantar fascia and reduce tension at its calcaneal attachment. A combination of arch support, mild heel elevation, ice, and antiinflammatory medication in the form of oral nonsteroidal antiinflammatory drugs or injected cortisone successfully treats most heel and arch pain.

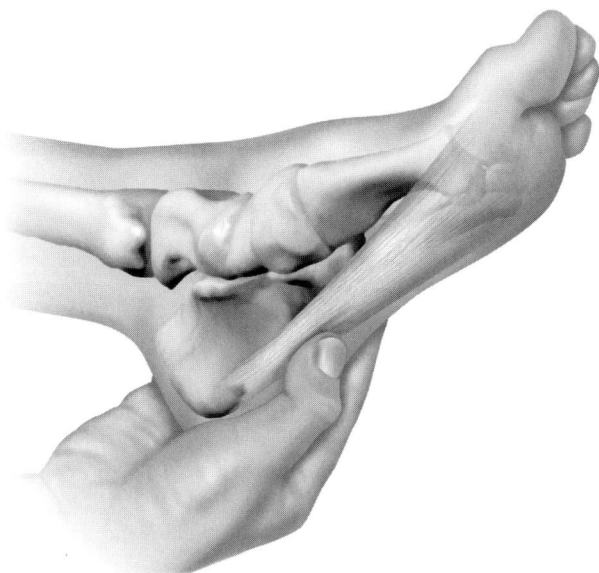

Figure 18-2   Painful plantar fasciitis with an associated heel spur.

BUNION AND HAMMERTOE FORMATIONS

Painful feet are an extremely common problem among older women and increase the risk of falls and hamper mobility (Dawson et al, 2002). Younger women need to be informed about the relationship between footwear, occupation, and the development of foot problems in later years.

Bunion and hammertoe formations are mechanically induced and are often painful (Figure 18-3). Excessive pronation and increased weight bearing on the inside of the foot cause bunions and lead to dorsiflexion, adduction, and hypermobility of the first metatarsal. The hallux abducts as the first metatarsal adducts, and the joint becomes malaligned. Bunion pain presents as either "bump" pain or joint pain. A distinction between these two types of pain is important. Bump pain is superficial pain or irritation caused by shoe pressure; it is treated with shoe modification or padding to reduce

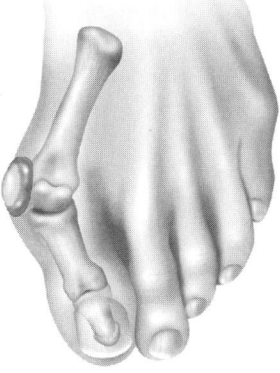

Figure 18-3   A, Bunion with painful callosity and bursitis.

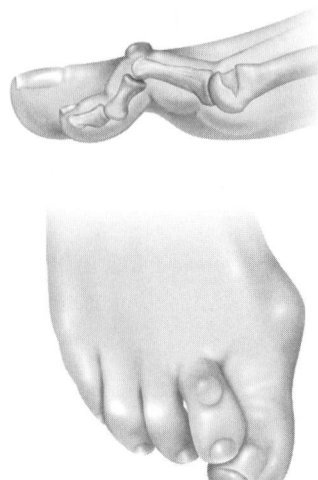

Figure 18-3,   cont'd **B,** Hammering of the second toe with dorsal proximal interphalangeal callosity secondary to bunion.

local pressure. Joint pain is associated with inflammation within the first metatarsal-phalangeal joint (MPJ); this inflammation is created by the malalignment. Joint pain is improved with pronation reduction and antiinflammatory medication.

Hammertoe formation is generally the product of wearing high-heeled shoes. Toes assist in balance. When a person leans back, the toes elevate. When a person leans forward, the toes grip the ground. When a person stands erect, the toes should be relaxed. High-heeled shoes push weight forward onto the forefoot, and as a result the toes grip the ground in hammertoe formation, which involves hyperextension of the MPJ, hyperflexion of the proximal interphalangeal joint (PIPJ), and hyperextension of the distal interphalangeal joint (DIPJ). Hammertoes can create joint inflammation at the hyperextended MPJ and shoe pressure irritation at the dorsally prominent PIPJ.

Treatment of hammertoe formation is based on the degree of rigidity. Flexible hammertoes will reduce and realign with significant heel reduction and adequate arch support. Rigid hammertoe treatment depends on the location of the pain. Dorsal shoe irritation can be accommodated by extradepth shoes that have a higher toe box. Inflamed, hyperextended MJPs require antiinflammatory medication and adequate arch support.

Severely hyperextended MPJs cause plantar-flexed and plantarly prominent metatarsal bones. This condition, in association with fat-pad atrophy of the plantar forefoot, causes a painful condition that the patient describes as a feeling of "walking on my bones." Treatment for this painful, chronic condition involves application of a cushioned pad beneath the metatarsal heads and proximal to the metatarsal heads so that pressure is redistributed to the metatarsal necks and away from the prominent metatarsal heads (Ferarri et al, 2001).

DERMATOLOGIC CHANGES

An examination of the dermatologic status of the older person's foot provides information about the foot's circulation, function, and shoe fit. Corns and calluses are areas of thickened epidermis caused by intermittent pressure on a broad area (*callus*) or focal area (*corn*). Pressure pushes the local circulation away from the skin, causing blanching and pallor. A rebound hyperemic response occurs when pressure is removed. Over time this repetitious, intermittent, hyperemic response causes epidermal thickening.

A thickened epidermis can cause two potential problems. As the epidermis thickens, it loses softness and flexibility. As a result, it can crack, causing a painful fissure and a potential infection risk.

Focal epidermal thickening (e.g., a corn) causes focal, painful pressure to the underlying tissue. Advanced corns can cause subepidermal bleeding or ulceration.

Because rebound hyperemia in response to ischemic pressure is responsible for thickening of the skin, well-formed corns and calluses suggest the presence of good skin circulation. A poorly formed callus or the absence of a callus on a pressure area is a sign of limited skin circulation because an adequate hyperemic response to pressure does not occur. This explains why patients with poor arterial circulation cannot tolerate firm, supportive shoes. The pressure from a shoe holding the foot in a mechanically proper position causes ischemic pain, and therefore these patients need soft, accommodating shoes.

The treatment of painful corns and calluses requires debridement and pressure removal. Debridement can be accomplished by mechanical or chemical means. Mechanical debridement by a skilled health care provider should be performed with a sharp blade or scalpel. Patients can perform routine mechanical debridement with a pumice stone. Chemical debridement can be accomplished with over-the-counter corn-remover pads that contain salicylic acid. The primary care provider should monitor this treatment, and it should not be used on patients with diabetes or peripheral vascular disease. Pressure removal can be accomplished by shoe modification, padding, or surgical intervention.

NAIL PROBLEMS

Nail problems account for most foot problems in older adults. With age, the toenails undergo predictable changes to varying degrees; they thicken, incurvate, and become more susceptible to nail fungus. Various digital deformities cause added shoe, floor, and adjacent toe pressures that further deform the nails and cause them to become dystrophic and difficult to manage. Often people either injure their feet by attempting to cut their nails with scissors or wire cutters or neglect their nails until they cause a problem. Common nail problems include painful hypertrophic nails, mycotic nails, periungual calluses, and ingrowing nails.

Onychomycosis

Onychomycosis, or nail fungus, is often encountered in older patients. Fungus thrives in a dark, warm, wet environment. Shoes cause darkness; socks keep feet warm; and foot perspiration, foot soaks, showers, baths, and closely positioned toes all contribute to chronic foot moisture. These factors create a favorable environment for fungal growth. Peripheral vascular disease and age-related, slowed nail growth maintain nail tissue on the toes for a longer time, increasing the chances of infection.

Onychomycosis has four common presentations: superficial white, distal subungual, proximal, and candidal (Beiser and Shuman, 1998). It causes nail discoloration, hypertrophy, and dystrophy, which often result in painful conditions. The extent of treatment for onychomycosis depends on a person's symptoms, degree of pedal circulation, and overall health. Treatment options include routine nail debridement, temporary or permanent nail removal, topically applied antifungal medication, oral antifungal medication, or a combination of these options. Routine nail debridement is the sole treatment for patients with extensive peripheral vascular disease and multiple medical problems. Permanent nail removal is used for patients who have an isolated chronic problematic nail and who have the circulation to heal a matrixectomy. Temporary nail removal is used for patients who have chronic or acute problematic nails and lack the circulation to heal a matrixectomy. Topical antifungal medications are effective for superficial nail fungal infections such as white superficial onychomycosis.

Oral antifungal therapy, which is used for more extensive mycotic nails, is becoming commonplace because of the introduction of newer and safer oral antifungal medications. Oral treatment for older patients, however, should be reserved for painful nail conditions, not for cosmetic reasons. It should also be reserved for healthy patients with no history of liver disease. Mild to moderately infected toenails require 3 months of therapy, whereas severely infected toenails often need 5 to 6 months of therapy. Temporary nail removal should be combined with oral antifungal therapy for most infected nails. With oral therapy, the proximal aspect of the nail grows in thin and clear compared with the distal, hypertrophic, infected, fungal nail tissue. Occasionally the fungal infection can spread from a distally infected nail to an uninfected proximal nail while the patient is undergoing oral therapy. Removing severely infected nails before initiating oral therapy eliminates this problem.

Ingrown Nails

Ingrown nails are a problem for both younger and older populations (Figure 18-4). Ingrown nails occur when the nail groove skin is pushed into the way of the normal growing nail because of confining shoes or when the nail plate is deformed and grows errantly into the skin. In general, older patients suffer from the second scenario. Incurvated, mycotic, dystrophic nails are usually the cause of the ingrown nail. Incurvated, dystrophic, ingrown nails may or may not puncture the skin. Chronic nail pressure often creates significant callus buildup in the nail groove, which causes pain and the feeling of an ingrown nail. Patients may relate gaining some relief from soaking their feet because the macerated callus softens and produces less pressure. Debridement of the nail groove callus and the offending nail edge brings instant relief. Excision of an ingrown nail should be referred to a podiatrist or a health care provider with expertise, training, and experience in the procedure.

Diabetes and the Foot

A significant percentage of patients over 55 years of age have diabetes. Diabetes is responsible for most nontraumatic lower-extremity amputations, a feared complication of diabetes that in many cases is preventable. Prevention begins with a careful foot assessment and patient education (Bowker and Pfeifer, 2001).

ASSESSMENT

Assessment of the foot of a patient with diabetes involves evaluation of the foot's circulation, bony prominences, corn and callus formation, skin condition, nail dystrophy, shoe-gear fit, and sensation loss. Any abnormal finding or combination of abnormal findings can cause a skin break and infection risk. Diminished circulation can cause skin atrophy, breakdown, and ulceration. A bony prominence from a bunion or hammertoe can cause shoe irritation and blister formation. Thick calluses can crack, and thick corns can create subepidermal ulcers. Chronic wet or dry skin can result in skin cracks. Dry skin can develop a fissure, whereas wet skin can promote a fungal infection that can cause blistering or fissuring. Dystrophic nails can cause infected, ingrown nails. Poorly fitting footwear can create dangerous pressure sores.

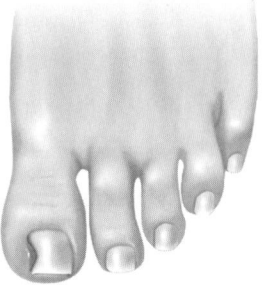

Figure 18-4   Ingrown toenail of the great toe.

The loss of sensation can result in delayed detection and the escalation of any of these problems. For example, severe circulation impairment, which typically causes extreme ischemic pain, goes unnoticed in the presence of significant numbness. The first sign of poor circulation to a diabetic patient with numbness may be gangrene and subsequent amputation. Sensation loss should be evaluated and classified as loss of superficial pressure sensation, loss of deep pressure sensation, or loss of bone sensation by using a 10-g Semmes-Weinstein monofilament, a 75-g Semmes-Weinstein monofilament, and a tuning fork, respectively.

PREVENTION

Preventive treatment addresses any abnormal findings. Diminished circulation needs to be carefully monitored. Corns, calluses, and dystrophic nails should be regularly debrided by a podiatrist. The patient needs to use footwear that provides support and accommodates bony prominences. Excessively wet or dry skin should be treated. Dry skin is best treated with 20% urea or 10% to 12% lactic acid cream or lotion. Excessive skin moisture, often found between the toes, can be "acutely" treated with povidone-iodine (Betadine) solution, a drying agent that reduces the risk of bacterial infection. It should be used for only a short period and for an acute episode. Chronic treatment includes interdigital powder, topical antifungal medication, and toe spacers.

Knowing the depth of sensation loss helps the primary care provider make treatment decisions and educate patients about their condition. Loss of superficial pressure sensation predisposes the patient not to recognize shoe irritation and superficial skin ulceration. This degree of sensory loss also prevents recognition of the "itch" sensation caused by a developing fungal infection. Corns and calluses may thicken to a dangerous level, and skin cracks go unnoticed. Patients should be educated to wear less stylish shoes and pay daily attention to the skin condition of their feet.

A loss of deep pressure sensation puts the patient at risk for not noticing objects in their shoes, ingrown nails, deeper ulcers, and excessive hot or cold temperatures. This degree of numbness warrants special footwear. For nondystrophic feet, an orthopedic shoe with a Plastizote lining is indicated; a custom-molded shoe with a Plastizote lining is indicated for dystrophic feet. Patients should be told to check inside their shoes and socks before putting them on, avoid going barefooted, inspect their feet daily, and have their toenails treated by a podiatrist.

With a loss of sensation, the patient can develop an undetected ulceration down to the bone, causing osteomyelitis. The patient is also at risk for developing a Charcot joint that can create a limb-threatening skeletal breakdown of the foot. This condition occurs in the presence of profound numbness and excessive pedal blood flow and is initiated by undetected chronic microtrauma or acute foot or ankle macrotrauma. In either case, the uneducated patient feels no pain and probably will continue to ambulate on the injured foot until a joint in the foot literally dislocates. Prevention of chronic microtrauma requires prescription footwear and firm arch support. Prevention of a Charcot joint after an acute trauma requires immediate immobilization and no weight bearing as well as appropriate diagnostic imaging studies to determine the extent of injury. The patient should be instructed to look daily for signs of discoloration, warmth, and swelling in the feet, using a mirror if necessary, and to seek medical attention for these changes.

The keys to preventing diabetic amputations for patients with diabetes are understanding, recognition, and treatment of the multiple amputation risks by the provider as well as daily foot inspections by the informed patient, spouse, or friend.

Summary

Foot problems in older adults are common; these problems develop for several reasons, and the appropriate footwear and treatments are important. An understanding of how common problems develop gives the provider foresight, which increases clinical acumen and enables the practice of preventive health care. For example, understanding that a diabetic foot callus is prone to crack compels the primary care provider to treat the callus instead of treating the forthcoming fissure or foot infection. Knowing that a patient with diabetes has superficial pressure loss around the toes and cannot feel an "itch" persuades the provider to look between the patient's toes for fungal infections. A patient who has an area of chronic shoe pressure and pain and has no corn or callus formation should be evaluated for peripheral vascular disease. If a patient presents with developing bunions and hammertoes, the patient should be evaluated for excessive foot pronation, and arch support should be considered.

With the exception of routine nail debridement, preventive foot care practices are rare. The immense number of mechanically induced foot problems in older adults justifies the use of custom-molded orthotics more frequently and sooner. The excessive number of amputations among the diabetic population demands more aggressive implementation of preventive treatment. Preventive foot-care practices will keep older adults on their feet longer and, as a result, they will be healthier.

Resources

Foot and Ankle Link Library
www.footandankle.com/podmed

Foot Care 4 U
www.footcare4u.com

References

Beiser IH, Shuman CJ: Foot care. In Yoshikawa TT, Cobbs EL, Brummel-Smith K, editors: *Practical ambulatory geriatrics*, ed 2, St Louis, 1998, Mosby.
Bowker JH, Pfeifer MA, editors: *Levin and O'Neal's the diabetic foot*, ed 6, St Louis, 2001, Mosby.
Dawson J et al: The prevalence of foot problems in older women: a cause for concern, *J Public Health Med* 24(2):77-84, 2002.
Ferrari J et al: Interventions for treating hallux valgus and bunions. *Cochrane Database Syst Rev* 2:CD000964, PMID 10796404, 2000.
Lebowitz B, Kern D: Common problems of the feet. In Barker LR et al, editors: *Principles of ambulatory medicine*, ed 6, Philadelphia, 2003, Lippincott Williams & Wilkins.

19

Falls

Falls are a major cause of death and a significant source of morbidity for people over 65 years of age. In the United States, accidents represent the sixth leading cause of death in this age group, with falls a major contributor. Stair falls account for more than 10% of fatal falls (Startzell et al, 2000). Falls also cause 90% of hip fractures, and the current cost of hip fractures in the United States is estimated to be 10 billion dollars (Carter, Kannus, and Khan, 2001).

Prevalent, dangerous, and often difficult to predict or prevent, falls are and have been the focus of clinicians and researchers alike. The search has been for either a strong predictive equation that would prevent falls or an equally strong intervention that would protect elderly patients from the harm of falling. Neither search has found the "silver bullet" or magic intervention that would cure every aspect of this enigma. Unless we find a replacement for ambulation or even movement (because older, frail people do fall out of bed), our task is to prevent and minimize the harm incurred in falling. One third of falls result in injury, but only 5% of falls result in fracture (Lyons et al, 2002; Nurmi and Luthje, 2002). Even if falls have not occurred or have not resulted in injury, the fear of falling is a serious detriment to the functioning of the older person and may severely reduce quality of life.

Falls occur in all settings–home, hospital, and long-term care facility—although 85% of falls occur in the home (Rosedale, 2001). Up to 30% of community-dwelling older Americans suffer from falls; 50% of those are over 80 years of age, and one of four of those who fall sustain an injury (Lyons et al, 2002). Of the estimated 1.7 million nursing home residents in the United States, about half fall each year—twice the rate for people dwelling in the community—and 11% sustain a serious fall-related injury (Ray et al, 1997).

Age-related Risk Factors

The causes of falls in older adults are multifactorial, with both intrinsic and extrinsic contributory factors. Balance and ambulation require complex interaction of the older person's cognitive and neuromuscular functions to react to an ever-changing environment. At times the capacity of the older person may be overwhelmed by environmental factors, such as rainy weather, a chipped sidewalk, a poorly lighted staircase, or a small animal sleeping in the hallway. On the other hand physical problems that are not diagnosed, such as pneumonia or myocardial infarction, may precipitate a fall.

Intrinsic factors include any impairment of sensory input, judgment, blood pressure regulation, reaction time, gait and balance, and any problems or diseases that affect the person's ability to maintain mobility. Chronic medical problems such as Parkinson's disease, stroke, arthritis, and anemia are associated with a higher risk of falls as well as symptoms of dizziness, weakness, and visual disturbances.

Extrinsic factors include the effects of medications, which have been studied extensively; although not all findings are identical, general agreement exists regarding an increased risk of falls for patients who are taking any psychotropic drug, long-acting benzodiazepines, opioids, phenothiazines, vasodilators, and diuretics (Cumming, 2002; Lyons et al, 2002). Medications and the use of alcohol are common significant and reversible causes of falls (Lyons et al, 2002). Frequency of falls substantially increases in the first month after hospitalization (Mahoney et al, 2000). Potential environmental causes include pedestrian walkways, relocation of living space, crowds in stores, glare, floor surfaces, clutter, lighting, accessibility of objects, bathroom equipment, and the appropriateness and integrity of assistive devices. Box 19-1 lists the identified risk factors for falls in all settings.

Assessment
HISTORY

If a fall has occurred, the details of events surrounding the fall should be ascertained as much as possible. Questions to be asked include the following:
- What was the patient doing when he or she fell?
- Was there an aura (suggesting seizure)?
- Was there a loss of vision (suggesting syncope)?
- Did the patient experience any dizziness (sensation of movement)?
- Was there a loss of consciousness?
- In what direction did the patient fall (e.g., forward or backward)?
- Did the patient break the fall (suggests alertness versus syncope)?

Box 19-1

Risk Factors for Falls

Intrinsic
Advanced age
Female sex
Caucasian race
Chronic medical conditions
Neuromuscular dysfunction
Cognitive impairment
ADL, dependence
Impaired vision and hearing

Extrinsic
Medications
Environmental hazards
Improper assistive devices
Gait and balance disorders

Source: Herndon JG et al: Chronic medical conditions and risk of fall injury events at home in older adults; *J Am Geriatr Soc* 45:739-743, 1997; and Ray WA et al: A randomized trial of a consultation service to reduce falls in nursing homes, *JAMA* 278(7):557-562, 1997.

- Was he or she using any prescribed assistive devices appropriately?
- Did witnesses notice any seizure activity?

It is important to determine whether falls are recurrent or whether they have recently increased, which might suggest a more acute underlying cause, such as an infection. A thorough history should be obtained regarding any history of falls, medical problems, medications (including any recent changes), and the use of alcohol or medications for pain. It is also important to ask about the patient's fear of falling, even if no previous falls have occurred. Patients often do not volunteer information about previous falls, and this history might be obtained only if the practitioner asks the question. This history is especially important when assessing a patient who is frail or has impaired balance or mobility. Table 19-1 outlines the possible differential diagnoses for various findings.

It is important to assess the patient's environment. Whether the patient is at home or in a health care facility, assessment of the surroundings for risk factors such as clutter, poor lighting, and throw rugs can prove critical in preventing falls. If the provider is not able to make a visit to the home, a visiting nurse or social worker can perform the assessment. If none of these options is feasible, the patient, a family member, or a caregiver can perform the assessment with a tool such as the Home Safety Checklist, developed by the National Safety Council (1982) (Figure 19-1). The patient can bring this information to the next appointment for review and discussion, and the practitioner can make recommendations based on the findings.

TABLE 19-1 **Possible Differential Diagnoses Based on Findings**

Historical Factors and Symptoms	*Possible Differential Diagnoses*
Historical Factors	
Change in position	Orthostatic hypotension
"Trip or slip"	Gait instability
	Balance problems
	Visual disturbance
	Environmental hazard
"Drop attack" with loss of consciousness	Vertebrobasilar insufficiency
Looking up or sideways	Arterial or carotid sinus compression
Loss of consciousness	Syncope or seizure
Symptoms Near Time of Fall	
Dizziness or giddiness	Orthostatic hypotension
	Vestibular problems
	Hypoglycemia
	Arrhythmia
	Drug side effect
Palpitation	Arrhythmia
Incontinence	Seizure
Tongue biting	Seizure
Asymmetric weakness	Cerebrovascular disease
Chest pain	Myocardial infarction
	Coronary insufficiency
Loss of consciousness	Any cause of syncope

Home Safety Checklist

Kitchen

- Do you use a step stool or utility ladder to reach high cabinets and shelves? Don't try to use chairs or other dangerous makeshifts.
- Do you store frequently used items on shelves that are within easy reach?
- Do you wipe or pick up spilled water, grease, or food peelings *immediately*?
- Do you keep kitchen cabinet doors and drawers closed?

Bathroom

- Does your tub or shower have a slip-resistant surface to stand on?
- Are grab bars securely fastened? Use long screws anchored directly in wall studs, not in plaster, tile, or wallboard.
- Do you store breakable bottles and jars where they can't be shattered?
- Have you installed night-lights in the bathroom?
- Do you use a rubber mat or nonslip decals in the tub or shower?
- Do you have a nonskid rug on the bathroom floor?
- Do you keep soap in an easy-to-reach receptacle?

Bedroom

- Is there a lamp or a light switch within reach of each bed?
- Are there bedroom night-lights? Are those night-lights a safe distance from bedding, curtains, or other materials that could catch fire?

Stairways and Halls

- Are stairs clearly lighted? Are there switches at the tops and the bottoms of stairways?
- Do all steps and stairways have a sturdy handrail on both sides?
- Do you keep stairways free of any obstructions or storage material?
- Are the treads, risers, and carpeting on stairways in good shape? Keep them free of tears and protruding nails that can catch a foot. Remove all scatter rugs.
- Is there plenty of light in hallways and passageways? Make sure there are no dark shadows that can hide tripping hazards.
- Are exits and passageways kept free of boxes, furniture, and other tripping hazards?
- Have you eliminated small rugs at the tops and bottoms of stairways?

Traffic Lanes

- Can you walk across every room in your home, and from one room to another, without detouring around furniture?
- Is the traffic lane from your bedroom to the bathroom free of obstacles?

Ladders and Step Stools

- Are ladders in good shape? Check for loose rungs, worn ladder shoes, and frayed ropes on extension ladders. Keep ladders away from overhead power lines.
- Do you always set up your ladder or step stool on a firm, level base that is free of clutter?
- Before you climb a ladder or step stool, do you always make sure it is fully open and that the stepladder spreaders are locked?
- When you use a ladder or step stool, do you face the steps and keep your body between the side rails?
- Do you avoid standing on top of a step stool or climbing beyond the second step from the top on a stepladder?

Figure 19-1   Home safety checklist. (Modified from National Safety Council: Falling—the unexpected trip. A safety program for older adults, *Program leader's guide*, 1982, and National Safety Council: *Your safety checklist*, 1992.)

Home Safety Checklist—cont'd

Outdoor Areas
- Do you put garden tools and game equipment back in place after you use them?
- Are your walks and driveway in good shape?
- Do you keep your yard free of broken glass, nail-studded boards, and other litter?
- Do you keep outdoor walkways, steps, and porches free of wet leaves and snow?
- Do you sprinkle icy outdoor areas with de-icers as soon as possible after a snowfall or freeze?
- Do you have mats at doorways on which people wipe their feet?
- Do you know the safest way of walking when you cannot avoid walking on a slippery surface?

Footwear
- Do your shoes have soles and heels that provide good traction?
- Do you wear house slippers that fit well and do not fall off?
- Do you wear low-heeled oxfords, loafers, or good quality sneakers when you work in your house or yard?
- Do you replace boots or galoshes when their soles or heels are worn too smooth to keep you from slipping on wet or icy surfaces?

Personal Precautions
- If young grandchildren visit, are you alert for children playing on the floor and toys left in your path?
- If you have pets, are you alert for sudden movements across your path and pets getting underfoot?
- Do you always move deliberately and avoid rushing to answer the phone or doorbell?
- Do you take time to get your balance when you change position from lying down to sitting and from sitting to standing?
- Do you keep yourself in good condition with moderate exercise, good diet, adequate rest, and regular medical checkups?
- If you live alone, do you have daily contact with a friend or neighbor?
- Do you keep emergency phone numbers (police, fire, doctor, poison control center, and local utilities) next to each phone?

Figure 19-1, cont'd

PHYSICAL EXAMINATION

The physical examination should be comprehensive, with a special focus placed on the following aspects:

1. Orthostasis: blood pressure and pulse checks with the patient in the supine, sitting, and standing positions; systolic changes of 20 mm Hg or more indicate orthostasis, especially if the patient is symptomatic
2. Cardiovascular system: arrhythmia, murmurs, carotid bruits
3. Sensory system: visual or hearing impairments
4. Musculoskeletal system: arthritic changes, limitations in joint motion, deformities, fractures, foot problems, strength of lower extremities
5. Neurologic: nystagmus, neuropathy, tremors, rigidity, focal deficits, weakness
6. Cognitive status: Mini-Mental State Examination
7. Mood: Geriatric Depression Scale

Special attention must be given to the patient's gait and balance by simply observing ambulation with and without any assistive devices (e.g., canes, walkers) that may normally be used (Edwards and Lee, 1998). Footwear must be assessed for stability, fit, and appropriateness. Assistive devices should be checked for size, fit, integrity, and the patient's knowledge of its correct use. Tests for clinical assessment of gait and balance are listed in Table 19-2.

Diagnostic studies to consider are listed in Box 19-2. As always, the decision to perform a test is based on the presenting symptoms and the anticipated benefits for the individual patient.

| TABLE 19-2 | Tests to Assist in the Clinical Assessment of Gait and Balance | | |

Test	Description	Administration	Norms
Functional reach	Single item: scored in inches change while forward reaching using a fixed base of support. Extended arm is parallel to yardstick at shoulder level	3 min Yardstick, tape	*Age (yr)* *Inches* 20–40 14–17 41–69 13–15 70–87 10–13
Berg balance test	14-item categorical scale: sit to stand, stand to sit, transfer chair to chair, stand eyes open and closed, reach forward, pick object up from floor, single leg stance, tandem stance, look over shoulders, turn 360 degrees, alternate foot on stool	10–15 min Stopwatch, chair with armrest and bed or second chair with no arms, ruler, shoe, stool	Score < 45 predicted multiple faller
Timed get-up and go test	Categorical scale and timed scoring Sit to stand from chair with armrests, walk 3 meters, turn, walk back to chair, sit down One trial run before timed test	1–2 min Measuring tape, arm chair, stopwatch	< 10 seconds = freely mobile < 20 seconds = mostly independent 20–29 seconds = variable mobility > 29 seconds = impaired mobility
Problem-oriented mobility assessment	18 items with categorical scale and timed scoring *Balance subscale*: stand to sit, sitting, sit to stand, immediate standing, side-by-side standing, backward waist pull, single leg stance, semi-tandem stance, pick up object off floor, toe standing, heel standing *Gait subscale*: gait initiation, path deviation, missed step, turning while walking, stepping over obstacle	10 min Stopwatch, chair without arms, pen, two shoes, belt	≤19 = high risk of falling 20–25 = intermediate risk > 25 = no unusual risk

Fink H et al: Falls. In Tallis RC, Fillit HM, editors: *Brockhehurst's textbook of geriatric medicine and gerontology,* ed 6, London, 2003, Churchill Livingstone.

Box 19-2

Diagnostic Studies in the Evaluation of Falls

CBC: rules out anemia or infection
Urinalysis: rules out infection
Serum chemistry screen: rules out electrolyte imbalance
TSH
Vitamin B$_{12}$
Sedimentation rate
Drug levels as indicated
ECG
Chest x-ray examination
Holter monitor: if transient arrhythmia is suspected
Head CT scan: if mental status or neurologic changes are present

CBC, Complete blood count; *CT*, computed tomography; *ECG*, electrocardiogram; *TSH*, thyroid-stimulating hormone

Interventions

Interventions are focused on correcting reversible causes, preventing future falls and injury, and alleviating the patient's fear of falling. See Table 19-3 for targeted intervention for risk factors. A patient's risk of falling should be assessed annually (if not more often), and approaches must be tailored for the patient's individual needs on the basis of underlying risk factors. It is important to include family members or caregivers in education and intervention planning. Physical therapy

TABLE 19-3 **Fall Risk Factors and Targeted Interventions**

Risk Factor	Targeted Intervention
Postural hypotension (> 20 mm Hg drop in systolic BP, or systolic BP < 90 mm Hg)	Behavioral recommendations, such as hand clenching, elevation of head of bed; discontinuation or substitution of high-risk medications
Use of benzodiazepine or sedative-hypnotic	Education about sleep hygiene, discontinuation or substitution of medications
Use of over three prescription medications	Review of medications
Environmental hazards	Appropriate changes; installation of safety equipment (e.g., grab bars)
Gait impairment	Gait training, assistive devices, balance or strengthening exercises
Impairment in transfer or balance	Balance exercises, training in transfers, environmental alterations (e.g., grab bars)
Impairment in leg or arm muscle strength or limb range of motion	Exercise with resistance bands or putty, with graduated increases in resistance

From Lyons W et al: Geriatric medicine. In Tierney LM et al, editors: *Current medical diagnosis and treatment: adult ambulatory and in-patient management*, ed 41, New York, 2002, Lange Medical Books/McGraw Hill.

often provides excellent benefits through balance training, gait training, and strengthening. The benefits of weight training and a regular exercise program for older adults are now widely recognized, and it appears to be a useful tool in fall prevention in older adults (Burbank et al, 2002; Carter, Kannus, and Khan, 2001; Hurley and Roth 2000). Evidence from research studies has consistently showed that physical activity is associated with a 20% to 40% reduced risk of hip fracture relative to sedentary older adults (Gregg, Pereira, and Caspersen, 2000).

Tai chi is a moderate-intensity strength and endurance training that is promising. It has been found to improve flexibility and balance control and reduce the risk of falls (Cumming, 2002; Li et al, 2001; Wu, 2002).

Anatomically designed external hip protectors have been introduced as a method of preventing hip fractures. Highlighting this international concern, studies have been conducted in Finland, Japan, Australia, Switzerland, Great Britain, and the United States; and the evidence from these studies has reported conflicting results (Cameron et al, 2001; Harada et al, 2001; Hubacher and Wettstein, 2001; Kannus et al, 2000; Parker et al, 2000). The hip protectors may be beneficial and may reduce hip fractures within a select high-risk population. Acceptance of the hip protector by the users is a problem because of discomfort and practicality (Parker et al, 2000).

Assistive devices such as a cane or walker may provide additional stability for patients while they ambulate or transfer. Table 19-4 outlines issues in prescribing assistive devices for the older person (Wasson et al, 1990).

General interventions include the following:
1. Minimize medications and dosages; eliminate high-risk drugs, if possible.
2. Prevent and treat osteoporosis.
3. Recommend proper footwear.
4. Recommend an obstacle-free, glare-free, and well-lit environment.
5. If necessary, raise toilet seats and chair heights and provide armrests.
6. Remove home hazards.
7. Install grab bars in bathrooms and other appropriate sites.
8. Provide physical therapy for flexibility, strength, gait, and balance training.
9. Add assistive devices as appropriate.

Even with close supervision and minimized risk factors, some patients may continue to experience falls. For these patients, perhaps the best outcome is the prevention of injury related to falls. In such instances, innovative approaches (e.g., mattresses placed on the floor for patients who fall out of bed) may help to prevent harm while maximizing freedom of movement. Plans for such situations should be created by a multidisciplinary team of nurses, physicians, and therapists, with input and agreement from family members, caregivers, and the patient, if appropriate. These plans can be tailored for any setting, including the hospital, long-term care facility, or home.

Establishment of a primary goal of maximum mobility and independence, with acceptance of the inevitability of the risks and dangers of falls, may need to be negotiated with the family. Restraints must be avoided at all costs. Restraints can cause both physical and psychological harm to patients and thus have been highly regulated and monitored in hospitals and long-term care facilities. Restraints include any equipment, medication, or intervention designed to prevent or limit movement. This definition goes beyond Posey vests and wrist restraints to include such devices as seatbelts and wedge pillows in wheelchairs, locked tray tables on recliners, and even raised bed rails.

Summary

Falls by older persons are prevalent and costly, not only financially but also in terms of quality of life. Many falls are preventable, and they should never be assumed to be a natural outcome of the aging process. The cause of a fall is often multifactorial, and every effort must be made to address as many of these causes as possible. A multidisciplinary approach is often necessary to accomplish this task successfully. The practitioner may need to treat medical problems and adjust medications. Physical

TABLE 19-4 Assistive Devices for Common Disabilities of the Elderly

Device	Indications	Limitations	Comments
Upper Extremity			
"Soap on a rope," long-handle back sponge, tub seat, shower bench, toothbrush grip, electric razor with rotary edges, and reaching devices (see also lower extremity)	Bathing, oral care, and grooming	Some grip or thumb opposition and range of motion required	
Splints	Wrist pain or instability, carpal metacarpal arthritis	Patient compliance	
Balance/Back/Lower Extremities			
Reaching device(s), long shoehorns, back sponges, elastic shoelaces, Velcro straps	Dressing and grooming	Dexterity necessary	
Canes[†]	Articular pain, mild weakness	Upper extremity weakness	Four-legged canes can be cumbersome
Crutches[†]	Significant weakness or pain of one or both lower extremities	Upper extremity weakness or incoordination	Forearm crutches preferable for chronic use; platform attachment for elbow, wrist, or hand disease
Walkers[†]	Significant imbalance or weakness	Cumbersome	Wheel and platform attachments available
Braces*[†]	Isolated severe joint or muscle dysfunction	Difficult to put on	
Wheelchair*[†]	Limited endurance or inability to walk	Poor access to house, weight of chair	
Bathroom grab bars, raised toilet seat, tub seat, commode	Transferring; weak or limited hip or knee motion; imbalance	Installation problems	Prescription should be individualized

From Wasson JH et al: The prescription of assistive devices for the elderly: practical considerations, *J Gen Intern Med* 5:48-49, 1990.
*Consultation is usually indicated.
[†]Medicare coverage when prescribed by a physician as medically necessary.

and occupational therapists can provide strengthening exercises and education regarding the proper use of assistive devices and adaptive equipment. A regular exercise program to include weight training for older adults has proven beneficial in enhancing strength and mobility. Social work can assist patients in obtaining support and resources for personal care and homemaking services. A coordinated management plan is often successful in preventing costly and dangerous falls in all settings.

Resources

AGENET Falls Prevention
www.agenet.com/fall_prevention.html

American Academy of Orthopaedic Surgeons
www.aaos.org/wordhtml/pat_educ/fallsbro.htm

References

Burbank PM et al: Exercise and older adults: changing behavior with the transtheoretical model, *Orthop Nurs* 21(4):51-61, 2002.

Cameron ID et al: Hip protectors in aged-care facilities: a randomized trial of use by individual higher-risk residents, *Age Ageing* 30(6):477-481, 2001.

Carter ND, Kannus P, Khan KM: Exercise in the prevention of falls in older people: a systematic literature review examining the rationale and the evidence, *Sports Med* 31(6):427-438, 2001.

Cumming RG: Intervention strategies and risk-factor modification for falls prevention: a review of recent intervention studies, *Clin Geriatr Med* 18(2):175-189, 2002.

Edwards BJ, Lee S: Gait disorders and falls in a retirement home: a pilot study, *Ann Long Term Care* 6(4):140, 1998.

Gregg EW, Pereira MA, Caspersen CJ: Physical activity, falls and fractures among older adults: a review of epidemiologic evidence, *J Am Geriatr Soc* 48(8):883-893, 2000.

Harada A et al: Hip fracture prevention trial using hip protectors in Japanese nursing homes, *Osteoporosis Int* 12(3):215-221, 2001.

Hubacher M, Wettstein A: Acceptance of hip protectors for hip fracture prevention in nursing homes, *Osteoporos Int* 12(9):749-799, 2001.

Hurley BF, Roth SM: Strength training in the elderly: effects on risk factors for age-related diseases, *Sports Med* 30(4):249-268, 2000.

Kannus P et al: Prevention of hip fracture in elderly people with use of a hip protector, *N Engl J Med* 343(21):1506-1513, 2000.

Li JX et al: Tai chi: physiological characteristics and beneficial effects on health, *Br J Sports Med* 35(3):148-56, 2001.

Lyons W et al: Geriatric medicine. In Tierney LM et al, editors: *Current medical diagnosis and treatment:* adult ambulatory and in-patient management, ed 41, New York, 2002, Lange Medical Books/McGraw-Hill.

Mahoney JE et al: Temporal association between hospitalization and rate of falls after discharge, *Arch Intern Med* 160(18):2788-2795, 2000.

Nurmi I, Luthje P: Incidence and costs of falls and fall injuries among elderly in institutional care, *Scand J Prim Health Care* 20(2):118-122.

Parker MJ et al: Hip protectors for preventing hip fractures in the elderly, *Cochrane Database Syst Rev* 4:CD001255, 2000.

Ray WA et al: A randomized trial of a consultation service to reduce falls in nursing homes, *JAMA* 278(7):557-562, 1997.

Rosedale M: Catching falls: a synthesis of recent research, *Caring* 20(1):14-19, 2001.

Startzell JK et al: Stair negotiation in older people: a review, *J Am Geriatr Soc* 48(5):567-580, 2000.

Wasson JH et al: The prescription of assistive devices for the elderly: practical considerations, *J Gen Intern Med* 5(1):46-54, 1990.

Wu G: Evaluation of the effectiveness of Tai Chi for improving balance and preventing falls in the older population—a review, *J Am Geriatr Soc* 50(4):746-754, 2002.

20

Genitourinary/Male: Benign Prostatic Hyperplasia and Erectile Dysfunction

Benign Prostatic Hyperplasia
BACKGROUND

Benign prostatic hyperplasia (BPH) is a nearly ubiquitous development in men who have testes and live long enough for it to develop. The condition is characterized by regional nodular growth in the transition zone of the prostate gland that may impinge on the function of the urinary tract and lead to symptoms of obstruction and irritation. The condition is not a premalignant state, nor is it related to the development of cancer in any way. It is defined in a variety of ways: by postmortem weight of the prostate, by digital palpation, by suggestive urinary symptoms, and by objective measures based on urinary flow rate or transrectal ultrasonography (TRUS). The prevalence of BPH rises from about 20% in men 41 to 50 years of age, to 50% in men 51 to 60 years of age, and to greater than 90% in men over 80 years of age (Tierney, McPhee, and Papadakis, 2003). Figure 20-1 describes the anatomy of the prostate gland.

As a man ages, the prostate gland undergoes two periods of growth. The first is a period of normal growth and maturation during puberty, which continues until around 20 years of age. At the end of this growth episode, the average gland weighs around 20 g. Many men have an abnormal pattern of excessive growth that begins around 40 years of age. This is a result of the presence of testosterone and the normal process of aging. The enlargement associated with BPH takes place in the transition zone of the prostate gland and results in the formation of nodules. After the nodules form, they begin to enlarge, leading to compression of the surrounding tissue and urethra, which passes through the transition zone. Simultaneously, growth of the fibromuscular stroma causes the transition zone to enlarge. The combination of these two processes varies in extent from patient to patient, but together they lead to compression of the urethral lumen and obstructive urinary symptoms. This pattern of growth continues and eventually results in overall hypertrophy of the gland that is palpable on digital rectal examination. Surprisingly, the size of the prostate is not directly related to the presence or degree of obstruction and cannot be used to predict the presence or

449

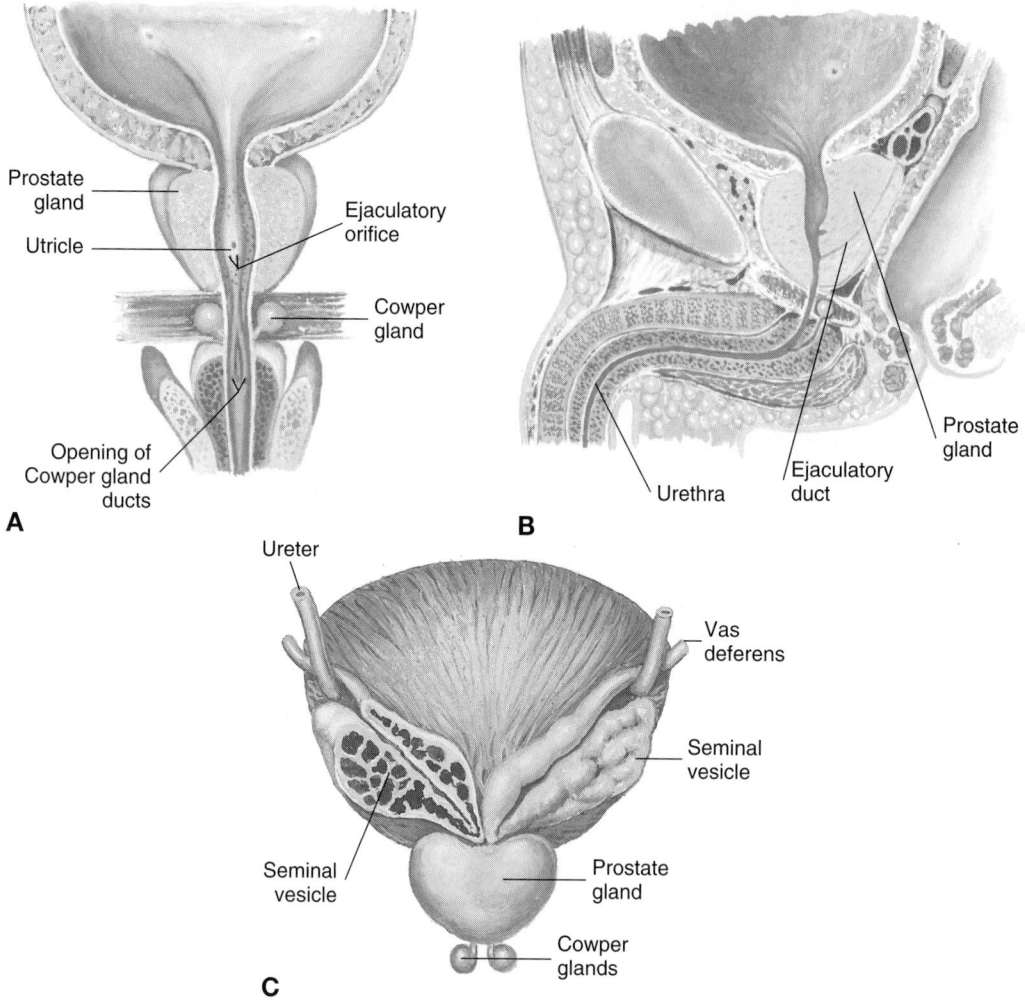

Figure 20-1   Anatomy of the prostate gland and seminal vesicles. **A,** Cross section. **B,** Lateral view. **C,** Posterior view. (From Seidel HM et al: *Mosby's guide to physical examination,* ed 5, St Louis, 2003, Mosby.)

absence of symptoms in an individual man. Not all men with BPH develop symptoms; some, with minimal enlargement, experience severe disturbances in function. Therefore the size and growth of the prostate are considered irrelevant as independent predictors of urinary flow rates.

Risk factors for the development of BPH are poorly understood. Some studies have suggested a genetic predisposition, and some have noted racial differences. About 50% of men under 60 years of age who undergo surgery for BPH may have a heritable form of the disease. This form is most likely an autosomal dominant trait, and first-degree male relatives of such patients carry an increased relative risk of about fourfold (Tierney, McPhee, and Papadakis, 2003.) The development of BPH is not related to sexual activity, vasectomy, improper diet, substance abuse, socioeconomic status, or unhealthy lifestyle.

The etiology is not completely understood, but the disorder seems to be multifactorial. In BPH the glandular cells and myofibroblasts of periurethral and transition zones proliferate excessively. This excessive growth of tissue mass physically compresses the urethra, leading to urinary obstruction and lower urinary tract symptoms (LUTS). Another major factor that contributes to LUTS in BPH is the increase in smooth muscle tone, a dynamic component. Contraction of the prostate gland is primarily under the control of the autonomic system and is mediated through alpha$_1$-adrenoceptors. In addition to alpha$_1$-adrenoceptors, many other components influence growth and contraction on the prostate gland, resulting in the development of BPH and LUTS. The prostate gland is contracted on stimulating 5-hydroxytryptamine (serotonin, 5-HT), endothelin, tachykinin, and muscarinic cholinergic receptors. Growth of the prostate is under the control of androgens, endothelin growth factor, vasoactive intestinal peptide, nerve growth factor, and growth hormone. The combination of excessive growth and the tone produced by different components results in LUTS and BPH (Thiyagarajan, 2002).

BPH is truly a hyperplastic process, resulting from an increase in cell numbers. Microscopic evaluation reveals a nodular growth pattern consisting of varying amounts of stroma or epithelium. Stroma is composed of varying amounts of collagen and smooth muscle. This variation explains the potential responsiveness to medical therapy. Thus, alpha-blocker therapy may result in excellent responses in men with BPH where there is a significant component of smooth muscle, whereas hyperplasia composed predominantly of epithelium might respond better to 5-alpha-reductase inhibitors. Patients with significant components of collagen in the stroma may not respond to either form of medical therapy. One cannot reliably predict the responsiveness to specific therapy (Tierney, McPhee, and Papadakis, 2003). Studies are under way to evaluate whether the efficacy of alpha-blocker therapy might be predicted by determining the area density of the smooth muscle of the prostate by ultrasound (Hayami et al, 2002).

Studies have also demonstrated that BPH is under endocrine control because orchiectomy results in the regression of established disease and improvement in urinary symptoms. Administration of a luteinizing hormone-releasing hormone analog in men reversibly shrinks established BPH, resulting in objective improvement in flow rate and subjective improvement in symptoms (Tierney, McPhee, and Papadakis, 2003.)

The cost for treatment of BPH is influenced by the two major factors: the patient and the health care system. Medical intervention for 2 years costs $2,000 compared with surgical intervention, such as a transurethral resection of the prostate (TURP), for $9,000 or an open prostatectomy for $13,000. The other salient factors influencing cost are the age, medical condition, and socioeconomic status of the patient.

HISTORY

Most men who seek treatment for BPH do so because symptoms interfere with their activities or their quality of life. For some this interference means the inability to complete a game of golf or to engage in any other long-term activity without devising a strategy for voiding at intervals throughout the afternoon or evening. For others, multiple trips to the bathroom during the night lead to sleep disturbances. The partners of men with BPH also experience significant morbidity because of the condition, including sleep disturbance, disruption of social life, psychological burden, inadequate sex life, and fears regarding prostate cancer and the need for surgery (Mitropoulos et al, 2002).

The characteristic complex of symptoms associated with BPH is known as *prostatism,* and these symptoms have been characterized as irritative or obstructive. The incidence rate of lower urinary tract symptoms increases linearly with age and reaches its maximum at the age of 79 years (Verhamme et al, 2002). Symptoms that develop initially in the course of BPH are usually caused by obstruction of the flow of urine from the bladder. The growth of the prostate gland exerts pressure on the urethra, which passes through it, and symptoms include a decreased force of stream, urinary hesitancy, dribbling at the end of urination (terminal dribbling), double voiding, and straining to urinate. These symptoms generally occur earlier in the course of the condition than do irritative urinary symptoms, which include nocturia, urinary frequency, urinary urgency, dysuria, and urge incontinence. As the urethra and bladder neck occlusion continues, the bladder must overcome increasing resistance to empty; it may begin to hypertrophy and gradually fail to function. Should this occur, one of two clinical scenarios often develops: the bladder may fail to empty, leading to increased postvoid residual (PVR) volumes, or it develops a condition known as *detrusor hyper-reflexia,* in which it begins to contract involuntarily at a set volume, leading to urge incontinence. Needless to say, not all men with BPH report all symptoms or develop them equally from each category, and men frequently report a waxing and waning of symptom severity.

Questioning men with BPH may elicit information about strategies used to compensate for certain symptoms. For example, sitting on the toilet, which appears to promote an increased volume voided, may reduce urinary frequency. Many men reduce their intake of liquids on days when they have to be out of the house, and some men resort to wearing dark-colored pants to disguise slight incontinence following urination. Finally, men avoid ingesting certain substances, such as caffeine or over-the-counter (OTC) cold medications, which frequently exacerbate symptoms.

A short questionnaire devised by the American Urological Association (AUA) assesses the severity of the reported symptoms. The AUA Symptom Index is the preferred instrument to gauge an individual patient's level of adjustment to symptoms and to guide decision making about interventions. The self-administered tool has seven questions about the symptoms of prostatism, and the scoring system classifies symptoms as mild, moderate, or severe. It helps the practitioner decide on the level of intervention to be used in each individual case: from watchful waiting to surgical intervention (Table 20-1).

PHYSICAL EXAMINATION

The physical examination focuses on the abdomen and genitalia and includes evaluation of the kidneys, bladder, penis, and scrotal contents. The bladder is palpated to assess the presence of distention and the need for further upper urinary tract evaluation. Men with BPH commonly suffer from incomplete emptying of the bladder, but residual urine volume does not necessarily correlate with the reported severity of symptoms, and percussion is generally not revealing.

A digital rectal examination (DRE) is mandatory to assess the size of the prostate and to identify any induration or nodules that might indicate the presence of cancer. The most important information obtained from the rectal examination is the consistency of the prostate gland (Stutzman, 2003). Prostate size does not correlate with the severity of symptoms or the degree of obstruction (Tierney, McPhee, and Papadakis, 2003). During the examination, the rectum is examined for polyps or internal hemorrhoids; the posterior and lateral lobes and borders of the prostate are examined for size, consistency, symmetry, and mobility; and the presence of nodules or masses is noted. The gland is not tender unless prostatitis is present (Stutzman, 2003). The normal gland feels smooth and rubbery and does not extend into the rectum more than 1 cm. A gland with BPH often feels enlarged, smooth, and firm but somewhat elastic, and it protrudes further into the rectum. Induration, if detected, must alert the provider to the possibility of cancer, and further evaluation is needed (i.e., prostate-specific antigen [PSA], TRUS, and biopsy).

A focused neurologic examination, particularly of the anal sphincter tone; genital and perineal sensation; and motor, sensory, and reflex activity of the lower extremities may disclose abnormalities that suggest a neurogenic bladder as the cause of the patient's symptoms (Stutzman, 2003).

DIAGNOSTICS

Baseline diagnostics include urinalysis to rule out infection and hematuria and also blood urea nitrogen and creatinine levels to assess renal function. Renal insufficiency may be observed in 10% of patients with prostatism and, if observed, warrants imaging of the upper tract structures (Tierney, McPhee, and Papadakis, 2003).

Prostate-specific antigen is believed to leak from the prostatic ductal system into the prostatic stroma and then the bloodstream via capillaries and lymphatics after the prostate gland is damaged by trauma or disease. The role of PSA in the routine workup of BPH is controversial. According to the guidelines developed by the Agency for Health Care Policy and Research (AHCPR), a PSA study

TABLE 20-1 American Urological Association Symptom Index for Evaluating Benign Prostatic Hyperplasia

Questions	Not at All	Less Than 1 Time in 5	Less Than Half the Time	About Half the Time	More Than Half the Time	Almost Always	Score
Over the past month, how often have you had a sensation of not emptying your bladder completely after you finished urinating?	0	1	2	3	4	5	——
Over the past month, how often have you had to urinate again less than 2 hours after you had finished urinating?	0	1	2	3	4	5	——
Over the past month, how often have you found you stopped and started again several times when you urinated?	0	1	2	3	4	5	——
Over the past month, how often have you found it difficult to postpone urination?	0	1	2	3	4	5	——
Over the past month, how often have you had a weak urinary stream?	0	1	2	3	4	5	——
Over the past month, how often have you had to push or strain to begin urination?	0	1	2	3	4	5	——
Over the past month, how many times did you most typically get up to urinate from the time you went to bed at night until you got up in the morning?	0	1	2	3	4	5	——
						TOTAL SCORE	——

From Barry MJ et al: The American Urological Association Symptom index for benign prostatic hyperplasia, *J Urol* 148:1549-1557, 1992.
Scoring Key: Mild symptoms: 0 to 7 total points; moderate symptoms: 8 to 19 total points; severe symptoms: 20 to 35 total points.

should be optional, although the agency concedes that, when used with DRE, PSA tests improve the detection of cancer. Routine PSA is not recommended by AHCPR because serum levels overlap in BPH and organ-confined prostate cancer, leading to a large number of false-positives and false-negatives. A man 45 to 50 years of age should have a PSA of less than 2.5 ng/ml, whereas an older man of 75 years of age may have an acceptable level of 6.5 ng/ml. Because similar PSA levels are possible in patients with BPH and in those with early prostate cancer, screening can result in unnecessary prostate biopsies and other tests; however, it is generally accepted that a level above 10 mg/ml is suggestive of cancer. Periodic PSA levels that are trending upward should also be suspect. PSA velocity takes into account that as men age the natural tendency is for the PSA to rise because of benign processes; however, if the PSA rises too rapidly it is suggestive of an increased suspicion for cancer.

Because of the discovery that several molecular forms of PSA exist in serum, the ability to differentiate between BPH and cancer may be improved. It has been demonstrated that the ratio of two of these molecular forms, free and unbound (f-PSA) and total (t-PSA), increased the diagnostic specificity of the PSA test. In fact, prostate cancer detection by a f-PSA:t-PSA ratio of less than 18% increased the diagnostic specificity by 20% compared with the diagnostic efficacy of the total serum PSA concentration alone (Figure 20-2).

The position of the AHCPR is in contrast to that of the AUA and the American Medical Association, which advocate annual PSA tests for all men over 50 years of age and for men in high-risk populations (i.e., African-American men and those with a family history) after 40 years of age. In practice, PSA testing is usually limited to men with a life expectancy of more than 10 years and those in whom a diagnosis of prostate cancer would change the treatment plan. It is not uncommon at autopsy, in fact, that some degree of prostate cancer is detected that was previously unsuspected and totally unrelated to the cause of death.

Further tests and procedures are reserved for men whose initial evaluation evokes suspicion of complications beyond simple BPH. Urethrocystoscopy is not recommended in the initial evaluation

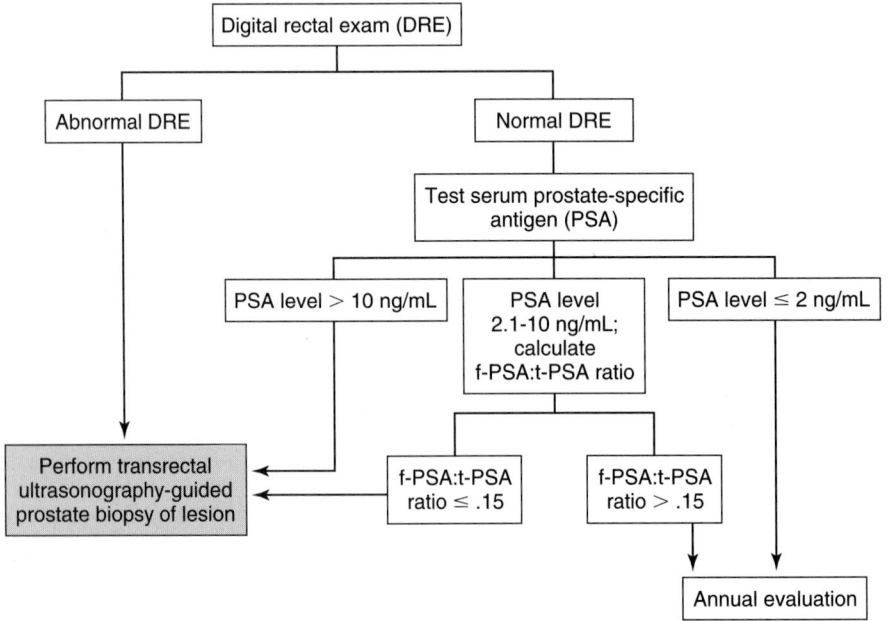

Figure 20-2   Prostate cancer detection algorithm. (From Oesterling JE: Molecular PSA: the next frontier in PCA screening, *Intern Med* 1(5 suppl):52-68, 1996.)

to determine the need for treatment of BPH, although it may assist in determining the surgical approach for patients opting for invasive therapy. Upper-tract imaging (i.e., intravenous pyelogram or renal ultrasound) is recommended only in the presence of concomitant urinary disease or complications from BPH (i.e., hematuria, urinary tract infection, renal insufficiency, history of stone disease) (Tierney, McPhee, and Papadakis, 2003).

Needle biopsy of the prostate is usually done in a urologist's office or in an utrasound suite, most commonly in conjunction with TRUS. No anesthesia or sedation is required. Aspirin and nonsteroidal antiinflammatory drugs (except cyclooxygenase-2 [COX-2] inhibitors) should be stopped for 1 week, and anticoagulants should be stopped until the effect has diminished. Only 30% to 40% of prostatic nodules that have biopsies done because of suspicion for carcinoma are positive on histologic examination (Stutzman, 2003).

DIFFERENTIAL DIAGNOSIS

The differential diagnosis for BPH includes a number of conditions. Disorders such as poorly controlled diabetes, peripheral edema, and diuretic use often manifest with urinary frequency but typically are not associated with obstructive symptoms. Other obstructive conditions of the lower urinary tract include urethral stricture, bladder-neck contracture, bladder stone, or carcinoma of the prostate. A history of prior urethral instrumentation, urethritis, or trauma should be elucidated to exclude urethral stricture or bladder-neck contracture (Tierney, McPhee, and Papadakis, 2003). Urinary infections have irritative symptoms, and urethral stricture causes both irritative and obstructive symptoms. Although BPH commonly causes hematuria, it is also associated with bladder cancer. Neurogenic bladder causes urinary frequency, urgency, and retention but not obstructive symptoms; it is associated with diabetes, cerebral infarction, Parkinson's disease, back injury, or spinal abnormalities. Finally, certain drugs and substances exacerbate prostatism, including alcohol, caffeine, and antihistamines. Anticholinergic agents, antispasmodics, antiparkinsonian drugs, and many antidepressant drugs depress bladder-muscle contractility; sympathomimetic agents (e.g., ephedrine and other decongestants found in OTC cold remedies), beta-blocking agents, and levodopa increase bladder outlet resistance (Stutzman, 2003). Table 20-2 lists selected pharmacologic agents with known influence on bladder function.

TREATMENT

The treatment goals of clinical BPH are to improve symptoms, relieve obstruction, improve bladder emptying, prevent urinary tract infection, and avoid renal deterioration (Beduschi, Beduschi, and Oesterling, 1998). The range of treatment options for men with BPH include watchful waiting, medication, surgery, and nonsurgical treatment. The presence of multiple disease processes in an individual patient is often a limiting factor in the development of a treatment plan, and involvement of the patient in the decision-making process is essential for the success of the intervention. The AHCPR has recommended that men with BPH should take a more active role in choosing treatment strategies and that facilitating their participation could result in a lower number of surgeries without sacrificing outcomes, ultimately reducing Medicare costs. Many urologists agree that watchful waiting is an appropriate strategy for men with mild symptoms (AUA symptom score of less than 7) (Clinical Practice Guidelines, 1998). (See Figure 20-3 for the management of BPH.) Progression is not inevitable, and some men undergo spontaneous improvement or resolution of their symptoms (Tierney, McPhee, and Papadakis, 2003).

Because BPH is characterized by a waxing and waning pattern of symptom severity, lifestyle changes can often reduce the bothersome factors. Suggested modifications include eating dinner early in the evening; avoiding fluids after 7 p.m.; taking time to void properly; avoiding excessive salt and diuretics (when possible); reducing caffeine, alcohol, and spices that tend to exacerbate symptoms; and avoiding OTC cold medications that contain adrenergic decongestants.

Phytotherapy is the use of plants or plant extracts for medicinal purposes. Although many "natural" remedies are touted for the relief of urinary symptoms, only saw palmetto, by acting as a

TABLE 20-2	**Selected Pharmacologic Agents with Known Influence on Bladder Function**

Drugs that Increase Bladder Tone and Contractility
Bethanecol (Urecholine)

Drugs that Decrease Bladder Contractility
Anticholinergic drugs (e.g., Pro-Banthine, Donnatal, Ditropan)
Antihistamines
Calcium antagonists (verapamil, nifedipine, diltiazem)
Prostaglandin inhibitors (e.g., ibuprofen)
Tricyclic antidepressants (e.g., imipramine, nortriptyline)
β_2-Adrenergic antagonists (e.g., terbutoline)

Drugs that Increase Bladder Outlet Resistance
Adrenergic agonists (e.g., ephedrine, Sudafed)
Antiparkinsonian drugs (e.g., levodopa, Sinemet)
β-Adrenergic antagonists (e.g., propranolol)
Estrogens

Drugs that Decrease Outlet Resistance
Antispasticity drugs (e.g., diazepam, Baclofen)
α-Adrenergic antagonists (e.g., doxazosin, prazosin, phenoxybenzamine, terazosin)

Drugs that Increase Urinary Volume
Diuretics

From Stutzman RE: Bladder outlet obstruction. In Barker LR, Burton JR, Zieve PD, editors: *Principles of ambulatory medicine*, ed 6, Philadelphia, 2003, Lippincott Williams & Wilkins.

5-alpha-reductase inhibitor, is believed by some to provide any benefit in BPH. Others that have become popular include the bark of the *Pygeum africanum,* the roots of *Echinacea purp*urea and *Hypoxis rooperi,* pollen extract, pumpkin seeds (Dreikorn, 2002), and the leaves of the trembling poplar. One study (Preuss at al, 2001) found that a combination of cernitin, saw palmetto, B-sitosterol, and vitamin E significantly lessened nocturia and frequency and diminished the overall symptoms of BPH (as indicated by an improvement in the total AUA Symptom Index score) and caused no significant adverse side effects. The benefits and risks of these substances are not well documented, however, and issues concerning the long-term beneficial and adverse effects of herbal therapy, prevention of complications, standardization of extracts, and concomitant use with "mainstream" medications need further study (Dvorkin and Song, 2002).

Prescription Medications

Two types of medication are currently approved for treatment of symptomatic BPH. The 5-alpha-reductase inhibitors are represented by a single drug, finasteride (Proscar), and act by inhibiting the conversion of testosterone to the prostatic androgen dihydrotestosterone, leading to a suppression of androgenic stimulation to the prostate gland, a reduction in size, and decreased resistance to urinary flow. Because of its action on testosterone, its side effects potentially include reduced libido, impotence, and ejaculatory disorders. Finasteride provides symptomatic improvement only in men with enlarged prostates (>40 ml) and exerts its action slowly, with only mild improvement in symptoms after 6 months of treatment, but continuing efficacy over time. Serum PSA is reduced by about

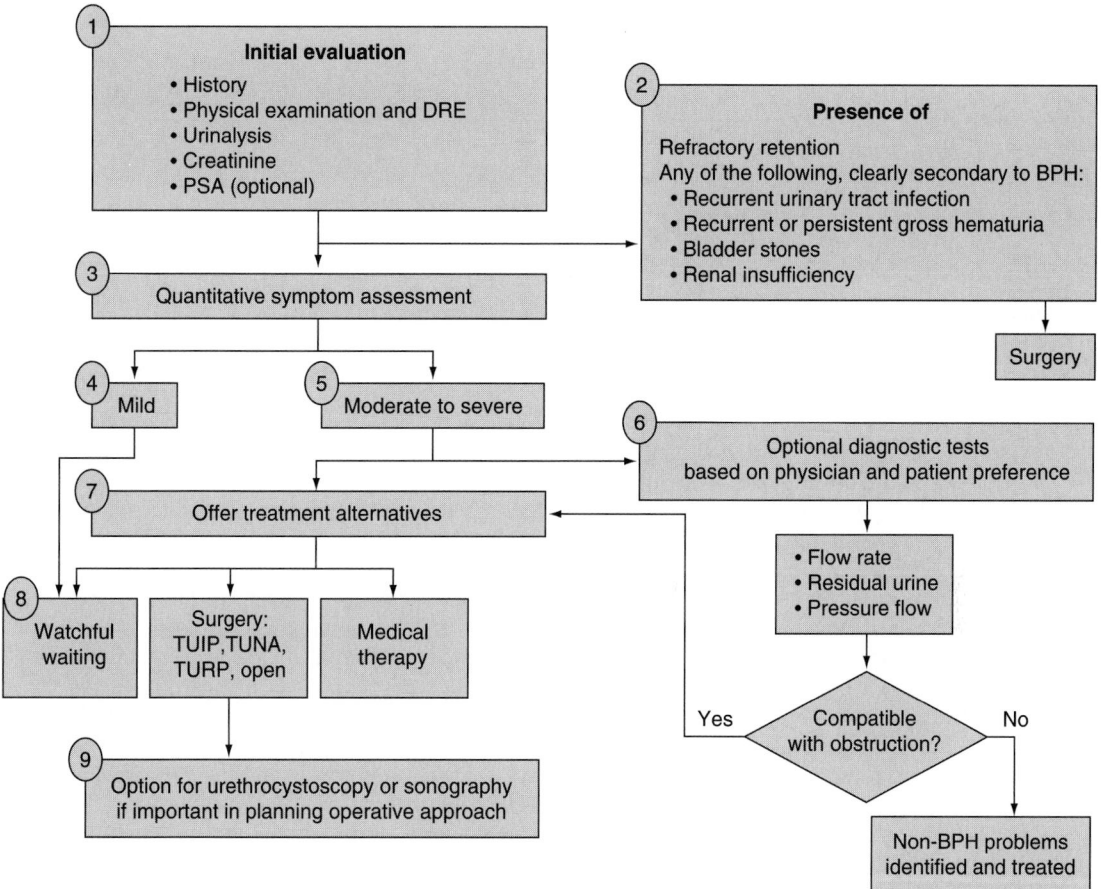

Figure 20-3 Benign prostatic hyperplasia decision diagram. BPH, benign prostatic hyperplasia; DRE, digital rectal examination; TUIP, transurethral incision of the prostate; TURP, transurethral resection of the prostate; TUNA, transurethral needle ablation of the prostate. (From Stoller M et al: Urology. In Tierney LM et al, editors: *Current medical diagnosis and treatment: adult ambulatory and in-patient management, ed 41,* New York, 2002, Lange Medical Books/McGraw-Hill.)

50% for patients receiving finasteride therapy; however, individual values can vary, thus complicating cancer detection (Tierney, McPhee, and Papadakis, 2003).

The second class of drugs used to treat BPH is the alpha-adrenergic antagonist group (see Table 20-3). These drugs decrease the smooth-muscle tone of the bladder neck and prostate, resulting in increased relaxation and decreased resistance to urine flow through the urethra and a reduction in the symptoms of outflow obstruction. Symptom relief is achieved quickly, often within hours of the first dose, but a trial of 4 to 6 weeks is recommended to assess response. Terazosin (Hytrin) is widely used for BPH, but doxazosin (Cardura) and prazosin (Minipress) are also used, especially in patients with coexisting hypertension. The most commonly encountered side effects of these drugs include initial dizziness and postural hypotension. Patients should be cautioned to take them at bedtime as they are preparing to turn out the light (bedside dosing) to reduce the risk of falls. Doxazosin is not associated with the occurrence of erectile dysfunction (ED) compared with other agents (Flack, 2002). Although about 10% of patients find it necessary to stop taking these medications because of side effects, initiating therapy with low dosages and careful titrating can reduce their

TABLE 20-3	Alpha Blockade for Benign Prostatic Hyperplasia	
Agent	**Action**	**Dose**
Phenoxybenzamine	α_1 and α_2 blockade	5-10 mg twice daily
Prazosin	α_1 blockade	1-5 mg twice daily
Terazosin	α_1 blockade	1-10 mg daily
Doxazosin	α_1 blockade	1-8 mg daily
Tamsulosin	α_{1a} blockade	0.4 or 0.8 mg daily

From Tierney LM, McPhee SJ, Papadakis MA: Benign prostatic hyperplasia. In *Current medical diagnosis and treatment*, ed 42, New York, 2003, Lange Medical Books/McGraw-Hill.

severity. It has also been noted that longer-acting agents have a more gradual onset of action, thus decreasing the risk of postural hypotension.

In 1995 the American Foundation for Urologic Disease reported findings of a study comparing the efficacy of finasteride and terazosin. By the AUA Symptom Index, symptoms were significantly reduced in patients given terazosin, but those taking finasteride did not show any significant improvement over a placebo. The study concluded that terazosin was an effective therapy but finasteride was not, whether used alone or in combination with an alpha-blocker. Prostate size was not a consideration in this study, however, and participants tended to have smaller prostates. A meta-analysis of six previous studies of finasteride concluded that the effect of this drug is restricted largely to patients with prostates of at least 40 ml, thus explaining in part the poor showing of finasteride in the Veterans Administration Cooperative Study (Eri and Kjell, 1997). Comparative studies focusing on prostate size and duration of therapy are now under way, and their results should be helpful in clarifying the confusion over appropriate drug therapy.

Patients who do not improve significantly after 6 months on finasteride or 2 to 3 months on an alpha-blocker should be referred to a urologist for further evaluation. Other indications for referral include an abnormal DRE, hematuria, or a finding of 300 ml or more on PVR evaluation.

Nonsurgical Treatments

Numerous minimally invasive therapies have been studied in the last decade for the treatment of lower urinary tract symptoms attributable to BPH. Minimally invasive therapies are particularly useful in patients taking anticoagulants (in whom anesthesia is contraindicated) and in men with an active sex life (Tunuguntla and Evans, 2002). Nonsurgical, minimally invasive treatment options include balloon dilation, urethral stents, microwave thermotherapy, and laser ablation. These options have the advantage of less risk than surgical intervention, require only outpatient treatment, and involve less blood loss. Disadvantages include unknown long-term effects and the use of unproven devices.

Transurethral balloon dilation involves the intraurethral placement and expansion of a balloon that was designed to split the anterior commissure of the prostate. This technique is most effective in small prostates (< 40 ml). Although symptomatic improvement has been shown to range from 50% to 70%, peak urinary flow rates tend to return to baseline levels by 1 year after treatment.

Intraurethral stents are used on a temporary basis in patients with obstruction who are at high risk for developing complications from surgery. Although many patients report symptomatic relief, reports of urinary frequency and incontinence are not uncommon after the procedure. Laser therapy uses two main energy sources of lasers: neodymium:yttrium-aluminum-garnet (Nd:YAG) and Holmium-YAG (Hurle et al, 2002). Several different coagulation necrosis techniques have been described. Transurethral laser-induced prostatectomy (TULIP) is performed under transrectal ultrasound guidance. Visual coagulative necrosis is performed under cystoscopic control. Coagulative techniques do not create an immediate effect on the prostatic urethra; tissue is sloughed over the course of several weeks, up to 3 months after the procedure. Advantages of laser surgery include minimal blood loss, rare occurrence of transurethral resection syndrome, the ability to treat patients while on anticoagulation therapy, and outpatient surgery (Tierney, McPhee, and Papadakis, 2003). Transurethral resection syndrome, which is an infrequent complication of the TURP procedure (occurring in about 2% of cases), is water intoxication of the body that results in hyponatremia and other acid-base imbalances. The consequences are increased intravascular volume, cellular edema, and hypothermia (Chambers, 2002).

Transurethral needle ablation of the prostate (TUNA) uses a specially designed urethral catheter that deploys interstitial radiofrequency needles, which pierce the mucosa of the prostatic urethra. Radiofrequencies are then used to heat the tissue, resulting in coagulative necrosis. Transurethral electrovaporization of the prostate uses a modified resectoscope to deliver high current densities, which result in heat vaporization of the tissue, creating a cavity in the prostatic urethra.

Microwave hyperthermia is delivered with a transurethral catheter. Symptom score and flow rate improvement are obtained, but (as with laser surgery) large randomized studies with long-term follow-up are needed to assess durability and cost-effectiveness.

High-intensity focused ultrasound (HIFU) is another means of performing thermal tissue ablation using a dual-function ultrasound probe placed in the rectum to allow imaging of the prostate and also to deliver short bursts of high-intensity focused ultrasound energy, which heats the prostate tissue and causes coagulative necrosis.

Surgery

For more than 50 years, the traditional operative approaches for BPH have been TURP and open prostatectomy; however, several simpler and less invasive surgical therapies have been developed or are being investigated. Table 20-4 provides indications for surgery in patients with BPH.

The gold standard of BPH treatment remains TURP because of its high success rate in relieving symptoms; these success rates are almost as high as those associated with an open prostatectomy, yet with much lower morbidity and mortality rates. In the United States 400,000 resections are performed each year, with a success rate of 80% to 90%. This procedure requires hospitalization for 1 to 2 days, although occasionally it is done as an outpatient procedure; general or spinal anesthesia is used. Despite this, complications such as bleeding, infection, stricture, retrograde ejaculation, impotence, and incontinence are associated with the surgery, making the decision to undergo it a serious one. Indications for this surgery include symptoms that are severe (a high "bother factor") and the presence of clinical conditions such as progressive azotemia, episodes of acute urine

---

TABLE 20-4   **Indications for Surgery in Patients with Benign Prostatic Hypertrophy**
Intractable symptoms not satisfactorily controlled by medical therapy
Urinary retention
Frequently recurrent or persistent urinary tract infection
Recurrent gross bleeding
Unacceptably high postvoid residual urine (e.g., >400-500 mL) not controlled with medical therapy
Bladder calculi
Evidence of obstruction affecting the ureters or kidneys

From Stutzman RE: Bladder outlet obstruction. In Barker LR, Burton JR, Zieve PD, editors: *Principles of ambulatory medicine*, ed 6, Philadelphia, 2003, Lippincott Williams & Wilkins.

retention or bladder stones, PVR of 300 ml or more, or recurrent urinary tract infections secondary to bladder outlet obstruction.

Transurethral incision of the prostate and bladder neck (TUIP) is simpler than a TURP and requires only an incision along the urethra from the bladder neck downward through the prostate. This procedure involves no tissue removal, and it can be used only in patients with glands weighing 30 g or less. Because it uses telescopically guided technology, recovery is more rapid in most cases. TUIP has fewer complications, and the postoperative flow rates and relief of symptoms are comparable with TURP. The only major disadvantage of TUIP is the potential for missing major localized prostate cancer; for this reason, some urologists advocate either a biopsy of the prostate or at least one loop incision (similar to that done in TURP) for tissue at the time of TUIP (Stutzman, 2003).

Open prostatectomy requires a longer hospitalization and recovery period. This approach is used when, in addition to having a large prostate, the patient has a bladder condition that can be repaired at the same time (e.g., bladder diverticulum, bladder stone). Erectile impotence occurs in about 5% to 15%, and urinary incontinence occurs in 3% to 5% of men who undergo this surgery. Because the entire gland is not removed, these patients have a risk equal to that of the general population of ultimately developing prostatic carcinoma (Stutzman, 2003).

Follow-up

Because BPH does not progress in a predictable manner, careful follow-up is required to assess the ongoing efficacy of the chosen treatment regimen. Patient monitoring is guided by the AUA Symptom Index, which should be administered every 6 months, or with reports by the patient of changes in symptoms. Changes in a patient's score indicate the need to consider a revision in the treatment plan and also signal the appropriate time to involve a specialist in treatment planning. The DRE is mandatory on an annual basis, and the prudent provider will order a PSA at the same visit, despite the current conflict about its usefulness. Complications associated with BPH include urinary tract infection, bladder stones, and renal failure, and the patient should be assessed for these conditions during routine visits.

EDUCATION

Patient education is a critical component of the treatment process, especially with the current emphasis on patient involvement in decision making. The patient and family should be assured that the presence of BPH is in no way associated with the development of cancer. Further, they should be assured that BPH is a normal part of aging, much as menopause is for a woman, and that many treatment options are available to relieve the symptoms of prostatism. The patient and family should be aware of the possible complications of BPH and what symptoms require immediate attention. Relevant patient education information may be discussed at routine clinic visits, but numerous written resources are available and should be provided for the patient's later reference.

Summary of Benign Prostatic Hyperplasia

The significant prevalence of BPH makes it inevitable that practitioners caring for adult men will evaluate and treat this condition. It is important to know how to proceed with evaluation and to be able to distinguish BPH from cancer of the prostate. Treatment options have grown in recent years, and patients will need and expect information and assistance in choosing an intervention that is appropriate for them to maintain function and quality of life. Ongoing monitoring is also important to evaluate the efficacy of the treatment.

Erectile Dysfunction

Sexuality remains a vital aspect of life despite aging. Although ED is not life threatening, it may result in withdrawal from sexual intimacy and reduced quality of life (Fink et al, 2002). Erectile functioning is a complex neurovascular, physiologic response requiring intact psychologic, neural, and vascular components (Nehra and Kulaksizoglu, 2002b). Advances in impotence research and increased knowledge of the pathophysiology of erection have completely changed the treatment of ED (Wespes, 2002).

Erectile dysfunction is defined as the persistent "inability to achieve or maintain an erection for satisfactory sexual performance" (Archer, 2002; Fink et al, 2002). In clinical practice, many male patients have mild forms of ED, such as weak erections, premature ejaculations, and occasional erectile failures (Dey and Shepherd, 2002).

EPIDEMIOLOGY

Erectile dysfunction is a worldwide health issue that affects nearly half the men over 40 years of age. Although prevalence estimates for ED vary, up to 30 million men in the United States may be affected. One study found that 7% of men aged 18 to 29 years of age have trouble achieving or maintaining an erection, with prevalence rising to 18% for men aged 50 to 59 years of age (Fink et al, 2002). It is a well-accepted fact that ED is far more prevalent than the estimated 10% of patients who seek medical therapy. The predominant reasons suggested for the low rate of reporting are the complexity of sexuality, taboos, cultural restrictions, lack of satisfactory treatment, and acceptance of the situation as a normal sequence of aging (Nehra and Kulaksizoglu, 2002b).

NORMAL PHYSIOLOGY

Penile erection occurs in response to visual, olfactory, imaginative, and tactile stimuli initiated within the brain or on the periphery. Blood flow into the paired corpora cavernosa and the bulbus spongiosum engorges the cavernosal spaces. The raised intracavernosal pressure in turn occludes the emissary veins, leading to further engorgement. High levels of intrapenile nitric oxide (NO) act as a local neurotransmitter to facilitate relaxation of intracavernosal trabeculae, thereby maximizing blood flow and penile erection. NO works by promoting the generation of cyclic guanosine monophosphate (cGMP), which facilitates smooth-muscle relation, and inflow of blood. Detumescence (loss of erection) occurs when NO-induced vasodilation subsides because of metabolism of cGMP, which is primarily mediated by intracavernosal type 5 cGMP phosphodiesterase (PDE5). Sildenafil and related compounds exert their role on erectile physiology by inhibiting PDE5 (Dey and Shepherd, 2002).

Initiation of the erectile process requires autonomic neural input to direct the blood flow into the corpora cavernosae. Psychogenic erections begin in response to erotic stimuli or sexual fantasy. The centrally perceived sensual stimuli are relayed through the spinal thoracolumbar erection center (T11-L2) to the pelvic vascular bed. Reflex erections are initiated by tactile stimuli to the penis or genital area, which activate a reflex arc with sacral roots originating at the sacral erection center (S2-4) (Dey and Shepherd, 2002).

Testosterone is needed to maintain intrapenile NO synthase levels, which may mediate local vasodilation by increased production of NO. Testosterone replacement in hypogonadal men restores libido and erectile function. Other hormones, including prolactin, thyroid hormone, and adrenal steroids, play a secondary by important role in facilitating and maintaining male sexual functioning (Dey and Shepherd, 2002).

ASSOCIATED CONDITIONS

Age in itself has proven to be the strongest correlate of ED in many studies around the world; but aging also carries increased medical comorbidity, such as cardiovascular disease, hypertension, and cerebrovascular disease, which are also associated with increased risk of ED (Nehra and Kulaksizoglu, 2002b). Diabetes has been another factor closely associated with ED. Diabetes has been associated with a twofold increase in the incidence rate of ED compared with the nondiabetic population (Nehra and Kulaksizoglu, 2002b). The severity and prevalence of ED increase with poor glycemic control, age, cigarette smoking, diabetic neuropathy, duration of disease, type 2 diabetes, diabetic nephropathy, and hypertension. Obesity and lack of exercise may contribute to diabetes-related ED (Dey and Shepherd, 2002).

The incidence of ED in patients with cardiovascular disease and cardiac risk factors has been reported to be as high as 80%. Some reports state that ED might be the first sign of serious cardiovascular disease. An association between chronic renal failure and ED has been established since 1975, and studies estimate that about 50% of such patients are affected (Nehra and Kulaksizoglu, 2002b).

Erectile dysfunction is associated with pelvic surgical procedures, especially radical prostatectomy, cystectomy, and rectal surgeries. A significant improvement has occurred in preserving the erectile function of men after radical prostatectomy with the introduction of nerve-sparing techniques; however, the number of patients eligible for these techniques remains limited. Other causes include structural penile lesions such as Peyronie's disease and trauma.

ASSOCIATED MEDICATIONS

Sexual dysfunction associated with medications may impact the ability of patients to remain on the prescribed therapy and can lead to deterioration in quality of life (Ferrario and Levy, 2002). Therefore, it is important for practitioners to become familiar with the wide variation in sexual side effects produced by medications and to discuss the potential occurrence of these side effects with patients. In many cases, a change in the drug regimen may help patients to overcome specific side effects experienced with certain treatments.

Medications that have been associated with ED include thiazide and non-thiazide diuretics, beta-blockers, calcium channel blockers, angiotensin-converting enzyme (ACE) inhibitors, benzodiazepines, digitalis, nitrates, 3-hydroxy-3-methylglutaryl coenzyme A reductase inhibitors, and histamine-2 receptor antagonists (Nehra and Kulaksizoglu, 2002b). Some findings have suggested that both statins and fibrates may cause ED in some cases (Rizvi, Hampson, and Harvey, 2002). Other common offenders are cimetidine, nicotine, alcohol, and opiates (Dey and Shepherd, 2002).

Angiotensin II antagonists can prevent or even correct erectile dysfunction in patients with hypertension. The favorable effects of these agents on sexual function may be related in part to their ability to block angiotensin II, which was recently recognized as an important mediator of detumescence and possibly ED (Ferrario and Levy, 2002).

PSYCHOSOCIAL ISSUES

Lifestyle has been found to be a strong determinant of the prevalence of ED. Men who are separated, divorced, or widowed seem to have a higher rate of ED than those who are married. Educational level seems to have a positive effect on the erectile capacity of men, with the risk being lower in those with some graduate school or a graduate degree than in men with a high school degree or less education (Nehra and Kulaksizoglu, 2002b). The prevalence of ED also increases with factors such as anxiety and depression.

EVALUATION

Clinical evaluation must include a thorough history and physical examination. The physical examination should include a search for signs of hypogonadism, such as small testes, gynecomastia with or without galactorrhea, decreased virilization, and eunuchoid proportions. The state of peripheral arterial supply as evidenced by distal pulsations, capillary refill, and peripheral arterial bruits should be documented. Signs of cauda equina syndrome include saddle anesthesia, lack of bulbocavernous reflex, and lax anal sphincter and may suggest an intraspinal mass lesion or intervertebral disk prolapse. External genitalia must be examined for the presence of any congenital or acquired structural lesion. The length of the corpora should be palpated to rule out fibrotic plaques as seen in Peyronie's disease. A prostate examination is useful to record the size and lack of suspicious nodularity before testosterone therapy is initiated for hypogonadism (Dey and Shepherd, 2002).

Biochemical evaluations to rule out secondary causes like hypogonadism and thyroid abnormalities are suggested. Laboratory testing includes complete blood cell count, chemistries, total testosterone levels, and thyroid stimulating hormone. Laboratory tests in diabetic men with ED should include appropriate studies to monitor glycemic control and assess complications of diabetes. Urinary microalbumin and serum cholesterol levels may suggest vascular atherosclerosis and endothelial dysfunction in the penile vasculature (Dey and Shepherd, 2002).

Specialized diagnostic testing may be used in select patients. Nocturnal penile tumescence studies, intracavernosal injection, arteriography, and duplex penile ultrasonography can help in clarifying the etiology and in guiding therapy (Dey and Shepherd, 2002; Yilmaz et al, 2002).

Once ED is diagnosed, the distinction must be made between psychogenic and organic ED. Psychogenic ED may begin suddenly after some stressful life event. Early morning, self-stimulated, and spontaneous nocturnal erections are often preserved. Psychogenic ED may be intermittent, depending on the patient's partner. The patient may report normal erection during masturbation. Organic ED may be due to neurogenic, vasculogenic, endocrinologic, drug-induced, or other causes. Clues to a vasculogenic origin may be insidious onset, no morning or nocturnal erections, intermittent claudication, history of smoking, and poor pulsations in distal arteries. Endocrinologic impotence usually is associated with a loss of libido, the lack of spontaneous sexual fantasies, feminization, gynecomastia, and decreased facial hair growth (Dey and Shepherd, 2002).

TREATMENT

A broad range of options are currently available for the management of ED. They include oral agents (PDE5 inhibitors, dopamine agonists, and alpha-receptor blocking drugs), intracavernosal injection (papaverine, phentolamine, prostaglandin E_1 [PGE_1] vasoactive intestinal peptide), transurethral vasoactive agents (PGE_1), vacuum erection devices, vascular surgery, and penile prostheses (Kalsi et al, 2002). Appropriate referrals to urology, endocrine, psychiatric, surgical, and cardiovascular disease specialists are encouraged.

Phosphodiesterase type 5 inhibitors sildenafil citrate (Viagra; Pfizer, Inc, New York, NY) affects erectile function by selectively inhibiting PDE5, the enzyme responsible for degradation of cyclic GMP in the corpora cavernosa. This enhances the effect of endogenous nitric oxide, producing penile smooth-muscle relaxation, arterial dilation, and inflow of blood, leading to penile engorgement. Sildenafil use does not enhance libido or normal erectile function, and it rarely produces erections in the absence of sexual stimulation. The recommended treatment dose is 50 to 100 mg taken 30 to 60 minutes before desired sexual activity (Fink et al, 2002).

Despite the proven efficacy of oral therapy for ED, some patients are unable to take these medications because of drug interactions (e.g., sildenafil and nitroglycerin) or a lack of response (Yap and McVary, 2002). Adverse effects associated with sildenafil include flushing, headache, dyspepsia (as a result of relaxation of the smooth muscle of the gastroesophageal sphincter with reflux), and visual disturbances (Fink et al 2002; Lim, Moorthy, and Benton, 2002). Sildenafil should not be prescribed to men taking any form of nitrate therapy because it may potentiate vasodilation and hypotension. In men with known coronary artery disease, exercise stress testing or another measure of cardiac reserve should be performed to determine whether they can safely achieve the physiologic workload of 4 to 6 metabolic equivalents associated with sexual activity (Dey and Shepherd, 2002).

Vacuum-constriction devices combine the twin effects of negative-pressure mechanism to induce an erection by increasing corporeal blood flow and an occlusive constriction ring around the base of the penis to prolong erection by decreasing corporeal venous drainage. The procedure involves placing a cylinder over the flaccid penis, creating an airtight seal, and generating suction via a vacuum pump to effect penile engorgement. One or more elastic bands are slipped over the base of the penis to maintain tumescence, and the cylinder is then removed. Bands should not be left in place continuously for more than 30 minutes because of the risk of ischemia (Dey and Shepherd, 2002).

A certain amount of mechanical dexterity is required to use the vacuum-constriction devices. Complications are reported to be minimal, with pain and lack of satisfactory ejaculation the most common problems (Dey and Shepherd, 2002).

Intraurethral suppository-PGE_1 is available as an intraurethral suppository, which has been reported to have an at-home successful sexual intercourse rating of about 60% (Dey and Shepherd, 2002).

Although PGE$_1$ is less invasive and easier to use than intracavernosal injection, it may reduce sexual spontaneity. Men must remain standing after the pellet is inserted to increase penile blood flow, and the time to erection is 15 to 30 minutes. Patients may complain of penile pain, minor urethral bleeding, testicular pain, and dizziness. Female partners may report vaginal burning or itching. PGE$_1$ is contraindicated in men with abnormal penile anatomy and those with hyperviscosity syndromes. Men cannot use PGE$_1$ if they have intercourse with pregnant women who are not using barrier contraceptives (Dey and Shepherd, 2002).

Intracavernosal injections of smooth-muscle relaxing agent such as a synthetic form of PGE$_1$ (alprostadil) allow a predictable clinical effect by specifically targeting the penile vasculature; the success rate is reported to be about 70% to 80% (Dey and Shepherd, 2002). Although this lessens the chances of adverse effects because of systemic absorption, local adverse effects include painful penile sensation, penile fibrotic changes, and priapism. Other agents (papaverine, moxisylyte, and phentolamine) also have been used with variable success rates. Combination therapy with the use of smaller amounts of synergistic compounds is generally preferred over single agents because of increased efficacy and a more favorable adverse-effect profile. If an erection lasts longer than 60 minutes or is painful, 30 mg of pseudoephedrine can be taken orally to ensure detumescence. Patients with priapism that does not respond promptly to oral therapy should be treated with an intracavernosal injection of alpha-agonists in a monitored and emergent setting (Dey and Shepherd, 2002).

Topical Therapies

Topical therapy has the potential to become a first-line treatment for ED because it acts locally and is easy to use (Montorsi et al, 2002). In contrast to oral agents such as sildenafil, agents such as PGE$_1$ act directly on the trabecular smooth muscle, binding to specific e-prostanoid receptors and increasing cAMP synthesis. For this reason, the direct-acting agents do not require sexual stimulation for efficacy (Nehra and Kulaksizoglu, 2002a). Testosterone has also been found to have some effect when used transdermally (Thomas, 2002).

Other Therapies

Phentolamine and yohimbine are alpha-adrergic blockers that have shown relatively modest efficacy in the treatment of ED but have not been used widely in the United States because of the lack of availability and the potential adverse effects, including palpitations and hypertension. Trazodone has been shown to improve premature ejaculation and ED in men with psychogenic ED but had only a marginal effect in men with organic ED (Dey and Shepherd, 2002). Korean red ginseng (*Panax ginseng*) has been found to enhance the ability to maintain an erection sufficient for intercourse safely and at a significantly lower cost than sildenafil (Price and Gazewood, 2003).

A surgically implanted penile prosthesis may be considered in selected patients. Adverse effects include those related to anesthesia, local wound infections, and mechanical failure necessitating surgical removal. Penile prostheses are now typically reserved for patients in whom less invasive therapies fail (Dey and Shepherd, 2002).

AREAS OF RESEARCH

Research in the field of ED has continued to expand rapidly. Several compounds are being researched for the treatment of ED. The two new PDE5 inhibitors vardenafil and IC351, sublingual apomorphine, and the combination of yohimbine and L-arginine are in phase 3 clinical trials. Early clinical and preclinical studies are investigating new PDE inhibitors, cyclic adenosine monophosphate activators, alpha-adrenergic antagonists, dopamine agonists, melanocyte-stimulating hormone, potassium channel modulators, endothelin antagonists, and nitric acid donors. Cloning of penile-inducible nitric oxide synthase (NOS) reflects the potential use of gene therapy for ED (Dey and Shepherd, 2002) and also may focus on augmenting potassium channel expression by gene transfer (Archer, 2002). Finally, preventive strategies, such as prevention of cavernosal degeneration or to restore cavernosal function, will be an important focus in the future (Andersson and Hedlund, 2002).

Summary of Erecticle Dysfunction

Although considerable advances have been made in the diagnosis and treatment of ED in the past decade, most men with ED are not treated because they do not seek medical attention or their primary care providers do not provide them an opportunity to discuss sexual problems during their visits. In the ultimate resolution of a patient's sexual dysfunction, practitioners must open a free and sympathetic dialogue and offer a full spectrum of treatment modalities tailored to the individual patient and his partner (Carson, 2002). Appropriate referral to urologists and other specialists will be an important step in obtaining appropriate treatment of erectile dysfunction.

Resources

American Urological Association
www.auanet.org

Virginia Urology Center website
www.uro.com/prostate.htm

References

Andersson KE, Hedlund P: New directions for erectile dysfunction therapies, *Int J Impot Res* 14(Suppl 1): S82-S92, 2002.

Archer SL: Potassium channels and erectile dysfunction, *Vasc Pharmacol* 38(1):61-71, 2002.

Beduschi R, Beduschi M, Oesterling J: Benign prostatic hyperplasia: use of drug therapy in primary care, *Geriatrics* 53(3):24-40, 1998.

Carson CC: Erectile dysfunction in the 21st century: whom we can treat, whom we cannot treat and patient education, *Int J Impot Res* 14(Suppl 1):S29-S34, 2002.

Chambers A: Transurethral resection syndrome – it does not have to be a mystery, *AORN J* 75(1):156-164, 2002.

Clinical Practice Guidelines: Benign prostatic hyperplasia: diagnosis and treatment, *J Am Geriatr Soc* 46:1163-1165, 1998.

Dey J, Shepherd MD: Evaluation and treatment of erectile dysfunction in men with diabetes mellitus, *Mayo Clin Proc* 77(3):276-282, 2002.

Dreikorn K: The role of phytotherapy in treating lower urinary tract symptoms and benign prostatic hyperplasia, *World J Urol* 19(6):426-435, 2002.

Dvorkin L, Song KY: Herbs for benign prostatic hyperplasia, *Ann Pharmacother* 36(9):1443-1452, 2002.

Eri LM, Kjell JT: Treatment of benign prostatic hyperplasia: a pharmacoeconomic perspective, *Drugs Aging* 10(2):107-118, 1997.

Ferrario CM, Levy P: Sexual dysfunction in patients with hypertension: implications for therapy, *J Clin Hypertens* 4(6):424-432, 2002.

Fink HA et al: Sildenafil for male erectile dysfunction: a systematic review and meta-analysis, *Arch Intern Med* 162(12):1349-1360, 2002.

Flack JM: The effect of doxazosin on sexual function in patients with benign prostatic hyperplasia, hypertension, or both, *Int J Clin Practice* 56(7):527-530, 2002.

Hayami S et al: The value of power Doppler imaging to predict the histologic components of benign prostatic hyperplasia, *Prostate* 53(2):168-174, 2002.

Hurle R et al: Holmium laser enucleation of the prostate combined with mechanical morcellation in 155 patients with benign prostatic hyperplasia, *Urology* 60(3):449, 2002.

Kalsi JS et al: Current oral treatments for erectile dysfunction, *Expert Opin Pharmacother* 3(11):1613-1629, 2002.

Lim PH, Moorthy P, Benton KG: The clinical safety of viagra, *Ann NY Acad* Sci 962:378-388, 2002.

Mitropoulos D et al: Symptomatic benign prostate hyperplasia: impact on partners' quality of life, *Eur Urol* 41(3):240-244, 2002.

Montorsi F et al: Current status of local penile therapy, *Int J Impot Res* 14(Suppl 1):S70-S81, 2002.

Nehra A, Kulaksizoglu H: Combination therapy for erectile dysfunction: where we are and what's in the future, *Curr Urol Rep* 3(6):467-470, 2002a.

Nehra A, Kulaksizoglu H: Global perspectives and controversies in the epidemiology of male erectile dysfunction, *Curr Opin Urol* 12(6):493-496, 2002b.

Preuss HG et al: Randomized trial of a combination of natural products on symptoms of benign prostatic hyperplasia, *Int Urol Nephrol* 33(2):217-225, 2001.

Price A, Gazewood J: Korean red ginseng effective for treatment of erectile dysfunction, *J Family Pract* 52(2):20-21, 2003.

Rizvi K, Hampson JP, Harvey JN: Do lipid-lowering drugs cause erectile dysfunction? A systematic review, *Fam Pract* 19(1):95-98, 2002.

Stutzman RE: Bladder outlet obstruction. In Barker LR, Burton JR, Zieve PD, editors: *Principles of ambulatory medicine*, ed 6, Philadelphia, 2003, Lippincott Williams & Wilkins.

Thiyagarajan M: Alpha-adrenoceptor antagonists in the treatment of benign prostate, *Hyperplasia Pharmacol* 65(3):119-128, 2002.

Thomas JA: Pharmacological aspects of erectile dysfunction, *Jpn J Pharmacol* 89(2):101-112, 2002.

Tierney LM, McPhee SJ, Papadakis MA: Benign prostatic hyperplasia. In *Current medical diagnosis and treatment*, ed 42, New York, 2003, Lange Medical Books/McGraw-Hill.

Tunuguntla R, Evans CP: Minimally invasive therapies for benign prostatic hyperplasia, *World J Urol* 20(4):197-206, 2002.

Verhamme K et al: Incidence and prevalence of lower urinary tract symptoms suggestive of benign prostatic hyperplasia in primary care—the triumph project, *Eur Urol* 42(4):323, 2002.

Wespes E: Intracavernous injection as an option for aging men with erectile dysfunction, *Aging Male* 5(3):177-180, 2002.

Yap RL, McVary KT: Topical agents and erectile dysfunction: is there a place? *Curr Urol Reports* 3(6):471-476, 2002.

Yilmaz E et al: Comparison of nocturnal penile tumescence monitoring and cavernosal smooth muscle content in patients with erectile dysfunction, *Int Urol Nephrol* 34(1):117-120, 2002.

21

Genitourinary/Female: Menopause

Menopause is a normal physiologic transition that happens in women at an average of 51 years of age, earlier for smokers. Menopause occurs when the ovulation and the menstrual cycle end, circulating estrogen and progesterone levels fall, and serum follicle-stimulating hormone and luteinizing hormone levels rise. This transition *(perimenopause)* develops over a period of typically 2 to 8 years in which there is a progressive loss of ovarian function, although variations exist in the estrogen production of postmenopausal women (Miller, 2003). The intervals between menses lengthen, and the postmenopausal period begins after menses cessation has lasted for at least 12 consecutive months.

Age-related Changes

The physical changes that result from the decrease in estrogen include thinning of the vaginal mucosa, a decrease in vaginal secretions, and often urogenital atrophy. Vasomotor instability or hot flashes occur in 75% of postmenopausal women, and for some women these symptoms can be quite severe. Because of the nighttime occurrence of vasomotor symptoms, many women experience sleep difficulties. There are nonpharmacologic treatments that alleviate some of these symptoms, but for most women estrogen eliminates vasomotor symptoms and has been widely used.

Postmenopausal women who are 50 years of age and older are at risk for osteoporosis and cardiovascular disease. Significant evidence has been found of an increase in loss of bone mass during the first 5 years after menopause. The incidence of death from cardiac disease for postmenopausal women equals that of men of the same age. The time of menopause marks a significant change in the ratio between men and women in terms of cardiac deaths, which led to the premise that estrogen provides a protective function from cardiac disease in women. One rationale for past use of estrogen-replacement therapy (ERT) was the assumed protective function in terms of development of cardiovascular disease and osteoporosis.

Psychological symptoms that may occur during menopause have reinforced a negative view of a normal physiologic transition period in the lives of older women. Within the youth-oriented culture of the United States are multiple negative images of older women (Gannon and Stevens, 1998). No consensus has been reached on the subject of menopausal causes of mood changes. Clinicians have differing views. Some believe that the physical changes associated with menopause, such as hot flashes, are responsible for mood changes; others fault coincident life events. Physiologic and socio-cultural influences, as well as personality traits, affect how an individual woman responds to these symptomatic changes. Providers must be aware of nonscientific influences on their abilities to provide appropriate evidence-based care for older women.

Epidemiology

Worldwide population aging is one of the most important demographic events of the recent century. The shift in age structure, which is most pronounced in the developed countries, has an impact on a broad range of social and economic conditions (Economic and Social Affairs, United Nations, 2002). Increased longevity can result in rising demands for health services and treatments that seem to delay the aging process. In the late 1990s more than 10 million postmenopausal women world-wide were taking some form of estrogen, accounting for sales figures of $2 billion. Even though only 10% of postmenopausal women in Europe and 20% in the United States were taking estrogen at that time, it was one of the world's best-selling drugs (Calif and Alsina, 1997; Ettinger, 1998; Rees, 1997). No doubt, postmenopausal women are a large market population. As we suggested in our first edition, clinicians need to approach the use of ERT with up-to-date evidence from clinical trials that investigate the benefits and risks associated with ERT. Symptoms may be extremely bothersome to some women, and short-term (6 months to one year) ERT is appropriate and effective; but we urge the need for evidenced-based prescribing practices related to the claim of the protective function of ERT. Recent federal supported clinical trials have demonstrated the risks associated with ERT.

History of Estrogen Replacement Therapy Use in the United States

In the 1960s unopposed estrogen was in wide use at a rate of one of every five prescriptions sold to American women; estimates were that a third of women over 50 years of age were prescribed the drug. In 1975 it was found that estrogen was a causal link to cancer of the uterus, and sales decreased by 40% (Voda, 1992). This risk was again confirmed in the 1990s by the Postmenopausal Estrogen/Progestin Interventions [PEPI] trials.

The 1980s found estrogen in use again, with the addition of progestin as a protective function against the effects of estrogen on uterine cancer. This new combined therapy was widely reported to protect women from heart disease and osteoporosis. The following quotation, taken from a respected textbook, reflects the prevailing view of the medical profession during the 1980s and most of the 1990s. The statement was footnoted with six medical journal articles:

Epidemiological studies reveal clear evidence for a reduced risk of cardiovascular disease (CVD) in women receiving hormone replacement therapy....Not only is the patient with previous myocardial infarction not at increased risk of developing complications from hormone replacement therapy but these women obtain the greatest CV benefit from estrogen replacement therapy (Marshburn and Carr, 1994).

The newly developed drugs in the 1990s for specific treatment of osteoporosis gave women an alternative to ERT for bone mass protection. The 1990s brought new focus to the old but newly recognized threat of dementia. A few studies reported that estrogen therapy may have a protective function against cognitive decline (Mortel and Meyer, 1995).

On May 21, 2002, the Data and Safety Monitoring Board of the National Institutes of Health (NIH), which funded the Women's Health Initiative randomized controlled trial of 16,608 postmenopausal women 50 to 79 years of age, recommended stopping the trial of estrogen plus progestin versus placebo because the risk of invasive breast cancer exceeded any benefit (Writing Group for the Women's Health Initiative Investigators, 2002). In July 2002 the estrogen/progestin arm of the study was halted because of the increased risks of cardiovascular disease and breast cancer that outweighed any benefit of the therapy (U.S. Food and Drug Administration [FDA], 2003).

The duration of the study was to be 8.5 years, but it was halted at 5.2 years. Study resu. reported that for participants taking the estrogen plus progestin, in addition to the risk of breast cer, the risk of stroke, heart attack, and pulmonary emboli were increased, and the risk of hip fracture and colorectal cancer was decreased. In November 2002 the Wyeth drug company reported that sales of Prempro, the estrogen-plus-progestin hormone combination used in the study, had dropped from 2.7 million users to 1.5 million (Kolata, 2002b). In January 2003 the FDA approved new labeling and new advice for the use of ERT. See Box 21-1.

Clinical Trials

HEART DISEASE

The Heart and Estrogen/Progestin Replacement Study (HERS) was a randomized, placebo-controlled trial involving 2763 women with coronary artery disease (CAD) in 20 centers. The primary objective of the study was nonfatal myocardial infarction (MI) and coronary heart disease (CHD) death. No significant decrease was seen in the ERT users in terms of CHD or secondary events. Therefore the ERT provided no protective benefit for cardiac events. The conclusion of the study was that ERT should not be used to reduce risk for CHD events in women with CHD (Grady et al, 2002a). Another objective of the study was to examine the effect of long-term postmenopausal

---

Box 21-1

New Labeling and New Advice to Postmenopausal Women Who Use or Are Considering Using Estrogen and Estrogen With Progestin

FDA's Actions

- FDA has carefully reviewed data from the Women's Health Initiative (WHI) study to ensure that the labels of Prempro and similar estrogen, and estrogen with progestin, products are accurate.
- FDA has revised the labeling of Prempro, Premphase and Premarin for patients and physicians to reflect the WHI study's findings of increased risk from these products.
- For two uses, FDA has revised the professional and consumer labels to include consideration of alternative therapies that may provide benefits to postmenopausal women.
- When these products are being prescribed solely for symptoms of vulvar and vaginal atrophy, the new label recommends that topical products be considered.
- When these products are only used for osteoporosis prevention, the new label specifies that the risks for osteoporosis must outweigh the risk of estrogen or estrogen with progesterin.
- FDA is asking all manufacturers to update their labeling with the results of the WHI, because all estrogen and progestin products are believed to have similar risks.
- FDA will soon revise its formal guidances for the industry in two related areas: labeling for all estrogen and estrogen with progestin products for postmenopausal women, and recommendations for conducting clinical trials to develop new products for postmenopausal women.

FDA's Advice to Women

- Estrogens provide valuable therapy for many women but carry serious risks, and therefore postmenopausal women who use or are considering using estrogen or estrogen with progestin treatments should discuss with their physicians whether the benefits outweigh the risks.
- For hot flashes and symptoms of vulvar and vaginal atrophy, these products are the most effective approved therapies.
- Estrogen and progestins should be used at the lowest doses for the shortest duration to reach treatment goals, although it is not known at what dose there may be less risk of serious side effects.

From US Food and Drug Administration, FDA Factsheet, January 8, 2003, Department of Health & Human Services.

hormone therapy on common noncardiovascular disease outcomes. Study conclusions were that after 6.8 years of treatment with ERT the rates of venous thromboembolism and biliary tract surgery increased (Hulley et al, 2002).

Heart disease is the leading cause of death in older women. The lifetime probability of a woman developing CAD is 46% (LaCharity, 1997). The primary and secondary protective effects of estrogen on heart disease have been a major reason for prescribing ERT. In analyses of the PEPI trial data, the documented cardioprotective effects of ERT are on the lipid profile (Barrett-Connor et al, 1977; Espeland et al, 1998). Changes in the lipid profiles were associated with increased high-density lipoprotein (HDL) cholesterol, decreased low-density lipoprotein (LDL) cholesterol, and decreased total cholesterol in all treatment arms. The only trend to gain statistical significance was a larger increase in HDL cholesterol in the treatment arm of estrogen 0.625 mg daily, only with no added drug (Barrett-Connor et al, 1997). Again the risks outweigh the benefit, and more specific drugs are available to treat lipid disorders.

The 1998 clinical trial of "estrogen plus progestin for secondary prevention of CHD in 2763 postmenopausal women" reported by Hulley et al (1998) does not support the claim of secondary protection from heart disease:

In a 4.1-year treatment with oral conjugated equine estrogen plus medroxyprogesterone acetate, the overall rate of CHD events in postmenopausal women with established coronary disease was not reduced. The treatment did increase the rate of thromboembolic events and gallbladder disease. (p. 605)

On the basis of these results, the recommendation was not to start ERT for the purpose of secondary prevention of CHD (Hulley et al, 1998).

In the Nurses Health 14-year study of 80,082 women, which included 658 cases of nonfatal MIs and 281 fatal cases, investigators reported interesting findings, including the following:
- The risk of CAD increased by 17% with each increase of 5% of energy from saturated fat than from carbohydrates.
- High intake of folate and vitamin B6 halved the risk of disease and death.
- One multivitamin a day had the same effect as long-term ERT.
- These dietary primary prevention therapies are considerably less expensive and incur less risk than ERT (Hu, 1997; Rimm et al, 1998; Verhoef et al, 1998).

OSTEOPOROSIS

Older postmenopausal women have an increased risk of sustaining hip fractures and compression fractures of the vertebrae because of the accelerated loss of bone mass during the early years of menopause. Bone loss in women is twice as great as that in men (Rosenthal, 1998).

In the 2002 report of the Women's Health Initiative study, evidence was found of a reduction in the occurrences of hip fractures in the treatment group (Writing Group for the Women's Health Initiative Investigators, 2002).

In the 3-year PEPI clinical trial, women assigned to the treatment arms of the protocol had significantly greater increases in hip and spinal bone density (3.5% to 5%) than those assigned to the placebo group, who lost bone density (spinal loss of 1.8% and hip loss of 1.7%) (Writing Group for PEPI, 1996). Bone-density treatment by ERT does provide a protective function and a decreased risk of hip fracture. Recent use of ERT provides protection, and the longer the duration of the therapy, the greater the decrease in risk. Five years after therapy is discontinued, however, the risk of fractures rises to the same level as would have occurred without therapy (Michaelsson et al, 1998). Use of ERT for longer than 5 years is not recommended, and therefore the risks outweigh the benefit; also, other drugs can provide protection without the same level of risk. Therapies for osteoporosis are addressed in Chapter 15.

COGNITIVE FUNCTION

The hope that ERT may provide a protective function for cognitive loss was never as well established or even supported by any significant study as the protective cardiac or osteoporosis functions.

Results from the HERS demonstrates that among older women with coronary disease 4 years of treatment with ERT did not result in better cognition as measured on six standardized tests (Grady et al, 2002b). This study also reports that high LDL and total cholesterol levels are associated with cognitive impairment and calls for research between statin use and better cognitive function (Yaffe et al, 2002).

A meta-analysis of studies dealing with cognitive function, dementia, and ERT counted five observational studies and eight trials that addressed cognitive function in healthy postmenopausal women, and there is no clear finding of benefit. Ten observational studies measured the risk of developing dementia. Analysis suggests a 29% decrease in risk among estrogen users, but the findings are not uniform. The conclusion of the meta-analysis was that all studies had substantial methodologic problems and produced conflicting results. The recommendations were not to prescribe ERT because of the known risks and the need for adequate trials to investigate the relationship of ERT and cognition (Yaffe and Grady, 1998). Yaffe (1998) then reported on a prospective cohort study of 532 women with an average follow-up of 5 years who were enrolled in the ongoing Study of Osteoporetic Fractures. Three cognitive tests were administered at year 1 and then repeated in 5 years. The conclusions reached were that endogenous estrogens are not consistently associated with cognitive performance or risk of cognitive decline.

PSYCHOLOGICAL SYMPTOMS

No support or relevant studies show that the use of ERT alleviates psychological symptoms that may occur at menopause. Furthermore, no scientific evidence has been established of a causal link between the physiologic changes associated with menopause and psychological symptoms; rather, a reaction to negative life events or a depressive episode may have been treated with ERT (Holte, 1998).

SYMPTOM DEFINITION

Many perimenopausal and postmenopausal women seek medical care for symptom relief. Estrogen is the most effective treatment for the alleviation of symptoms that result from the physiologic hormonal changes associated with menopause. In January 2003 the FDA published "Guidance for Industry Estrogen and Estrogen/Progestin Drug Products to Treat Vasomotor Symptoms and Vulva and Vaginal Atrophy Symptoms—Recommendations for Clinical Evaluation: Draft Guidance." The draft document outlines future study parameters with the dual objectives of safety from adverse effects and efficacy in the reduction of symptoms. The document is distributed for comment purposes and is available on the FDA web site.

An interesting aspect for practitioners is the preliminary definition of two troublesome postmenopausal symptoms: hot flashes and genital irritations. The vasomotor experiences referred to as *hot flashes* is usually described as a sudden feeling of warmth that increases in intensity in the area of the upper chest, neck, and face, followed for many women by profuse sweating or a visible erythema. The severity of vasomotor effects is clinically defined as follows:

Mild	Sensation of heat without sweating
Moderate	Sensation of heat with sweating, able to continue activity
Severe	Sensation of heat with sweating, causing cessation of activity (Center for Drug Evaluation and Research, CDER, 2003)

Vulvar and vaginal atrophy symptoms reported by women in the HERS study were vaginal dryness (26% of study participants) and genital irritation (10%). Another frequent problem was sleep disturbances, both early awakenings (53%) and trouble sleeping (55%) (Barnabei et al, 2002).

Moderate to severe symptoms of vulvar and vaginal atrophy associated with menopause include the following:
- Vaginal dryness
- Vaginal or vulvar irritation or itching
- Dysuria

- Vaginal pain associated with sexual activity
- Vaginal bleeding associated with sexual activity (Center for Drug Evaluation and Research, 2003)

Even though sleep disturbances are reported by postmenopausal women, treatment of the vasomotor symptoms would most likely alleviate sleep problems associated with menopause.

Clinical Examination

HISTORY

History should focus on the following:
- Menstrual and reproductive history
- Sexual history
- Sleep disturbances
- Risk assessment for:
    Breast cancer
    Gynecologic cancer
    Cardiovascular disease
    Osteoporosis
- Review of systems
- Family history
- Lifestyle assessment

The family history should review breast cancers, gynecologic cancers, osteoporosis, and cardiovascular disease. Necessary lifestyle information includes smoking history, alcohol intake, dietary habits, and level of exercise. Current sexual activity is an important consideration for the practitioner to ascertain because postmenopausal women are at increased risk for contracting sexually transmitted human immunodeficiency virus; vaginal mucosa that is atrophic is easily torn.

PHYSICAL EXAMINATION

The physical examination should include the following:
- Weight, height and body mass index
- Posture
- Breast examination
- Pelvic and rectal examination

Baseline height should be recorded for future tracking of loss of height due to osteoporetic vertebral fractures. Breasts and cardiovascular status need to be examined. The pelvic examination evaluates for enlargement of the uterus and ovaries, the presence of cystocele or rectocele, and the condition of the vaginal mucosa.

Management

In light of the recent published research findings, the action of the FDA in regard to labeling of hormonal drugs and the 2003 Guidance for Industry, most practitioners will need to rethink their management of postmenopausal patients. At present the protective cardiovascular function of estrogen is not valid. The protection for bone density by estrogen products carries long-term risk, and other alternatives are effective and available. Therefore the only valid reason to start hormonal therapy may depend on the severity of the symptoms that a woman is experiencing.

The opportunity for counseling and patient education will arise because each patient will need to assimilate new findings in light of her own needs and understanding of the risk-to-benefit profile of estrogen and estrogen/progestin products. The opportunity for health professionals to review how they come to know the risk benefit of new and old drugs will also be present. Additionally, health professionals will have the opportunity review what types of monitoring of drugs are essential to ensure the health and well-being of patients.

TREATMENT MANAGEMENT

Alternatives to consider for alleviating hot flashes include safe lifestyle activities such as daily exercise, relaxation practices, cotton clothing, layered clothing, and avoidance of caffeine and alcohol (MacKay, 1997; Miller 2003). Some women prefer an herbal remedy to alleviate the vasomotor symptoms. Black cohosh is a North American herb used by Native Americans. A 1998 review of eight studies concluded that black cohosh is safe and may be effective in alleviating vasomotor postmenopausal symptoms (Lieberman, 1998). Issues of dosage and bioavailability of herbs confound the findings of effectiveness because standardization is not enforced (Miller, 2003).

If the patient decides to use ERT for vasomotor relief, it is prudent to explain to the patient that hot flashes may return on termination of ERT. At present treatment should be considered for only short-term therapy. Persistent breakthrough bleeding on ERT needs to be evaluated to rule out endometrial cancer. Annual mammograms are a necessity for all older women.

Lower doses of estrogen are needed for the relief of genitourinary symptoms than for vasomotor symptoms, although topical estrogen preparations have the same risks and contraindications as do all other forms of drug preparations. Vaginal atrophy can be alleviated somewhat by continued sexual activity or use of lubricants, such as estrogen cream (Premarin) or a water-based lubricant such as KY lubricant. Because all types of preparations of topical estrogen preparation have comparable effectiveness, patient preference is the defining factor in therapy choice. The practitioner should mention that creams and pessaries may be difficult for some patients to administer. Also, because of the low dosage, there is no benefit for bone density that occurs during systemic administration of estrogen (Miller, 2003). Preparations of topical estrogen are listed in Table 21-1.

ALTERNATIVE PHARMACOLOGIC AGENTS

A relatively new class of drugs is the selective estrogen receptor modulators (SERMs); these drugs are an alternative for some women who are unwilling to take estrogen. These drugs have both estrogen receptor agonist and antagonists effects, depending on the target organ. Tamoxifen was one of the first SERMs, and it is used primarily for prevention of breast cancer recurrence. As with all drugs there is a risk-to-benefit profile.

Raloxifene, a recently developed SERM, has been used as an alternative to estrogen. Raloxifene is approved for the prevention and treatment of postmenopausal osteoporosis (Cauley et al, 2001).

The Multiple Outcomes of Raloxifene Evaluation (MORE) trial is a 4-year randomized double-blind, placebo-controlled trial conducted between 1994 to 1997 in 25 countries at 180 sites with

TABLE 21-1	**Therapies for Vaginal Dryness and Genitourinary Symptoms**	
Preparation	**Estrogen (brand)**	**Dose**
Lubricants	No estrogen (Replens)	Use liberally or as needed with intercourse
Cream	Conjugated estrogens (Premarin)	0.5-2.0 g qd for 3 wk each mo 2-4 g qd ×
	Estradiol (Estrace)	2 wk then decrease dose 2-4 g qd for
	Estropipate (Ogen)	3 wk each month 1-2 applicators qd for
	Dienestrol (Ortho Dienestrol)	1-2 wk then decrease dose
Ring	Estradiol (Estring)	Insert and replace every 90 days
Tablet	Estradiol (Vagifem)	1 tablet vaginally qd × 2 wk, then 1 tablet 2 × per wk

From Miller RG: Menopause and beyond. In Barker LR, Burton JR, Zieve PD, editors: *Principles of ambulatory medicine,* ed 6, New York, 2003, Lippincott Williams & Wilkins.

7705 postmenopausal women as subjects of the study. Raloxifene, as estrogen, is effective in protecting bone density and is an approved drug for this purpose. Although not as effective as estrogen, lipid levels are lowered (Miller, 2003). Raloxifene use has shown a significant reduction in estrogen receptor-positive invasive breast cancer (Cauley et al, 2001). The multiple-year treatment with raloxifiene (60 or 120 mg) had no effect on overall cognitive scores (Yaffe et al, 2001). Adverse effects of raloxifene are worsening of hot flashes, leg cramps, and a threefold increase over estrogen in the development of thromboembolic disease (Davies et al, 1999; Miller, 2003). Further study is necessary to investigate long-term adverse effects. A study is under way that is investigating the effect of raloxifene on the risk of CHD events. Results of this trial, the Raloxifene for the Heart (RUTH), have not yet been published (Wenger et al, 2002).

Summary

A sea of change has developed in regard to the use of estrogen for treatment of postmenopausal women. New labeling on estrogen products and new approaches to symptom and disease prevention have caused reassessment of practice for most primary care providers, but not every professional or lay persons will accept the study results. The following represents two opposing viewpoints:

In a July 9, 2002, article in the *New York Times*, Dr. Victoria Kusiak, vice president of clinical affairs and North America director of Wyeth, the largest maker of hormones, was quoted as follows: "Eighty five percent of women do have symptoms. The hot flushes, the night sweats, are not just annoying—they can interfere with your life." She went on to comment, "For the longer term, particularly beyond the four-year point we would advise that it has to be an individualized risk-benefit analysis."

In the same article Dr. Deborah Grady, who directs the University of California San Francisco/Mount Zion Women's Health Clinical Research Center, commented as follows: "This is a dangerous drug." She did go on to talk about how some women can stop the drug without any return of symptoms. For women who have symptom recurrence, she said to resume treatment but to stop again within a short time. Dr. Nannette Wegner, a cardiologist at Emory University, said the only reason to take hormones was for temporary relief of severe symptoms. She added, "I would not tell anyone to start taking it" (Kolata, 2002a). It is important for all primary care practitioners to follow the FDA labeling practices to protect patients from the serious adverse effects of long-term use of estrogen.

Resources

The North American Menopause Society
P.O. Box 94527
Cleveland, OH 44101
(216) 844-8748
www.menopause.org

OBGYN Net
www.obgyn.net

References

Barnabei VM et al: Menopausal symptoms in older women and the effects of treatment with hormone therapy, *Obstet Gynecol* 100(6):1209-1218, 2002.

Barrett-Connor E et al: The postmenopausal estrogen/progestin intervention study: primary outcomes in adherent women, *Maturitas* 27(3):261-274, 1997.

Calif I, Alsina J: Benefits of hormone replacement therapy: overview and update, *Int J Fertil Womens Med* 42(Suppl 2):329-346, 1997.

Cauley JA et al: Continued breast cancer risk reduction in postmenopausal women treated with raloxifene: 4-year results from the MORE trial: Multiple outcomes of raloxifene evaluation, *Breast Cancer Res Treat* 65(2):125-134, 2001.

Center for Drug Evaluation and Research: Guidance for industry estrogen and estrogen/progestin drug products to treat vasomotor symptoms and vulva and vaginal symptoms—recommendations for clinical evaluation: draft guidance, Rockville, MD, 2003, U.S. Food and Drug Adminstration.

Davies GC et al: Adverse events reported by postmenopausal women in controlled trials with raloxifene, *Obstet Gynecol* 93(4):558-565, 1999.

Economic and Social Affairs Department: *World population ageing: 1950-2050*, New York, 2002, United Nations.

Espeland M et al: Effect of postmenopausal hormone therapy on lipoprotein (a) concentration: PEPI investigators, postmenopausal estrogen/progestin interventions, *Circulation* 97(10):979-986, 1998.

Ettinger B: Overview of estrogen replacement therapy: a historical perspective, *Proc Soc Exp Biol Med* 217:2-5, 1998.

Gannon L, Stevens J: Portraits of menopause in the mass media, *Women's Health* 27(3):1-15, 1998.

Grady D et al: Cardiovascular disease outcomes during 6.8 years of hormone therapy: Heart and Estrogen/progestin Replacement Study follow-up (HERS), *JAMA* 288(1):49-57, 2002a.

Grady D et al: Effect of postmenopausal hormone therapy on cognitive function: the Heart and Estrogen/Progestin Replacement Study, *Am J Med* 113(7):543-548, 2002b.

Holte A: Menopause, mood, and hormone replacement therapy: methodological issues, *Maturitas* 29(1):5-18, 1998.

Hu FB: Dietary fat intake and the risk of coronary heart disease in women, *N Engl J Med* 337:1491-1499, 1997.

Hulley S et al: Randomized trial of estrogen plus progestin for secondary prevention of coronary heart disease in postmenopausal women and estrogen/progestin replacement study (HERS) research group, *JAMA* 280(7):650-652, 1998.

Hulley S et al: Noncardiovascular disease outcomes during 6.8 years of hormone therapy: Heart and Estrogen/Progestin Replacement Study follow-up (HERS II), *JAMA* 288(1):58-66, 2002.

Kolata G: Citing risk, US will halt study of drugs for hormones. *New York Times*, July 9, 2002a.

Kolata G: Menopause without pills: rethinking hot flashes. *New York Times*, November 12, 2002b.

LaCharity L: The experience of postmenopausal women with coronary artery disease, *West J Nurs Res* 19(5):583-602, 1997.

Lieberman S: A review of the effectiveness of *Cimicifuga racemosa* (black cohosh) for symptoms of hot flashes among women with a history of breast cancer, *J Womens Health* 7:525, 1998.

MacKay H: Gynecology. In Tierney LM, McPhee SJ, Papadakis MA, editors: *Current medical diagnosis and treatment*, ed 36, Stamford, Conn, 1997, Appleton & Lange.

Marshburn P, Carr B: The menopause and hormone replacement therapy. In Hazzard WR et al, editors: *Principles of geriatric medicine and gerontology*, ed 3, New York, 1994, McGraw-Hill.

Michaelsson K et al: Hormone replacement therapy and the risk of hip fracture; population based case-control study: The Swedish Hip Fracture Study Group, *BMJ* 316(7148):1858-1863, 1998.

Miller RG: Menopause and beyond. In Barker LR, Burton JR, Zieve PD, editors: *Principles of ambulatory medicine*, ed 6, New York, 2003, Lippincott Williams & Wilkins.

Mortel KF, Meyer JS: Lack of postmenopausal estrogen replacement therapy and the risk of dementia, *J Neuropsychiatry* 7(3):334-337, 1995.

Rees M: The need to improve compliance to HRT in Europe, *Br J Obstet Gynecol* 104:1-3, 1997.

Rimm EB et al: Folate and vitamin B6 from diet and supplements in relation to risk of coronary heart disease among women, *JAMA* 279:359-364, 1998.

Rosenthal R: Osteoporosis, *Arch Am Acad Orthop Surg* 1:52, 1998.

U.S. Food and Drug Administration: FDA approves new labeling and provides new advice to postmenopausal who use or who are considering using estrogen and estrogen with progestin. FDA Fact Sheet, January 8, 2003.

Verhoef P et al: Folate and coronary heart disease, *Curr Opin Lipidol* 9(1):17-22, 1998.

Voda A: Menopause: a normal view, *Clin Obstet Gynecol* 35(4):923-933, 1992.

Wenger NK et al: Baseline characteristics of participants in the Raloxifene Use for the Heart (RUTH) trial. *Am J Cardiol* 90(11):1204-1210, 2002.

The Writing Group for the Women's Health Initiative Investigators. Risks and benefits of estrogen plus progestin in healthy postmenopausal women: principal results from the Women's Health Initiative randomized controlled trial. *JAMA* 288(3):321-33, 2002.

The Writing Group for the PEPI: Effects of hormone therapy on bone mineral density: results from the postmenopausal estrogen/progestin interventions (PEPI) trial, *JAMA* 276(17):1389-1396, 1996.

Yaffe K: Estrogen therapy in postmenopausal women: effects on cognitive function and dementia, *JAMA* 279(9):688-695, 1998.

Yaffe K, Grady D: Serum estrogen levels, cognitive performance, and risk of cognitive decline in older community women, *J Am Geriatr Soc* 46(7):816-821, 1998.

Yaffe K et al: Serum lipoprotein levels, stain use and cognitive function in older women, *Arch Neurol* 59(3):378-384, 2002.

Yaffee K et al: Cognitive function in postmenopausal women treated with raloxifene, *N Engl J Med* 344(16):1207-1213, 2001.

22

Genitourinary: Incontinence

Urinary incontinence (UI) knows no national or social boundaries and can affect both healthy and frail men and women. Also known as *lower-urinary-tract dysfunction,* UI is defined as the involuntary loss of urine that is objectively demonstrable or a social or hygiene problem (Scientific Committee of the First International Consultation on Incontinence, 2000). At least 13 million or more Americans are affected by UI at an annual cost of $11.2 billion. It is well known that a significant number of those with UI do not seek treatment either because of their own or their health provider's discomfort in discussing the condition (Vapnek, 2001).

As the country continues to experience a growing aging population, these numbers are expected to increase (Abdelghany et al, 2001). Advanced age by itself is not the cause of UI, although 15% to 30% of community-dwelling older persons, up to one third of older patients in acute-care settings, and about 50% of residents in long-term care facilities are affected. Multiple factors contribute to UI; and age, although significant, is not the sole cause. Other contributing factors that predispose an older person to develop UI are neuromotor loss, loss of cognitive abilities, infection, drugs, depression, and restricted mobility (Lyons et al, 2002).

The consequences of UI are formidable and can have an impact on the physical, psychological, social, and financial realms, not only for the patient but also for the caregiver. Every primary care provider (PCP) must be aware of the burden that UI imposes, but each PCP also must educate patients to the reality that treatment is available and prevention is possible.

Genitourinary Anatomy and Physiology

Anatomically, the lower urinary tract is composed of the bladder; the detrusor muscle, which is best thought of as a large, trainable muscle; and the sphincter mechanism (Figure 22-1). The two parts of the urinary sphincter are the internal urethral sphincter, which is composed of both smooth and striated muscle and surrounds the urethra; and the external striated muscle sphincter, which is part of the pelvic floor. The bladder and the sphincters need to be intact to maintain urine control. Strengthening the external sphincter may compensate for damage to the sphincter mechanism.

Bladder function is primarily a spinal reflex mediated at S2 to S4. If central nervous system centers are not intact, the bladder empties as a spinal reflex. Stretch receptors are triggered as the bladder fills, and messages are sent to the sacral micturition center and the brain via autonomic pathways. The supraspinal centers either inhibit or facilitate voiding. The micturition center in the brainstem coordinates detrusor contraction and sphincter relaxation. Centers in the cerebral cortex

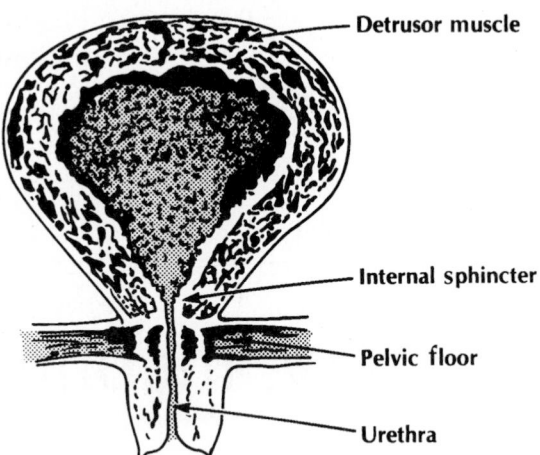

Figure 22-1   The urinary bladder. (From Burke MM, Walsh MB: *Gerontologic nursing: wholistic care of the older adult,* ed 2, St Louis, 1997, Mosby.)

inhibit detrusor contractions to delay voiding. Voiding occurs when detrusor contraction and sphincter relaxation are coordinated. As increasing amounts of urine collect in the bladder, the sphincters increase their resistance and the cortex inhibits detrusor contractions. Micturition occurs when the inhibition is released, the sphincters relax, and parasympathetic stimulation causes detrusor contractions.

Physical Changes

Age-related changes in the genitourinary system make maintaining control of urine more challenging for older adults. Differences in age-related changes exist between women and men. With aging women, detrusor instability is increased and contributes to the occurrence of urge incontinence. Detrusor instability in both sexes is associated with lower bladder capacity. Both older women and older men have changes in their voiding patterns. The most significant and most frequent change in voiding is incomplete emptying of the bladder, which leads to higher residual urine volumes. This residual urine can contribute to the older person's increased risk of UTIs. Reduced bladder sensation, which leads to a delayed onset of the desire to void when the bladder capacity has been reached, has been associated with impaired cognition (Malone-Lee, 2003).

For men, some degree of prostatic hypertrophy occurs as a normal part of aging, which, depending on the degree of enlargement, can influence bladder patterns (such as hesitancy in starting the stream). For women, urethral tissues are affected by the estrogen changes associated with menopause and become less robust with aging, making the external sphincter less competent. Upper motor neuron and lower motor neuron disease affects bladder function. Stroke, cord injury, and multiple sclerosis can cause loss of inhibition of reflexes and can lead to spasticity; diabetic neuropathy can cause a flaccid bladder (Finucane and Wright, 2003).

An older person is more vulnerable to incontinence than a younger person, but it is difficult when assessing causality to separate normal age-related changes from changes resulting from disease.

Social and Psychological Changes

Psychologically, an older person who is incontinent may experience isolation, a loss of self-esteem, and even depression as he or she withdraws from social settings and becomes more reliant on caregivers to maintain continence and hygiene. Socially, incontinence is likely to lead to the older person's restriction of social engagements to avoid the embarrassment associated with UI. Incontinence is also burdensome because of the expense of incontinence supplies and the management of laundry and other cleaning costs.

Providing care for an incontinent older person can be both physically and emotionally demanding. The amount of time needed to provide appropriate assistance to an older person with UI may be more than most people can easily manage. Going to the toilet is a 24-hour-a-day need. Many older people with UI need aid in transferring to a commode or in taking care of personal hygiene, and they require assistance throughout the day and night. Laundry and cleaning responsibilities are likely to fall to the caregiver. When the assistance needed by an incontinent older adult is more than the caregiver alone can provide, caregivers often must hire home health aides or similar staff to assist them in providing care. Caregivers often cite UI as one of the reasons for placing an older loved one in a nursing home. This problem is significant for older adults, and primary health care providers need to offer assistance in managing it.

INCONTINENCE

Incontinence is a clinical syndrome; therefore the guiding principle of treatment is a response to the patient's reported symptoms. The UI diagnostic categories do not fit all patients. The recent development of overactive bladder dysfunction as a new diagnosis of an ancient problem may be an indication of an appreciation of the complexity of the condition.

URGE INCONTINENCE

The major reported symptom of urge incontinence is the sudden irresistible urge to void accompanied by an inability to inhibit bladder contractions until a toilet is reached. Usually the patient will report a large amount of urine lost, but others may not experience the same type of urine loss but report a fear of potential loss. It is well to remember that it is quite common for normal healthy young women to experience, at times, involuntary loss of small amounts of urine (Finucane and Wright, 2003). Urge incontinence is the most common and accounts for more than two thirds of geriatric cases (Lyons et al, 2002). Urge incontinence can be worsened by infection, irritation by stone, or tumor.

Frequency, urgency, and nocturnal enuresis are symptoms associated with unstable contractions of the bladder (Malone-Lee, 2003). The term most commonly used to describe the contraction is *detrusor instability*. The multiplicity of terms to describe the bladder contractions that lead to urge incontinence can cause confusion for the PCP. Uninhibited, spastic, hyperactive, overactive, and unstable bladder are terms found frequently in the extant literature to describe the same contraction that leads to urge continence.

STRESS INCONTINENCE

Stress incontinence is characterized by leakage of urine that is associated with coughing, sneezing, and other physical activity. The leakage is related to reduced sphincter function, also described as *urethral incompetence* (Malone-Lee, 2003). The acquired urethral deficiency may be related to surgical damage, trauma, radiation therapy, or a sacral cord lesion. In women it is commonly associated with postmenopausal tissue changes and previous childbearing.

OVERFLOW INCONTINENCE

Overflow incontinence is the loss of small or large amounts of urine at times when the bladder is excessively full. In this condition the outflow of urine is disrupted related to low pressure in the bladder or high pressure in the urethra. High intraurethral pressure in men is associated with prostatic enlargement, but in women the most common cause is prior surgery. Low intravesical (bladder) pressure is most frequently caused by diabetic neuropathy (Finucane and Wright, 2003). In overflow incontinence the pressure in an overdistended bladder builds until it is sufficient to overcome the outflow resistance and allow the involuntary passage of urine.

OVERACTIVE BLADDER

Overactive bladder (OAB) dysfunction can be considered a result of poor functioning of neuromuscular control of the lower urinary tract. At times the cause of the OAB will be obscured and will be referred to as *idiopathic* OAB (Ahlberg et al, 2002). This disorder encompasses frequency, urgency, and urge incontinence, singly or in combination. Furthermore a significant negative impact on the quality of life occurs, and the affected person's activities become limited. The prevalence increases with age and is more common in women than men (Milsom et al, 2000). Chronic medical and psychiatric illness, multiple medications, cognitive impairment, and impairments of the lower urinary tract contribute to the diagnosis and management of OAB (Ouslander, 2002).

RECENT-ONSET INCONTINENCE

Recent-onset incontinence usually occurs in a previously continent person and may be reversible. The causative factors usually are associated with acute changes in cognition, limited mobility, undue stress on the bladder, or a temporary condition that causes temporary genitourinary dysfunction. Many times the older person first experiences incontinence while hospitalized (Palmer et al, 2002). The treatment is not to insert a catheter. Finding the causative condition and treating the underlying problem will resolve the incontinence.

Common contributing causes to recent-onset incontinence include delirium, infection, medications, fecal impaction, vaginitis, and emotional causes (Finucane and Wright, 2003; Palmer, 1996). UI is often cited as a side effect of several medications. Particular attention should be given to any newly prescribed medications. Medications that can cause urinary retention and overflow incontinence include anticholinergics, antidepressants, antipsychotics, alpha-adrenergic agonists, beta-adrenergic agonists, and calcium channel blockers. Diuretics cause polyuria, which can overwhelm the bladder of an older person. Bladder infections, which are common in older people, are often associated with incontinence.

An adequate amount of fluid must be consumed for the bladder to function correctly. Chronic fluid restriction results in the formation of concentrated urine, which irritates bladder tissue and does not provide adequate stimulus for normal bladder functioning. Older adults should drink at least six glasses of noncaffeinated liquid in a 24-hour period. Older people sometimes restrict fluids to control their incontinence, but this actually tends to increase UI and can lead to a UTI, in itself a common cause of UI.

URINARY TRACT INFECTIONS

In an older person, incontinence is often one of the first symptoms of a UTI, the prevalence of which increases with age. Residual urine provides a breeding ground for the development of infections. Restriction of fluids in an attempt to prevent urine loss leads to a decreased urine flow, and as a result the urinary tract is not washed out as frequently. Another cause of UTI in an older person is an indwelling catheter; indwelling catheters should be avoided or at least removed as soon as possible.

UTIs may manifest as urinary frequency with incontinence, urgency, and dysuria. Hematuria and fever may be present but often are not. Infections in older people are often atypical; any change in behavior from baseline, including lethargy, agitation, flu-like symptoms, and delirium, may result from a UTI and warrants evaluation. Pyuria revealed by urinalysis should be treated with a full course of an appropriate antibiotic; however, bacteriuria without symptoms is probably colonization and should not be treated, lest the risk of antibiotic resistance be increased. Patient education regarding taking the full course of the antibiotic and increasing fluid intake is important. Symptoms often subside shortly after the patient begins the medication, and an older person may try to save money by hoarding some of the pills for a future infection.

FUNCTIONAL INCONTINENCE

Functional incontinence is caused by factors outside the genitourinary system that result in an inability to reach the toilet before urine is lost. Functional problems that prevent normal toilet behaviors include environmental restraints, mobility restriction, cognitive difficulties, and psychiatric disorders. A person who is unable to get to a bathroom or commode in sufficient time will experience episodes of incontinence. Impaired mobility may result from arthritis, pain, clutter, side rails, or other mechanical or pharmacologic agents.

Primary Care Evaluation of Urinary Incontinence

The purpose of the initial evaluation is to confirm objectively the presence of UI, to identify the presumptive cause of the UI, to rule out potentially reversible conditions, and to distinguish between patients appropriate for initial behavioral intervention and patients suitable for referral. The International Consultation on Incontinence developed algorithms for the assessment and management of five major client groups, three of which are presented in Figures 22-2 through 22-4. The algorithm for women is presented in Figure 22-2, the algorithm for men in Figure 22-3, and the algorithm for frail, disabled older patients in Figure 22-4.

HISTORY

The history of UI begins with a focused medical history that includes an assessment of risk factors, a review of medications, and a detailed exploration of the patient's symptoms and understanding of all associated symptoms. Of course, if appropriate and with the patient's approval, caregiver input has the potential to add clarity to somewhat vague presentation of the condition. Many times frail older patients will have difficulty remembering all the significant facts associated with their UI.

History should include the following:

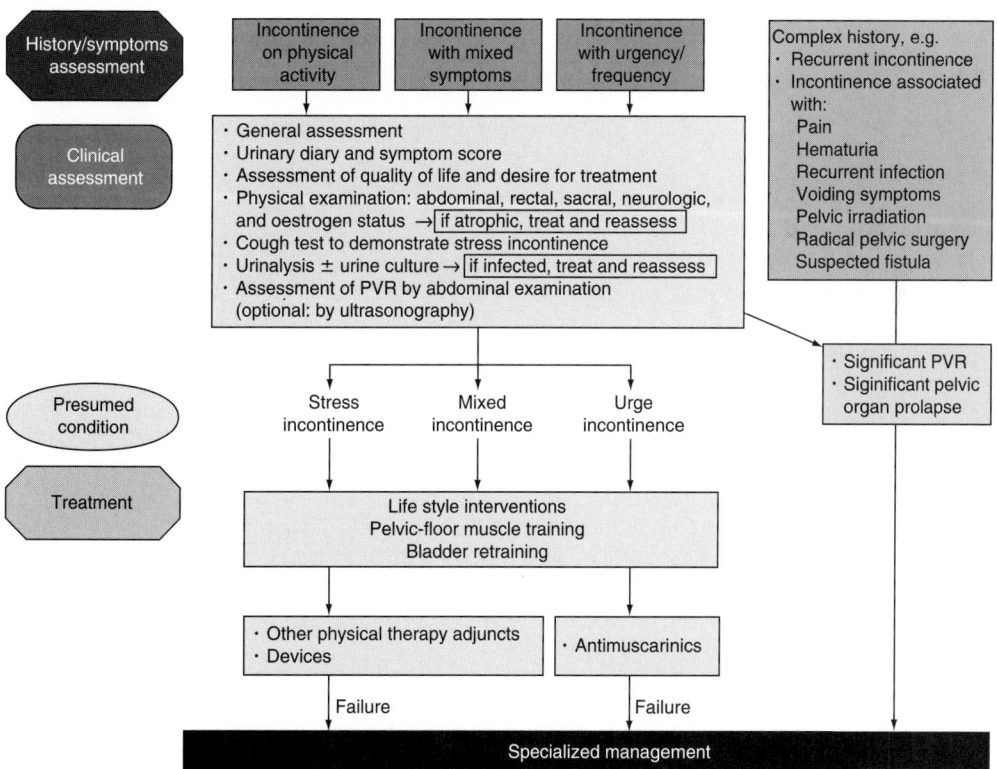

Figure 22-2 Initial management of urinary incontinence in women. (From Scientific Committee of the First International Consultation on Incontinence: Assessment and treatment of urinary incontinence, *Lancet* 355(9221):2153-2158, 2000.)

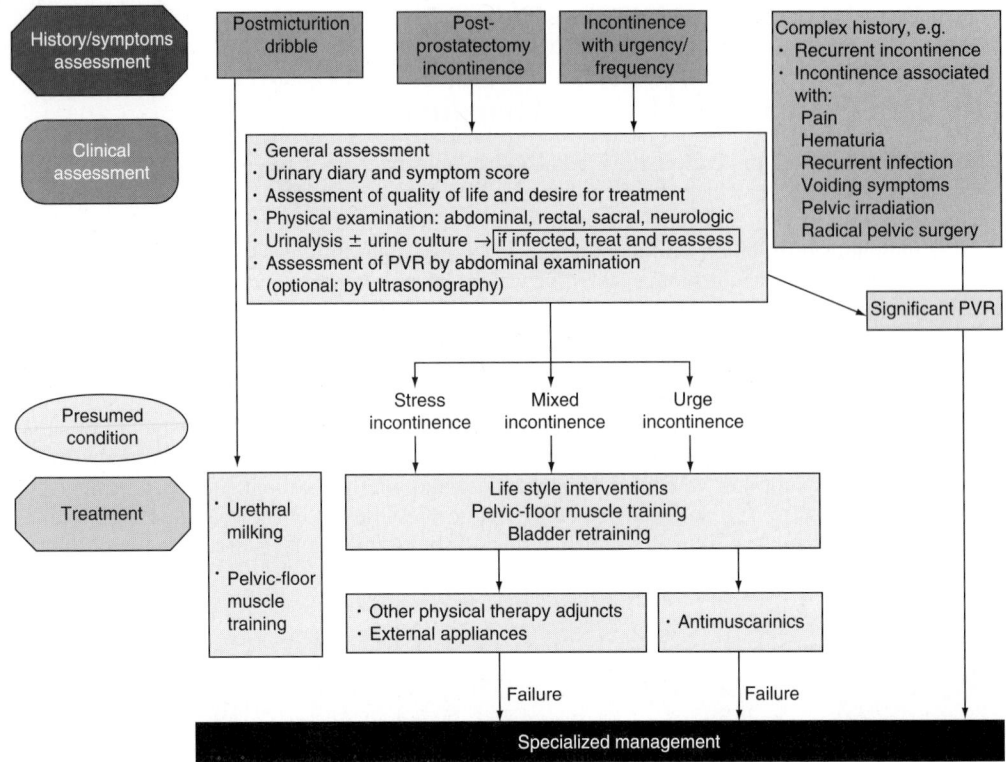

Figure 22-3 Initial management of urinary incontinence in men. (From Scientific Committee of the First International Consultation on Incontinence: Assessment and treatment of urinary incontinence, *Lancet* 355(9221):2153-2158, 2000.)

- Medical history
- Physical symptoms
  - First recognition of UI as a problem
  - Acute/chronic/recurrent
  - Daily pattern (bladder record Figure 22-5) with the following specific details:
    - Number of wetting episodes
    - Usual times of wetting episodes
    - Amounts of urine lost each time
    - Activities before and after wetting episodes
    - Presence of leakage
    - Amount and type of pads or protective devices
    - Precipitants of incontinence (e.g., situational antecedents such as coughing, laughing, or exercising; "on way to the bathroom")
    - Incontinence associated with (e.g., recurrent infection, nocturia, dysuria, hesitancy, enuresis, straining, poor or interrupted stream, pain)
    - Surgery, trauma or injury, radiation therapy, recent illness
    - Medications: prescriptions and over-the-counter (new and old)

When reviewing medications it is well to remember that certain medications can either cause or contribute to UI. Especially important is asking about the intake of antihistamine-decongestant cold remedies because many of these preparations can cause urinary retention. Also narcotics and calcium channel blockers may cause UI.

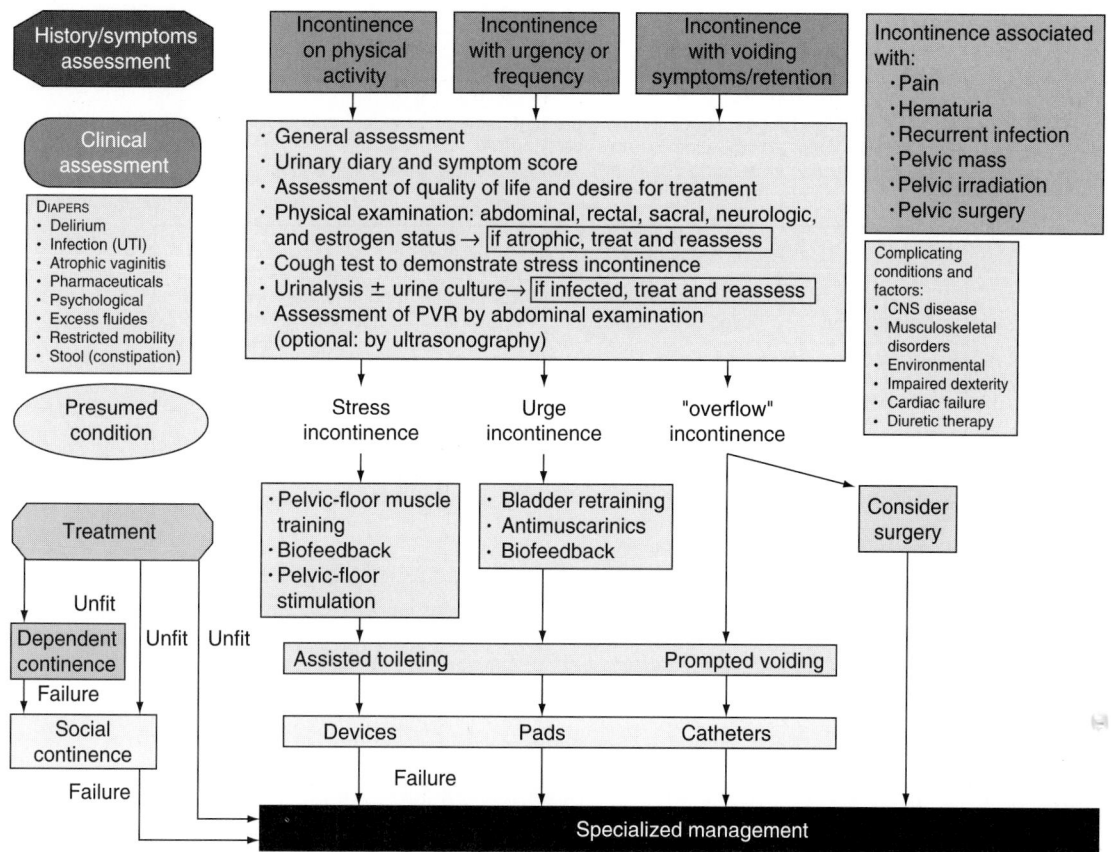

Figure 22-4 Initial management of urinary incontinence in frail, disabled older adults. (From Scientific Committee of the First International Consultation on Incontinence: Assessment and treatment of urinary incontinence, *Lancet* 355(9221):2153-2158, 2000.)

PSYCHOSOCIAL AND ENVIRONMENTAL FACTORS

- Home-environment toileting conditions
- Effects on family and social activities
- Presence of potential or actual caregiver
- Previous self-care treatments and effects on UI
- Previous treatments from formal health care providers and effects on UI
- Bowel habits
- Alteration in sexual function
- Expectation of treatment
- Motivation to self-toilet
- Depressive symptoms
- Cognitive ability

If possible, an environmental assessment should include a visit to the patient's living arrangement; if not, certain information would assist the PCP in developing appropriate treatments:

- Access (to include obstacles) and distance to toilets or commode
- Chair or bed that allows ease when rising
- Lighting in bathroom

NAME: _____

DATE: _____

INSTRUCTIONS: Place a check in the appropriate column next to the time you urinated in the toilet or when an incontinence episode occurred. Note the reason for the incontinence and describe your liquid intake (for example, coffee, water) and estimate the amount (for example, one cup).

Time interval	Urinated in toilet	Had a small incontinence episode	Had a large incontinence episode	Reason for incontinence episode	Type/amount of liquid intake
6–8 AM					
8–10 AM					
10–noon					
Noon–2 PM					
2–4 PM					
4–6 PM					
6–8 PM					
8–10 PM					
10–midnight					
Overnight					

No. of pads used today: _____ No. of episodes: _____

Comments: _____

Figure 22-5 Sample bladder record. (From Fantl JA et al: *Urinary incontinence in adults: acute and chronic management: clinical practice guideline 2, 1996 update.* AHCPR Pub 96-0682, Rockville, Md, 1996, US Department of Health and Human Services, Public Health Service, Agency for Health Care Policy and Research.)

change takes approximately 1 week. Relaxation techniques to divert attention from the older person's full bladder are helpful (Box 22-2). It should be emphasized that the bladder is a large muscle that can be trained to hold more urine in the same way that frequent voidings have resulted in a bladder that holds less urine.

A behavioral management study that combined pelvic-muscle exercise with feedback, self-monitoring, and bladder training as the treatment in a controlled study of older rural women found that after 2 years the treatment group had decreased UI severity by 61% and the controlled group (no treatment) had increased UI severity by 184% (Dougherty et al, 2002). When possible, behavioral intervention is usually the treatment of choice for uncomplicated UI.

Biofeedback/Toileting Program

The problem is usually related to cognitive impairment or mobility problems, and in both instances the older person requires assistance to maintain continence. Individualized scheduled toileting (IST) involves identifying the person's usual bladder patterns and developing a toilet schedule based on these patterns. An IST program provides reminders to toilet in a timely fashion. When appropriate, encouragement and praise should be given while the patient is toileting. An adequate amount of fluid must be taken on a regular basis to maintain bladder patterns. The key to a successful IST program is the consistency with which it is provided. Routine scheduled toileting (RST) is similar to an IST program, but it differs in that the schedule is not individualized to the person's usual bladder patterns. RST is often adopted in nursing homes where staffing and ward routines prevent individualization of toileting schedules. The success of these programs usually depends on the consistency of the caregiver.

CONTAINMENT STRATEGIES

Absorbent products should be used for chronic UI or in combination with other treatments to provide protection (Fantl et al, 1996). Most older people with UI already use these products, but the PCP should address the issue in a way that prevents undue embarrassment to the older person. The discussion should center on product differences in availability, ease of use, and cost.

When feasible, intermittent catheterization is the preferred alternative to indwelling catheters. Indwelling urethral catheters (IUCs) are recommended for containment in older adults whose UI results from obstruction or when other interventions are not feasible (Fantl et al, 1996). IUCs should be the treatment of last resort; all other approaches, including the use of absorbent products and toileting programs, should be considered before an IUC is used. It is inappropriate to use an IUC as a convenient way to contain the urine loss. IUC may be the appropriate treatment choice for a patient for whom changing absorbent padding is painful; such a patient's urinary output needs to be strictly measured.

Box 22-2

Relaxation Techniques

Divert attention away from bladder.
Use quick, rapid contractions of pelvic muscles.
Avoid strenuous activities.
Keep self busy with sedentary activities.
Take some deep breaths and concentrate on diversional music.
Avoid stimuli such as running water or putting hands in water.
Use absorbent padding in clothes to help relaxation.
Avoid any stimuli that increase bladder contraction.

PHARMACOLOGIC TREATMENT

Pharmacologic interventions for UI have been effective in some cases. Most of the focus of the pharmacologic interventions has been urge incontinence and OAB by treating detrusor instability, thereby preventing unstable bladder contractions (Hay-Smith et al, 2002; Malone-Lee, 2003). Antimuscarinic drugs that are effective in the treatment of urge incontinence are oxbutynin and tolterodine.

Oxybutynin (Ditropan) is thought to be most effective and is considered the first drug of choice for most patients with urge incontinence and overactive bladder. The efficacy of Ditropan has been improved by the new controlled-release preparation Ditropan XL (Appell, 2002; Malone-Lee, 2003). The most significant reason for drug withdrawal is reflux esophagitis, although the most common side effect is dry mouth.

Tolterodine (Detrusitol, Detrol) is a recently developed drug that is effective in the treatment of urge incontinence and OAB. The extended-release formulation of tolterodine increases efficacy by reducing the severity and frequency of dry mouth, the most common side effect. The once-daily dose increases the compliance of many patients. The most significant reason for drug withdrawal is blurred vision or headache (Crandall, 2001). Low doses at 2 mg are appropriate; 4 mg twice daily can cause urinary retention (Malone-Lee, 2003). It is important to remind the patient that the full therapeutic effect can take up to 8 weeks.

Imipramine (Tofranil), a tricyclic antidepressant, has also been used to treat urge UI. It is less effective than either oxbutynin or tolterodine, and side effects are similar but also may cause postural instability and drowsiness (Finucane and Wright, 2003; Malone-Lee, 2003).

Propantheline (Pro-Banthine) has been used in the past, and some providers may still prescribe this drug. Therapeutic levels are difficult to maintain, and efficacy is limited. There seems little reason or evidence to use this drug to treat incontinence.

Urogenitial atrophy, along with atrophic vaginitis, is a common disorder that affects many postmenopausal women. Oral or vaginal estrogen has been used as a pharmacologic treatment for stress incontinence. Current opinion regarding the risks inherent in the use of estrogen suggest caution before prescribing this intervention. In study of 1525 subjects, oral estrogen with progestin was associated with worsening urinary incontinence in older postmenopausal women (Grady et al, 2001).

One-month application of estrogen cream by the vaginal route has been effective for treating atrophic vaginitis. One half to one applicator of estrogen cream every night for 1 to 2 weeks is followed by application every other night for 1 to 2 weeks (Bachmann and Nevadunsky, 2000). A 1-month trial with all the precautions is a sufficient period to evaluate efficacy for treating the patient's symptoms of stress incontinence (Finucane and Wright, 2003). See Table 22-1 for a summary of pharmacologic drugs used to treat UI.

SURGICAL TREATMENTS

Surgical procedures for incontinence have had varied success, and many have been abandoned for lack of satisfaction. Measuring outcomes is hampered by a lack of standardization. Most older patients should have a significant trial of behavioral and medical therapy before any surgical referral is made. Before making the referral, the PCP together with the patient needs to consider the following:

- Impact of incontinence on the patient's quality of life
- Expected outcome of the surgery
- Patient's understanding of the risks
- Patient's understanding of the state of the art
- Physical health and stamina of the patient
- Local surgical expertise

The potential risks for older women contemplating surgery for treatment of incontinence include injury to the bladder, urethra, ureters, and the bowel. Changes in bowel and sexual functions could

TABLE 22-1	Drug Treatment for Urinary Incontinence

		Dose and Frequency			
	Drug Name	**Initial**	**Usual**	**Max**	**Comments**
Urge incontinence	Oxybutinin	2.5 mg b.i.d.	5 mg t.i.d.	5 mg q.i.d.	Dry mouth, constipation, other anticholinergic effects, glaucoma
	Tolterodine	1 mg q.i.d.	1 mg b.i.d.	2 mg b.i.d.	Less toxic, expensive
	Oxybutinin extended release	5 mg q.d.	10 mg q.d.	30 mg q.d.	Same as oxybutinin regular release
Alternative with limited efficacy data	Imipramine	10 mg h.s.	25 mg b.i.d.	25 mg t.i.d.	Anticholinergic effects, especially dry mouth
	Propantheline	7.5 mg q.d.	7.5 mg t.i.d.	15 mg q4h	Anticholinergic effects, especially constipation
Stress incontinence (limited data available)	Imipramine	10 mg h.s.	25 mg b.i.d.	25 mg t.i.d.	Anticholinergic effects, especially dry mouth

Adapted from Finucane T, Wright J: Urinary incontinence. In Barker et al, editors: *Principles of ambulatory medicine*, ed 6, Philadelphia, 2003, Lippincott Williams & Wilkins.
b.i.d., Twice daily; *t.i.d.*, three times daily; *qd*, each day; *h.s.*, at bedtime; *q4h*, every 4 hours.

be adversely affected by some procedures (Finucane and Wright, 2003). See Table 22-2 for current surgical procedures.

Summary

Urinary incontinence is not a normal consequence of aging and can be the cause of loss of self-esteem and loss of function and at times can threaten the physical health of the older adult. Knowledge of the genitourinary anatomy and physiology is necessary to understand the pathophysiology of the various types of incontinence. A patient history, including bladder records, and a physical examination will help the practitioner to determine which type of incontinence the patient is exhibiting, and therefore the treatment plan. Although much of the evaluation and intervention can be carried out in the primary care setting, referral to a urologist may be necessary to explore certain causes and modalities.

Resources

Bladder Health Foundation
c/o American Foundation for Urologic Disease
300 West Pratt Street, Suite 401
Baltimore, MD 21201
www.afud.org
(800) 242-2383

TABLE 22-2 Current Surgical Procedures Used to Treat Urinary Incontinence

Procedure	Indication	Hospitalization	"Cure" rate (%)	Special complications	Comment
Retropubic colposuspension	Stress in women	2-4 days	up to 85 at 10 yr	Voiding dysfunction 20%, usually transient (3 wk to 3 mo)	Restricted activity of 4-8 wk is typical
Laparoscopic colposuspension	Stress in women	1-2 days	30-80	Same as above but less	
Pubovaginal or suburethral slings (includes tension-free vaginal type)	Stress in women	1-2 days	80-85 at 3-7 yr 60-70 if preoperative symptoms included urgency	Retention up to 7%; frequency/urgency 10%-12%	
Urethral bulking agents: collagen	Stress in women and men	Outpatient	50-60 after an average of two injections improve but only 15-30 are cured	Transient (1-3 days) retention; embolization and material migration in men, minimal in women; must be tested for allergy to collagen used	Typically requires two or more injections at 4-6 wk; typically used when more invasive surgery cannot be done; treatment usually lasts 2-4 yr and can be repeated
Artificial urinary sphincter	Stress in women		Limited use	Infection, erosion, mechanical failure	Occasionally used in women with difficult-to-manage recurrent incontinence and a rigid (pipestem) urethra
Artificial urinary sphincter	Stress in men	1 day	90-95	Infection, malfunction, erosion of cuff in 2%-7%	Uses a Silastic reservoir, cuff and in-line pump; patient mechanically pumps fluid from cuff to reservoir to void so requires dexterity and adequate recognition

				of the need to void; often used if incontinence has resulted from prostate surgery
Sacral neuromodulation	Urge	Outpatient local anesthesia for temporary or permanent placement is required	About 80% of patients achieve 50% or greater reduction in incontinent episodes	Low-level pulsed electrical stimulation to appropriate sacral nerves; requires at first an external stimulator for 2-7 days of adjustment; this temporarily stimulator is replaced permanently if effective; permanent implantation requires surgical implantation and the battery lasts 5-7 yr
Bladder augmentation	Urge		Improves urge incontinence in about 70%	Goal is to increase bladder capacity and weaken contractions; a patch of intestine is added to bladder or a mucosal diverticular is created; up to 75% of patients require subsequent intermittent catheterization

From Finucane T, Wright J: Urinary incontinence. In Barker et al, editors: *Principles of ambulatory medicine*, ed 6, Philadelphia, 2003, Lippincott Williams & Wilkins.

References

Abdelghany S et al: Biofeedback and electrical stimulation therapy for treating urinary incontinence and voiding dysfunction: one center's experience, *J Urol Nurs* 21(6):401-405, 410, 2001.

Ahlberg J et al: Neurological signs are common in patients with urodynamically verified "idiopathic" bladder overactivity, *Neurourol Urodyn* 21(1):65-70, 2002.

Appell RA: The newer antimuscarinic drugs: bladder control with less dry mouth, *Cleve Clin J Med* 69(10):765-766, 768-769, 2002.

Bachmann GA, Nevadunsky NS: Diagnosis and treatment of atrophic vaginitis, *Am Fam Physician* 61:3090, 2000.

Crandall C: Tolterodine: a clinical review, *J Womens Health Gender Based Med* 10(8):735-743, 2001.

Dattilo J: A long-term study of patient outcomes with pelvic muscle re-education for urinary incontinence, *J Wound Ostomy Continence Nurs* 28(4):199-205, 2001.

Dougherty MC et al: A randomized trial of behavioral management for continence with older rural women, *Res Nurs Health* 25(1):3-13, 2002.

Fantl JA et al: *Urinary incontinence in adults: acute and chronic management: clinical practice guideline 2, 1996 update.* AHCPR Pub 96-0682, Rockville, Md, 1996, US Department of Health and Human Services, Public Health Service, Agency for Health Care Policy and Research.

Finucane T, Wright J: Urinary incontinence. In Barker L et al, editors. *Principles of ambulatory medicine*, ed 6, Philadelphia, 2003, Lippincott Williams & Wilkins.

Grady D et al: Postmenopausal hormones and incontinence: the Heart and Estrogen/Progestin Replacement Study, *Obstet Gynecol* 97(1):116-120, 2001.

Hay-Smith J et al: Anticholinergic drugs versus placebo for overactive bladder syndrome in adults, *Cochrane Database Syst Rev* 3:CD003781, 2002.

Lyons WL et al: Geriatric medicine. In Tierney LM et al, editors: *Current medical diagnosis and treatment: adult ambulatory and inpatient management*, New York, 2002, Lange Medical Books/McGraw-Hill.

Malone-Lee J: Urinary incontinence. In Tallis RC, Fillit H, editors: *Brocklehurst's textbook of geriatric medicine and gerontolgy*, ed 6, London, 2003, Churchill Livingstone.

Milsom I et al: The prevalence of overactive bladder, *Am J Manag Care* 6(11 suppl):S565-S573, 2000.

Ouslander JG: Geriatric consideration in the diagnosis and management of overactive bladder, *Urology* 60 (5 suppl 1):50-55, 2002.

Palmer M et al: Risk factors for hospital-acquired incontinence in elderly female hip fracture patients, *J Gerontol Biol Sci Med Sci* 57(10):M672-M677, 2002.

Porro D et al: Impact of early pelvic floor rehabilitation after transurethral resection of the prostate, *Neurourol Urodyn* 20(1):53-59, 2001.

Scientific Committee of the First International consultation on Incontinence: assessment and treatment of urinary incontinence, *Lancet* 355(9221):2153-2158, 2000.

Vapnek JM: Urinary incontinence: screening and treatment of urinary incontinence, *Geriatric* 56(10):25-29, 2001.

23

Neurologic: Parkinson's Disease

Parkinson's disease (PD) is a progressive neurodegenerative disorder that most often affects people older than 65 years of age. About 200 per 100,000 persons in the United States older than 70 years of age will develop PD (Miller, 2002). Onset of symptoms usually occurs between the ages of 60 and 69, although in 5% of patients the first signs are seen before 40 years of age. The disease occurs throughout the world, in all ethnic groups, and affects both genders equally, with only a slight predominance in men.

PD is costly in terms of medications and care. Antiparkinsonian medications alone cost $5,000 per year (Feinberg, 1998). This cost increases dramatically for patients who experience motor complications with progressive disease. In addition, the indirect costs of care are high in the loss of productivity for both the patient and the caregiver.

Pathophysiology

PD was first described in 1818 by James Parkinson, a British physician who published a paper on what he called "the shaking palsy." PD results from the degeneration of neurons involved in motor control. The nature and severity of symptoms and the pattern of symptom progression vary greatly from one individual to another.

The exact cause of PD is unknown; however, a combination of factors is thought to be responsible, including environmental factors, free radicals, aging, and genetic susceptibility (Scott, 2002). The degeneration of dopaminergic neurons may be caused by encephalitis, carbon-monoxide poisoning, cerebrovascular accident, or metabolic and degenerative disorders. A rural environment is thought to be associated with an elevated risk of PD, with the factors of herbicide, pesticide, and well-water exposure as possible causes (Miller, 2002).

Genetic factors are being closely studied (Kruger et al, 2002). Some evidence supports an autosomal dominant inheritance of PD, and a major breakthrough in this field occurred with the identification of two distinct gene mutations. Other studies have failed to detect mutations, suggesting that they only rarely cause PD (Miller, 2002). The discovery of the [alpha]-synuclein *(PARK1)* and parkin *(PARK2)* genes have shown that genetic mutations can lead to the development of phenotypes of PD. It is not yet clear whether the known gene mutations contribute most of the genetic risk of developing PD or whether new genes remain to be found (Foltynie et al, 2002).

Some studies implicate iron in the pathophysiology of PD. Iron levels have been found to be elevated in the brains of patients with PD, and the levels of iron-binding proteins are abnormal. Iron

493

has been suspected to contribute to PD because Fe(II) is known to promote oxidative damage. Recent studies suggest that an additional mechanism by which iron might contribute to PD is by inducing aggregation of alpha-synuclein, which is a protein that accumulates in Lewy bodies in PD (Wolozin and Golts, 2002).

The brain cell degeneration in PD occurs primarily in the midbrain region called the *substantia nigra*. Normally, the brain cells of the substantia nigra communicate to another region of the brain, the striatum, and through the neurotransmitter dopamine. In PD, nigral cell loss results in declining levels of striatal dopamine (Miller, 2002). An 80% to 90% loss of dopamine-producing cells has occurred by the time the patient becomes symptomatic. The result is an excessive inhibitory output from the basal ganglia to the thalamus. This change leads to decreased stimulation from the thalamus to the motor cortex, resulting in the characteristic bradykinesia of the disease (Feinberg, 1998). Imbalance between the levels of dopamine and acetylcholine, together with the loss of the dopamine receptor sites, affects the refinement of voluntary movement and causes the primary symptoms of PD: bradykinesia, resting tremor, and postural instability. The seven cardinal features of PD are tremor at rest, rigidity, bradykinesia, hypokinesia, flexed posture, loss of postural reflexes, and the freezing phenomenon.

Up to 30% of people diagnosed with PD will present with dementia, particularly in the later stages of the disease. People with the disease are less able to cope with mixed messages of sarcasm or double meanings; they have difficulty in "doing two things at once"; for example, talking and walking at the same time will create difficulties. Thinking processes are slower, and rapid thought-shifting is problematic (Scott, 2002).

Secondary PD may be caused by several medications, such as antipsychotic medications, antiemetic medications, antihypertensives, antianginals, antineoplastics, and antiepileptics (Table 23-1). Drugs and toxins such as 1-methyl-4-phenyl-1,2,3,6 tetrahydropyridine (MPTP), carbon monoxide, manganese, and alcohol withdrawal can also cause parkinsonian symptoms. Another cause of parkinsonian symptoms is multiinfarcts to the substantia nigra. In this case symptoms are usually unresponsive to Parkinson's medication. Other possible causes of secondary parkinsonism to consider are parathyroid abnormalities, hypothyroidism, hepatocerebral degeneration, brain tumors, and normal-pressure hydrocephalus. Depression often accompanies PD (Zesiewicz and Hauser, 2002) and can mimic or enhance its symptoms. Parkinson-plus syndromes are similar to PD but have additional neurologic abnormalities. Examples are progressive supranuclear palsy, Shy-Drager syndrome, and olivopontocerebellar palsy. Discussion of these diseases is beyond the scope of this chapter, but Table 23-2 summarizes symptoms associated with each condition.

TABLE 23-1	Drugs That May Cause Parkinsonian Symptoms

Drug Category	*Specific Drug*
Antipsychotics	Haloperidol (Haldol), thioridazine (Mellaril), risperidone (Risperdal), chlorpromazine (Thorazine), lithium (Lithobid)
Antiemetics	Prochlorperazine (Compazine), metoclopramide (Reglan)
Antihypertensives	Methyldopa (Aldomet), verapamil (Calan), captopril (Capoten), reserpine
Antianginals	Diltiazem (Cardizem)
Antineoplastics	Cytarabine (Cytosar), vincristine (Oncovin)
Antiepileptics	Valproate (Depakote), phenytoin (Dilantin)

Modified from Kollar W, Montgomery E: Issues in the early diagnosis of Parkinson's disease, *Neurology* 49(suppl 1): 10-25, 1997; and Moreau D: *Nursing 96 drug handbook*, Springhouse, PA, 1996, Springhouse.

TABLE 23-2	Distinguishing Features

Neurologic Disorder	Distinguishing Features
Essential tremor	Kinetic tremor plus instability
	Frequent family history
Drug-induced parkinsonism	Antidopaminergic exposure
	Bilateral onset
	Reversibility
Progressive supranuclear palsy	Voluntary vertical gaze palsy
	Axial rigidity
	No tremor
Multiple system atrophy	Prominent dysautonomia (Shy-Drager syndrome)
	Cerebellar dysfunction (usually hereditable cerebellar atrophy) or peripheral neuropathy with brainstem/cerebellar atrophy
Striatal nigral degeneration	Akinetic-rigid
	No tremor
	Minimal or no benefit from levodopa
Alzheimer's disease with parkinsonism	Dementia more prominent than parkinsonism
	Dementia and parkinsonism probably related to the same pathologic process
Cortical basal ganglionic degeneration	Alien limb
	Dystonia
	Myoclonus
	Supranuclear gaze palsy
	Parietal sensory loss
	Asymmetric
Huntington's disease	Younger patient
	Positive family history
	No tremor
	Positively distinguished by DNA triplet code (CAG) repeat length
Toxin-induced parkinsonism	Exposure to carbon monoxide, manganese, cyanide, carbon disulfide, 1-methyl-4-phenyl-1,2,3,6 tetrahydropyridine (MPTP), n-hexane, methanol, or lacquer thinner

From Uitti RJ: Tremor: how to determine if the patient has Parkinson's disease, *Geriatrics* 53(5):34, 1998.

Clinical Examination

HISTORY

For many, onset of the disease is insidious, which delays treatment. In early stages of the disease, the most common complaint is tremor. The PD tremor is most commonly a pill-rolling motion of the forefinger and thumb at rest, but tremor can also be seen in the head and feet.

The patient may also complain of changes in handwriting, trouble with speech volume, stiffness, unusual fatigue, slowness of movement, difficulty in walking, falling, and difficulty in rising to a standing position or turning in bed. Symptoms increase over time as the disease progresses. A patient in stage 3 or 4 of the Unified Parkinson's Disease Rating Scale (UPDRS) is considered a late

PD patient (Askenasy, 2001). Those with severe disease may become bedridden and require complete assistance with activities of daily living (Box 23-1).

PHYSICAL EXAMINATION

Neurologic examination includes looking for evidence of the primary symptoms of PD: bradykinesia, resting tremor, and postural instability. In early disease, patients exhibit bradykinesia (slowness of movement). They have masked facies, decreased blink rate, a monotonous tone, and low-volume speech. Frequent postural adjustments are not made; they seem to sit absolutely still. Muscular rigidity or cogwheeling can be found in all extremities and the neck. Testing for muscle tone can be followed by testing for cogwheeling: one hand is placed on the elbow or knee and the limb is moved; a cogwheeling or ratcheting of the limb is felt. Table 23-3 describes a diagnostic evaluation for PD.

Tremor

Resting tremor may be noted in the hands, feet, or head. During movement the tremor diminishes. For example, during finger-to-nose testing, the tremor in the hand diminishes. This tremor is distinguished from an essential tremor because it diminishes with movement of the affected limb. Tremor can also be temporarily aggravated during stress (such as an argument) or with fatigue. Micrographia is present; handwriting is small and cramped. It may also be affected by tremor. Samples of handwriting in the chart are useful to monitor the progress of the disease or the effectiveness of medication.

Differentiation of tremors is an important aspect of securing a differential diagnosis because one of the common errors in clinical practice is to diagnose PD on the basis of tremor alone. Frequently an essential tremor with a family history is mistaken for a resting tremor of PD (Table 23-4).

Tremor is defined as a rhythmic oscillation of a body part. The two most frequently encountered tremors in primary care are essential tremor and the tremor associated with PD. The characteristic tremor of PD is tremor at rest with pill rolling. A tremor maximally activated during maintenance of a posture is characteristic of essential tremor, and a tremor maximally activated during movement, a kinetic or intention tremor, is generally synonymous with cerebellar disease (i.e., secondary to trauma, tumor, multiple sclerosis, or stroke) (Reich, 1998).

Postural Instability

Postural instability is easily examined by first watching the patient move from the waiting room. Patients have difficulty rising from a chair without pushing themselves up. Gait is difficult to initiate, slow and shuffling, with decreased arm swing. Posture is flexed, with a stooped trunk and arms semiflexed (Figure 23-1).

Turning is accomplished en bloc with small steppage in a circle (marche à petits pas). *Propulsion* (an inability to stop forward movement) or *retropulsion* (an inability to stop backward movement) is present. Freezing of movement occurs as the disease advances. When negotiating a curb or a doorjamb or turning in a tight circle, patients are unable to lift their feet to walk. Freezing can be interrupted by initiating movement other than walking, such as touching another's arm, or taking a large step or marching step. One patient in the study had severe freezing, walked with the aid of a walker, and was able to walk by only kicking a small cigar box while walking. If the box was taken away, the patient was unable to walk.

Psychosis

Psychosis is seen in PD as an apparent complication of treatment; however it is also present in some patients on either no or very low doses of medication, the latter being suggestive of dementia with Lewy bodies (Tintner and Jankovic, 2002). It is thought that the psychosis is due to stimulation of dopamine receptors. Treatment in the past has used conventional antipsychotics, which typically block D2 dopamine receptors and tend to worsen primary PD features. Atypical antipsychotics have

Box 23-1

Unified Parkinson's Disease Rating Scale

I. MENTATION, BEHAVIOR AND MOOD

1. Intellectual Impairment

0 = None.
1 = Mild. Consistent forgetfulness with partial recollection of events and no other difficulties.
2 = Moderate memory loss, with disorientation and moderate difficulty handling complex problems. Mild but definite impairment of function at home with need of occasional prompting.
3 = Severe memory loss with disorientation for time and often to place. Severe impairment in handling problems.
4 = Severe memory loss with orientation preserved to person only. Unable to make judgements or solve problems. Requires much help with personal care. Cannot be left alone at all.

2. Thought Disorder (Due to dementia or drug intoxication)

0 = None.
1 = Vivid dreaming.
2 = "Benign" hallucinations with insight retained.
3 = Occasional to frequent hallucinations or delusions; without insight; could interfere with daily activities.
4 = Persistent hallucinations, delusions, or florrid psychosis. Not able to care for self.

3. Depression

1 = Periods of sadness or guilt greater than normal, never sustained for days or weeks.
2 = Sustained depression (1 week or more).
3 = Sustained depression with vegetative symptoms (insomnia, anorexia, weight loss, loss of interest).
4 = Sustained depression with vegetative symptoms and suicidal thoughts or intent.

4. Motivation/Initiative

0 = Normal.
1 = Less assertive than usual; more passive.
2 = Loss of initiative or disinterest in elective (nonroutine) activities.
3 = Loss of initiative or disinterest in day to day (routine) activities.
4 = Withdrawn, complete loss of motivation.

II. ACTIVITIES OF DAILY LIVING (for both "on" and "off")

5. Speech

0 = Normal.
1 = Mildly affected. No difficulty being understood.
2 = Moderately affected. Sometimes asked to repeat statements.
3 = Severely affected. Frequently asked to repeat statements.
4 = Unintelligible most of the time.

6. Salivation

0 = Normal.
1 = Slight but definite excess of saliva in mouth; may have nighttime drooling.
2 = Moderately excessive saliva; may have minimal drooling.
3 = Marked excess of saliva with some drooling.
4 = Marked drooling, requires constant tissue or handkerchief.

Continued

Box 23-1

Unified Parkinson's Disease Rating Scale—cont'd

7. Swallowing

0 = Normal.
1 = Rare choking.
2 = Occasional choking.
3 = Requires soft food.
4 = Requires NG tube or gastrotomy feeding.

8. Handwriting

0 = Normal.
1 = Slightly slow or small.
2 = Moderately slow or small; all words are legible.
3 = Severely affected; not all words are legible.
4 = The majority of words are not legible.

9. Cutting food and handling utensils

0 = Normal.
1 = Somewhat slow and clumsy, but no help needed.
2 = Can cut most foods, although clumsy and slow; some help needed.
3 = Food must be cut by someone, but can still feed slowly.
4 = Needs to be fed.

10. Dressing

0 = Normal.
1 = Somewhat slow, but no help needed.
2 = Occasional assistance with buttoning, getting arms in sleeves.
3 = Considerable help required, but can do some things alone.
4 = Helpless.

11. Hygiene

0 = Normal.
1 = Somewhat slow, but no help needed.
2 = Needs help to shower or bathe; or very slow in hygienic care.
3 = Requires assistance for washing, brushing teeth, combing hair, going to bathroom.
4 = Foley catheter or other mechanical aids.

12. Turning in bed and adjusting bed clothes

0 = Normal.
1 = Somewhat slow and clumsy, but no help needed.
2 = Can turn alone or adjust sheets, but with great difficulty.
3 = Can initiate, but not turn or adjust sheets alone.
4 = Helpless.

13. Falling (unrelated to freezing)

0 = None.
1 = Rare falling.
2 = Occasionally falls, less than once per day.
3 = Falls an average of once daily.
4 = Falls more than once daily.

Continued

Box 23-1

Unified Parkinson's Disease Rating Scale—cont'd

14. Freezing when walking

0 = None.
1 = Rare freezing when walking; may have start hesitation.
2 = Occasional freezing when walking.
3 = Frequent freezing. Occasionally falls from freezing.
4 = Frequent falls from freezing.

15. Walking

0 = Normal.
1 = Mild difficulty. May not swing arms or may tend to drag leg.
2 = Moderate difficulty, but requires little or no assistance.
3 = Severe disturbance of walking, requiring assistance.
4 = Cannot walk at all, even with assistance.

16. Tremor (Symptomatic complaint of tremor in any part of body.)

0 = Absent.
1 = Slight and infrequently present.
2 = Moderate; bothersome to patient.
3 = Severe; interferes with many activities.
4 = Marked; interferes with most activities.

17. Sensory complaints related to parkinsonism

0 = None.
1 = Occasionally has numbness, tingling, or mild aching.
2 = Frequently has numbness, tingling, or aching; not distressing.
3 = Frequent painful sensations.
4 = Excruciating pain.

III. MOTOR EXAMINATION

18. Speech

0 = Normal.
1 = Slight loss of expression, diction and/or volume.
2 = Monotone, slurred but understandable; moderately impaired.
3 = Marked impairment, difficult to understand.
4 = Unintelligible.

19. Facial Expression

0 = Normal.
1 = Minimal hypomimia, could be normal "Poker Face".
2 = Slight but definitely abnormal diminution of facial expression
3 = Moderate hypomimia; lips parted some of the time.
4 = Masked or fixed facies with severe or complete loss of facial expression; lips parted 1/4 inch or more.

20. Tremor at rest (head, upper and lower extremities)

0 = Absent.
1 = Slight and infrequently present.
2 = Mild in amplitude and persistent. Or moderate in amplitude, but only intermittently present.
3 = Moderate in amplitude and present most of the time.
4 = Marked in amplitude and present most of the time.

Continued

Box 23-1

Unified Parkinson's Disease Rating Scale—cont'd

21. Action or Postural Tremor of hands

0 = Absent.
1 = Slight; present with action.
2 = Moderate in amplitude, present with action.
3 = Moderate in amplitude with posture holding as well as action.
4 = Marked in amplitude; interferes with feeding.

22. Rigidity (Judged on passive movement of major joints with patient relaxed in sitting position. Cogwheeling to be ignored.)

0 = Absent.
1 = Slight or detectable only when activated by mirror or other movements.
2 = Mild to moderate.
3 = Marked, but full range of motion easily achieved.
4 = Severe, range of motion achieved with difficulty.

23. Finger Taps (Patient taps thumb with index finger in rapid succession.)

0 = Normal.
1 = Mild slowing and/or reduction in amplitude.
2 = Moderately impaired. Definite and early fatiguing. May have occasional arrests in movement.
3 = Severely impaired. Frequent hesitation in initiating movements or arrests in ongoing movement.
4 = Can barely perform the task.

24. Hand Movements (Patient opens and closes hands in rapid succesion.)

0 = Normal.
1 = Mild slowing and/or reduction in amplitude.
2 = Moderately impaired. Definite and early fatiguing. May have occasional arrests in movement.
3 = Severely impaired. Frequent hesitation in initiating movements or arrests in ongoing movement.
4 = Can barely perform the task.

25. Rapid Alternating Movements of Hands (Pronation-supination movements of hands, vertically and horizontally, with as large an amplitude as possible, both hands simultaneously.)

0 = Normal.
1 = Mild slowing and/or reduction in amplitude.
2 = Moderately impaired. Definite and early fatiguing. May have occasional arrests in movement.
3 = Severely impaired. Frequent hesitation in initiating movements or arrests in ongoing movement.
4 = Can barely perform the task.

26. Leg Agility (Patient taps heel on the ground in rapid succession picking up entire leg. Amplitude should be at least 3 inches.)

0 = Normal.
1 = Mild slowing and/or reduction in amplitude.
2 = Moderately impaired. Definite and early fatiguing. May have occasional arrests in movement.
3 = Severely impaired. Frequent hesitation in initiating movements or arrests in ongoing movement.
4 = Can barely perform the task.

Continued

Box 23-1

Unified Parkinson's Disease Rating Scale—cont'd

27. Arising from Chair *(Patient attempts to rise from a straightbacked chair, with arms folded across chest.)*

0 = Normal.
1 = Slow; or may need more than one attempt.
2 = Pushes self up from arms of seat.
3 = Tends to fall back and may have to try more than one time, but can get up without help.
4 = Unable to arise without help.

28. Posture

0 = Normal erect.
1 = Not quite erect, slightly stooped posture; could be normal for older person.
2 = Moderately stooped posture, definitely abnormal; can be slightly leaning to one side.
3 = Severely stooped posture with kyphosis; can be moderately leaning to one side.
4 = Marked flexion with extreme abnormality of posture.

29. Gait

0 = Normal.
1 = Walks slowly, may shuffle with short steps, but no festination (hastening steps) or propulsion.
2 = Walks with difficulty, but requires little or no assistance; may have some festination, short steps, or propulsion.
3 = Severe disturbance of gait, requiring assistance.
4 = Cannot walk at all, even with assistance.

30. Postural Stability *(Response to sudden, strong posterior displacement produced by pull on shoulders while patient erect with eyes open and feet slightly apart. Patient is prepared.)*

0 = Normal.
1 = Retropulsion, but recovers unaided.
2 = Absence of postural response; would fall if not caught by examiner.
3 = Very unstable, tends to lose balance spontaneously.
4 = Unable to stand without assistance.

31. Body Bradykinesia and Hypokinesia *(Combining slowness, hesitancy, decreased armswing, small amplitude, and poverty of movement in general.)*

0 = None.
1 = Minimal slowness, giving movement a deliberate character; could be normal for some persons. Possibly reduced amplitude.
2 = Mild degree of slowness and poverty of movement which is definitely abnormal. Alternatively, some reduced amplitude.
3 = Moderate slowness, poverty or small amplitude of movement.
4 = Marked slowness, poverty or small amplitude of movement.

IV. COMPLICATIONS OF THERAPY (In the past week)

A. DYSKINESIAS

32. Duration: What proportion of the waking day are dyskinesias present? *(Historical information.)*

0 = None
1 = 1-25% of day.
2 = 26-50% of day.
3 = 51-75% of day.
4 = 76-100% of day.

Continued

Box 23-1

Unified Parkinson's Disease Rating Scale—cont'd

33. Disability: How disabling are the dyskinesias? (Historical information; may be modified by office examination.)

0 = Not disabling.
1 = Mildly disabling.
2 = Moderately disabling.
3 = Severely disabling.
4 = Completely disabled.

34. Painful Dyskinesias: How painful are the dyskinesias?

0 = No painful dyskinesias.
1 = Slight.
2 = Moderate.
3 = Severe.
4 = Marked.

35. Presence of Early Morning Dystonia (Historical information.)

0 = No
1 = Yes

B. CLINICAL FLUCTUATIONS

36. Are "off" periods predictable?

0 = No
1 = Yes

37. Are "off" periods unpredictable?

0 = No
1 = Yes

38. Do "off" periods come on suddenly, within a few seconds?

0 = No
1 = Yes

39. What proportion of the waking day is the patient "off" on average?

0 = None
1 = 1-25% of day.
2 = 26-50% of day.
3 = 51-75% of day.
4 = 76-100% of day.

C. OTHER COMPLICATIONS

40. Does the patient have anorexia, nausea, or vomiting?

0 = No
1 = Yes

41. Any sleep disturbances, such as insomnia or hypersomnolence?

0 = No
1 = Yes

Continued

Box 23-1

Unified Parkinson's Disease Rating Scale—cont'd

42. Does the patient have symptomatic orthostasis? (Record the patient's blood pressure, height and weight on the scoring form)

0 = No
1 = Yes

V. MODIFIED HOEHN AND YAHR STAGING

STAGE 0 = No signs of disease.
STAGE 1 = Unilateral disease.
STAGE 1.5 = Unilateral plus axial involvement.
STAGE 2 = Bilateral disease, without impairment of balance.
STAGE 2.5 = Mild bilateral disease, with recovery on pull test.
STAGE 3 = Mild to moderate bilateral disease; some postural instability; physically independent.
STAGE 4 = Severe disability; still able to walk or stand unassisted.
STAGE 5 = Wheelchair bound or bedridden unless aided.

VI. SCHWAB AND ENGLAND ACTIVITIES OF DAILY LIVING SCALE

100% = Completely independent. Able to do all chores without slowness, difficulty or impairment. Essentially normal. Unaware of any difficulty.
90% = Completely independent. Able to do all chores with some degree of slowness, difficulty and impairment. Might take twice as long. Beginning to be aware of difficulty.
80% = Completely independent in most chores. Takes twice as long. Conscious of difficulty and slowness.
70% = Not completely independent. More difficulty with some chores. Three to four times as long in some. Must spend a large part of the day with chores.
60% = Some dependency. Can do most chores, but exceedingly slowly and with much effort. Errors; some impossible.
50% = More dependent. Help with half, slower, etc. Difficulty with everything.
40% = Very dependent. Can assist with all chores, but few alone.
30% = With effort, now and then does a few chores alone or begins alone. Much help needed.
20% = Nothing alone. Can be a slight help with some chores. Severe invalid.
10% = Totally dependent, helpless. Complete invalid.
0% = Vegetative functions such as swallowing, bladder and bowel functions are not functioning. Bedridden.

From Fahn S et al, editors: *Recent developments in Parkinson's disease*, vol 2, Florham Park, NJ, 1987, MacMillan Health Care Information.

the advantage of not worsening the Parkinson's motor symptoms. Clozapine is the best medication for this; however, the tendency (albeit low) to cause agranulocytosis makes its use problematic. Olanzapine can be effective without worsening motor features in patients with PD, and amoxapine carries a relatively low risk of parkinsonism but has been shown to cause deterioration in PD motor features when used as an antipsychotic (Tintner and Jankovic, 2002).

DIAGNOSTIC TESTING

For diagnostic testing, elimination of other causes of the patient's symptoms should be considered first. Computed tomography (CT) or magnetic resonance imaging of the brain can rule out vascular disease, tumor, hydrocephalus, and other structural abnormalities. Repeat scanning during the course of the disease is indicated only when there has been a marked change in the patient's

TABLE 23-3	Diagnosis Evaluation; Parkinson's Disease

History

- Explore onset and progression of signs and symptoms, with focus on tremor, rigidity, dyskinesia, postural instability, manifestations related to autonomic dysfunction, and mental status changes.
- Ask patient which symptoms are most bothersome.
- Determine patient's ability to perform physical activities of daily living (ADLs), such as bathing, dressing, toileting, and eating.
- Determine patient's ability to perform instrumental ADLs.
- Assess for depression.
- Carefully ask about medication history, focusing on neuroleptic, gastrointestinal, and antihypertensive medications.
- Inquire about occupational, recreational, and environmental history to uncover exposure to toxins, such as carbon monoxide, manganese, cyanide, licit and illicit drugs.
- Obtain complete past medical history, social history, and family history with a focus on any dementing illnesses or hereditary disorders.

Physical Examination

- Take time to complete history and physical, which require patience with a PD patient because of bradykinesia and bradyphrenia. Hurrying the patient will exacerbate symptoms.
- Observe for characteristic posture (simian) and gait (difficulty turning, absent arm swing, slow shuffling gait, tendency to ward propulsion or retropulsion).
- Observe for tremor, "pill-rolling" motion (also may affect jaw, tongue, and lips or may be absent).
- Take orthostatic blood pressure and pulse readings to assess for autonomic dysfunction.
- Perform mental status examination; cognitive impairment is common.
- Assess cranial nerves:
  —Sense of smell often lost or reduced
  —Blink reflex and facial expression diminished; faces may become mask-like
  —Extraocular movements normal except for impairment in upward gaze
- Test motor and extrapyramidal systems:
  —Passively move limbs, noting characteristic rigidity
  —Observe for hand and foot posturing, which is common; pill-rolling motion often noticeable
  —Ask if handwriting has become smaller (micrographia)
- Check reflexes, which usually are normal but may be slightly hyperactive or difficult to elicit because of tremors and rigidity. Postural reflex losses cause the body to fall forward or backward unless supported.
- Examine sensory system for common peripheral neuropathies.
- Examine skin for scaly, greasy lesions characteristic of seborrhea; check for excessive perspiration.

Plan/Management

- Consult with a neurologist when the PD diagnosis is made. The neurologist can help develop a treatment plan; the primary care provider, nurse, occupational therapist, physical therapist, and patient also are essential to the development of a holistic plan of care.
- Individualize treatment by basing it on several important factors with management implications:
  —Age, severity of disease or degree of functional impairment, existing or potential support systems, and expected benefits and risks of pharmacologic agents
  —Guiding principle of care: keep patient functioning independently as long as possible
  —Key to long-term success is to continue to control symptoms but limit complications of pharmacotherapy

Continued

TABLE 23-3	Diagnosis Evaluation; Parkinson's Disease—cont'd

- Ascertain benefits and risks of available pharmacologic agents:
  —Levodopa: Patients respond to this drug almost immediately, but almost all patients develop dyskinesia or motor fluctuations within 5 years of starting therapy.

From Miller JL: Parkinson's disease primer, *Geriatric Nursing* 23(2): 69-75, 2002.

TABLE 23-4	Parkinson's Disease Versus Essential Tremor

	Parkinson's Disease	*Essential Tremor*
History		
Age of onset	60, with limited variability	Variable, more common after 50
Duration of symptoms from prior presentation	Months-year	Years-decades
Family history	Generally negative	Generally positive (autosomal dominant)
Response to alcohol (small amount)	None	Improvement
Physical Examination		
Position of maximal activation	Rest	Maintenance of a posture
Frequency	3-6 Hz	6-12 Hz
Morphology	Pill rolling	Flexion and extension at shoulder, wrist
Anatomic	Unilateral	Bilateral, may be onset asymmetric
Body part affected	Upper limb > lower limb > chin = lips	Upper limbs > head > voice > chin = lips > lower limbs
Associated parkinsonian signs	Yes	No
Handwriting	Small, nontremulous	Normal size, tremulous
Natural history	Progressive	Insidiously progressive

Adapted from Reich SG: "Doctor, I shake." Presentation at Current Topics in Geriatrics, American Geriatric Society, Baltimore, 1998.

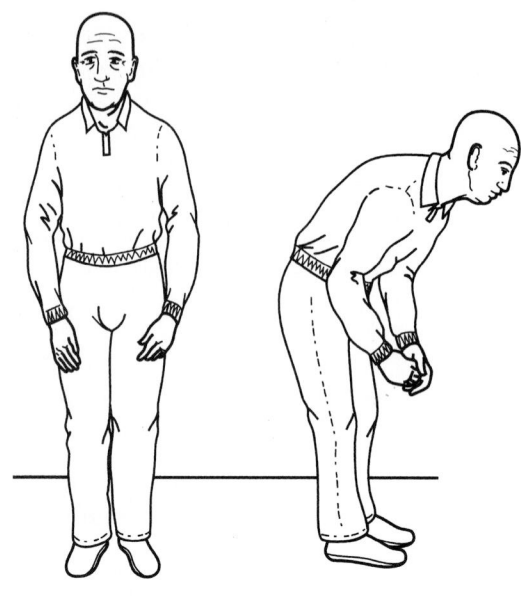

Anterior view   Lateral view

Figure 23-1 Parkinson's patient body posture.

condition; other causes should be considered. For instance, a person with PD who frequently falls may need to have a CT scan to rule out subdural hematoma. Complete blood count, chemistries, liver function testing, thyroid testing, and a drug screen should be obtained as necessary. Refer to Table 23-1 for drugs that can cause parkinsonian symptoms.

After the diagnosis of PD is made, no further diagnostic testing is necessary unless there is a major change in the patient's status. For instance, an increase in falling may be caused by orthostatic hypotension, development of hydrocephalous, or subdural hematoma. Appropriate diagnostic testing after examination should be ordered. The patient should continue to have annual physical examinations to monitor other age-related conditions or concurrent illness.

Consultation

A person in whom PD is suspected should always have a neurologic consultation to determine or confirm the diagnosis. If distance or availability impedes the care of a neurologist, the primary care provider can follow recommendations for treatment. When treatment is ineffective, new problems arise, or there is a marked change in the patient's condition, the neurologist should be consulted or the patient reevaluated. Again, the diagnosis is based on history, neurologic examination indicating the clustering of the primary symptoms of PD (rigidity, tremor, bradykinesia, loss of postural reflexes), and elimination of other causes. Box 23-2 lists the differential diagnoses.

Treatment

PD is a chronic, progressive neurologic disease. Treatment goals are twofold: short-term treatment to alleviate symptoms and reverse functional disability and long-term treatment to maintain effectiveness and limit pharmacologic complications (Miller, 2002). Disease management can be subdivided into three categories: protective, symptomatic, and restorative.

Box 23-2
Differential Diagnosis

- Drug-induced parkinsonism, phenothiazines, vestibular sedatives, neuroleptics; prolonged use or misuse of neuroleptic drugs and anti-emetic drugs might cause Parkinson's disease-like symptoms. Withdrawal of the drugs reduces the symptoms but can take many months to settle
- Vascular encephalopathy history of strokes, arterial hypertension; often lower body parkinsonism symptom, that is, gait disturbance with start hesitations
- Trauma: pugilistic encephalopathy; repeated blows to the head might precipitate Parkinson's disease-like symptoms
- Viral brain infections: post-encephalitis lethargica, AIDS encephalopathy
- Toxin induced: manganese, cyanide poisoning
- Parkinson's plus syndromes: multiple system atrophy, Shy-Drager syndrome, progressive supranuclear palsy, olivopontocerebellar atrophy (OPCA)
- Essential tremor
- Wilson's disease: a rare metabolic (copper) disorder; usually affects younger adults

From Scott S: Understanding the challenge of Parkinson's disease, *Nursing Standard* 16(41):48-55, 2002.

Experimental therapeutics in PD has focused on prevention of levodopa complications, treatment of dyskinesias associated with levodopa therapy, surgical intervention, and neuroprotection (Tintner and Jankovic, 2002). Pharmacotherapy must be individualized, and the patient's age at diagnosis is an important consideration. Differences exist in treatment goals for patients younger than 60 and those older. The goals for younger patients are symptom control, sparing levodopa use, and neuroprotective consideration. For patients 60 and older, improved functional impairment is the foremost goal. Special concern must be taken to avoid inducing or exacerbating cognitive impairment (Miller, 2002).

THERAPEUTIC

Many medications are available to treat PD and several pending Food and Drug Administration (FDA) approval. The pharmacologic management of PD is a complex and dynamic task; there is no one "right" strategy indicating which drugs should be used at a particular stage of the disease (Korczyn and Nussbaum, 2002). When deciding among them, one must first consider the impact of the disease and symptoms on the person to determine which medication to use. Another important aspect of PD medication is compliance. Patients get the most benefit from their medications if they are taken on a regular schedule. Frequently symptoms improve when patients are asked to take their medications consistently at the same time, thus avoiding additional medication. See Table 23-5 for major drug classes used to treat PD.

None of the available protective treatments have been shown to slow the progression of PD, although the monoamine oxidase (MAO) inhibitor selegiline and high doses of the antioxidant vitamin E are thought to be useful. Symptomatic therapy, primarily levodopa, remains the best treatment for PD. Although levodopa is effective, patients generally begin to lose their response to the drug within 5 to 7 years. Its early use may result in earlier development of complications. The wearing off of the drug's effect can be managed in a variety of ways, including more frequent doses, controlled-release forms, the addition of a dopamine agonist, or a catechol-O-methyltransferase (COMT) inhibitor (Miller, 2002). The complex clinical pharmacokinetics of levodopa are due to several factors: erratic absorption, short half-life, peripheral O-methylation, and facilitated transport across the blood-brain barrier (Deleu, Northway, and Hanssens, 2002).

TABLE 23-5	Parkinson's Medications

Medications	Action	Dosage	Side Effects
Anticholinergics			
Trihexyphenidyl (Artane)	Blocks acetylcholine,	2-20 mg/d	Dry mouth, blurred
Benztropine (Cogentin)	thus promoting	0.5-7 mg/d	vision, constipation,
	balance between		orthostatic
	orthostatic		hypotension,
	acetylcholine and		confusion and
	dopamine		hallucinations
Symmetrel (amantadine)	Increases endogenous	100 mg bid	Mottling of skin,
	dopamine, prevents		confusion
	neuronal uptake of		
	natural dopamine		
Levodopa			
Carbidopa (Lodosyn)	Levodopa crosses the	25-75 mg/d	Nausea and vomiting,
Levodopa (L-dopa)	blood-brain barrier and	400-1000 mg/d	orthostatic
Carbidopa-levodopa	converts to dopamine	100-150/1000-	hypotension, and
(Sinemet, Sinemet CR)	inside the brain;	1500 mg/d	confusion and/or
	carbidopa blocks		hallucinations.
	conversion of levodopa		Long-term
	outside the brain.		complications:
			dyskinesia,
			dystonias, motor
			fluctuations
Dopamine Agonists			
Bromocriptine (Parlodel)	Dopamine synaptic	2.5-100 mg/d	Dyskinesias,
Pergolide (Permax)	agonists, decrease	0.05-5 mg/d	orthostatic
Pramipexole (Mirapex)	dopamine turnover.	0.1-5 mg/d	hypotension,
Ropinirol (Requip)		3-24 mg/d	confusion and
			hallucinations
MAO Inhibitor			
Selegiline (Eldepryl)	Inhibits MAO-B,	5-10 mg/d	
	thereby inhibiting		
	dopamine metabolism		
COMT Inhibitors			
Tolcapone (Tasmar)	Prolongs the effect	100-200 mg/d	Mild headache, nausea,
	of levodopa		loose stools, changes
			in urine color,
			transient increase
			in dyskinesias

MAO, Monoamine oxidase; *COMT*, catechol-O-methyltransferase.

Anticholinergics

Anticholinergics are used primarily for the treatment of tremor and for treatment early in the course of the disease. They block the action of the neurotransmitter acetylcholine, promoting a balance between acetylcholine and dopamine. The most commonly used anticholinergics are trihexyphenidyl (Artane), benztropine (Cogentin), and procyclidine (Kemadrin). The most common side effects of these medications are dry mouth, blurred vision, constipation, orthostatic hypotension, confusion, and hallucinations.

Amantadine

Early in PD amantadine is also useful, but its usefulness tends to last only several months. It has anticholinergic and mild dopaminergic activity. Side effects include ankle edema, urinary retention, psychosis, confusion, and mottling of the skin, particularly in older adults. When discontinuing amantadine therapy, the patient must be weaned to avoid a sudden increase in PD symptoms.

Levodopa or Carbidopa-Levodopa

Levodopa is the precursor to dopamine, the lacking neurotransmitter in PD. Levodopa crosses the blood-brain barrier and then is converted to dopamine inside the brain. Carbidopa blocks conversion of the levodopa outside the brain, decreasing the side effect of nausea and allowing more levodopa to enter the brain. Although dopamine replacement therapy improves the symptoms, it does not inhibit the degeneration of dopamine neurons in the substantia nigra (Kitamura, Kakimura, and Taniguchi, 2002). Levodopa is available in several formulations, including "regular" tablets or slow or controlled-release preparations, and it can also be dissolved in an aqueous solution. Patients usually respond to carbidopa-levodopa (Sinemet) and can feel the onset within 60 minutes. Regular carbidopa-levodopa should be taken on an empty stomach, if tolerated, for the best absorption. Patients who cannot tolerate this should begin taking the drug with food and then change to taking it on an empty stomach later. Time-release carbidopa-levodopa (Sinemet CR) was developed to reduce motor fluctuations and results in relatively constant plasma levels for about 6 hours in a normal gastrointestinal tract (Tinter and Jankovich, 2002). To switch from Sinemet to Sinemet CR, amount of levodopa is increased by 10%. Changes in Sinemet CR may take 7 to 10 days to take effect; it is important to remind patients of this wait factor because they will be accustomed to receiving an immediate response to regular carbidopa-levodopa. Also, patients do not feel this form "kick in" after 30 minutes, and they may think it is ineffective. The time-release form should be taken on a full stomach and should not be crushed. Common side effects are nausea and vomiting, orthostatic hypotension, confusion, and hallucinations.

Long-term complications of this therapy are dyskinesias, dystonias, and motor fluctuations (the wearing-off phenomenon and the on-off phenomenon). As many as 50% of patients on L-dopa for 5 years experience motor fluctuations and dyskinesias (Tarsy, 2002). Dyskinesias are the most common side effect; they are caused by too much dopamine in the brain and create symptoms opposite to the slow- and poor-moving patient with PD. Dyskinesias are choreoathetoid movements usually of the head, trunk, or extremities. They may be expressed as mild turning or tapping of the foot or hand or a twitching of the mouth, or they may be as dramatic as flinging of the extremities and trunk. When given a choice, most patients prefer to be mildly dyskinetic instead of bradykinetic. Dystonias are painful sustained muscle contractions that may occur with dyskinesias. They are difficult to treat but may respond to a decrease in levodopa-carbidopa or to an addition of the time-release form at bedtime to avoid early morning dystonias.

Motor fluctuations may manifest in two different ways: the wearing-off phenomenon or the on-off phenomenon. The wearing-off phenomenon occurs after several years of levodopa-carbidopa treatment. The drug's effectiveness begins to wear off before the next dose is due. As the frequency of doses is increased, the on-off phenomenon begins to occur. The patient has periods of immobility lasting minutes to hours ("off"), followed by periods of mobility ("on").

These changes are not associated with medication doses. This phenomenon can be dramatic; the patient may enter the office in a wheelchair, unable to move. Then, during the appointment, the patient gradually begins to move more freely and eventually walks out of the office unassisted.

Dopamine Agonists

Dopamine agonists act directly on the dopamine synapses and are useful adjunctive therapies to levodopa-carbidopa. They are effective in helping control motor fluctuations and can reduce the total amount of levodopa-carbidopa dosage. A variety of direct dopamine receptor agonists have been developed and licensed over the years: bromocriptine, lisuride, pergolide, cabergoline, pramipexole, and ropinirole are currently marketed oral agents, although not in all countries. New dopamine agonist patch preparations, developed to avoid problems with pharmacokinetics and bioavailability, have been effective in reducing levodopa dosage in all trials and have shown efficacy as initial monotherapy (Tintner and Jankovic, 2002). The most common side effects are orthostatic hypotension, confusion, and hallucinations.

Monoamine Oxidase Inhibitor

The type B MAO inhibitor selegiline (Eldepryl) delays the need for levodopa-carbidopa in the treatment of early disease and is helpful in treating motor fluctuations. It stops the metabolism of dopamine. Patients do not need to follow the tyramine-free diet (or "cheese diet") recommended with the MAO inhibitor antidepressants because of its selectivity of MAO inhibition. It is given in a twice-daily dosage, one tablet in the morning and one at noon, because more MAO is available in the morning. This dosage also helps with the common side effect of insomnia. Other side effects are nausea, dizziness, dry mouth, abdominal pain, confusion, and hallucinations.

Catechol-O-Methyltransferase Inhibitors

Catechol-O-methyltransferase (COMT) is involved in the metabolism of levodopa and dopamine. Inhibition of this enzyme causes a decreased concentration of levodopa metabolite, 3-O-methyldopa, which may cause levodopa motor fluctuations. Also, levodopa blood levels are maintained for a longer time, resulting in a smoother effect from levodopa. Two COMT inhibitors are currently available: tolcapone (Tasmar), which acts both centrally and peripherally, and entacapone (Comtan), which acts only peripherally (Tintner and Jankovic, 2002). The starting dose of tolcapone is 100 mg three times a day, and the clinical effect is evident immediately. The dose of entacapone is one 200-mg tablet with each dose of L-dopa, up to a maximum of eight doses per day (Tarsy, 2002). Side effects are headache, dizziness, nausea, orthostatic hypotension, loose stools, change in urine color, and a transient increase in dyskinesias. Tolcapone has been implicated in possible liver damage in a very small number of patients, which has resulted in a dramatic reduction in its use, to the point of cessation in some countries, including Canada. It has been argued, however, that tolcapone has some advantages over entacapone and that it still has utility in the treatment of PD patients with motor fluctuations (Tintner and Jankovic, 2002).

The drug therapies aim to control the symptoms and the progression of the disease. Many important nonpharmacologic and educational interventions are available that can assist the patient in maintaining maximum function and preventing or alleviating disability (Boxes 23-3 and 23-4).

SURGICAL PROCEDURES

Enthusiasm for surgery in PD has been growing. Procedures include thalamotomy (unilateral and bilateral), pallidotomy (unilateral and bilateral), deep brain stimulation (DBS), adrenal implant, and fetal implant (Tarsy, 2002). Surgical interventions have targeted the Vim (ventral intermediate) nucleus of the thalamus, subthalamic nucleus (STN) or globus pallidus internum (GPi), directly by an ablative procedure or indirectly by high-frequency DBS (Pollack et al, 2002; Tintner and Jankovic, 2002).

Box 23-3

Parkinsonism Teaching Plan

1. Assess the patient's and family's knowledge of, misconceptions about, and experiences with Parkinson's disease (PD).
2. Identify areas of concern to the patient and family regarding the disease, its treatment, and its impact on their lives.
3. Describe the incidence, etiology, pathophysiology, and primary and secondary symptoms of PD.
4. Describe the medical management of PD, including the various drug therapies.
5. Describe the common side effects of the drug therapies, their manifestations and measures that minimize the side effects.
6. Discuss common self-care deficits of PD patients, and identify those the patient now has.
7. Teach methods to minimize or overcome the identified self-care deficits, and provide written information as needed.
8. Discuss common safety hazards faced by PD patients, and identify those presently existing for the patient.
9. Discuss measures to minimize or eliminate the identified safety hazards of the PD patient.
10. Instruct and provide information on a protein-restriction diet, as appropriate, to manage parkinsonism symptoms.
11. Provide written information regarding available PD community and national resources and organizations.
12. Assess the need for further education of the patient and family, and develop learning objectives if necessary.

Unilateral thalamotomy and DBS of the thalamus are effective for tremor, but do not help other features of PD. DBS of the GPi and STN, however, may offer benefits by improving parkinsonian symptoms, smoothing out motor fluctuations and reducing dyskinesias by allowing a decrease in daily levodopa dose.

Unilateral pallidotomy is effective and relatively safe in patients with severe dyskinesias and on-off fluctuations. The effect on bradykinesia is limited. A review of this procedure found that the risk of permanent adverse effects was 14% with symptomatic infarction or hemorrhage occurring in 4% and an associated mortality of 1% (Tarsy, 2002).

Human fetal mesencephalic cell transplants for the treatment of bradykinesia are promising but still investigational.

Box 23-4

Guidelines for Managing Common Problems

1. If a patient is having a poor response to the medications, make sure the patient is taking the medications at regular intervals. Many times poor compliance with the prescribed regimen is the reason for inadequate medication response.
2. Educating the patient about the benefits of following the prescribed regimen (e.g., avoiding increased dosages or an increase in the number of drugs) is an early goal.
3. If the patient is experiencing confusion, hallucinations, or increasing memory problems, first review the patient's medication list to determine if these symptoms are a side effect.
4. Exercise is as important as medication in treating Parkinson's disease.
5. Stressful situations, such as anxiety or an argument, can increase symptoms temporarily.

Interventions for Managing Common Problems

Symptoms associated with PD, such as postural hypotension, depression, anxiety, sexual dysfunction, and hallucinations, are of particular concern in the patient's plan of care. Education of patients and family members is a critical aspect of care. Patient-oriented books, support groups, websites, and PD clinics are often helpful. Complementary therapies to enhance physical and emotional wellness include massage therapy, tai chi, relaxation, visual imagery, and music therapy.

- *Inability to Perform Activities of Daily Living*
  - Encourage regular exercise within limitations.
  - Encourage realistic independence with activities of daily living.
  - Encourage use of affected hand unless tremor is extreme.
  - Provide nutritional counseling (e.g., protein redistribution diet), if indicated.
  - The patient who is not taking a decarboxylase inhibitor should omit any multivitamin containing B_6 and should limit intake of foods high in B_6 (e.g., milk, eggs, meat).
  - Avoid phenothiazines for nausea because they block dopamine action.
  - Evaluate effectiveness of drugs for rigidity, tremor, and bradykinesia.
  - Evaluate the need for devices to assist the patient or for physical and occupational therapy consultation, as needed.
- *Poor Speech*
  - Encourage diaphragmatic speech.
- *Poor Handwriting*
  - Encourage face and tongue exercises and massage.
  - Explore alternate methods of written communication.
  - Evaluate choreiform and athetoid movements (e.g., head dropping, facial grimacing, tongue protrusion, opening and closing mouth) in relation to medication.
- *Constipation*
  - Provide nutritional counseling (e.g., high-residue diet, increased fluid intake).
  - Encourage exercise.
  - Establish defecation pattern.
  - Use stool softeners, laxatives, suppositories, and enemas, as needed.
  - Use warm liquids to stimulate peristalsis.
  - Evaluate constipation in relation to medication.
  - Monitor for signs of impaction or bowel obstruction.
- *Impaired Gait (Freezing, Propulsion, Retropulsion)*
  - Evaluate symptoms (shuffling, tremor, freezing) in relation to medication.
  - Teach methods to facilitate rising from bed or chair (rocking back and forth before standing up).
  - Teach methods to assist with freezing (e.g., stepping over imaginary line, rocking).
  - Assess potential safety hazards in home.
  - Encourage regular exercise.
  - Physical therapy consultation for gait training and muscle-strengthening exercises, as needed.
- *Poor Sleep*
  - Causative factors include the aging process, anti-PD medications, the disease process itself, and concomitant factors such as nocturia, anxiety and immobility (Crabb, 2001).
  - Teach methods to promote a regular sleep pattern (e.g., daytime stimulus, exercise, quiet environment).
  - Sleep medication, as needed.
  - Evaluate sleep disturbance in relation to medication.
- *Dysphagia*
  - Provide nutritional counseling (e.g., semisoft diet).
  - Teach measures that minimize problems associated with dysphagia (e.g., avoid thin liquids, cut food into small pieces, sit upright for meals).

- Evaluate medication in relation to dysphagia.
- *Overweight or Underweight*
  - Provide nutritional counseling, referral to nutritionist, as needed.
  - Increase activity as appropriate.
  - Establish short- and long-term goals for weight change.
- *Urinary Hesitancy, Urgency, and Incontinence*
  - Establish bladder-emptying schedule.
  - Stimulation techniques to initiate voiding (Credé's reflex, Valsalva maneuver).
  - Use incontinence devices, as needed.
  - Evaluate urinary problems in relation to medication and to mobility.
- *Risk of Injury*
  - Assess potential safety hazards in home.
  - Teach measures to minimize or eliminate safety hazards.
  - Evaluate need for supervision of patient.
  - Provide physical or occupational therapy consultation, as needed.
- *Poor Memory, Confusion, Hallucinations, Dementia*
  - Evaluate symptoms in relation to medication.
  - Evaluate memory deficit, dementia symptoms, and disease progression through mental status tests, as needed.
  - Teach cognitive remediation techniques for memory problems.
  - Teach family and caregivers help strategies for specific dementia symptoms (such as confusion and hallucinations).
  - Evaluate need for family counseling, caregiver support, and community resources.
- *Depression*
  - Assess the presence and degree of depressive symptoms.
  - Evaluate depressive symptoms in relation to medication.
  - Provide psychiatric consultation, as needed.
  - Educate about the disease and medications.
  - Provide written information regarding the disease and current regimens.
  - Provide information on community and national resources and organizations.

Palliative Care

The palliative stage aims to relieve the distress that arises from symptoms and side effects, not just for patients but also for families and caregivers. Maintaining dignity is paramount, along with morbidity relief. The need for reassessment and access to a specialist remain priorities. Advice on drug administration, progressive dopaminergic withdrawal and appropriate use of analgesia predominate. The nursing role is complex and aims to provide appropriate information about care, avoidance of pressure ulcers, continence management and stress management (Scott, 2002).

Advance Care Planning

Patient and family counseling should include a discussion of health care directives in an ongoing fashion and should begin relatively early in the course of the disease. Specific issues include the desire for feeding tube when swallowing becomes too difficult, as well as preferences regarding attempts at resuscitation and ventilator support.

Summary

PD is a costly, disabling disorder that can be difficult to diagnose, especially early in its onset. The history and a skillful neurologic examination can provide the clues to detecting this problem.

Appropriate diagnostic testing and referral to a neurologist are important in establishing the diagnosis and treatment plan. Pharmacologic intervention is important, but focused education and therapies for managing problems common to PD can enhance successful management of the patient's overall functioning and well-being.

Resources

American Parkinson Disease Association
1250 Hylan Boulevard, Suite 4B
Staten Island, NY 10305
(718) 981-8001
(800) 223-APDA
www.APDAParkinson.com

National Parkinson Foundation, Inc.
1501 NW 9th Avenue (Bob Hope Road)
Miami, FL 33136-1494
(305) 547-6666
(800) 327-4545
(800) 433-7022 (in Florida)
www.parkinson.org

Parkinson's Disease Foundation
710 West 168th Street
New York, NY 10032
(800) 457-6676
www.pdf.org

Parkinson Society Canada
4211 Yonge Street Suite 316
Toronto, Ontario M2P 2A9
Canada
(800) 565-3000
www.parkinson.ca/home.html

The Parkinson's Institute
1170 Morse Avenue
Sunnyvale, CA 94089-1605
(408) 734-2800
(800) 786-2958
www.parkinsonsinstitute.org

United Parkinson Foundation
360 West Superior Street
Chicago, IL 60610
(312) 664-2344

References

Askenasy JJ: Approaching disturbed sleep in late Parkinson's disease: first step toward a proposal for a revised UPDRS, *Parkinsonism & Related Disorders* 8(2):123-131, 2001.
Crabb L: Sleep disorders in Parkinson's disease: the nursing role, *Br J Nursing* 10(1):42-47, 2001.
Deleu D, Northway MG, Hanssens Y: Clinical pharmacokinetic and pharmacodynamic properties of drugs used in the treatment of Parkinson's disease, *Clin Pharmacokinetics* 41(4):261-309, 2002.

Feinberg M: The role of COMT inhibitors in improving levodopa therapy in elderly patients with Parkinson's disease, *Annals of Long Term Care* 6(suppl F), 1998.

Foltynie T et al: The genetic basis of Parkinson's disease, *J Neurol Neurosurg Psychiatry* 73(4):363-370, 2002.

Kitamura Y, Kakimura J, Taniguchi T: Antiparkinsonian drugs and their neuroprotective effects, *Biological & Pharmaceutical Bulletin* 25(3):284-290, 2002.

Korczyn AD, Nussbaum M: Emerging therapies in the pharmacological treatment of Parkinson's disease, *Drugs* 62(5):775-786, 2002.

Kruger R et al: Parkinson's disease: one biochemical pathway to fit all genes? *Trends in Molecular Medicine* 8(5):236-240, 2002.

Miller JL: Parkinson's Disease primer, *Geriatric Nursing* 23(2):69-75, 2002.

Pollak P et al: Treatment results: Parkinson's disease, *Movement Disorders* 17(suppl 3):S75-S83, 2002.

Reich SG: "Doctor, I Shake" presentation at Current Topics in Geriatrics, Johns Hopkins Geriatrics Center and the American Geriatrics Society, Baltimore, October 1998.

Scott S: Understanding the challenge of Parkinson's disease, *Nursing Standard* 16(41):48-55, 2002.

Tarsy D: Treatment of advanced Parkinson's disease. Available at www.uptodate.com, 2002.

Tintner R, Jankovic J: Treatment options for Parkinson's Disease, *Curr Opin Neurol* 15(4):467-476, 2002.

Uitti RJ: Tremor: how to determine if the patient has Parkinson's disease, *Geriatrics* 53:30-36, 1998.

Wolozin B, Golts N: Iron and Parkinson's disease, *Neuroscientist* 8(1):22-32, 2002.

Zesiewicz TA, Hauser RA: Depression in Parkinson's disease, *Current Psychiatry Reports* 4(1):69-73, 2002.

24

Neurologic: Stroke and Stroke Prevention

Stroke is the third leading cause of death and a major cause of disability among persons 70 years of age and older. A stroke occurs every 53 seconds in North America (Gladstone, Black, and Hakim, 2002). The incidence in persons under 65 years of age is less than 2 per 1000 annually, but the incidence increases with age for men and women, respectively: 4.6 and 3.8 per 1000 for ages 65 to 74; 9.4 and 7.4 for ages 75 to 84 (Weinberger, 2002).

Stroke is the leading cause of brain damage in adults. The damage results from destroyed neurons following either disruption of cerebral blood supply or hemorrhage into or around the brain. This destruction of brain tissue results in decreased brain function and, for the patient, reduced independence, a loss of self, and even death.

Dramatic decreases in stroke morbidity and mortality rates over the past 25 years have been largely due to hypertension control, atherosclerosis prevention, therapy for cardiac disease to eliminate sources of emboli, and surgical therapy for stroke prevention.

Costs can be divided into direct and indirect components. *Direct costs* include the dollar burden of all medical care received in response to a stroke as well as nonmedical costs, such as those for caregiver services and home modification. *Indirect costs* include the dollar value of lost productivity due to stroke. The annual health costs of stroke are estimated at $18.6 billion. The total cost, including lost wages and care of the disabled, approximates $45 billion (Ramirez-Lassepas, 1998). The average cost per case of stroke is about $50,000. From a Medicare perspective, the largest proportion of the cost is hospital readmission, reflecting the comorbidities associated with stroke. A major cost not reflected directly in Medicare data (because it is typically not covered) is nursing home care. This cost is especially great for stroke patients with more severe disability. Stroke prevention is one of the most effective ways to reduce this public health and economic burden.

Thrombolytic therapy with tissue plasminogen activator (t-PA) within 3 hours of event onset can significantly improve outcomes in selected ischemic stroke patients (Weinberg, 2002). Most patients are ineligible for intravenous t-PA because of delays in obtaining treatment (Meschia, Miller, and Brott, 2002). Because of the improvements in this and other treatments of acute stroke in recent years, great effort is being made by leaders in the field to instill in the minds of persons the need for urgent evaluation and treatment at the first onset of stroke symptoms. One method of achieving

517

this goal is by renaming stroke "brain attack." This is being done in an effort to attach the same urgency in seeking treatment that has been achieved with heart attack over the years.

Age-related Changes

Cerebral blood flow decreases with advancing age. This is caused in part by a loss of neuronal connections that results in loss of neurons and glial cells with resulting brain atrophy. Atherosclerosis of extracranial and intracranial arteries, heart disease, and hypertension further decrease cerebral blood flow. The major determinants of cerebral perfusion are age and status of the vascular system.

Pathophysiology

The two basic mechanisms for stroke are occlusion and hemorrhage. Ischemic strokes, caused by occlusion of an artery, account for 80% to 85% of cerebrovascular events, and hemorrhagic strokes, caused by a ruptured artery, account for 15% to 20% (Weinberger, 2002). The signs and symptoms of stroke may include unilateral weakness or paralysis, a sagging of one side of the face, double or blurred vision, vertigo, numbness or tingling, and language disturbances (Zerwic, Ennen, and DeVon, 2002).

The three main causes of ischemic stroke are atherosclerotic disease of large extracranial and intracranial vessels, occlusion of intracranial vessels by emboli from a cardiac source (cardioembolic stroke), and small-vessel intracranial occlusive disease resulting from hypertension and diabetes (Weinberger, 2002). When a major artery to the brain is occluded, the occurrence of ischemic symptoms depends on collateral circulation. If collateral circulation is immediately available, symptoms do not occur or are only short-lived; if it is not immediately available, the occurrence of cerebral infarction will depend on whether collateral circulation can be established in time to prevent irreversible neuronal damage.

The clinical result of an episode of transient focal cerebral ischemia is a *transient ischemic attack* (TIA), defined as an episode of focal neurologic deficit of sudden onset that lasts minutes, rarely hours, and always subsides in less than 24 hours (American Heart Association, 1994). Patients who experience TIAs and the associated transient symptoms—difficulty with speech, sudden weakness or numbness of the extremities, loss of balance, visual disturbance—are at increased risk for stroke. Without stroke prophylaxis, these patients have a 25% to 50% chance of experiencing a subsequent stroke that causes permanent neurologic deficits. Stroke is most likely to occur in the first 3 months after a TIA (Weinberger, 2002).

C-Reactive Protein

The pathophysiology of atherosclerosis is complex and multifactorial. The probability of the development of symptomatic coronary heart disease may be predicted by standard risk factor stratification involving hypertension, dyslipidemia, age, positive family history, and diabetes. Risk factor stratification, however, has been demonstrated to have significant limitations in the individual patient, which has generated a search for more specific and sensitive markers (Farmer and Torre-Amione, 2002). Evidence suggests that inflammation plays a key role in the pathogenesis of atherosclerosis. The chronic inflammatory process can develop to an acute clinical event by the induction of plaque rupture and therefore can cause acute coronary syndromes (Auer et al, 2002).

Recent investigations have shown an association between inflammatory markers (including C-reactive protein [CRP], modified low-density lipoprotein, homocysteine, tumor necrosis factor, and thermogenicity) and vascular events, which have been identified as emerging risk factors that may add prognostic information in patient management (Benzaquen, Yu, and Rifai, 2002; Case and Ballantyne, 2002; Farmer and Torre-Amione, 2002). Increased CRP concentration reflects the inflammatory condition of the vascular wall (Magadle et al, 2002). CRP has been found to be significantly increased in patients with acute myocardial infarction (MI) and unstable angina shortly after the onset of symptoms (after a period of 12 hours) (Auer et al, 2002). One study found that the risks for progression of atherosclerosis associated with high CRP levels were as high as those associated with the traditional cardiovascular risk factors high cholesterol, hypertension, and smoking (Van Der Meer et al, 2002). CRP level has been shown to be a stronger predictor of cardiovascular events than the low-density lipoprotein (LDL) cholesterol level (Ridker et al, 2002).

With the release of the third iteration of the National Cholesterol Education Programs Adult Treatment Panel guidelines (National Heart, Lung and Blood Institute web site, 2003; Stone and Van Horn, 2002), debate has been renewed about the appropriate use of pharmacologic therapies in individual patients, especially in primary prevention. CRP may have important implications for the optimal targeting of such interventions as statin therapy (Gotto, 2002). Although many uncertainties remain in using CRP in clinical practice (Zebrack and Anderson, 2002), measurement of this marker is becoming increasingly common in primary care and most certainly will be a focus of much discussion and research in the coming years.

Risk Factors

Everyone is at risk of stroke, regardless of age; however, advancing age is a major risk factor for ischemic stroke and intracerebral hemorrhage. Risk factors are categorized as modifiable or nonmodifiable. *Nonmodifiable* risk factors are characteristics inherent in a particular individual that cannot be changed. *Modifiable* risk factors have the potential to be controlled through lifestyle change or by medical intervention. See Box 24-1 for categories of risk factors.

Among the modifiable risk factors, hypertension is extremely important, as is atrial fibrillation, which becomes more prevalent with increasing age. Systolic blood pressure is at least as powerful a coronary risk factor as the diastolic blood pressure, and isolated systolic hypertension is now established as a major hazard for coronary heart disease and stroke (Hennekens, 2002). Chapter 11 discusses the new recommendations for classification and management of hypertension. Additional factors associated with risk of first stroke include diabetes, physical inactivity, obesity, cardiovascular

---

Box 24-1

Risk Factors for Ischemic Stroke

Nonmodifiable	**Modifiable**
Age	Hypertension
Gender	Atrial Fibrillation
Race/ethnicity	Cigarette smoking
Heredity	Hypercholesterolemia
Geographic location	Heavy alcohol use
	Asymptomatic carotid stenosis
	Transient ischemic attack
	Diabetes
	Physical inactivity
	Obesity
	Cardiovascular disease
	Hypercoagulability
	High-dose contraceptives
	Dietary factors
	Stress

diseases (coronary artery diseases, MI, cardiomyopathy, congestive heart failure [CHF]), aortic arch atheroma, hypercoagulability, and the use of high-dose contraceptives in younger women.

Research is ongoing to evaluate the role of insulin resistance as a risk factor for stroke. Resistance to insulin-mediated glucose uptake by peripheral tissues is a cardinal defect in type 2 diabetes mellitus, but insulin resistance is also common among nondiabetic prsons. The principal pathophysiologic defect is impaired intracellular signaling in muscle tissue leading to defective glycogen synthesis. Insulin resistance is associated with numerous metabolic, hematologic, and cellular events that promote atherosclerosis and coagulation. The adverse biologic events associated with insulin resistance include hypertension, dyslipidemia, abnormal fibrinolysis, hyperglycemia, hyper-insulinemia, systemic inflammation, altered vascular endothelial function, and atherogenesis. Insulin resistance may be a prevalent risk factor for stroke, and research is evaluating whether new drugs that can safely reduce insulin resistance also have a role in stroke prevention (Kernan et al, 2002).

The most common mechanism by which heart disease causes stroke is cardioembolism, most frequently caused by cardiac arrhythmia. Atrial fibrillation is the most common arrhythmia. Risk of stroke from untreated nonvalvular atrial fibrillation is 5% per year in patients over 70 years of age (Weinberger, 2002).

People who abstain from alcohol consumption and, to a greater extent, heavy drinkers are at greater risk for first stroke than are mild to moderate drinkers. Evidence suggests that one to two drinks per day may actually provide some protection against stroke. This benefit rapidly disappears when alcohol consumption exceeds two drinks per day. Of course, the other risks of alcohol consumption need to be weighed for each patient.

A high degree of carotid stenosis, even if asymptomatic, correlates with a high risk of stroke. About half of patients with TIAs exhibit greater than 50% stenosis at the bifurcation of the cervical carotid artery. The definitive test for measuring the degree of carotid stenosis is catheter angiography, but this procedure is associated with a 1% incidence of stroke or death in patients with atherosclerotic or cerebrovascular disease (Weinberger, 2002).

Transient ischemic attacks are associated with an 8% risk for first stroke in the first month after a TIA and a 12% risk within the first year after diagnosis of TIA. This risk of stroke may reach 30% within 5 years after a first TIA. The risk is higher in the first month and highest for patients with hemispheric TIA and more than 70% carotid stenosis (www.americanheart.org). Most TIAs have a duration of less than 1 hour, a median duration of 14 minutes in carotid-distribution ischemia, and 8 minutes in vertebrobasilar ischemia. Atherosclerosis of cerebrovascular arteries is the most common cause of transient ischemia in older patients with risk factors for stroke. A TIA should be promptly evaluated to institute therapy as soon as possible to decrease the risk of stroke.

Homocysteine (tHcy) is a toxic amino acid recently accepted as a risk factor for atherosclerosis and stroke (Cingozbay et al, 2002). Accumulation of tHcy occurs with certain enzyme deficiencies or with dietary deficiency of vitamin B_6, B_{12}, or folic acid and can be treated with dietary supplements. In current practice, tHcy levels are most commonly drawn in the evaluation of a low B_{12} level rather than as a primary assessment of stroke risk.

Studies have found that persons who eat more fruits and vegetables have a reduced risk of MI and stroke. The lowest risks have been observed with high consumption of cruciferous vegetables (e.g., cauliflower, broccoli, cabbage, brussel sprouts), green leafy vegetables, citrus fruits, and vitamin-C-rich fruit and vegetables. High-fiber intake is associated with a 40% to 50% reduction in the risk of heart disease and stroke compared with low intake of fiber. Regarding fat intake, the type of fat consumed appears to be more important than the amount of total fat; trans fatty acids increase risk, whereas polyunsaturated fat and monounsaturated fat decrease risk.

Atherosclerotic stroke, hypertension, and hyperglycemia have been documented as important predictors of early stroke recurrence. For late stroke recurrence, some studies have found that age, hypertension, atrial fibrillation, CHF, and diabetes are risk factors, as well as prior TIA or stroke (Weinberger, 2002). Care of certain patients in the primary care setting will include optimal management of risk factors to reduce risks of first or recurrent stroke. Table 24-1 provides a checklist for patient management in the prevention of stroke.

Assessment

The most important aspect of the assessment for stroke risk is a thorough history to assess for any of the potential contributing factors discussed, both modifiable and nonmodifiable (e.g., family history, alcohol use, activity level, hypertension, diabetes). Assessment should include regular blood pressure checks at the time of routine physical examination; auscultation of the neck and chest to check for carotid artery bruit and heart murmur (suggestive of valvular heart disease); electrocardiography, which can identify cardiac arrhythmias such as atrial fibrillation (a cause of cardioembolic stroke); serum lipid profiling; and questions about smoking history (Weinberger, 2002).

TABLE 24-1	Ischemic Stroke: Checklist for Patient Management

Review risk factors
Hypertension
Diabetes
Poor diet; no exercise
High serum cholesterol
Smoking
Atrial fibrillation
Carotid stenosis (TIA history)

Patient assessment
History and physical exam
Is patient high-risk? (e.g., has one or more of the risk factors above)
If high-risk, check for TIA history or TIA risk (auscultation, Doppler studies)
Rule out atrial fibrillation
Primary prevention
Patient education regarding stroke symptoms, signs

Risk-factor management
Maintain normotension
Tight glycemic control
Cholesterol lowering
Diet modification; exercise
Antithrombotic therapy (platelet antiaggregant therapy)

Primary/secondary prevention
Pharmacologic management of cardiac risk factors (e.g., atrial fibrillation, post MI)
Antithrombotic therapy (platelet antiaggregant therapy, anticoagulation)

Surgical Intervention*
Endarterectomy
Stent placement

From Weinberger J: Stroke and TIA: prevention and management of cerebrovascular events in primary care, *Geriatrics* 57(1):38-43, 2002.
*Consider for select patients

In the clinical setting the practitioner can order a variety of imaging procedures for the evaluation of patients at risk of stroke. New procedures have improved accuracy and lessened invasiveness but increased the complexity of decision making. When all the standard imaging techniques are available, a sequential choice must be made to optimize diagnostic yield, reduce the risk of harm to the patient, and minimize cost. The goals of imaging are to identify candidates for specific surgical or medical therapeutic modalities, determine prognosis, and exclude rare nonvascular causes.

Physical and diagnostic evaluation should include the areas listed in Boxes 24-2 and Box 24-3, respectively.

Noninvasive techniques allow study of carotid arteries with no risk to the patient. Carotid Doppler ultrasonography should be performed whenever carotid stenosis is suspected, as when carotid bruit is present or when cerebrovascular episodes have already occurred in the distribution of the carotid circulation.

Head CT is useful in detection of cerebral infarction in patients who have had a TIA and to exclude other lesions that may simulate stroke, such as subdural hematoma, brain tumor, arteriovenous malformation, or aneurysm.

Magnetic resonance imaging (MRI) of the head is used less often than CT for initial evaluation because it is more expensive, time-consuming, and less available; however, MRI has certain advantages, such as the ability to detect acute and small infarcts and "flow voids" in the carotid arteries. MRI may not be performed on patients with aneurysm clips, otic or cochlear implants, old prosthetic heart valves, pacemakers, or neurostimulators or when agitation and claustrophobia cannot be resolved.

Box 24-2

Physical Examination in Assessment of Stroke Risk

Weight
Blood pressure (annually)
Cardiovascular examination to include auscultation of carotids for bruits and assessment of peripheral circulation
Abdominal examination to assess for aortic bruit
Neurologic examination to establish any baseline deficits

Box 24-3

Diagnostic Studies for the Assessment of Stroke Risk (As Appropriate for Individual Patients)

- Complete blood count
- Lipid profile
- Electrocardiogram
- Echocardiogram
- Carotid Doppler study
- Computed tomography (CT)
- Magnetic resonance imaging
- Magnetic resonance angiography
- CT angiography

Magnetic resonance angiography (MRA) is a generic name for different approaches and variations of vascular imaging by MRI. MRA is useful in detecting arterial narrowing and sometimes the source vessel of ischemic attacks. Sensitivity and specificity of MRA is improved when used in conjunction with other studies such as ultrasound and CT.

Computed tomographic angiography is a high-resolution, contrast-enhanced CT scan of the cervical vessels that visualizes the arterial lumen wall, providing information about changes in the carotid artery that might precipitate a TIA. CT angiography reveals enough vascular detail to be useful as a diagnostic screening method in patients with presumed atherosclerosis of the carotid bifurcation.

Interventions

An important aspect of any risk factor modification program is that a given patient may have multiple risk factors that may lead to cumulative risks for stroke that require multitargeted interventions. Table 24-2 provides recommendations for risk intervention for the primary prevention of cardiovascular diseases. An emerging issue in stroke prevention and stroke treatment is that therapies shown to be effective in clinical trials are not being used or are being used suboptimally. For primary prevention of stroke, adequate blood pressure reduction, and treatment of hyperlipidemia, the use of antithrombotic therapy in patients with atrial fibrillation and of antiplatelet therapy in patients who have had an MI are effective and supported by evidence from several randomized trials. Effective strategies for the secondary prevention of stroke include treatment of hypertension and hyperlipidemia, antithrombotic therapy for patients with atrial fibrillation, antiplatelet therapy, and carotid endarterectomy in patients with severe carotid artery stenosis (Straus, Majumdar, and McAlister, 2002).

Table 24-3 discusses risk stratification and treatment of hypertension. Weight reduction in obese patients and a program of moderate physical activity may be generally recommended.

Use of the 3-hydroxy-3-methylglutaryl coenzyme A (HMG-CoA) reductase inhibitors or statin medications for the reduction of total cholesterol and LDL cholesterol concentrations has been shown to have some benefit for reduction of stroke. In addition to reducing LDL cholesterol, HMG-CoA reductase inhibitors prevent precipitation of vascular events by stabilizing atherosclerotic plaque and exerting beneficial effects on clotting.

Antiplatelet agents are the mainstays of ischemic stroke prevention (see Table 24-4). The therapies recommended for initial therapy include aspirin (50-325 mg daily), the combination of aspirin and extended-release dipyridamole (200 mg) twice daily, or clopidogrel (75 mg) daily. Ticlopidine 250 mg twice daily is approved for stroke prevention but is not considered a first-line therapy (Crawford and Talbert, 2001). Debate continues regarding the best dosing for prophylaxis, but it is generally adequate to start with a small dose ("baby aspirin," 81 mg). The dose may be increased (325 mg or 650 mg per day) in patients with high risk or who have experienced minor cerebrovascular episodes while on lower doses. Ticlopidine is useful for patients with TIA in whom aspirin therapy has not successfully eliminated the occurrence of symptoms or who are not able to take aspirin. Patients who have had an embolic stroke or are at high risk may require anticoagulation with warfarin (Coumadin). Anticoagulation with warfarin in patients with nonvalvular atrial fibrillation can reduce stroke risk by 70%, whereas platelet antiaggregate therapy using aspirin reduces the risk by 20% (Weinberger, 2002).

Patients with atrial fibrillation who are at high risk for stroke should receive warfarin. Warfarin therapy is monitored via the International Normalization Ratio (INR), which is reported with the prothrombin time. Used for many years in other countries, the INR has been adopted in the United States to monitor anticoagulation therapy with warfarin because of less variability in results. Stroke prophylaxis guidelines for patients over 70 years of age who have nonvalvular atrial fibrillation recommend warfarin administration that achieves a target INR of 2.5 (or within a range of 2.0 to 2.9). Patients over 85 years of age are at greater risk for complications of cerebral hemorrhage when

TABLE 24-2	American Heart Association Guide to Risk Intervention for the Primary Prevention of Cardiovascular Disease

Smoking

Goal: Complete smoking cessation. No exposure to environmental tobacco smoke.

Blood pressure control

Goal: < 140/90 mm Hg; < 130/85 mm Hg if renal insufficiency or heart failure is present; < 130/80 mm Hg if diabetes is present.

Dietary intake

Goal: An overall healthy eating pattern

Blood lipid management

LDL Cholesterol

< 100	Optimal
100-129	Near optimal/above optimal
130-159	Borderline high
160-189	High
≥190	Very high

Total Cholesterol

< 200	Desirable
200-239	Borderline high
≥240	High

HDL Cholesterol

< 40	Low
≥60	High (desirable)

Physical activity

Goal: At least 30 min of moderate intensity physical activity on most (and preferably all) days of the week.

Weight management

Goal: Achieve and maintain desirable weight (body mass index 18.5 to 24.9 kg/m^2). When body mass index is ≥25 kg/m^2 waist circumference at iliac crest level ≤40 in in men, ≤35 in in women.

Diabetes management

Goals: Normal fasting plasma glucose (< 110 mg/dl) and near normal HbA1c (< 7%). Treat other cardiovascular risk factors aggressively (e.g., change blood pressure goal to < 130/80 and LDL-C goal to < 100 mg/dl).

Aspirin

Goal: Low dose aspirin in persons at higher CHD risk (especially those with 10-year risk of CHD ≥10%).

[†]Adapted from Pearson TA, Blair SN, Daniels SR et al, *Circulation* 106:388, 2002; NIH: *Third report of the National Cholesterol Education Program on Detection, Evaluation, and Treatment of High Blood Cholesterol in Adults.* National Heart, Lung, and Blood Institute, May 2001.

warfarin is used; therefore their target INR should be kept close to 2.0. In patients with atrial fibrillation and mitral stenosis and those with mechanical cardiac valve replacement, anticoagulation should achieve a target INR range of 3.0 to 3.5. Anticoagulation with warfarin is beneficial as stroke prophylaxis during the first 3 months after an MI; it is particularly useful in patients with large anterior wall infarction and akinetic wall segments (Weinberger, 2002).

| **TABLE 24-3** | **Classification and Management of Blood Pressure for Adults*** |

| | | | | Initial drug therapy | |
BP Classification	SBP* mmHg	DBP* mmHg	Lifestyle Modification	Without Compelling Indication	With Compelling Indications
Normal	< 120	and < 80	Encourage		
Prehypertension	120–139	or 80–89	Yes	No antihypertensive drug indicated.	Drug(s) for compelling indications‡
Stage 1 Hypertension	140–159	or 90–99	Yes	Thiazide-type diuretics for most. May consider ACEI, ARB, BB, CCB, or combination.	Drug(s) for the compelling indications.‡ Other antihyper tensive drugs (diuretics, ACEI, ARB, BB, CCB) as needed.
Stage 2 Hypertension	≥160	or ≥100	Yes	Two-drug combination for most† (usually thiazide-type diuretic and ACEI or ARB or BB or CCB).	

Data from Joint National Committee: Seventh report of the Joint National Committee on Prevention. Detection Evaluation and Treatment of High Blood Pressure, National Institutes of Health, National Heart, Lung, and Blood Institute, NIH Publication No. 03-5233 May, 2003.

DBP, Diastolic blood pressure; *SBP,* systolic blood pressure.

Drug abbreviations: *ACEI,* Angiotensin-converting enzyme inhibitor; *ARB,* angiotensin receptor blocker; *BB,* beta-blocker; *CCB,* calcium channel blocker.

*Treatment determined by highest BP category.

†Initial combined therapy should be used cautiously in those at risk for orthostatic hypotension.

‡Treat patients with chronic kidney disease or diabetes to BP goal of < 130/80 mmHg.

| **TABLE 24-4** | **Antiaggregant Therapy for Prevention of Stroke*** |

Agent	Dosage
Aspirin	50 mg/d to 650 mg bid
Ticlopidine (Ticlid)	200 mg bid
Clopidogrel (Plavix)	75 mg/d
Aspirin/dipyridamole (Aggrenox)	25/100 mg bid

From Weinberger J: Stroke and TIA: prevention and management of cerebrovascular events in primary care, Geriatrics 57(1):38-43, 2002.

bid, Twice daily.

*For patients at risk of stroke and not scheduled for surgical intervention

Some older patients with atrial fibrillation may not be considered good candidates for anticoagulation. These may include patients who have a tendency to fall, patients who may not be able to manage medication regimens reliably (and have no assistance), or those who refuse or are unable to have blood drawn frequently. For these patients, the priority is adequate control of the heart rate. This may be accomplished with diltiazem or digoxin, which a cardiologist or other physician may administer intravenously with cardiac monitoring until initial control is achieved. Another option includes cardioversion with medication maintenance. These patients may also benefit from aspirin therapy at the 325-mg daily dose.

Patients with carotid stenosis of 70% to 99% should be evaluated by a vascular surgeon for possible endarterectomy. Although many surgeons may delay surgery until stenosis is 90% to 99%, it is beneficial to obtain the input of the vascular surgeon in the management of the patient whenever significant stenosis is present. At centers where the complication rate for endarterectomy is less than 2%, the intervention can reduce the risk of subsequent stroke from 25% to 50% in patients on aspirin therapy (Weinberger, 2002). Table 24-5 provides suggested treatment strategies for stroke prevention in patients with carotid stenosis.

For older patients who are not endarterectomy candidates, carotid artery stent placement is an option. The risk of stroke during the procedure is similar to that of carotid endarterectomy (2%-8%, depending on the center), but the systemic complications are reduced (Weinberger, 2002).

SMOKING CESSATION

Smoking causes 417,000 deaths each year (www.americanheart.org). The risk for stroke decreases among those who quit smoking and approaches that of nonsmokers within several years (Hennekens, 2002). Practitioners need to be familiar with various smoking cessation programs and tools to be prepared to help the patient with this difficult task. Two addictions are associated with smoking: the response behavior and nicotine. A patient who has smoked less than half a pack a day (10 cigarettes) may not require much more than moral support and assistance in substituting a different, healthier habit when the smoking "trigger" occurs. These triggers often include first thing on arising in the morning, commuting in the car, and after a meal. Substituting other behaviors such as going for a walk, brushing the teeth, or chewing gum may help to "break the habit" for lighter smokers. Heavier smokers probably will require a tapered nicotine replacement in addition to behavioral modifications. Several nicotine replacement systems are currently

TABLE 24-5   **Stroke Prevention in Patients with Carotid Stenosis**

Patient	Degree of Stenosis (%)	Treatment
Asymptomatic (identified by carotid artery bruit)	< 60	Antiaggregant therapy
	> 60	Consider endarterectomy
History of TIA	0 to 40	Antiaggregant therapy
	50 to 69	Antiaggregant therapy; endarterectomy in selected cases
	70 to 99	Endarterectomy (or stenting in high-risk patients), unless significant contraindications exist

From Weinberger J: Stroke and TIA: prevention and management of cerebrovascular events in primary care, *Geriatrics* 57(1):38-43, 2002.
TIA, Transient ischemic attack.

on the market, including gum and titrated patches. When considering a nicotine replacement patch, one must consider the number of cigarettes smoked in an average day. The patient who smokes irregularly, or less than half a pack per day, may actually be increasing the nicotine dose by using a patch and may benefit from one of the other replacements. One tool in smoking cessation is Zyban (Glaxo Wellcome), a short-term, low-dose bupropion course that helps to alleviate the craving for tobacco.

Patient Education

It is critical to educate patients regarding the devastating effects of stroke, especially their individual risk factors. Studies of acute intervention for stroke have shown that outcome is more favorable if the symptoms are recognized early. Many factors contribute to delays in seeking medical treatment for acute stroke, but one that should be remediable is public lack of knowledge about symptoms (Yoon and Byles, 2002). Patients should understand that stroke requires emergency medical treatment within 3 hours of onset for the best outcomes (Weinberger, 2002). At each visit the patient should be asked about smoking cessation, exercise, and attention to other modifiable risk factors, as appropriate. Patients and caregivers must also be educated regarding the signs of a TIA or stroke and importance of obtaining rapid medical attention. Delays in patients arriving at the hospital with suspected stroke can be reduced by the increased use of emergency services ("Call 911!") (Harraf et al, 2002). To improve the outcomes of stroke patients, public awareness of stroke must be increased and emergency medical services (EMS) response to stroke call optimized. Rapid response to stroke is key, as emphasized in the American Stroke Association's "Stroke Chain of Survival" (www.strokeassociation.org), which emphasizes four components: rapid recognition of and reaction to stroke warning signs through immediate use of the 911 system; rapid EMS assessment; priority transport with prenotification of the receiving hospital; and rapid and accurate diagnosis and treatment at the hospital (Brice et al, 2002). See Box 24-4 for warning signs of a stroke.

Summary

Prevention of stroke is an important task for those caring for persons of all ages because so many high-risk behaviors begin early in life. Because strokes tend to occur in the older population, however, this seems to be the time most providers and patients focus on the issue. Fortunately, interventions aimed at reducing risk are still effective and beneficial. In addition, many interventions, such as smoking cessation, exercise, and aspirin therapy, are neither difficult nor expensive. The practitioner must identify patients with risk factors so that appropriate education and intervention can begin before the first stroke causes disability and possibly death.

Box 24-4

Warning Signs of a Stroke

- Sudden numbness or weakness or face, arm, or leg, especially on one side of the body
- Sudden confusion, trouble speaking or understanding
- Sudden trouble seeing in one or both eyes
- Sudden trouble walking, dizziness, loss of balance or coordination
- Sudden, severe headache with no known cause

From American Heart Association website (www.americanheart.org) click on warning signs.

Resources

American Heart Association
www.americanheart.org

American Heart Association Stroke Connection
(800) 553-6321
Brain Attack Coalition
www.stroke-site.org

National Stroke Association
(800) STROKES
www.stroke.org

References

American Heart Association: Medical/scientific statement: guidelines for the management of transient ischemic attacks, *Stroke* 25:1320-1335, 1994.

Auer J et al: C-reactive protein and coronary artery disease, *Jpn Heart J* 43(6):607-619, 2002.

Benzaquen LR, Yu H, Rifai N: High sensitivity C-reactive protein: an emerging role in cardiovascular risk assessment, *Crit Rev Clin Lab Sci* 39(4-5):459-497, 2002.

Brice JH et al: Stroke: from recognition by the public to management by emergency medical services, *Prehospital Emergency Care* 6(1):99-106, 2002.

Case CC, Ballantyne CM: Statins and inflammatory markers, *Current Atherosclerosis Reports* 4(1):42-47, 2002.

Cingozbay BY et al: Role of homocysteine for thromboembolic complication in patients with non-valvular atrial fibrillation, *Blood Coagul Fibrinolysis* 13(7):609-613, 2002.

Crawford KM, Talbert RL: Antiplatelet therapy in secondary stroke prevention, *Expert Opin Pharmacother* 2(10):1609-1613, 2001.

Farmer JA, Torre-Amione G: Atherosclerosis and inflammation, *Curr Atherosclerosis Rep* 4(2):92-98, 2002.

Gladstone DJ, Black SE, Hakim AM: Toward wisdom from failure: lessons from neuroprotective stroke trials and new therapeutic directions, *Stroke* 33(8):2123-2136, 2002.

Gotto AM Jr: Statins and C-reactive protein: considering a novel marker of cardiovascular risk, *Prev Cardiol* 5(4):200-2003, 2002.

Harraf F et al: A multicentre observational study of presentation and early assessment of acute stroke, *BMJ* 325(7354):17, 2002.

Hennekens CH: Primary prevention of cardiovascular disease and stroke, Up To Date Web Site: www.uptodate.com, 2002.

Kernan WN et al: Insulin resistance and risk for stroke, *Neurology* 59(6):809-815, 2002.

Magadle R et al: C-reactive protein as a marker for active coronary artery disease in patients with chest pain in the emergency room, *Clin Cardiol* 25(10):456-460, 2002.

Meschia JF, Miller DA, Brott TG: Thrombolytic treatment of acute ischemic stroke, *Mayo Clin Proc* 77(6):542-551, 2002.

National Heart, Lung, and Blood Institute: *Third Report of the Expert Panel on Detection, Evaluation, and Treatment of High Blood Cholesterol in Adults (Adult Treatment Panel III)*. Available at www.nhlbi.nih.gov/guidelines/cholesterol/. Accessed 5/19/03.

Ramirez-Lassepas M: Stroke and the aging of the brain and arteries, *Geriatrics* 53(suppl 1):s44-s48, 1998.

Ridker PM et al: Comparison of C-reactive protein and low-density lipoprotein cholesterol levels in the prediction of first cardiovascular events, *N Engl J Med* 347(20):1557-1565, 2002.

Stone NJ, Van Horn L: Therapeutic Lifestyle Change and Adult Treatment Panel III: evidence then and now, *Curr Atherosclerosis Rep* 4(6):433-443, 2002.

Straus SE, Majumdar SR, McAlister FA: New evidence for stroke prevention, *JAMA* 288(11):1388-1395, 2002.

Van Der Meer IM et al: C-reactive protein predicts progression of atherosclerosis measured at various sites in the arterial tree: the Rotterdam study, *Stroke* 33(12):2750-2755, 2002.

Weinberger J: Stroke and TIA: prevention and management of cerebrovascular events in primary care, *Geriatrics* 57(1):38-43, 2002.

Yoon SS, Byles J: Perceptions of stroke in the general public and patients with stroke: a qualitative study, *BMJ* 324(7345):1065, 2002.

Zebrack JS, Anderson JL: Role of inflammation in cardiovascular disease: how to use C-reactive protein in clinical practice, *Prog Cardiovasc Nurs* 17(4):174-185, 2002.

Zerwic JJ, Ennen K, DeVon HA: Stroke: risks, recognition, and return to work, *AAOHN J* 50(8):354-359, 2002.

25

Neuro/Psychiatric: Dementia, Delirium, and Depression

The three D's—dementia, delirium, and depression—are common conditions in the older population. They often occur simultaneously in various combinations and they are often not adequately diagnosed. It is important to recognize each condition's uniqueness so that their common aspects will not hinder making an accurate diagnosis in a complicated older person. This chapter aims to provide information to assist the primary care provider in discerning between these conditions in the older adult and to confirm the diagnosis and treat the appropriate condition.

Dementia is a slowly progressive, generally irreversible loss of intellectual function. The disease affects both recent and remote memory, but a clear state of consciousness and alertness are maintained. Depression occurs in 20% to 30% of people with dementia. Because it can resemble cognitive impairment, it may not be readily identified. Depressive symptoms include weight loss, anhedonia, early morning arising, vague somatic complaints, and sleep disturbances. *Delirium* is characterized by disorganized thinking, a decreased attention span, lowered or fluctuating level of consciousness, disturbances in the sleep-wake cycle, disorientation, and changes in psychomotor activity (Henry, 2002). Unlike dementia, *delirium* has an acute onset and, if treated appropriately, is reversible. It can frequently be correlated to a specific cause, including a reaction to medications (particularly anticholinergics such as diphenhydramine), polypharmacy, or an acute illness (particularly infection or a metabolic disorder). Figure 25-1 provides an algorithm for the evaluation of underlying causes of delirium. Although delirium is most commonly thought to involve agitation and hyperactivity, researchers are finding that hypoactive symptoms such as lethargy and reduced psychomotor activity are actually more common but are less frequently identified. Those with dementia are more likely to develop delirium by twofold to fivefold. In addition, patients who develop delirium in the hospital are more likely to die within 3 years of hospital discharge, even when variables such as comorbid illness, age, and baseline functional status are controlled (Henry, 2002). Table 25-1 outlines the clinical features of delirium, dementia, and depression.

Delirium

Delirium in older patients is a medical emergency, and interventions to prevent it must be initiated for those at risk. It has been suggested that delirium develops when people made vulnerable by factors such as cognitive impairment, advanced age, severe illness, and sensory deficits are confronted with

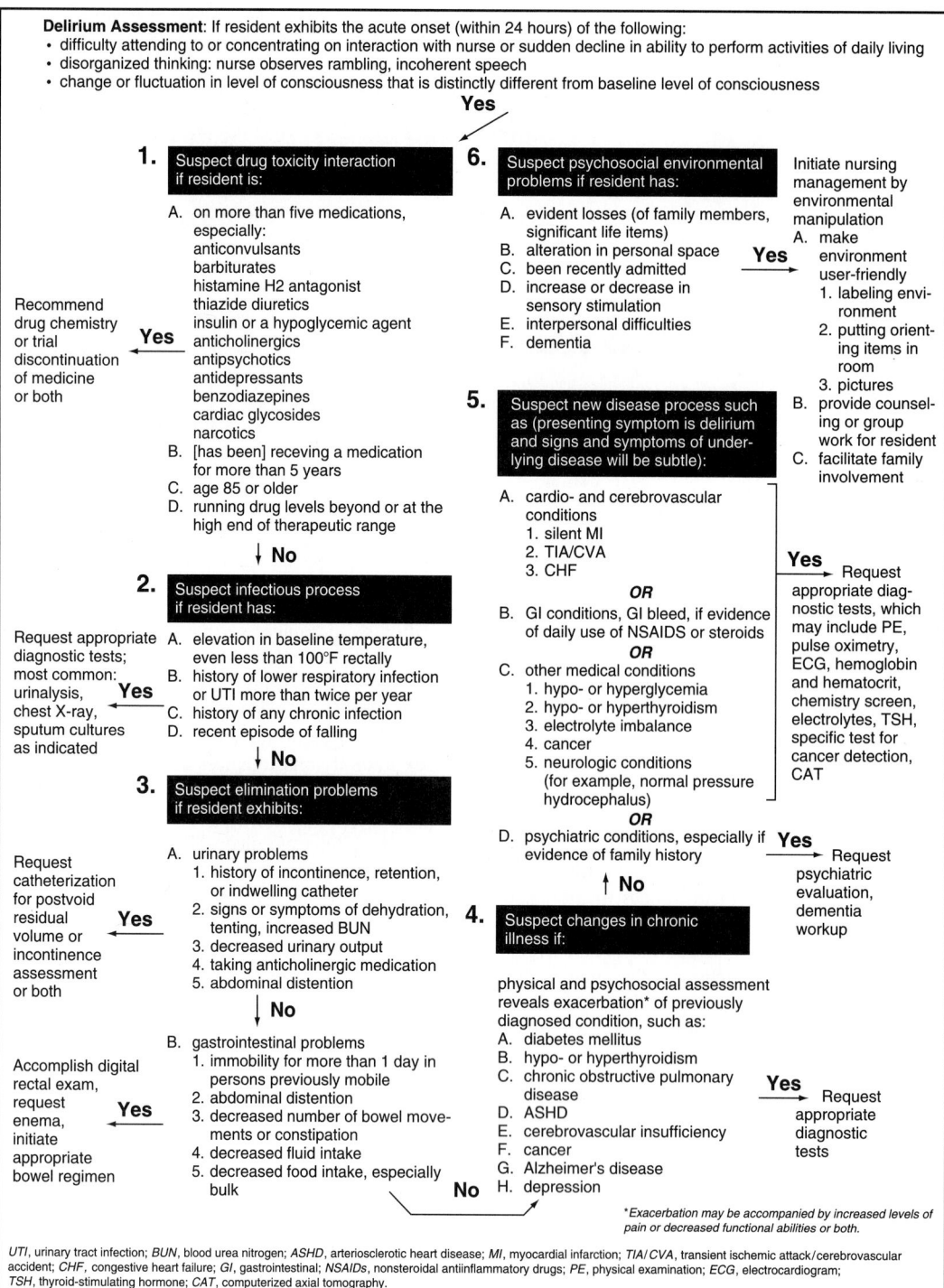

Delirium Assessment: If resident exhibits the acute onset (within 24 hours) of the following:
- difficulty attending to or concentrating on interaction with nurse or sudden decline in ability to perform activities of daily living
- disorganized thinking: nurse observes rambling, incoherent speech
- change or fluctuation in level of consciousness that is distinctly different from baseline level of consciousness

Yes

1. Suspect drug toxicity interaction if resident is:

Recommend drug chemistry or trial discontinuation of medicine or both ← **Yes**

A. on more than five medications, especially:
anticonvulsants
barbiturates
histamine H2 antagonist
thiazide diuretics
insulin or a hypoglycemic agent
anticholinergics
antipsychotics
antidepressants
benzodiazepines
cardiac glycosides
narcotics
B. [has been] receiving a medication for more than 5 years
C. age 85 or older
D. running drug levels beyond or at the high end of therapeutic range

↓ **No**

2. Suspect infectious process if resident has:

Request appropriate diagnostic tests; most common: urinalysis, chest X-ray, sputum cultures as indicated ← **Yes**

A. elevation in baseline temperature, even less than 100°F rectally
B. history of lower respiratory infection or UTI more than twice per year
C. history of any chronic infection
D. recent episode of falling

↓ **No**

3. Suspect elimination problems if resident exhibits:

Request catheterization for postvoid residual volume or incontinence assessment or both ← **Yes**

A. urinary problems
1. history of incontinence, retention, or indwelling catheter
2. signs or symptoms of dehydration, tenting, increased BUN
3. decreased urinary output
4. taking anticholinergic medication
5. abdominal distention

↓ **No**

Accomplish digital rectal exam, request enema, initiate appropriate bowel regimen ← **Yes**

B. gastrointestinal problems
1. immobility for more than 1 day in persons previously mobile
2. abdominal distention
3. decreased number of bowel movements or constipation
4. decreased fluid intake
5. decreased food intake, especially bulk

No

6. Suspect psychosocial environmental problems if resident has:

A. evident losses (of family members, significant life items)
B. alteration in personal space
C. been recently admitted
D. increase or decrease in sensory stimulation
E. interpersonal difficulties
F. dementia

Yes →

Initiate nursing management by environmental manipulation
A. make environment user-friendly
1. labeling environment
2. putting orienting items in room
3. pictures
B. provide counseling or group work for resident
C. facilitate family involvement

5. Suspect new disease process such as (presenting symptom is delirium and signs and symptoms of underlying disease will be subtle):

A. cardio- and cerebrovascular conditions
1. silent MI
2. TIA/CVA
3. CHF
OR
B. GI conditions, GI bleed, if evidence of daily use of NSAIDS or steroids
OR
C. other medical conditions
1. hypo- or hyperglycemia
2. hypo- or hyperthyroidism
3. electrolyte imbalance
4. cancer
5. neurologic conditions (for example, normal pressure hydrocephalus)
OR
D. psychiatric conditions, especially if evidence of family history

↑ **No**

Yes → Request appropriate diagnostic tests, which may include PE, pulse oximetry, ECG, hemoglobin and hematocrit, chemistry screen, electrolytes, TSH, specific test for cancer detection, CAT

Yes → Request psychiatric evaluation, dementia workup

4. Suspect changes in chronic illness if:

physical and psychosocial assessment reveals exacerbation* of previously diagnosed condition, such as:
A. diabetes mellitus
B. hypo- or hyperthyroidism
C. chronic obstructive pulmonary disease
D. ASHD
E. cerebrovascular insufficiency
F. cancer
G. Alzheimer's disease
H. depression

Yes → Request appropriate diagnostic tests

Exacerbation may be accompanied by increased levels of pain or decreased functional abilities or both.

UTI, urinary tract infection; *BUN*, blood urea nitrogen; *ASHD*, arteriosclerotic heart disease; *MI*, myocardial infarction; *TIA/CVA*, transient ischemic attack/cerebrovascular accident; *CHF*, congestive heart failure; *GI*, gastrointestinal; *NSAIDs*, nonsteroidal antiinflammatory drugs; *PE*, physical examination; *ECG*, electrocardiogram; *TSH*, thyroid-stimulating hormone; *CAT*, computerized axial tomography.

Figure 25-1 Six areas in which to search for underlying causes of delirium. (Mentes J (1995). A nursing protocol to assess for causes of delirium. Journal of Gerontological Nursing 21(2), 26-30.)

TABLE 25-1	**Clinical Features of Delirium, Dementia, and Depression**		

Feature	*Acute Confusion or Delirium*	*Dementia*	*Depression*
Onset	Acute or subacute, often at twilight	Chronic, generally insidious	Coincides with life changes; often abrupt
Course	Short, diurnal fluctuations in symptoms; worse at night, in the dark, and on awakening	Long, no diurnal effects, symptoms progressive yet relatively stable over time	Diurnal effects, typically worse in the morning; situational fluctuations but less than in delirium
Progression	Abrupt	Slow but even	Variable, uneven
Duration	Hours to less than 1 month, seldom longer	Months to years	At least 2 weeks, but can be several months to years
Awareness	Reduced	Clear	Clear
Alertness	Lethargic or hypervigilant; fluctuates	Generally normal	Normal
Attention	Impaired, fluctuates	Generally normal	Minimal impairment but is distractible
Orientation	Generally impaired; fluctuates in severity	May be impaired	Selective disorientation
Memory	Recent and immediate impaired	Recent and remote impaired	Selective or patchy impairment; "islands" of intact memory
Thinking	Disorganized, distorted, fragmented, slowed or accelerated; speech is incoherent	Difficulty with abstraction; thoughts impoverished; judgment judgment impaired; words difficult to find	Intact but with themes of hopelessness, helplessness, or self-deprecation
Perception	Distorted; illusions, delusions, and hallucinations; difficulty distinguishing between reality and misperceptions	Misperceptions often absent	Intact; delusions and hallucinations absent except in severe cases
Psychomotor Behavior	Variable, hypokinetic, hyperkinetic, or mixed	Normal, may have apraxia	Variable, psychomotor retardation or agitation
Sleep–Wake Cycle	Disturbed; cycle may be reversed	Fragmented	Disturbed, often early morning awakening
Associated Features	Variable affective changes; symptoms of autonomic hyperarousal; exaggeration of personality type; associated with physical illness	Affect superficial, inappropriate, and labile; attempts to conceal deficits in intellect; cality personality changes; aphasia; agnosia; lack of insight	Affect depressed; exaggerated and detailed complaints; preoccupation with personal thoughts; insight present; verbal elaboration
Mental Status Testing	Distracted from task	Failings highlighted by family; frequent "near miss" answers; struggles with test; great effort to find on appropriate reply	Failings highlighted by the patient; frequent "don't know" answers; little effort; frequently gives up; indifferent, does not care or attempt to find answer

From Henry M: Descending into delirium, *Am J Nurs* 102 (3):49-56, 2002.

one or more noxious insults; even a relatively benign insult may lead to delirium in the presence of multiple vulnerabilities (Henry, 2002). Preventive measures that have proven successful in decreasing the incidence of delirium in hospitalized older patients include compensating for sensory deficits by providing the patient with glasses and hearing aides; instituting ambulation or range-of-motion activities three times a day; avoiding multiple new medications; minimizing the use of immobilizing devices, such as indwelling catheters and physical restraints; encouraging fluid intake to maintain hydration; and using warm milk, herbal teas, relaxation tapes, music, and massage to induce sleep and relieve anxiety (Henry, 2002). Other helpful interventions include minimizing the number of invasive procedures and stimuli that may be misperceived by the patient, such as noise (from television, intercoms, floor buffers, and monitor alarms) or recently mopped floors, and not attempting to convince the patient that what he or she perceives is false. It is more helpful to join confused and agitated patients in their reality than to insist that they join ours; integrating simple orienting statements into conversations with the patient, such as "Isn't it beautiful this morning?" or "It sure seems warm for March"; allowing the patient to participate in his or her own care (brushing the teeth, washing his or her face); using a low, clear calming voice and maintaining eye contact; and maximizing nutrition and hydration. Other interventions include encouraging family visits, using bed alarms and wander guards, providing adequate analgesia, and creating a more familiar environment by having objects brought from home (Henry, 2002).

Antipsychotics and benzodiazepines are frequently used to control agitation, but they should be used at the lowest possible therapeutic dosages if at all because vulnerability to adverse effects, including worsening delirium, is high. Although the neuroleptic haloperidol has been used for years, risperidone is now gaining popularity because it produces less sedation and fewer extrapyramidal symptoms and anticholinergic effects, such as dry mouth, constipation, and urinary retention (Henry, 2002).

Dementia

Dementia is an organic disorder that entails a loss of intellectual abilities of sufficient severity to interfere with social or occupational functioning. The deficit is multifaceted and involves memory, judgment, and abstract thought. Behavioral and personality changes also occur in an alert person. An estimated 45% of persons experience some cognitive decline by 85 years of age (Sable, Dunn, and Zisook, 2002).

The main etiologic factor in the development of primary dementia is advanced age. At present no known definite cause of most dementia-type illnesses has been determined, although infections, medications, metabolic disorders, toxic chemicals, neurologic disorders, nutritional disorders, vascular disorders, and space-occupying lesions can cause or contribute to the development of dementia (Box 25-1).

ALZHEIMER'S DISEASE

Alzheimer's disease (AD) can be categorized into two types: *familial* AD, an inherited form, and *sporadic* AD, in which no obvious inheritance pattern is seen. Age of onset is used to categorize AD. Early onset AD occurs in persons younger than 65 years of age, whereas late-onset AD occurs in persons 65 years of age and older. Early onset AD is rare (5%-10% of all cases) and generally affects persons 30 to 60 years of age (Marin, Sewell, and Schlechter, 2002).

The hallmark neuropathologic signs of AD are beta-amyloid-rich plaques, tau-rich neurofibrillary tangles, and neuronal degeneration. Increasing numbers of plaques and tangles are seen with aging, and yet their cortical and limbic location and concentration in AD distinguishes the illness from normal aging (Marin, Sewell, and Schechter, 2002).

Neurotransmitter deficits are another hallmark of AD. Cholinergic deficits are ubiquitously observed and increase with dementia severity. The importance of acetylcholine in AD has been shown empirically by the efficacy of cholinesterase inhibitors for the treatment of the illness.

Box 25-1

Diseases and Disorders That Can Cause Dementia

Central Nervous System Disorders

Alzheimer's disease (primary degenerative dementia)
Huntington's disease
Pick's disease (primary degenerative dementia)
Parkinson's disease

Systemic Disorders

Cardiovascular disease
  Cerebral hypoxia or anoxia
  Vascular dementia (including multi-infarct dementia)
  Cardiac arrhythmias
  Inflammatory diseases of blood vessels
Deficiency states
  Cyanocobalamin deficiency
  Folic acid deficiency
Effects of drugs
Effects of toxins
Endocrine and metabolic disorders
  Thyroid disease
  Parathyroid disease
  Pituitary-adrenal disorders
Infectious processes
  Acquired immunodeficiency syndrome
  Creutzfeldt-Jakob disease
  Cryptococcal meningitis
  Neurosyphilis
Liver disease
  Chronic progressive hepatic encephalopathy
Neoplastic conditions
  Intracranial tumors
Pulmonary disease
  Respiratory encephalopathy
Urinary tract disease
  Chronic uremic encephalopathy
  Progressive uremic encephalopathy (dialysis dementia)

Miscellaneous Disorders

Hepatolenticular degeneration
Hydrocephalic dementia
Sarcoidosis

From Buckwalter K, Buckwalter J: Chronic cognitive dysfunction (dementia), *Arch Am Acad Orthop Surg* (1)20-32, 1998.

Other neurotransmitters, including norepinephrine, corticotropin-releasing factor, and glutamate, are also involved in cognition and AD (Marin, Sewell, and Schlechter, 2002).

Dementia patients frequently develop depression; the reported prevalence of clinically meaningful depressive symptoms in patients with AD ranges from 17% to 31% (Sable, Dunn, and Zisook, 2002). Distinguishing these symptoms from the "natural" course of AD is often difficult.

VASCULAR DEMENTIA

Vascular dementia is frequently associated with hypertension and cardiovascular disease. AD is characterized by degeneration and loss of neurons as well as the presence of amyloid plaques and neurofibrillary tangles within the brain. Whereas the deterioration seen in AD is gradually progressive, that of vascular dementia is often stepwise in response to vascular events such as subclinical strokes (Henry, 2002).

Age-related Changes

Cognitive ability is influenced by a person's state of health, genetic code, past experiences, educational background, cultural influences and beliefs, and current living conditions. Physical changes in the brain caused as a result of the normal process of aging and selected pathologic conditions may also affect the cognitive abilities of some older persons (Box 25-2). When cognitive abilities fall to a level that precludes a person's ability to care for himself or herself, health problems occur.

Scientists disagree about what universal changes occur in the human brain and how these changes relate to cognitive function. Agreement has been reached that the following changes do occur in association with aging: loss in brain volume and brain weight, enlargement of the ventricles, decrease in enzymes, loss of protein, loss of lipids, and alterations in the amount of and receptors for some neurotransmitters.

The extent of the contribution of these age-related changes to each aging person's cognitive abilities is unknown. The most significant functional loss related to neurologic change is the slowed response time to tasks and the increase in time needed to recover from physical exertion. Nonetheless, the ability of the human body to adjust to age-related alterations and the ability of the human spirit to be resilient in the face of physical loss must not be overlooked or devalued.

COGNITIVE CHANGES

Cognitive changes or declines do not develop uniformly, neither across all areas of cognitive functioning nor at the same rate in all persons. The diversity in older people is evident in this realm as loss begins from each person's level of acquired cognitive abilities.

Memory is the first area of cognition to be affected as the capacity of the brain to process, store, and retrieve information begins to function less efficiently. Because of this change, word finding becomes a slower and more difficult process for the individual patient.

Box 25-2

Normal Changes in the Brain with Aging

Neuron death in some brain regions (although not neurons important to learning)
Decline of neuron function, especially neurons important to learning, memory, and planning
Gradual accumulation of protein plaques and neurofibrillary tangles
Increased fragility of cellular mitochondria that results in diminished cell function
Increased inflammation
Increased oxidative stress

From Marin DB, Sewell MC, Schlechter A: Alzheimer's disease: accurate and early diagnosis in the primary care setting, *Geriatrics* 5(2):36-40, 2002.

Risk Factors

Just what constitutes lifetime risk for the development of a dementia-type illness is a matter of debate. The risk depends on life expectancy, gender, and disease incidence because of the ample probability of mortality from other competing illness or injury. The apolipoprotein E epsilon-4 allele, high cholesterol levels, and high systolic blood pressure all have been shown to increase independently the risk for AD (Kivipelto et al, 2002). Early onset AD has been frequently associated with genetic abnormalities. Although the overall number of familial AD cases is small, nearly half are linked with mutations in one of three genes: amyloid-precursor protein (APP), presenilin-1, and presenilin-2. The genes are found on chromosomes 21, 14, and 1, respectively. Presenilin-1 and –2 are known to cause the most aggressive form of familial AD.

Persons who inherit one or two copies of the apolipoprotein E epsilon-4 allele on chromosome 19 also are at higher risk for late-onset AD (although its presence does not ensure development of AD; so genetic testing is not routinely recommended for the diagnosis of AD) (Marin, Sewell, and Schlechter, 2002). All forms of AD share the same neuropathic features and treatment recommendations.

Several studies have demonstrated a higher age-specific prevalence of dementia, cumulative risk of AD, and incidence rates among African Americans compared with non-Hispanic whites (Green et al, 2002).

Atrial fibrillation is an independent risk factor for vascular dementia by association with the risk of silent cerebral infarction. Antithrombotic therapy may protect patients at risk. Disorders that worsen cerebral blood flow, such as head injury or coronary artery disease, are considered risk factors by those who suggest that the pathogenesis of AD is related to impaired vascular delivery of nutrients to the brain.

Predictors of shorter survival (i.e., at 3 and 7 years of a dementia-type disease) are older age, male, low education, comorbidity, and functional disability.

Epidemiology and Economics

Prevalence rates for dementia range from 6% to 8% in community-dwelling persons over 65 years of age to nearly 75% among residents in nursing homes and chronic care facilities. Of the four most common dementia types (AD, diffuse Lewy body dementia, frontotemporal dementia, and vascular dementia), about 50% of the cases are AD. Prevalence of dementia increases with age, doubling every 5 years after age 60, indicating that at least 30% of the U.S. population over 85 years of age have AD (Marin, Sewell, and Schlechter, 2002). These numbers are expected to increase dramatically, with projections that 1 in 45 older Americans will be affected by AD by 2050 (Marin, Sewell and Schlechter, 2002). This is occurring for two reasons:

1. Mortality rates in the older population have declined consistently over the past 30 years, leading to a major increase in the number of persons 75 years of age and older, particularly those 85 years of age and older.
2. Those who develop the disease are likely to be diagnosed and live longer because care is available to treat infections and other life-threatening conditions.

Mortality attributed to dementia-type disease has increased significantly during the last 20 years. In the United States dementia is an extremely frequent cause of morbidity and mortality. Rates vary widely, and death certificates grossly underestimate and underreport dementia as a cause of death.

The cost of dementia care in the United States is difficult to approximate because much of the care is done by the private and informal care-giving system of relatives and friends. It is clear that costs increase dramatically as the severity of the disease progresses. The ability to delay onset of the disease or to delay the progression could have a major impact on the cost of care. Effectiveness of interventions can be measured not only by costs but also by changes in the patient's cognitive functioning, years of life gained, and quality of life in those years.

Diagnostic Criteria

Although a definitive diagnosis of AD can be made only at autopsy, the primary care provider can make a highly accurate and reliable clinical diagnosis more than 90% of the time (Marin, Sewell, and Schlechter, 2002). The first goal is to rule out other causes of dementia. AD is often considered a diagnosis of exclusion.

The hallmark, classic first symptom of mild-stage AD is memory loss. Accompanying symptoms include aphasia, apraxia, agnosia, and impaired executive functioning. These deficits manifest in word-finding difficulty, difficulty performing familiar tasks, disorientation, and deficits in judgment and problem solving. Changes in personality and behavioral symptoms are common during the course of the illness. The onset of AD is gradual and is characterized by progressive decline in cognition and function. Sensory and motor functions typically are not significantly affected until well into disease progression (Marin, Sewell, and Schlecter, 2002).

Neuropsychiatric symptoms of dementia include noncognitive symptoms such as apathy, depression, or psychosis. *Apathy,* defined by the loss of drive, motivation, or lack of feeling or emotion, is the most common neuropsychiatric symptom in AD and increases with disease progression. Psychosis in dementia usually includes delusions (frequently persecutory) and hallucinations (mostly visual). Patients with frontotemporal dementia exhibit different behaviors, often including socially aberrant behavior. The frequency of delusions and visual hallucinations is increased in Parkinson's disease (PD) with dementia and in dementia with Lewy bodies, suggesting common mechanisms such as Lewy body pathology and cholinergic deficiency (Assal and Cummings, 2002).

The duration of AD averages 10 years, with a range of 3 to 20 years (Marin, Sewell, and Schlecter, 2002). Progression of the disease and the dimensions of any one symptom vary from person to person.

A. Development of multiple cognitive deficits manifests by the following:
   1. Memory impairment (short- and long-term memory impairment)
   2. One or more of the following cognitive disturbances:
      a. Aphasia: Difficulty with use of language, which may involve forgetting simple words or substituting one for another with a similar sound
      b. Apraxia: Difficulty in performing motor activities despite intact physical functioning
      c. Agnosia: Failure to recognize or identify objects in spite of intact sensory function
      d. Disturbance in executive functioning: Problem solving; the ability to plan, organize, or think in abstract terms (e.g., difficulty in defining words or detecting similarities, as in comparing a dog and a lion and clock drawing).
B. The cognitive deficits in A each cause significant impairment in social or occupational functioning and represent a significant decline from a previous level of functioning.
C. The course is characterized by gradual onset and continuing cognitive decline.
D. The cognitive deficits in A are not caused by any of the following:
   1. Other central nervous system conditions that cause progressive deficits in memory and cognition
   2. Systemic conditions that are known to cause dementia
   3. Substance-induced conditions
E. Deficits do not occur during the course of a delirium.
F. The disturbance is not better accounted for by another axis I disorder (major depression, schizophrenia).

COMMON BEHAVIORAL PROBLEMS

- Concealed memory losses (confabulation)
- Wandering
- Sleep disturbances
- Losing and hiding things
- Inappropriate sexual behavior
- Repeating questions and phrases (perseveration)

CRITERIA FOR VASCULAR DEMENTIA

In contrast to AD, in which there are few identifiable physical findings, multiinfarct dementia is identified by the following characteristics:

- A history of high blood pressure
- Recurrent strokes or emboli, which may have affected other organs
- Rapid, as opposed to slow and insidious, onset
- A fluctuating course, with stepwise deterioration (a period of decline in cognitive functioning may be followed by some degree of improvement as compensatory brain function occurs)
- Relative preservation of personality
- Nocturnal confusion compared with relative lucidity during the day
- Distinctive neurologic signs such as weakness of arms or legs, defects in the visual fields, or diminished reflexes (these vary from case to case, depending on the areas of the brain that have been affected)
- Same as A, B, and E under Diagnostic Criteria, plus focal neurologic signs and symptoms or laboratory evidence of cerebrovascular disease (multiple infarctions involving cortex and underlying white matter) that is judged to be etiologically related to the disturbance

INCLUSION CRITERIA

- Dementia established by clinical examination and documented by standardized mental status examination or neuropsychological tests
- Deficits in two or more areas of cognition
- Progressive worsening of memory and other cognitive functions
- No disturbance of consciousness
- Onset between 40 and 90 years of age
- Absence of systemic disorders or other brain diseases

SUPPORTING CRITERIA (PROBABLE DIAGNOSIS OF ALZHEIMER'S DISEASE)

- Progressive deterioration of specific cognitive functions
- Impaired activities of daily living (ADL) and altered patterns of behavior
- Family history of similar disorders
- Normal lumbar puncture
- Normal-pattern electroencephalogram
- Evidence of progression of cerebral atrophy documented by computed tomography

EXCLUSION CRITERIA

- Sudden, apoplectic onset
- Focal neurologic findings
- Seizures or gait disturbance early in the course of disease

DIAGNOSTIC WORKUP

- History and physical examination, preferably with a provider who knows the patient well.
- Neurologic examination, including assessment of focal findings, laterality, tremor, and gait changes. The presence of frontal release signs (reemergence of certain primitive reflexes such as grasping, sucking, or groping, that are normally present in infants) is useful in differentiating normal aging or vascular dementia from AD (Marin, Sewell, and Schlecter, 2002).
- Careful mental status examination, including brief standardized mental status tests
- Laboratory: Complete blood count; electrolytes, calcium level; thyroid-stimulating hormone; vitamin B_{12}, Venereal Disease Research Laboratories (VDRL), and other laboratory tests warranted by examination findings and risk assessment, including human immunodeficiency virus (HIV) and Lyme disease titers
- Lumbar puncture (not routinely recommended) may be useful to rule out metastatic disease or an unusual presentation; also may be done to rule out normal pressure hydrocephalus

- ADL assessment
- Instrumental ADL (IADL) assessment
- Depression screening
- Social assessment (home visit preferable)
- Drug review
- Nutritional evaluation
- Neurologic imaging assessments
- Magnetic resonance imaging/computerized tomography or structural imaging scans: Not recommended as routine by consensus groups; may demonstrate atrophy, which is not helpful in the diagnosis; white-matter changes, the significance of which has not been determined; space-occupying lesions; hydrocephalus, and vascular disease
- Single-photon emission computed tomography/positron emission tomography or functional imaging: Provides information on neuronal functioning by measuring cerebral blood flow and glucose uptake; can help differentiate AD from other dementias by revealing parietotemporal hypometabolism and right/left asymmetry; can reveal evidence for vascular dementias by identifying focal asymmetric cortical and subcortical deficits; currently being used in some clinical settings to increase the likelihood of specifically diagnosing AD in mild to moderately impaired persons.

   Neuropsychological testing is particularly helpful for distinguishing normal aging, early AD, or depression. A neuropsychological battery typically includes assessment of verbal and nonverbal memory, language, attention, visuospatial and executive functions, and speed of information processing. Neuropsychological testing also is useful for benchmarking the severity of dementia (Marin, Sewell, and Schlecter, 2002).

MINI-MENTAL STATUS EXAMINATION

For more than 25 years, the Mini-Mental State Examination (MMSE) has been the most widely used screening test for simple, rapid assessment of cognitive impairment. It provides a quick screen of cognitive function; however, it is not a diagnostic test for dementia. Items on the MMSE address seven cognitive performance areas totaling 30 points: orientation to place (5 points), orientation to time (5 points), registration (3 points), attention and concentration (5 points), recall (3 points), language abilities (8 points), visual construction (1 point). Points are given for correct responses to specific questions within each area. Strict cutoff scores for the 30-point instrument are not particularly helpful because education level, sensory deficits (especially hearing loss), and tremor can skew test results (Marin, Sewell, and Schlecter, 2002). A score of 24/30 or better is considered normal for those with at least a ninth-grade education. For those with fewer years of schooling, a score of 19 or better is within the normal range (Table 25-2). A decline in the MMSE of 1.8 to 3.2 points per year is typical for patients with Alzheimer's dementia (Likourezos and Lantz, 2001).

Interpretation of the MMSE score should take into account education, economic class, and physical impairments. Hearing, vision, or speech impairment as well as physical disability and frailty may cause a falsely low MMSE score in the absence of cognitive impairment (Likourezos and Lantz, 2001).

The addition of clock-drawing tests and questions that assess judgment when dealing with potentially dangerous situations will provide a more comprehensive clinical cognitive assessment. Having the patient draw the numbers and hands of a clock tests comprehension, planning, conceptualization of time, and visuospatial skills and complements the information obtained from the MMSE (Likourezos and Lantz, 2001).

Differential Diagnoses

- Normal age-related forgetfulness
- Alcohol abuse
- Polypharmacy or drug-related
- Hypothyroidism

TABLE 25-2	MMSE Score and Cognitive Status	

MMSE Score	Cognitive Status	Associated Factors
24 to 30	No cognitive impairment	For patients with at least a high school education, a cutoff of 25 to 28 may indicate impairment The scale is less sensitive in identifying very mild cognitive decline Hearing loss, vision loss, physical frailty may also cause lower scores
19 to 23	Mild cognitive impairment	For those with less than a ninth grade education, a score < 19 is more indicative of true cognitive loss Decline in ADL/IADL may be a problem Clinical correlation between MMSE score and functional status is extremely important
11 to 18	Moderate cognitive impairment	Clinical dementia is typically apparent Loss of ADL skills is common
0 to 10	Severe cognitive impairment	Dementia is advanced; the scale is limited by a floor effect in being unable to monitor decline in those patients who score 0 but maintain some cognition Clinical assessment should focus on functional skills

From Likourezos A, Lantz MS: MMSE: Interpreting mental status examination scores in cases of mild dementia, *Geriatrics* 56(6):55-56, 2001.

- Delirium
- Depression (pseudodementia)
- PD
- Sensory impairment(s)
- Compensatory actions by spouse/family delays diagnosis

Primary Care Issues

Alzheimer's disease is progressive and cannot be halted or reversed; yet some interventions can alleviate suffering, improve coping, and enhance patients' dignity as they live with the disorder. By answering the four clinical questions in Box 25-3, providers can help patients and families deal with behavioral problems that accompany AD (Cohen, 2002).

Other important aspects of care include the following:
- Communicate to the family and patient that judgment and memory impairment are key features.
- Dementia increases mortality; AD is not a benign disease.
- Multiple illnesses are common in older patients and complicated by the presence of AD.
- Medication management is a priority.
- Address advance directives early on.
- Minimize excess disability by identifying and treating other disorders.
- Always refer atypical presentations to a specialist.
- Family members will have multiple needs during the progression of the illness.
- Treatment plans must consider the health of and resources available to the caregiver members.

Clinical Questions to Answer When Managing Behavioral Problems in Alzheimer's Disease

1. Is pharmacologic intervention indicated? If so, what symptom should be targeted (e.g., delusions, depression, anxiety, etc.)?
2. What behavioral and psychosocial interventions could:
   - make the patient's environment less challenging (e.g., written reminders, night lights leading to the bathroom, etc.)?
   - provide structured activities the patient can perform and finds satisfying?
3. Which community services can provide supportive, structured, and supervised activities (e.g., day programs, home care aides)?
4. What interventions and supportive programs could reduce the family caregiver's burden and emotional strain?

From Cohen GD: Alzheimer's disease: managing behavioral problems in patients with progressive dementia, *Geriatrics* 57(2):53-54, 2002.

PHARMACOLOGIC DISEASE MANAGEMENT

Treatment of AD is characterized by two broad clinical goals: managing symptoms (cognitive enhancement) and slowing disease progression (neuroprotection). *Cognitive enhancers* primarily improve cognitive function; *neuroprotection* involves interfering with underlying AD pathology (Marin, Sewell, and Schlecter, 2002).

Cholinesterase inhibitors increase the concentration of acetylcholine to the brain by inhibiting the activity of acetylcholinesterase. They effectively moderate some symptoms and postpone, but do not prevent, cognitive decline; however, the cost savings and enhancement to quality of life that can be achieved by delaying nursing home placement for even 6 months are not insignificant. The U.S. Food and Drug Administration (FDA)-approved cholinesterase inhibitors include donepezil HCL (Aricept), revastigmine tartrate (Exelon), and galantamine hydrobromide (Reminyl). Donepezil has shown benefit not only in ameliorating cognitive deficits but also in relieving depression, anxiety, apathy, delusions, irritability, and disinhibition (Assal and Cummings, 2002).

Table 25-3 provides information about dosing and the side effects of cholinesterase inhibitors. Fifty percent of patients show some response, as measured by the MMSE and assessment of global change. Cholinesterase inhibitor treatment improves cognition in 6 to 12 months; after 6 months of treatment, a responding patient will perform at least one point better on the MMSE (Marin, Sewell, and Schlecter, 2002).

Behavioral problems such as agitation and psychosis associated with dementia may benefit from treatment with neuroleptic medications (Table 25-4)(Cohen, 2002). In addition, most patients with dementia (AD or stroke related) experience depression in the course of the disease and will benefit greatly from antidepressant therapy.

Disease Process

The disease process is marked by slow progression and decline of social and cognitive skills.

STAGE 1

Stage 1 is often indiscernible to all but spouses or those close to the patient on a daily basis. Attempts to hide memory loss are common; withdrawal and depression may be present. Judgment and intellectual and social functioning seem faulty.

TABLE 25-3	Cholinesterase Inhibitors for Treatment of Alzheimer's-type Dementia	
Drug	**Recommended Dosage**	**Side Effects**
Donepezil HCl Aricept	5 mg once daily at bedtime for 4 to 6 wk, then increase to 10 mg once daily	Vomiting, nausea, muscle cramps, diarrhea, asthenia
Rivastigmine tartrate Exelon	1.5 mg bid for at least 2 wk; increase gradually to maximum dose of 6 mg bid, if tolerated	Vomiting, anorexia, asthenia, weight loss
Galantamine hydrobromide Reminyl	4 mg bid for at least 4 wk; if tolerated, increase to 8 mg bid for at least 4 wk; attempt increase to 12 mg bid if tolerated	Nausea, vomiting, anorexia, weight loss

From Marin DB, Sewell MC, Schlecter A: Alzheimer's disease: accurate and early diagnosis in the primary care setting, *Geriatrics* 57(2):36-40, 2002.
bid, Twice daily.

TABLE 25-4	Common Medications Used for Treating Psychosis in Alzheimer's Disease
Medication	**Dose range**
Typical neuroleptics	
Haloperidol (Haldol)	0.25 to 2 mg/d
Perphenazine (Trilafon)	2 to 8 mg/d
Thioridazine HCl (Mellaril)	10 to 100 mg/d
Atypical neuroleptics*	
Olanzapine (Zyprexa)	2.5 to 15 mg/d
Quetiapine fumarate (Seroquel)	25 to 100 mg/d
Risperidone (Risperdal)	0.25 to 2 mg/d

From Cohen GD: Alzheimer's disease: managing behavioral problems in patients with progressive dementia, *Geriatrics* 57(2):53-54, 2002.
*Because they have fewer side effects, the newer atypical neuroleptics have generally replaced the older typical neuroleptics for the treatment of psychotic symptoms associated with AD.

Most Common Symptoms
- Short-term memory loss
- Difficulty learning and retaining new material, which leads to inability to follow directions
- Loss of thinking ability, judgment, and decision-making capacity
- Difficulty completing common tasks (cooking, driving)
- Disorientation; gets lost, cannot find way home
- Loss of time sense

- Loss of physical coordination
- Awareness of memory changes
- Communication loss: Includes forgetting events such as birthdays and names of acquaintances; long pauses between words and sentences; losing track and rambling; repetition; decreasing attention span
- Wandering
- Changes in personality; may become self-centered or passive
- Refusal to give up driving
- Loss of social inhibition
- Changes in emotion, including agitation, depression, and suspiciousness

Managing Communication

- Get the patient's attention in a calm environment.
- Avoid multiple distractions.
- Speak clearly.
- Use one-step commands when giving directions.
- Be willing to repeat and rephrase.
- Avoid traditional reality orientation; orient to season/holidays.

STAGE 2

In stage 2 a decrease in recall and word recognition occurs; attention span is even shorter; digressions increase. Closely related words are often substituted for forgotten words. The patient will have more difficulty understanding and following directions. The most common symptoms of stage 2 are the following:

- Delusions and hallucinations
- Impatience
- Wandering and pacing
- Striking out, physically or verbally
- Hiding things
- Resistance to help
- Intimacy/sexuality issues
- Decreased tolerance for stress
- Catastrophic reactions
- Purposeless behavior
- Motor apraxias
- Compulsive repetitive behavior

Managing Delusions and Hallucinations

- Check eyesight and hearing.
- Use glasses or hearing aid, if needed.
- Avoid confusing noises (e.g., pagers, background radios, television).
- Ignore the delusion/hallucination if it is not frightening.
- Avoid contradicting or arguing about the delusion or hallucination.
- Distraction sometimes helps.
- False accusations (e.g., of unfaithfulness) may represent a need for reassurance.
- Recognize the underlying emotions. Give comfort if you can.
- Find new ways to deal with the problem. Example: If the patient is anxiously awaiting the arrival of her mother (long dead), do not tell her that her mother died 10 years ago. This type of reality is harmful to a distressed person who has lost intellectual capacity. Deal with the anxiety in a caring manner. If you are comfortable with saying, "Mother called to say she isn't coming today," consider saying that. Otherwise reassure her as best you can by saying, "Your mother isn't here right now, but I can help."

- Remember that delusions/hallucinations may be the symptoms of infection or other disease. When they arise, evaluate for other illnesses.

Other Potential Stage 2 Management Situations

- Promote function; allow patient to do as much as he or she can safely do.
- Control social situations.
- Determine when patient is no longer able to competently manage finances and legal matters.
- To control agitation try white noise, music, nature sounds, dimmed lighting.

STAGE 3

Almost all ability to communicate is lost, and the patient becomes nonverbal. Many patients are bedridden or chairbound and have the lost the ability to walk, talk, and care for themselves.

Management

- Continue speaking quietly with eye contact.
- Pat or stroke the patient. Touch with love.
- Smile.
- Comfort care is appropriate for this stage. The patient is no longer aware of what is happening.
- Long-term-care placement is often best for patients and caregivers at this time.
- Recognize that you have done all you can.
- Assist family members to recognize they have done the best they could. Help them to recall the positive memories of their relative or friend.

Day-to-Day Caregiving
GENERAL PRINCIPLES

- Promote as much function and independence as the patient and situation allow.
- Prevent as much excess disability as long as possible.
- Help, but do not do—as long as possible.

BATHING

- Keep it simple with regular routine. Bathing every day is not necessary.
- Patient may tolerate shower better than bath.
- For tub bathing, fill tub after patient is in the tub–about 6 inches of water.
- Do not use slippery oils or bubble bath.
- Provide support with handrails, tub bench, or chair.

GROOMING

- Hair: Keep in easy-to-care for style. The barber shop or beauty parlor may be the best solution for regular hair care.
- Shaving: Electric razors are easier. Let the patient shave himself or herself as long as possible. Female patients may need help with leg shaving and facial hair.
- Makeup: If a woman is used to wearing makeup, it will enhance her self-image.
- Hand and feet: Trim nails about once a month. It may help to distract the patient with television or music. Bunions and calluses may need care of a podiatrist. A visit every 6 months should be adequate.
- Teeth: Have the patient brush his or her own teeth as long as possible. Schedule visits to the dentist.

TOILETING

- Simplify the process.
- If the patient has trouble finding the bathroom, put a picture on the bathroom door.
- Have the patient wear loose-fitting, easy-to-remove clothing.

- Remind the patient after meals and before going out.
- Respect privacy.

CONSTIPATION

- Constipation can be caused by soft diet, inactivity, some medications, or inadequate fluid.
- Institute high-fiber diet, daily exercise, and five to eight glasses of water daily.
- Consider the need for laxatives.
- Be observant. The patient will not remember or be able to identify constipation symptoms.

URINARY INCONTINENCE

- First, rule out infection.
- Schedule toileting times: prompted voiding. Watch for nonverbal clues.
- Encourage the use of adult absorbency pads.

BOWEL INCONTINENCE

- Bowel incontinence usually develops at the later stages of the disease.
- Check for impaction, drug effect.
- Protective pads will be needed.
- Watch diet to avoid diarrhea-causing foods.
- Provide good skin care to the perianal area.

DRESSING

- Simplify clothing with Velcro, front fastenings, and loose-fitting elastic waistbands.
- Provide tube sox, lace-up, or Velcro shoes.
- Use comfortable fabrics such as cotton.
- If the patient has favorite clothing items, buy duplicates.
- Sort and arrange all clothing by type.
- Put out-of-season clothing away.
- Put accessories with the matching item of clothing.
- Do not offer too many choices.

GLASSES

- Keep more than one pair.
- Get plastic lenses.
- Keep a copy of the prescription.

EATING

- Planning and preparing meals
- Let the patient assist with meal preparation tasks as much as possible.
- Serve favorite foods often.
- Use contrasting colors of dishes and placemats.
- Add extra nutrients to the diet of a patient who is underweight.
- Serve portions to a patient who eats too much.
- Spoons are easier than forks.
- Finger foods are easiest of all.
- Eat together.
- Keep presentation of food simple.

EATING OUT

- Avoid the peak hours to avoid too much stimulation.
- Order for the patient; offer choice of two things.

- Tell the waiter your companion is confused.
- Consider takeout food.

RECREATION

- Recreation can be anything the patient can do and once enjoyed.
- Watching television may confuse some patients with AD.
- Encourage listening to music, especially old favorites.

SUGGESTED ACTIVITIES

- Looking at family photo albums
- Reminiscing
- Music and free form dancing
- Art therapies
- Playing with pets
- Walking the dog
- Stationary bicycle
- Tasks like arranging flatware, piling newspapers, folding clothes

SLEEPING

- Room temperature and bedding should be comfortable.
- Night-lights are invaluable in hallways and bathrooms.
- Encourage a dark room for sleeping.
- Limit daytime naps.

SLEEP-WAKE CYCLE DISTURBANCE

- Establish bedtime routine.
- Use bedroom only for sleep or sexual activity.
- Sexual intimacy depends entirely on agreement between parties. If one person does not want to continue intimacy, separate beds and bedrooms are a good idea.

HOME SAFETY

Accidents happen even in the home without an AD patient. A first-aid kit is a requirement.

Basic Concepts

- Do not change too much.
- Make changes over time as they are needed.
- Make changes that simplify.
- Make changes that make life easier for the caregiver.
- Make a kitchen and bathroom safety list.
- Turn off stoves, unplug them, and remove knobs.
- Put away matches and lighters.
- Unplug electrical equipment in kitchen at night. Use timers or circuit breakers to keep power off.
- Turn hot water temperature down.
- Remove locks from inside bathroom door.
- Be sure that smoke detectors are in working order.
- Remove weapons.
- Lock up potentially dangerous cleaning supplies.

GENERAL SAFETY

- Be sure there is adequate lighting, especially on stairs, entryways, and bathrooms.
- Clear the clutter off stairs. Put railings on both sides.

- Consider covering mirrors. Some patients are afraid of their images.
- Fasten small rugs securely to the floor; do not use high gloss on floors.
- Lock windows.
- Arrange furniture with clear pathways; furniture should be firm, not wobbly.
- Place locks on doors very high or very low to deter patients from wandering out of the house.
- Lock the garage.
- Do not allow driving; the car may have to be disabled.

COMMUNITY SUPPORTS AND RESOURCES

- Family and friends
- Support groups
- Alzheimer's Association (for all types of dementia)
- Church groups
- Caregiver support groups (often sponsored by hospitals, nursing facilities)
- Adult day care
- Professional support
- Registered nurses (RNs)
- Social workers
- Home health aids
- Homemakers
- Geriatric case managers (usually RNs or social workers)
- Adult homes, group homes, or assisted living facilities
- Hospitals and nursing homes
- Long-term care facilities
- Skilled nursing facility
- Long-term care facility (often combined with skilled care)
- Continuing care facility
- Assisted-living facility (may provide some ADL and medication management)

Depression and Suicide

Depression is the most common mental illness among persons over 60 years of age, and aging baby boomers are expected to have a higher risk of depression than older adults thus far. About 15% of older Americans suffer from significant depression, and most treatment occurs in the primary care setting. Depression contributes to increased medical morbidity and mortality, diminished quality of life, and increased health care costs (Sable, Dunn, and Zisook, 2002).

Depression is an affective illness characterized by disturbances in mood, cognition, and behavior. It is often associated with functional impairment and a reduced capacity for pleasure and enjoyment. Too often underdiagnosed and undertreated in the older population, depression contributes to increased medical morbidity and mortality, diminished quality of life, and increased health care costs. Three factors that complicate the diagnosis of depression in older adults are comorbid medical illness, cognitive impairment, and adverse life events (Sable, Dunn, and Zisook, 2002). Common comorbid psychiatric disorders are alcohol use, anxiety, and personality disorders. Older depressed adults are three to four times more likely to have an alcohol use disorder compared with nondepressed older persons, with a prevalence of 15% to 30% in patients with late-life depression (Devanand, 2002).

In older medical outpatients, the prevalence of depression ranges from 7% to 36%. Patients hospitalized for medical reasons experience depressive symptoms at a rate of 10% to 30%. In nursing home residents, the prevalence of major depression is about 10% (Sable, Dunn, and Zisook, 2002).

Depression in older persons increases the risk of subsequent development of AD. Although depressed mood can occur in AD, apathy is the most common mood observed. Major depression, on the other hand, complicates AD in about 11% of cases. Depression complicated by dementia is referred to as a *pseudodementia* or *dementia syndrome of depression*. With appropriate treatment, these cognitive deficits should be reversible. If a patient recovers from the depression and still has a cognitive impairment, the clinician should consider a comorbid memory disorder as well (Marin, Sewell, and Schlecter, 2002).

The consequences of failure to recognize and treat depression in this population are significant, including increased rates of institutional placement, physical illness, and suicide. About two thirds of suicides in the older population are associated with depression, and 25% of all U.S. suicide victims are over 60 years of age. The completed ratio of suicide is 4:1 in older persons compared with 200:1 in the younger population. Older people typically use more lethal and reliable means of suicide such as guns, asphyxiation, and hanging.

Depression in older persons results from a variety of factors, including psychological stress, polypathology, and biochemical changes in the brain. In turn, depression can contribute to increased symptoms from medical illness, higher utilization of health care services, and increased rates of suicide and nonsuicide mortality. Depression may also be caused by various drugs. Overall, however, the pathogenesis of geriatric depression is not well understood (Gareri, De Fazio, and De Sarro, 2002). The leading theory to explain the biologic basis of depression is the monoamine hypothesis. This theory proposes that depression is due to a deficiency in one or more of three monoamines, namely, serotonin, norepinephrine, and dopamine. It is clear, however, that social and emotional factors affect brain chemistry and must be addressed in designing an effective treatment plan.

RISK FACTORS

Female gender is a risk factor for major depression throughout the life cycle, although the gender gap narrows with increasing age (Sable, Dunn, and Zisook, 2002). Other risk factors for depression in the older adult include being single or widowed; the presence of chronic illness; financial strain; lack of social supports; a personal or family history of affective illness; recent admission to a long-term care facility; loss of a body part (i.e., amputation); loss of autonomy, privacy, or functional status; and poorly controlled pain (Greenberg and Lantz, 2002). Alcohol or other substance abuse can play an important role as can the use of other (often prescription) medications.

Comorbid medical illnesses, including PD, AD, and stroke, also are associated with an increased risk of depression (Tables 25-5 and 25-6). Certain medications are also associated with an increased risk of depression (Table 25-7). It is important to evaluate whether any of these associated factors may be contributing to the depressive presentation and to treat them, if possible. Remember that the presence of these illnesses or conditions does not preclude treatment of the depressive syndrome.

Several factors increase the risk of suicide for an older person: personal or family history of mood disorders, living alone, recent death of a spouse or friend, alcohol use or abuse, physical illness and pain, and the feeling of being a burden. Others include recent admission to a long-term care facility; loss of autonomy, privacy, or functional status; expectation of death from some cause; and being a white male (higher rate of suicide than any other group). See Box 25-4 for risk factors associated with suicide.

ASSESSMENT

Depression must always be differentiated from other underlying medical conditions, including dementia. As mentioned before, another condition may not preclude the need to treat the depression as a separate but important entity.

The Diagnostic and Statistical Manual of Mental Disorders, fourth edition (American Psychiatric Association, 1994) provides specific diagnostic criteria for a major depressive disorder (Box 25-5). Table 25-8 compares the DSM-IV criteria with alternate presentations that may be seen in older adults. Key signs of depression include being discouraged or sad; frequently complaining; and being anxious, irritable, agitated or slow, and self-effacing or demanding. There are several mnemonics for remembering the symptoms and behavior changes associated with depression. One of these is SIGECAPS:

TABLE 25-5	Medical Conditions Associated with Depression

Body System	Condition
Neurologic	Alzheimer's disease
	Acquired immunodeficiency syndrome dementia complex
	Brain mass or tumor
	Multiple sclerosis
	Stroke
	Parkinson's disease
Cardiovascular	Congestive heart failure
	Myocardial infarction
	Hypertension
Autoimmune	Rheumatoid arthritis
	Systemic lupus erythematosus
Metabolic	Addison's disease
	Cushing's disease
	Diabetes mellitus
	Hypothyroidism
	Hyperthyroidism
	Hyperparathyroidism
Others	Malignancies (especially pancreatic, lung, colorectal, ovarian, lymphoma)
	Infectious disease
	Malnutrition
	Pancreatic disease
	Metabolic abnormalities
	Pernicious anemia
	Chronic pain syndrome
	Chronic obstructive pulmonary disease
	Rheumatoid arthritis
	Renal dialysis
	Hearing loss

Adapted from Butler RN, Lewis MI: Late-life depression: when and how to intervene, *Geriatrics* 50(8):44-55, 1995.

S = **S**leep disturbance (insomnia or hypersomnia)
I = lack of **I**nterest
G = feelings of **G**uilt
E = decreased **E**nergy
C = decreased **C**oncentration
A = change in **A**ppetite (increased or decreased)
P = **P**sychomotor retardation or agitation
S = **S**uicidal ideation

The initial manifestation of the older person with depression may differ somewhat from that of the younger person. Older adults seem to have more somatic complaints (although some authorities would disagree with this) and an increase in psychotic or delusional symptoms, especially if onset is after age 60 years. Frequently these delusions are of a somatic (cancer), persecutory, or nihilistic

TABLE 25-6	Coexistence of Major Depression and Common Medical Illnesses

Medical illness	*Reported prevalence of major depression*
Stroke	22 to 50%
Cancer	18 to 39%
MI	15 to 19%
Rheumatoid arthritis	13%
Parkinson's disease	10 to 37%
Diabetes mellitus	5 to 11%

From: Sable JA, Dunn LB, Zisook S: Late-life depression: how to identify its symptoms and provide effective treatment, *Geriatrics* 57(2):18-31, 2002.

TABLE 25-7	Medications Associated with Depression*

Antihypertensives	Digoxin	Antimicrobials
Beta blockers*	Analgesics	Ethambutol
Calcium-channel blockers*	NSAIDs	Sulfonamides
ACE inhibitors*	Opiates	Progesterone*
Methyldopa*	L-Dopa	Corticosteroids*
Reserpine*	Benzodiazepines	Barbiturates
Guanethidine	H_2 blockers	Anticholesterolemic
Tamoxifen*	Cyclosporine	agents
Metoclopramide	Disulfiram	HMG-CoA reductase
Baclofen	Interferon-alfa*	inhibitors

From Sable JA, Dunn LB, Zisook S: Late life depression: how to identify its symptoms and provide effective treatment, *Geriatrics* 57(2):18-31, 2002.
*Indicates medications for which the association with depression is more strongly supported by empiric data

nature. Older patients are more likely to experience weight loss, but they may tend to minimize their depressed mood. Other prominent symptoms, such as decreased appetite, sleep, energy, and pleasure, may be attributed to physical illness or to social or economic problems by both the patient and the practitioner. Depressed older persons frequently have concurrent symptoms of anxiety or comorbid anxiety disorders. Such comorbidity is associated with a more severe presentation of depressive illness, including greater suicidal tendencies (Lenze et al, 2002). On obtaining the history, the practitioner often discovers that older patients have had a previous episode of depression at some time in their earlier years.

Primary anxiety disorders are uncommon in later life, and onset in late life is rare. Therefore the newly anxious older patient with a diminished self-attitude, vague "vital sense changes" ("I'm sick, something's wrong"), and a low mood should be suspected of having depression. Older adults may also have a dementia-like syndrome of depression known as *pseudodementia*. One distinguishing factor is that, unlike true dementia, poor performance is usually neither

---

Box 25-4

Risk Factors Associated with Suicide

Sociodemographic Risk Factors

Male sex
Age 60 or older
Widowed or divorced
Caucasian or Native American
Living alone
Unemployed or having financial problems
Recent adverse events, such as job loss or death of someone close

Clinical Risk Factors

Clinical depression or schizophrenia
Substance abuse
History of suicide attempts or ideation
Feeling of hopelessness
Panic attacks
Severe anxiety, particularly if combined with depression
Severe anhedonia

Data from Hirschfeld RMA, Russell JM: Assessment and treatment of suicidal patients, *N Engl J Med* 337(13):910-915, 1997.

Box 25-5

DSM-IV Criteria for Major Depressive Disorder

A. Five or more of the following symptoms for 2 weeks.
   Must include 1 or 2.
   1. Depressed mood
   2. Loss of interest or pleasure
   3. Weight loss or gain
   4. Insomnia or hypersomnia
   5. Psychomotor agitation or retardation
   6. Fatigue
   7. Worthlessness or inappropriate guilt
   8. Decreased concentration or indecisiveness
   9. Thoughts of death or suicidal ideation
B. Not a mixed episode
C. Impaired social, occupational, or other important area of functioning
D. Not secondary to substance abuse or a medical condition
E. Not better accounted for by bereavement

From American Psychiatric Association: *Diagnostic and statistical manual of mental disorders*, ed 4, Washington, DC, 1994, American Psychiatric Association.

---

global nor consistent. Attention and concentration are markedly affected, and the patient usually exhibits less confabulation. For example, when asked what the date is, a demented person might say with confidence that it is 1942, whereas a patient with pseudodementia classically answers, "I don't know." Other distinguishing characteristics of dementia versus pseudodementia follow:

TABLE 25-8	Comparison of DSM-IV Criteria for Major Depression and Alternate Presentations That May Be Seen in Older Adults
DSM-IV criteria for major depression	**Alternate presentations seen in older adults[†]**
Five or more of the following symptoms have been present most of every day for at least 2 weeks and represent a change from previous functioning:[*] Depressed mood Loss of interest or pleasure Weight loss or gain Insomnia or hypersomnia Psychomotor agitation or retardation Fatigue or loss of energy Worthlessness or excessive guilt Decreased concentration/indecisiveness Thoughts of death/suicidal ideation	Irritability Agitation/anxiety/worrying Somatic complaints Cognitive impairment Diminished initiative and problem-solving capacities Deterioration in self-care Alcohol or substance abuse Social withdrawal Excessive guilt Paranoia Obsessions and compulsions Marital discord

Source: Prepared for Geriatrics by Jeremy A. Sable, MD, Laura B. Dunn, MD, and Sidney Zisook, MD, from American Psychiatric Association: *Diagnostic and statistical manual of mental disorders,* ed 4, Washington, DC, 1994, American Psychiatric Association.
[*]At least one of the symptoms is depressed mood or loss of interest or pleasure
[†]Any one of these presentations is a red flag for further evaluation. The combination of irritability, somatic complaints, and social withdrawal is especially suggestive of depression in patients age 85 and older.

Dementia	Pseudodementia
Cognitive changes happen first.	Mood changes occur first.
Mood is labile.	Mood is consistently dysphoric.
Cooperative but inaccurate on Mini-Mental State Examination (MMSE).	Uncooperative or does not try on MMSE.
Aphasia is present.	Aphasia is absent.
Can enjoy things.	Cannot enjoy things.

Simply questioning a patient about mood may be adequate to reveal symptoms of depression. Often, however, it is helpful to use a standardized screening tool such as the Geriatric Depression Scale (short form) to elicit information (Box 25-6). The presence of other medical conditions besides dementia must be determined, as well as the impact of the presenting symptoms on the patient's ability to function on a daily basis. Diagnostic studies for the evaluation of depression are listed in Box 25-7.

TREATMENT

Treatment of depression in older adults begins with the assumption that symptoms may be complicated by physical and cognitive disorders and external stressors (Sable, Dunn, and Zisook, 2002). Several therapies are known to be effective, either alone or in combination, for the treatment of depression including psychotherapy, medications, and electroconvulsive therapy (ECT). Usually the primary care provider can initiate treatment in an outpatient setting. People who do not respond to initial therapy or who have complicated needs such as psychotic or delusional symptoms should be referred to a psychiatrist, preferably one with experience working with the older population.

If the risk of suicide seems imminent, immediate hospitalization is usually required. If the risk of suicide is high but not imminent, it may be helpful to try to involve a family member or another

---

Box 25-6

Yesavage Geriatric Depression Scale (short form)

1. Are you basically satisfied with your life?	Y	N
2. Have you dropped many of your activities and interests?	Y	N
3. Do you feel that your life is empty?	Y	N
4. Do you often get bored?	Y	N
5. Are you in good spirits most of the time?	Y	N
6. Are you afraid that something bad is going to happen to you?	Y	N
7. Do you feel happy most of the time?	Y	N
8. Do you often feel helpless?	Y	N
9. Do you prefer to stay at home, rather than going out and doing a few things?	Y	N
10. Do you feel you have more problems with memory than most?	Y	N
11. Do you think it is wonderful to be alive now?	Y	N
12. Do you feel pretty worthless the way you are now?	Y	N
13. Do you feel full of energy?	Y	N
14. Do you feel that your situation is hopeless?	Y	N
15. Do you think that most people are better off than you are?	Y	N

Score 1 point for each "depressed" answer (no on 1,5,7,11,11,13; yes on others)

Normal:	3 ± 2
Mildly depressed:	7 ± 3
Very depressed:	12 ± 2

Adapted from Sheikh JI, Yesavage JA, Brooks JO III et al: *Int Psychogeriatr* 3:23, 1991.

Box 25-7

Diagnostic Studies for the Evaluation of Depression

- Complete blood count
- Chemistry profile (electrolytes, blood urea nitrogen, creatinine, glucose)
- Serologic test for syphilis (rapid plasma reagin)
- Thyroid studies (thyroid stimulating hormone, T_3, T_4)
- Vitamin B_{12} level (methylmalonic acid/homocysteine if low)
- Folate level
- Human immunodeficiency virus testing
- Urinalysis
- Chest x-ray
- Electrocardiogram

---

person who is close to the patient (with the patient's permission). Increased vigilance and a collaborative approach to dealing with the problem can be suggested and inquiries made about (and document) the availability of firearms and ammunition, potentially lethal medications, and other means of suicide. Contact with the patient, including phone calls and visits, should be increased. Communication of one's commitment to help the patient may be lifesaving. If a psychiatric disorder is present, referral for treatment is crucial, as is referring a patient who is abusing alcohol or any other substance to a comprehensive treatment program.

PSYCHOTHERAPY

For many years it was thought that older patients did not benefit from psychotherapy because they were, as Freud stated in 1904, "no longer educable and, on the other hand, the mass of material to be dealt with would prolong the duration of the treatment indefinitely." Studies have shown, however, that older people do benefit from psychotherapy, either alone or in combination with medications, especially patients with specific stressors or maladaptive personality factors. Unfortunately, because of the social stigma (and sometimes financial issues), many older patients may be unwilling to accept this treatment modality.

PHARMACOTHERAPY

Practitioners must remember that the response to antidepressant therapy may be delayed in this population; so any treatment regimen must be given an adequate trial (4 to 6 weeks). Life-long treatment at full therapeutic doses may be necessary because of the high risk of relapse, recurrence, and suicide in this population.

The decision regarding an initial pharmacotherapeutic agent depends on the following factors:

- The patient's presenting symptoms (e.g., one of the more sedating medications at bedtime might be appropriate for a patient with associated insomnia)
- Coexisting illnesses
- Concurrent medications
- Alterations of pharmacokinetics in older persons
- Side-effect profile of the antidepressant being considered
- Response to prior treatment

If a patient had a positive response in the past to a particular antidepressant, generally that drug should be the initial therapy for subsequent depressive episodes; however, in the case of an older person who has been successfully treated with a tricyclic antidepressant (TCA), increased age and the concomitant prescription of other medications will increase the risk for adverse effects from a TCA. A newer agent may be preferable. If the patient did not respond to a particular antidepressant in the past, an antidepressant from another class should be prescribed initially for subsequent episodes. Whichever drug is used, the average geriatric patient is taking between six and eight medications already, which increases the risk of drug-drug interactions. The geriatric medicine adage of "start low, go slow" should be the rule for dosage.

Pharmacologic treatment of depression in old age is associated with an increased risk of adverse pharmacokinetic and pharmacodynamic drug interactions. Older patients may have multiple disease states and therefore may require a variety of other drugs. In addition to polypharmacy, other factors such as age-related physiologic changes, diseases, genetic constitution, and diet may alter drug response and therefore predispose older patients to adverse effects and drug interactions.

Antidepressant drugs currently available differ in their potential drug interactions. In general, older compounds such as TCAs and monoamine oxidase inhibitors (MAOIs), have a higher potential for interactions than newer compounds, such as selective serotonin reuptake inhibitors (SSRIs) and other relatively novel agents with a more specific mechanism of action (Spina and Scordo, 2002).

Every known antidepressant increases neurotransmission of serotonin, norepinephrine, or dopamine, either alone or in combination. Six classes of antidepressants accomplish this effect by blocking one or more of the reuptake pumps or receptors for these three monoamines. One inhibits an enzyme, namely, monoamine oxidase (MAO) and the remaining class acts as monoamine-releasing agents (central nervous system stimulants). See Table 25-9 for classes and examples of antidepressants.

Increased monitoring for falls is warranted during the acute treatment of late-life depression. When treating these patients, providers should be especially watchful of those with memory impairments or these who develop orthostatic blood pressure changes (Joo et al, 2002).

In treating patients who have anxiety secondary to major depression, antidepressants, not anxiolytics, are the treatment of choice. Remember, however, that patients who may have been taking

TABLE 25-9	Classes of Antidepressants

Class	Antidepressant Medication
Tricyclics (TCA)	Amitriptyline (Elavil)
	Desipramine (Norpramin)
	Doxepin (Sinequan)
	Imipramine (Tofranil)
	Nortriptyline (Pamelor)
Monoamine oxidase inhibitors	Phenelzine (Nardil)
	Tranylcypromine (Parnate)
Selective serotonin reuptake inhibitors	Fluoxetine (Prozac)
	Paroxetine (Paxil)
	Sertraline (Zoloft)
Dual serotonin and norepinephrine reuptake inhibitor (SNRI)	Venlafaxine (Effexor)
Serotonin-2 antagonist/reuptake inhibitors	Nefazodone (Serzone)
	Trazodone (Desyrel)
Norepinephrine and dopamine reuptake inhibitor	Bupropion (Wellbutrin)
Noradrenergic and specific serotonergic antidepressants	Mirtazepine (Remeron)
Psychostimulants	Dextroamphetamine (Dexedrine)
	Methylphenidate (Ritalin)
	Methamphetamine (Desoxyn)
	Pemoline (Cylert)

From Richardson JP, Gallo JJ: Geriatrics for the clinician: treatment of depression in the elderly, *Md Med J* 45(7), 1996; Stahl SM: Basic psychopharmacology of antidepressants, part 1: antidepressants have seven distinct mechanisms of action, *J Clin Psychiatry* 59(4), 1998; Hay DP, Rodriguez MM, Franson KL: Treatment of depression in late life, *Clin Geriatr Med* 14(1), 1998.

benzodiazepines for "anxiety" for several weeks to months are psychologically and physiologically dependent. To treat depression successfully, an antidepressant can be added without changing the benzodiazepine dose initially. Once the antidepressant has had the opportunity to become effective, the patient will be feeling better, and the benzodiazepine can then be tapered and stopped.

Serotonin syndrome is a potentially life-threatening complication of psychopharmacologic drug therapy. The syndrome is produced most often by the concurrent use of two or more drugs that increase brainstem serotonin activity, and it is often unrecognized because of the varied and non-specific nature of its symptoms. Serotonin syndrome is characterized by alterations in cognition, behavior, autonomic nervous system function, and neuromuscular activity. Patients with serotonin syndrome usually respond to discontinuation of drug therapy and supportive care alone, but they may require treatment with a specific antiserotonergic drug. Tables 25-10 and 25-11 discusses several common antidepressants, their dosages, pharmacologic profiles, advantages and disadvantages.

ELECTROCONVULSIVE THERAPY

Electroconvulsive therapy (ECT) is recognized as an effective treatment for depression; however, it is not often used among older patients because of the increased comorbid medical problems and fear of complications (Alao, 2002). ECT can be a safe and effective treatment modality for the psychiatrist to use for older patients with severe depression, those who have psychotic features, those who cannot tolerate or do not have a response to antidepressant medications, or those who have

TABLE 25-10   Tricyclic and SSRI Antidepressants for Use in Older Patients

Drug	Dosage (mg)	Half-life (hr)	Pharmacologic profile	Advantages	Disadvantages
Tricyclics					
Desipramine Norpramin	Initial: 10 Target: 20 to 100	12 to 24	Moderate histaminic, muscarinic, adrenergic (α1) affinity	Least sedating TCA; least anticholinergic TCA; can be activating for daytime use; safety and compliance monitoring with serum levels ≤125 ng/mL	↓ tolerability; risk of cardiotoxicity; narrow therapeutic index; overdose can be lethal
Nortriptyline Aventyl Pamelor	Initial: 10 Target: 20 to 100	20 to 50	Moderate histaminic, muscarinic, adrenergic (α1) affinity	Most extensively studied antidepressant in older patients; lowest rate of orthostatic hypotension; safety and compliance monitoring with serum levels 80 to 120 ng/mL	↓ tolerability; risk of cardiotoxicity; narrow therapeutic index; lethality in overdose
SSRIs				SSRIs as a class Tolerability, safety in overdose; once-daily dosing	SSRIs as a class GI and sexual side effects; agitation or insomnia; discontinuation syndrome; risk of serotonin syndrome; SIADH (rare)

Continued

TABLE 25-10 Tricyclic and SSRI Antidepressants for Use in Older Patients—cont'd

Drug	Dosage (mg)	Half-life (hr)	Pharmacologic profile	Advantages	Disadvantages
Citalopram Celexa	Initial: 10 Target: 10 to 40	36	Most selective affinity for serotonin	May be used IV; minimal drug interactions	See class effects (above)
Fluoxetine Prozac	Initial: 5 to 10 Target: 10 to 80	48 to 72	Active, long-acting metabolites; 21 to 60 days to steady state; higher plasma levels in older patients	Minimal withdrawal symptoms after discontinuation or missed doses; activating	Prolonged side effects and drug interactions due to long half-life
Paroxetine Paxil	Initial: 5 to 10 Target: 10 to 50	24	Moderately adrenergic in high doses; no active metabolites; 7 to 14 days to steady state; higher plasma levels in older patients	Established safety in heart disease	See class effects (above)
Sertraline Zoloft	Initial: 25 Target: 25 to 150	24 to 36	Mildly dopaminergic; 7 to 14 days to steady state; plasma levels comparable in older and younger patients	Tends to be neither activating nor sedating	See class effects (above)

From Sable JA, Dunn LB, Zisook S: Late-life Depression: how to identify its symptoms and provide effective treatment, *Geriatrics* 57(2): 18-31, 2002. *TCA*, Tricyclic antidepressant; *SSRI*, selective serotonin reuptake inhibitor; *SIADH*, syndrome of inappropriate secretion of antidiuretic hormone.

TABLE 25-11	Atypical Antidepressants for Use in Older Patients				
Drug	**Dosage (mg)**	**Half-life (hrs)**	**Pharmacologic profile**	**Advantages**	**Disadvantages**
Bupropion SR Wellbutrin SR	Initial: 100 Target: 100 to 400	21	Norepinephrine/ dopamine reuptake inhibitor; negligible serotonin effect	SR formulation for convenient dosing and fewer side effects; minimal antihistaminic, anticholinergic, and antiadrenergic side effects; benign cardiovascular profile; minimal drug-drug interactions; safety in overdose; no interference with REM sleep; may augment sexual performance; may induce weight loss, improve focus and attention	CNS side effects; headaches, insomnia; agitation, small risk of hypertension
Mirtazapine Remeron	Initial: 7.5 to 15 Target: 15 to 45	20 to 40	α2 antagonist/5-HT$_2$ and 5-HT$_3$ antagonist; strong affinity for histaminic receptors (inversely related to dose); mild affinity for adrenergic receptors	Safety in overdose; minimal drug-drug interactions; ↓ nausea, anxiety, and minimal sexual side effects; increases appetite, sedation for insomniac, medically ill patients	Sedation (especially (at lower doses), increased appetite and weight gain, dizziness, dry mouth, constipation; rare adverse event of agranulocytosis/ neutropenia
Nefazodone Serzone	Initial: 100 Target: 100 to 400	2 to 4	5-HT$_2$ antagonist and serotonin reuptake/ norepinephrine inhibitor; moderate adrenergic receptor affinity	↑ REM sleep; anxiolytic properties; minimal sexual side effects; safety in overdose	Dizziness, sedation, constipation; inhibits cytochrome P450-3A4 isoenzyme; contraindicated with pimozide, cisapride; caution with alprazolam, triazolam

Continued

TABLE 25-11   **Atypical Antidepressants for Use in Older Patients—cont'd**

Drug	Dosage (mg)	Half-life (hrs)	Pharmacologic profile	Advantages	Disadvantages
Venlafaxine XR Effexor XR	Initial: 37.5 Target: 75 to 225	4 to 10	Serotonin/ norepinephrine reuptake inhibitor; dose-dependent pharmacology (i.e., serotonergic effect at low doses, norepinephrine effect at medium-high doses)	XR formulation for dosing convenience and fewer side effects; potency of a TCA with safety and tolerability of an SSRI; safety in overdose; minimal drug-drug interactions	Dose-related elevation in diastolic BP; risk of serotonin syndrome and sexual side effects (similar to SSRIs)

From Sable JA, Dunn LB, Zisook S: Late-life depression: how to identify its symptoms and provide effective treatment, *Geriatrics* 5(2):18-31, 2002.
SR, Sustained-release; *CNS*, central nervous system; *REM*, rapid eye movement; *XR*, extended release; *TCA*, tricyclic antidepressant; *SSRI*, selective serotonin reuptake inhibitor.

medical conditions that contraindicate such treatment. It is usually performed two or three times per week for a total course of 6 to 12 treatments once a complete evaluation and anesthesia consult have been performed. Maintenance treatments may continue as warranted by the history.

Contraindications to this treatment include the following:

- Any patient who cannot withstand general anesthesia
- Space-occupying intracerebral lesion
- Cardiovascular problems such as recent myocardial infarction, unstable aneurysm, or risk of bradyarrhythmia
- Recent cerebral vascular accident (increased risk of bleeding for weeks to months)
- Seizure disorder (relative contraindication)
- Medication interactions (e.g., MAO inhibitors increase the risk of elevating blood pressure)

The possible adverse effects of this treatment include the following:

- Delirium (usually short-lived)
- Prolonged cardiac arrhythmia
- Prolonged apnea
- Oral trauma
- Retrograde amnesia

EVALUATION AND FOLLOW-UP

Response to treatment should be monitored with frequent telephone contact and visits. During follow-up calls and visits, family members may need special attention to any burden they may be experiencing because living with a depressed person is a great challenge. In addition, a formal evaluation of the therapy and response should be conducted after about 6 weeks. This evaluation can be accomplished through subjective reports from the patient and family members regarding symptoms, evaluation of sleep patterns, or objective signs such as affect and weight gain or loss. The goal is to determine whether the original diagnosis is still appropriate and to evaluate the extent of success of the treatment modalities thus far. Decisions regarding change in dose or medication should be made at this time. Also, the possible need to augment the original therapy with an additional modality or to refer for further consultation and treatment will be evident at this time. Because of the high incidence of recurrence and the chronicity of depression in this population, continued follow-up and monitoring for persistent or recurrent episodes are as important as recognizing and treating the initial depression in the older patient.

SUICIDE

Suicide is the most serious consequence of depression. More than 32,000 people in the United States kill themselves every year. Suicide accounts for 1.4% of all U.S. deaths and is the ninth leading cause of death. A person commits suicide about every 15 minutes, but it is estimated that an attempt is made about once a minute. The suicide rate in older persons is about twice that of younger age groups (Sable, Dunn, and Zisook, 2002). The highest rates of suicide are in men 50 years of age and older. This 10% of the population represents 33% of all suicides. For women the rate of suicide peaks between 40 and 54 years of age and again after 75 years of age. Sixty to 90% of patients over 75 years of age who commit suicide have clinically diagnosable depression (Sable, Dunn, and Zisook, 2002). Older adults who commit suicide are more likely to have cancer, ischemic heart disease, chronic pulmonary disease, peptic ulcer, prostatic disorder, and other psychiatric illnesses in addition to depression (Quan et al, 2002).

The practitioner must recognize a patient who is at risk of committing suicide. Numerous warning signs should prompt the health care provider to ask whether the patient has ever considered suicide as an option. A "yes" answer should be taken seriously. Patients who are at risk may exhibit certain behaviors that offer clues to their intentions: talking about suicide; statements about hopelessness, helplessness, or worthlessness; preoccupation with death; becoming suddenly happier or calmer; loss of interest in things they cared about; visiting or calling people they care about; making arrangements and setting their affairs in order; and giving things away. A patient who is being treated for depression is actually at higher risk for suicide as the depression lifts. There is no need to be concerned that asking about suicide will "put the idea into someone's head" who previously had not considered it. It can be a great relief for the patient to bring the subject out in the open.

The San Francisco Suicide Prevention Crisis Team (1998) has developed a screening tool (PLAID-PALS) to help determine the degree of suicide risk for a patient:

Plan: Do they have one?

Lethality: Is it lethal? Can they die?

Availability: Do they have the means to carry it out?

Illness: Do they have mental or physical illness?

Depression: Have there been chronic or specific incidents?

Previous Attempts: How many? How recent?

Alone: Are they alone? Do they have a support system?

Loss: Have they suffered a loss? Death, job, relationship, self-esteem?

Substance Abuse: Drugs, alcohol, medicine? Current or chronic?

If the patient is thought to be at imminent risk for suicide, immediate referral to a psychiatrist or inpatient hospitalization is warranted. If the patient is at moderate to high risk, certain measures should be put in place to minimize this risk. The patient should not be left alone; a supportive friend or family member should stay with him or her. The home, hospital room, or nursing home room should be cleared of all potential means (pills, plastic bags, sharp implements), and close follow-up by the psychiatrist and primary care provider is important. It is advisable to be in daily contact with these patients either through office visits or by telephone to monitor their response to therapy.

Summary

Dementia, delirium, and depression are common problems among older patients. Accurate diagnosis can be complicated by overlapping of these three conditions as well as by concomitant medical illness. Because these patients will most commonly consult their primary care providers with these conditions, it is important that practitioners are able to distinguish accurately between them and be able to detect potentially reversible underlying conditions. Appropriate referral to specialty providers and community resources will enhance the demented or depressed patient's function and quality of life.

Primary care providers also have an expanded role in providing continuous care throughout the course of a dementia-type illness. Much can be done in the early and mild stages of this disease to improve quality of life for the patient and his or her family. It is important to remember all that can be done rather than emphasizing the decline. As the disease progresses in severity and as institutional placement becomes an option, acknowledging the difficulties is an important element in the provider's ability to continue to assist family members as they make decisions regarding provision of care.

Depressive symptoms in late life are a major concern because they increase disability and aggravate existing medical conditions. Depression is underrecognized and undertreated because of a variety of factors, including somatic symptoms, comorbid physical illness or anxiety, or because it is accepted as a normal feature of aging (Montgomery, 2002). Appropriate treatment and support of the depressed older person can significantly reduce the risk of suicide in this susceptible population.

Resources

Alzheimer's Association
919 N. Michigan Ave.
Suite 1000
Chicago, IL 60611-1676
www.Alz.org

American Association of Suicidology
(202) 237-2280
www.suicidology.org

American Foundation for Suicide Prevention
(888)-333-2377
www.afsp.org

Children of Aging Parents
1609 Woodbourne Rd.
Levittown, PA 19057
(215) 945-6900

The National Alliance for the Mentally Ill (NAMI)
Colonial Place Three
2107 Wilson Boulevard, Suite 300
Arlington, VA 22201
(800) 950-NAMI
www.nami.org

National Council on the Aging
409 Third St., Suite 200
Washington, DC 20024
(202) 479-1200

The National Crisis Helpline
(800) 999-9999

National Institute of Mental Health
NIMH Clinical Center, Bldg. 103N234
Bethesda, MD 20892
(800) 647-2642 (Publication ordering line)

National Mental Health Association (NMHA)
1021 Prince St.
Alexandria, VA 22314-2971
(800) 969-NMHA
www.NMHA.org

Senate Special Committee on Aging
Dirksen Senate Office Bldg.
Room 623
Washington, DC 20510

U.S. Department of Health and Human Services
www.aoa.dhhs.gov
The website of the Department of Health and Human Services is an excellent site to link to many types of information.

References

Alao AO: ECT in the medically ill elderly: a case report, *Int J Psychiatry Med* 32(2):209-213, 2002.
American Psychiatric Association: *Diagnostic and statistical manual of mental disorders*, ed 4, Washington, DC, 1994, American Psychiatric Association.
Assal F, Cummings JL: Neuropsychiatric symptoms in the dementias, *Curr Opin Neurol* 15(4):445-450, 2002.
Cohen GD: Alzheimer's disease: managing behavioral problems in patients with progressive dementia, *Geriatrics* 57(2):53-54, 2002.

Devanand DP: Comorbid psychiatric disorders in late life depression, *Biol Psychiatry* 52(3):236-242, 2002.

Gareri P, De Fazio P, De Sarro G: Neuropharmacology of depression in aging and age-related diseases, *Ageing Res Rev* 1(1):113-134, 2002.

Green RC et al: Risk of dementia among white and African American relatives of patients with Alzheimer's disease, *JAMA* 287(3):329-336, 2002.

Greenberg LS, Lantz MS: Recognition and management of depression in patients with terminal illness, *Clin Geriatr* 10(7):26-32, 2002.

Henry M: Descending into delirium, *Am J Nurs* 102(3):49-56, 2002.

Hirschfeld RMA, Russell JM: Assessment and treatment of suicidal patients, *N Engl J Med* 337(13):910-915, 1997.

Joo JH et al: Risk factors for falls during treatment of late-life depression, *J Clin Psychiatry* 63(10):936-941, 2002.

Kivipelto M et al: Apolipoprotein E epsilon4 allele, elevated midlife total cholesterol level, and high midlife systolic blood pressure are independent risk factors for late-life Alzheimer's disease, *Ann Intern Med* 137: 149-155, 2002.

Lenze EJ et al: Anxiety symptoms in elderly patients with depression: what is the best approach to treatment? *Drugs Aging* 19(10):753-760, 2002.

Likourezos A, Lantz MS: MMSE: interpreting mental status examination scores in cases of mild dementia, *Geriatrics* 56(6):55-56, 2001.

Marin DB, Sewell MC, Schlechter A: Alzheimer's disease: accurate and early diagnosis in the primary care setting, *Geriatrics* 57(2):36-40, 2002.

Montgomery SA: Late-life depression: rationalizing pharmacological treatment options, *Gerontology* 48(6): 392-400, 2002.

Sable JA, Dunn LB, Zisook S: Late life depression: how to identify its symptoms and provide effective treatment, *Geriatrics* 57(2):18-32, 2002.

Spina E, Scordo MG: Clinically significant drug interactions with antidepressants in the elderly, *Drugs Aging* 19(4):299-320, 2002.

Quan H et al: Association between physical illness and suicide among the elderly, Social Psychiatry Psychiatr *Epidemiol* 37(4):190-197, 2002.

26

Sleep Disorders

Sleep disorders affect almost everyone sometime during his or her life span. It is estimated that chronic sleep–wake disorders affect at least 40 million Americans, and most of these disorders go unreported and untreated (Neubauer, Smith, and Earley, 2003). The changes in the quality and structure of sleep are now recognized as an integral aspect of the aging experience. The prevalence of insomnia increases with age and is reported by up to one in every three persons 65 years of age and older. Dissatisfaction with sleep is more common in older women than in older men and is higher among low-income and lower-education groups (Barthlen, 2000; Morgan, 2003).

Insomnia is a perception of inadequate or poor-quality sleep, usually related to the patient's subjective description of one or more of the following: difficulty falling asleep, waking up frequently during the night with difficulty returning to sleep, waking up too early, and not feeling rested after a night's sleep (National Center on Sleep Disorders Research [NCSDR], 1995). Sleep disturbances usually can be divided into the categories of *sleep-onset problems* (trouble getting to sleep), *sleep maintenance* (trouble staying asleep), and early morning awakening. These symptoms may occur singly or in combination and may be either transient or chronic. Frequent geriatric sleep disorders include obstructive sleep apnea (OSA) and restless legs syndrome (RLS). Nocturnal leg cramps are quite common in older adults, and the symptoms are severe enough to disturb sleep (Barthlen, 2002; Butler et al, 2002). Severe sleep disturbances, if not treated, can lead to depression, cognitive impairments, deterioration of quality of life, reduced productivity, an increased need for health services, and increased health care costs (Montgomery and Dennis, 2002; Simon and VonKorff, 1997).

Normal Sleep Characteristics

Most people have a normal pattern of living that involves a daily division of the 24-hour day into about 16 hours of daytime alertness and 8 hours of nighttime sleep. This human sleep–wake cycle is maintained with some regularity by the individual patient's circadian rhythm, which modulates core temperature and a large number of physiologic functions. Light exposure during the daytime and darkness at night are factors that influence the rhythm (Neubauer, Smith, and Earley, 2003).

Normal sleep has two major physiological states: rapid eye movement (REM) and non–rapid eye movement (NREM). During the period of normal sleep, a person experiences a pattern of three to five sleep cycles consisting of four distinct stages of either REM or NREM sleep. See Box 26-1 for characteristics of stages of sleep.

Box 26-1

Sleep Stage Characteristics

Stage I (NREM)

Lightest sleep stage

Presence of theta waves on the EEG

Transitional state between wakefulness and deeper sleep

Lasts only a few minutes in normal persons

Person very easily awakened by sensory stimulation such as touch or noise

Slow, rolling eye movements

Sensation of drowsiness and relaxation

Vital signs (pulse, blood pressure, and respirations) gradually decrease

Body temperature and metabolism declining

Constitutes about 5% of normal sleep time

Increases in those with chronic illness and in the elderly

Stage 2 (NREM)

Light sleep stage

Presence of sleep spindles and K complexes on the EEG

Person not as easily awakened

Vital signs (pulse, blood pressure, and respirations) decreased

Body temperature and metabolism continue to decline

Constitutes about 50%-55% of normal sleep time

Stage 3 (NREM)

Deep sleep stage

Presence of some delta waves on the EEG

Person is difficult to arouse

Vital signs (pulse, blood pressure, and respirations) decreased

Body temperature and metabolism low

Constitutes about 10%-15% of normal sleep time in young adults

Reduced or absent in chronic illness and in the elderly

Stage 4 (NREM)

Deepest sleep stage

Delta waves predominant on the EEG

Person very difficult to arouse

Vital signs (pulse, blood pressure, and respirations) lowest

Body temperature very low

Constitutes about 5%-10% of normal sleep time in young adults

Reduced or absent in chronic illness and in the elderly

REM

Fast, low-amplitude random EEG waves, similar to the awake state

Normally first occurs about 90 minutes after falling asleep

Occurs earlier than 90 minutes in the elderly and in those with major depression

Occurs at onset of sleep in persons with narcolepsy

REM periods normally get longer and closer together as the night progresses

Rapidly darting eye movements visible

Visible twitching of small facial muscles

Skeletal muscle paralysis

Periods of oxygen desaturation in persons with diminished respiratory muscle function (i.e., chronic obstructive pulmonary disease)

Vivid dreaming reported if awakened from this stage

Vital signs increase and widely fluctuate

Hypothalamus unable to regulate body temperature (cannot thermoregulate)

Probably responsible for mental alertness and memory recall

Constitutes about 20%-25% of normal sleep time in adults

Constitutes more than 50% of normal sleep time in newborns and infants

Adapted from Lee KA: Rest and sleep. In Lindeman CA, McAthie M, editors: *Fundamentals of contemporary nursing practice*, Philadelphia, 1998, Saunders.

NREM, Non–rapid eye movement; *EEG*, electroencephalogram; *REM*, rapid eye movement.

Normal Age-related Changes

Age-related sleep changes include alterations in the *continuity, duration, and depth of sleep.* Continuity of sleep is negatively influenced by frequent episodes of nocturnal wakefulness; sleep is more fragmented as a result of frequent shifts from one sleep stage to another. This lack of continuity of sleep is highly correlated with daytime sleepiness. The duration of sleep in the older adult decreases in the total time asleep and in sleep efficiency (time spent asleep divided by the amount of time in bed). The structural change that affects the depth of sleep is the progressive loss of deeper, slow sleep with the resulting increase in the lighter sleep stages. The most consistent age-related NREM sleep change is the progressive loss and, for some older people, the total disappearance of stage 4 sleep. Although not universal this change can result in a lower threshold of auditory awaking. See Figure 26-1 for differences between the sleep changes in young and older adults.

Studies have suggested that it is not the *need* for sleep but the *ability* to sleep that is reduced with age (Ancoli-Israel, 1997). Some evidence has been found that age-related changes occur in the circadian cycle as sleep changes. Older adults do not tolerate disturbances in the sleep–wake cycle brought on by shift work, travel, or sleep deprivation as well as younger adults. The average younger adult gets sleepy at around 10:00 or 11:00 PM, sleeps for about 8 to 9 hours, and wakes between 6:00 and 8:00 AM. The circadian clock advances with age, causing advanced sleep-phase syndrome. This is one of the primary reasons older adults wake early in the morning. People with an advanced sleep cycle get sleepy early in the evening (8:00 or 9:00 PM). If they go to bed at that time and sleep for 8 hours, they wake at 4:00 or 5:00 AM; however, when people with advanced sleep phase stay up until their customary 10:00 or 11:00 PM, their bodies still wake at 4:00 or 5:00 AM. Therefore, they get only 5 to 6 hours of sleep before their advanced sleep–wake cycle awakens them (Ancoli-Israel, 1997). Other factors associated with aging thought to interfere with the circadian mechanism include changes in daily social patterns, lack of mentally stimulating external environment, insufficient exercise, less exposure to sunlight (particularly nursing home residents), and irregular mealtimes.

INSOMNIA

Sleep disorders of older adults are caused not only by the structural changes of sleep that are experienced by most older adults. Although these changes do contribute to many of the sleep disorders, clear evidence has been found that medical illnesses, depression, emotional stress, and adverse effects

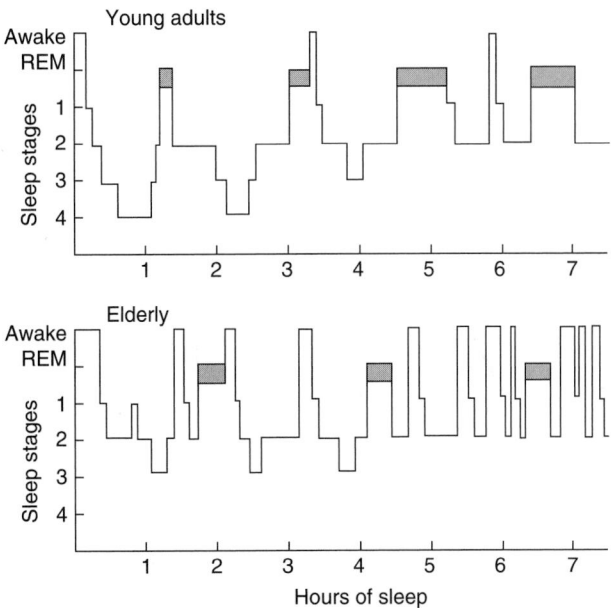

Figure 26-1   Normal sleep cycles in healthy young adults and older subjects. (From Morgan K: Sleep, aging and late life insomnia. In Tallis RC, Fillit HM, editors: *Brocklehurst's textbook of geriatric medicine & gerontology*, ed 6, London, 2003, Churchill Livingstone.)

of drugs are strongly associated with sleep problems in later life (Ancoli-Israel, 2000). Insomnia, as defined by the National Institutes of Health (NIH), includes perception by the patient of difficulty falling asleep, frequent awakenings during sleep, and waking up too early, all of which lead to the complaint of inadequate or poor-quality sleep. Symptoms may be in combination or may occur singly.

Insomnia is often associated with medical illnesses that cause pain, discomfort, difficulty breathing, or frequent need for urination; such illnesses include rheumatologic disorders, Parkinson's disease, congestive heart failure, human immunodeficiency virus (HIV), gastroesophageal reflux disease (GERD), and chronic obstructive pulmonary disease (COPD) (Brostrom et al, 2001; Nokes and Kendrew, 2001). Sleep disturbances are a frequent problem for patients and caregivers affected by dementia. A variety of medications are also known to disrupt sleep by various mechanisms: theophylline, diuretics, thyroxine, corticosteroids, alcohol, decongestants, and caffeine (Martin et al, 2000).

Caffeine, along with nicotine and alcohol, is one of the most widely used drugs worldwide. Unknown to many people, beverages, certain foods, and some over-the-counter drugs contain caffeine, leading many people to underestimate their actual drug intake. Low to moderate dosage of 30 to 200 mg can increase vigilance, but more than 500 mg can lead to anxiety, agitation, restlessness, and insomnia (Eisendrath, 2002).

Types of insomnia are explicitly defined in the Diagnostic and Statistical Manual of Mental Disorders (DSM-IV) and The International Classification of Sleep Disorders (ICSD). For primary care providers we have included a glossary of sleep-related terms in Table 26-1 and the ICSD classification in Box 26-2.

With more than 100 known sleep disorders, the question becomes what the role is of the primary care provider in managing the care of older persons with a chief complaint of a sleep disturbance. Clinical practice calls for the use of knowledge meshed with a practical and convenient system to

TABLE 26-1	Glossary of Sleep-related Terms
Actigraph	A biomedical instrument used to measure body movement.
Apnea	Cessation of airflow at the nostrils and mouth lasting at least 10 seconds. The three types of apnea are obstructive, central, and mixed. Obstructive apnea is secondary to upper-airway obstruction; central apnea is associated with a cessation of all respiratory movements; mixed apnea has both central and obstructive components.
Arousal	An abrupt change from a "deeper" stage of sleep to a "lighter" stage of sleep. Multiple arousals occurring during the night in association with sleep disorders can cause severe daytime sleepiness.
Central Sleep Apnea Syndrome (CSAS)	A disorder characterized by a cessation or decrease of ventilatory effort during sleep usually associated with oxygen desaturation. May be associated with nocturnal arousals and daytime sleepiness.
Deep Sleep	A common term for NREM stages 3 and 4 sleep (also called delta or slow wave sleep).
Excessive Daytime Sleepiness (EDS)	A subjective report of difficulty in maintaining the alert awake state.
Insomnia	Difficulty in initiating or maintaining sleep. This term is employed ubiquitously to indicate any and all gradations and types of sleep loss.
NREM Sleep	Non–rapid eye movement sleep; divided into four stages, 1 through 4, based on EEG wave forms.

TABLE 26-1	**Glossary of Sleep-related Terms—cont'd**
Multiple Sleep Latency Test (MSLT)	A series of measurements of the interval from "lights out" to sleep onset that is used in the assessment of excessive sleepiness. Subjects are allowed a fixed number of opportunities (typically four or five) to fall asleep during their customary awake period. Excessive sleepiness is characterized by short sleep latencies (< 10 minutes).
Obstructive Sleep Apnea Syndrome (OSAS)	A disorder characterized by repetitive episodes of upper airway obstruction that occur during sleep usually associated with a reduction in blood oxygen desaturation. May be associated with nocturnal arousal and daytime sleepiness.
Periodic Leg Movement (PLM)	A rapid partial flexion of the foot at the ankle, extension of the big toe, and partial flexion of the knee and hip that occurs during sleep. May be associated with nocturnal arousals and daytime sleepiness.
Periodic Leg Movement Disorder (PLMD)	A disorder characterized by periodic episodes of repetitive and highly stereotyped limb movements that occur during sleep.
Polysomnogram	The continuous and simultaneous recording of multiple physiologic variables during sleep (i.e., electroencephalogram, electrooculogram, electromyogram, electrocardiogram, respiratory air flow, respiratory movements, leg movements, and other electrophysiologic variables).
REM Sleep	Rapid eye movement sleep.
Restless Legs Syndrome (RLS)	A disorder characterized by disagreeable leg sensations that usually occur prior to sleep onset and that cause an almost irresistible urge to move the legs.
Sleep Architecture	The NREM-REM sleep-stage and cycle infrastructure.
Sleep Cycle	Synonymous with the NREM-REM cycle.
Sleep Efficiency (SE)	The proportion of sleep in the episode potentially filled by sleep (the ratio of total sleep time to time in bed).
Sleep Latency (SL)	The duration of time from "lights out" or bedtime to the onset of sleep.
Sleep Maintenance	The maintenance of sleep after sleep onset is achieved.
Total Sleep Time (TST)	The amount of actual sleep time in a sleep episode; this time is equal to the total sleep episode less the awake time.

From American Sleep Disorders Association: *The international classification of sleep disorders*, Rochester, Minn, 1997, The Association.

REM, Rapid eye movement, *NREM*, non–rapid eye movement.

recognize and manage insomnia and other sleep disorders that affect the health and quality of life of the patient and to recognize which of those problems need referral.

SLEEP-DISORDERED BREATHING

Sleep-disordered breathing (SDB) problems are estimated to affect up to 4% of Americans, with a higher prevalence among older persons in the community, of whom about 9% of men and 4% of women are affected (Ancoli-Israel, 1997; Dobbin and Strollo, 2002). SDB problems include upper-airway resistance syndrome, obstructive sleep hypopnea, and obstructive sleep apnea (OSA). All these conditions have an interruption in upper-airway airflow, ranging from narrowing to complete collapse of the upper airway. The major distinction between these conditions is that significant oxygen desaturations are more common in OSA, which is defined as cessation of airflow for 10 seconds or longer during sleep. Obstructive sleep hypopnea is a 30% to 50% reduction in airflow for 10

Box 26-2

The International Classification of Sleep Disorders

Dyssomnias

Intrinsic Sleep Disorders

Psychophysiologic insomnia
Sleep state misperception
Idiopathic insomnia
Narcolepsy
Recurrent hypersomnia
Idiopathic hypersomnia
Posttraumatic hypersomnia
Obstructive sleep apnea syndrome
Central sleep apnea syndrome
Central alveolar hypoventilation syndrome
Periodic limb movement disorder
Restless legs syndrome
Intrinsic sleep disorder NOS

Extrinsic Sleep Disorders

Inadequate sleep hygiene
Environmental sleep disorder
Altitude insomnia
Adjustment sleep disorder
Insufficient sleep syndrome
Limit-setting sleep disorder
Sleep-onset association disorder
Food allergy insomnia
Nocturnal-dependent sleep disorder
Stimulant-dependent sleep disorder
Alcohol-dependent sleep disorder
Toxin-induced sleep disorder
Extrinsic sleep disorder NOS

Circadian Rhythm Sleep Disorders

Time-zone change (jet lag) syndrome
Shift work sleep disorder
Irregular sleep-wake pattern
Delayed sleep phase syndrome
Advanced sleep phase syndrome
Non–24-hour sleep-wake disorder
Circadian rhythm sleep disorder NOS

Parasomnias

Arousal Disorders

Confusional arousals
Sleepwalking
Sleep terrors

Sleep-Wake Transition Disorders

Rhythmic movement disorder
Sleep starts

Sleepwalking
Nocturnal leg cramps

Parasomnias Usually Associated with REM Sleep

Nightmares
Sleep paralysis
Impaired sleep-related penile erections
Sleep-related painful erections
REM sleep-related sinus arrest
REM sleep behavior disorder

Other Parasomnias

Sleep bruxism
Sleep enuresis
Sleep-related abnormal swallowing syndrome
Nocturnal paroxysmal dystonia
Primary snoring
Congenital central hypoventilation syndrome
Benign neonatal sleep myoclonus
Other parasomnia NOS

Sleep Disorders Associated with Medical or Psychiatric Disorders

Associated with Mental Disorders

Psychoses
Mood disorders
Anxiety disorders
Panic disorder
Alcoholism

Associated with Neurologic Disorders

Cerebral degenerative disorders
Dementia
Parkinsonism
Fatal familial insomnia
Sleep-related epilepsy
Electrical status epilepticus of sleep
Sleep-related headaches

Associated with Other Medical Disorders

Sleeping sickness
Nocturnal cardiac ischemia
Chronic obstructive pulmonary disease
Sleep-related asthma
Sleep-related gastroesophageal reflux
Peptic ulcer disease
Fibrositis syndrome

Box 26-2

The International Classification of Sleep Disorders—cont'd

Proposed Sleep Disorders

Short sleeper
Long sleeper
Subwakefulness syndrome
Fragmentary myoclonus
Sleep hyperhidrosis
Menstrual-associated sleep disorder
Pregnancy-associated sleep disorder
Terrifying hypnagogic hallucinations
Sleep-related neurogenic tachypnea
Sleep-related laryngospasm
Sleep choking syndrome

From American Sleep Disorders Association: *International classification of sleep disorders: diagnostic and coding manual*, Rochester, Minn, 1990, The Association.
NOS, Not otherwise specified; *REM*, rapid eye movement.

seconds or longer during sleep, and upper-airway resistance is without hypopnea or apnea, accompanied by loud snoring. Upper-airway resistance may be caused by sinus congestion, large tonsils, or nasal septal deviation (Dobbin and Strollo, 2002).

OSA is caused by muscular relaxation of the throat or oral structures during sleep and results in a period of apnea that awakens the subject. This awakening period may last only a few seconds and is usually not remembered. Risk factors for development of OSA are male gender, obesity (especially neck size of more than 17 inches), alcohol, smoking, and nasal congestion (Young et al, 2002). OSA is associated with hypertension, heart disease, and cerebrovascular disease.

Symptoms of OSA include daytime sleepiness and a complaint of frequent nocturnal awakenings. The patient will have a long history of nightly loud snoring that is audible outside the bedroom. Both the patient and his or her bed partner will complain of sleep disturbances. Excessive daytime sleepiness is reported in up to 90% of patients with OSA. The impairment in daytime functioning is potentially dangerous because altered driving performance increases the risk for motor-vehicle accidents. In an older patient daytime sleepiness often manifests as confusion, depression, headaches, memory loss, and cognitive impairment. Sleep apnea, left untreated, can result in serious morbidity and is associated with an increased risk of death (Community Internal Medicine Division, Mayo Clinic, 2001).

Once the patient has been identified, a definitive diagnosis is made by an overnight sleep study (polysomnogram) performed in a sleep laboratory. Many patients experience apnea when they are in a supine position during sleep. Treatment for OSA has three modalities: behavior modification, medical treatment, and surgical intervention. Avoiding alcohol and sedatives, weight reduction, and change in sleeping position if indicated are aspects of a behavior-modification program. Medical treatment is continuous positive airway pressure (CPAP) delivered through a mask that keeps the airway open. Successful compliance with CPAP treatment eliminates snoring, hypopnea, and apneas, and daytime symptoms of excessive sleepiness and confusion improve. If the patient is unable to tolerate the CPAP, dental intraoral devices can be used. Patients with mild OSA generally can tolerate the dental devices. Surgical treatment is reserved for patients who are unable to tolerate the positive pressure and would benefit from restructuring of the airway (Dobbin and Strollo, 2002). See Figure 26-2 for CPAP bedside system.

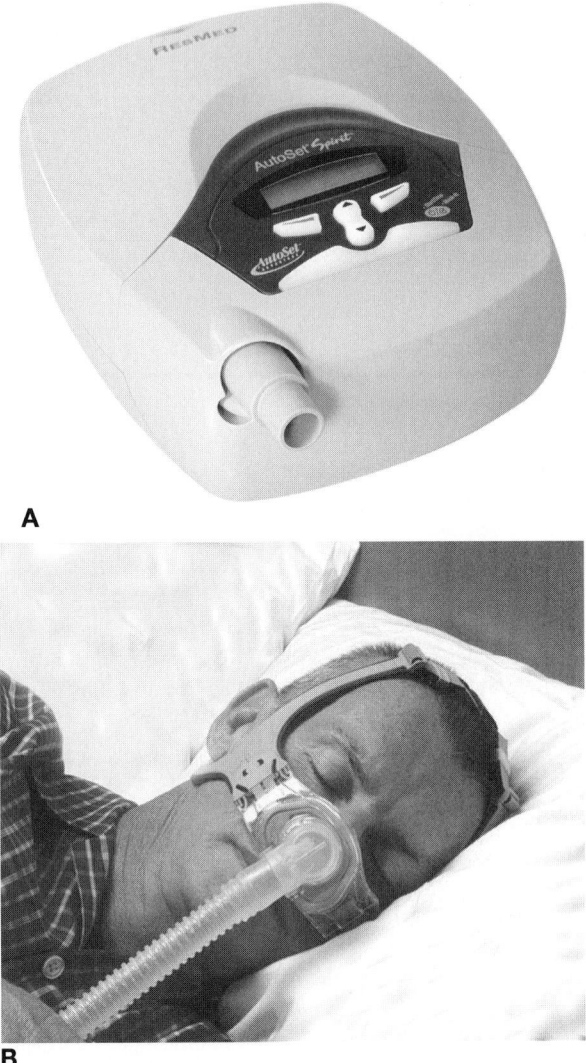

A

B

Figure 26-2   A, AutoSet Spirit. **B,** Mirage Vista mask. (Use of the text, images, drawings, and materials is made with the permission of ResMed Limited. ResMed Limited owns the copyright in the text, images, drawings, and materials, and ResMed Limited reserves all rights.)

RESTLESS LEGS SYNDROME

Restless legs syndrome (RLS) is a disorder of sensation of unknown etiology. It occurs in up to 10% to 15% of adults 65 years of age or older. Prevalence is increased in adults with iron deficiency, chronic renal failure, and peripheral neuropathy. The use of dopamine antagonists may aggravate existing RLS (Neubauer, Smith, and Earley, 2003). Symptoms include a sensation in one or both legs that are characterized as deep, uncomfortable aching, something moving, or crazy legs. Although the description varies, the patient usually has no pain. A need to move accompanies the feeling, and the urge to move is so strong that most patients describe the legs almost seeming to move by themselves. To relieve this sensation and the need to move, the patient reports a constant movement of walking and rubbing the legs. The sensation is brought on by sitting or lying that is relieved by walking and is worsened in the late evening or bedtime. The patient may be unable to relax long enough to watch a movie, read a book, or travel any distance without the need to move and to walk. At night, sleep is prevented for long periods while the patient walks to relieve the sensation, leading to all the deleterious effects of loss of sleep. The primary care provider must rule out arthralgia, myalgia, or sensory neuropathy.

Associated with RLS is the presence of semiinvoluntary leg movements, called *periodic limb movement* (PLM) disorder, which consists of rhythmic and stereotypic movements of the legs or arms that occur only during sleep. Incidence increases with age and is estimated to occur in 45% of community-dwelling people older than 65 years of age (Morgan, 2003). Typically patients have a normal neurologic examination while awake, with no evidence of seizure disorder on the electroencephalogram. During sleep, however, these patients demonstrate characteristic PLM that involves the anterior tibialis and lasts 0.5 to 5 seconds and occurs every 20 to 40 seconds, usually in clusters and without the person waking (Mendelson and Aikens, 1998), although the person experiencing PLM perceives sleep as restless and as not restorative.

The diagnosis of RLS is based on a clinical history and is differentiated from nocturnal seizures, sleep apnea, primary insomnia, myoclonus, and PLS. If the history is not adequate for this differentiation, the patient should be referred to a sleep disorder clinic. Nonpharmacologic treatment includes exercise, stretching, avoidance of caffeine, and prolonged soaking in a hot tub before sleep. The effectiveness is mixed. Pharmacologic treatments include benzodiazepines, dopamine agonists, and opioids. The initial drug of choice is carbidopa/levodopa (Sinemet 25/100 mg) at one half a tablet taken 1 hour before bedtime. The most common side effect of the dopamine agonist agents is augmentation of the symptoms (Neubauer, Smith, and Earley, 2003). Because of the vulnerability of older adults to the side effects of drugs, treatment of the RLS symptoms and referral to a sleep specialist may be appropriate.

INTENSIVE CARE DELIRIUM

Also known as *ICU psychosis*, intensive care delirium is commonly seen in patients who have been in the intensive care unit (ICU). It is worth mentioning because of the susceptibility of the older population to this disorder. Although its cause is unknown, it has been correlated with sleep deprivation, sensory deprivation, age, severity of illness, duration of surgery, and time spent on the heart–lung bypass machine (Lee, 1997). Symptoms can include those of sleep deprivation as well as hallucinations, psychosis, and paranoia. Regardless of the underlying etiology, this condition typically resolves with the patient's return to a more conducive sleep environment and a full night's sleep.

DEMENTIA

Sleep disturbances in Alzheimer's-type dementia are cause by multiple factors that include normal age-related physiologic changes, related medical illness, drug-induced sleep problems, primary sleep disorders, and poor sleep hygiene (Vitiello and Borson, 2002).

Nocturnal delirium, or sundowning, is one of the most important causes of institutionalization of demented patients and is thought to occur in 12% to 14% of nursing home residents. *Sundowning* is defined as the recurrent appearance or exacerbation of behavioral disturbances at night. These behaviors may include agitation, pacing, restlessness, confusion, aggression, and paranoid ideation (Brown, 1997).

Optimal clinical management of patients with dementia calls for systematic evaluation with assessment to include mood and cognitive ability, daytime behaviors, medical disorders, intensive drug review, pain, environment, and sleep hygiene.

Assessment of Insomnia
HISTORY

The first task of history taking should be to listen to the patient's chief complaint related to sleep and then to determine how long the symptom or symptoms have been present. It is wise to have the review of medications in hand because the recent addition of a medication could be part of the problem.

Early screening questions to consider include the following:

- Is the patient satisfied with his or her sleep? Does he or she feel rested on awakening?
- Is the patient experiencing unexplained fatigue? Does he or she fall asleep in the daytime when reading, watching television, or sitting in a car or a theatre?
- Does the bed partner or caregiver report loud snoring, breathing pauses, or abnormal movements during sleep?

Questions for a complete sleep history are listed in Box 26-3.

As sleep problems occur over time, assessment requires a compilation of serial self-reports of sleeping behavior recorded in a sleep diary. Therefore the practitioner needs to enlist the cooperation of the patient and bed partner or caregiver if warranted by symptoms or frailty of the patient. See Figure 26-3 for suggested aspects of a self-diary.

A complete review of prescription and over-the-counter drugs are pertinent to sleep problems. All alternative therapies used by the patient should be investigated to include all herbal preparations. The use and amount of alcohol and caffeine intake need to be ascertained. See Table 26-2 for the amount of caffeine in certain types of beverages and products.

A complete medical and psychological/psychiatric history needs to be obtained. Emphasis should be on conditions that would affect sleep, such as the following:

- Arthritis, myalgias, bursitis
- GERD, peptic ulcers
- Asthma, COPD, pulmonary disease
- Prostatism, urologic dysfunction
- Situational stress

Box 26-3

Questions for a Sleep History

- When did the current sleep problem start?
- Have you had a past history with sleep problems?
- How much sleep do you have during a 24-hour period?
- How long does it take you to go to sleep?
- What do you consider as a normal amount of time to sleep?
- What time do you retire?
- How many nights a week do you retire at the same time?
- Do you awaken frequently in the night? What wakes you?
- Are you able to go back to sleep after being awake in the night?
- What time do you awaken?
- How much time do you spend in bed?
- Do you feel rested when you awaken?
- Do you ever experience sleepiness during the day?
- Do you take a nap? How many naps during a day? How long do you nap?
- Has your bed partner told you that you have stopped breathing, snore, have abnormal movements, or talk or walk when you are asleep?
- Have you ever fallen asleep watching TV, driving, or during any quiet activity?
- Do you feel worried, sad, blue, or depressed?
- What do you think is causing your sleep problem?

Adapted from *Sleep disorders*. Geriatric Medicine Community Internal Medicine, Mayo Clinic, 2001.

- Depression, anxiety
- Dementia, cognitive disorders

  A social history and environmental history should include the following:
- Alcohol and smoking history
- Living space
- Bedroom use
- Work schedule
- Diet and eating habits
- Recent travel
- Driving experiences

  Physical examination is guided by history and may include the following:
- Weight, height, and vital signs
- A complete oral and facial examination (especially if apnea is suspected)
- Neck, including the thyroid
- Pulmonary examination
- Cardiovascular examination, including the abdomen and extremities, to evaluate signs of heart failure
- Musculoskeletal-neurologic examination to evaluate the ability to reposition oneself in bed
- Prostate (if nocturia is present)
- Urogynecologic examination (if appropriate to address incontinence)

A laboratory evaluation is usually not indicated, but if the patient reports symptoms of restless legs it is wise to obtain a complete blood count (CBC) to test for anemia. Any other laboratory tests will be guided by findings in the history and physical examination.

		1	2	3	4	5	6	7	8	9	10	11	12	13	14	15
Sleep latency (minutes)	120+															
	60															
	50															
	40															
	30															
	20															
	10															
Total sleep (hours)	8+															
	7															
	6															
	5															
	4															
	3															
	2															
	1															
Sleep quality	Very Good															
	Good															
	Average															
	Poor															
	Very poor															
Day		1	2	3	4	5	6	7	8	9	10	11	12	13	14	15
Start date																

Figure 26-3 Sleep diary. (From Morgan, K: Sleep, aging and late life insomnia. In Tallis RC, Fillit HM, editors: *Brocklehurst's textbook of geriatric medicine & gerontology,* ed 6, London, 2003, Churchill Livingstone.)

Continued

Name .... Date..................

1	At what time did you go to bed last night?
2	At what time did you settle down to sleep?
3	How long did it take you to fall asleep
4	How many times did you wake up?
5	What woke you up?
6	For how long do you think you were awake on each of these occasions?
7	At what time did you finally wake up?
8	How did you feel when you woke up this morning? (pick one) — Refreshed and alert ☐ Alert but not at peak ☐ Tired ☐ Absolutely shattered ☐
9	At what time did you get up?
10	How would you rate last night's sleep? (pick one) — Very good ☐ Good ☐ Average ☐ Poor ☐ Very poor ☐
11	What medicines did you take yesterday?
12	How much alcohol did you drink yesterday?

Figure 26-3,   cont'd

Treatment

The first step in the treatment of insomnia is to identify and treat any underlying medical, psychological, or psychiatric problems. Many times this will solve the sleep problem.

The objectives of treatment of sleep disorders is first to improve the patient's quality of life and that of the family and second to prevent morbidity and mortality. Because only OSA is associated with increased mortality, most treatments in this section are focused on improvement of the quality of life by alleviating the symptoms and improving the quality sleep. Interventions include the following:
- Management of sleep hygiene
- Behavioral management
- Pharmacologic management

MANAGEMENT OF SLEEP HYGIENE

Suggestions about managing sleep hygiene are beneficial to most patients with insomnia, regardless of their symptoms. The suggestions include the following:

- Bedroom environment should be comfortable, and an extra-warm room can disrupt sleep. The room temperature should be kept near 68° F, and fresh air through an open window, if possible, may help the quality of the air. The bedroom should be used only for sleep or intimacy. A bedroom clock is to be avoided. Watching television or listening to the radio in an attempt to fall asleep should be avoided because these tend to inhibit deep sleep and cause awakenings (Neubauer, Smith, and Earley, 2003).
- Minimize annoying noises or light.
- Eliminate stimulants (caffeine, nicotine, and late evening alcohol).
- Dietary habits: Late heavy meals can interfere with sleep, and a light bedtime snack can alleviate hunger.
- Regular exercise: Aerobic exercise 3 to 4 hours before bedtime should be avoided.
- A hot bath before bedtime may be helpful.

BEHAVIORAL MANAGEMENT

- Progressive relaxation, meditation, imagery training, or yoga
- Stimulus control therapy/sleep restriction therapy: To eliminate the nightly anxiety and arousal of patients with chronic insomnia that has been associated with the act of going to bed
- Going to bed only when tired
- Leaving the bedroom if sleep does not occur within 15 to 20 minutes
- Arising at a certain time to promote regularity in a circadian pattern
- Develop a relaxing evening routine that minimizes daily stress and concerns
- Maintaining a regular sleep–wake schedule

PHARMACOLOGIC MANAGEMENT

If behavioral approaches are not effective after a reasonable time and if the sleep disorder is disruptive to the patient's health or functional status, medications may be considered for *short-term* management of the problem. Pharmacologic treatment of insomnia in older patients is always considered a short-term solution. The chronic use of benzodiazepines is hazardous for older patients and is associated with falls and hip fractures, worsened insomnia, daytime sedation, and cognitive impairment. Pharmacologic treatment of older patients with insomnia should be the last resort after all other methods have been given a sufficient trial. Usually when prescribing drugs for temporary treatment of insomnia, drugs with a short half-life are preferred; long-acting drugs are to be avoided. The ideal drug has a rapid action, duration of action that lasts through the night, no residual daytime effect,

TABLE 26-2	**Amount of Caffeine**
Item	*Amount of Caffeine (mg)*
Coffee (8-oz cup)	80-140
Instant coffee	60-100
Decaffeinated coffee	1-6
Black leaf tea (8-oz cup)	30-80
Tea bags	25-75
Instant tea	30-60
Cocoa (8 oz cup)	10-50
Cola drink	30-65
Chocolate (1 oz)	8-25

and no adverse effects. Zaleplon (Sonata) has been demonstrated to be effective in improving sleep latency, duration, and sleep quality in older persons (Ancoli-Israel, 2000). Pharmacologic and behavior treatments should be used in combination. Another short-acting benzodiazepine is zolpidem (Ambien). It is well to remember that all these drugs have potential side effects of residual daytime sedation, which can be hazardous to the well-being of older patients. Other less common side effects include dizziness, headache, and confusion. When discontinuing benzodiazepine, a gradually tapered dose is useful to minimize withdrawal symptoms.

Antihistamines, such as diphenhydramine (Benadryl), are widely used by many older persons as a hypnotic. The drug is available over the counter at any drugstore in the United States, and many combination drug preparations that are highly advertised to assist with sleep problems contain diphenhydramine. These drugs may cause confusion, agitation, orthostatic hypotension, and urinary retention. Although they cause drowsiness, no scientific data exist to show that antihistamines either improve insomnia or prolong sleep (Ancoli-Israel, 1997). Furthermore they negatively affect the quality of sleep, and hangover results in daytime sleepiness. Antihistamines are not recommended for treatment of insomnia in older adults.

Antidepressants are sedating, and some can be useful as hypnotics. Desipramine (Norpramin 10-25 mg) and nortriptyline (Pamelor 10-25 mg) have few anticholinergic side effects and are the drugs of choice if antidepressants are to be used. A lower dose at bedtime is usually all that is needed to induce sedation.

Melatonin has been receiving a great deal of media attention as a sleep aid. Studies are insufficient, however, to demonstrate its effectiveness or determine its safety at this time.

Summary

It is important to assess and treat disordered sleep in the older patient to avoid associated morbidity and mortality and to improve the quality-of-life issues surrounding this common problem. Often sleep can be improved simply by addressing behavioral issues and minimizing the insult from comorbidities and medications. Occasionally, however, it may be necessary to treat older patients with sedative–hypnotic medications for limited periods. It is critical that the practitioner be familiar with these medications to ensure the safety and efficacy of the prescribed treatment and monitoring and to minimize untoward outcomes.

Resources

Doctor's Guide to Insomnia
www.pslgroup.com/insomnia.htm

National Center for Sleep Disorders (NCSDR)
Two Rockledge Centre
Suite 7024
6701 Rockledge Drive MSC 7920
Bethesda, MD 20892-7920
(301) 435-0199
(301) 480-3451 (FAX)

National Sleep Foundation
1367 Connecticut Ave. NW
Suite 200
Washington, DC 20036

Open Directory Project
dmoz.org/health/conditions_and_diseases/sleep_disorders/

References

Ancoli-Israel S: Insomnia in the elderly: a review for the primary care practitioner, *Sleep* 23:(suppl 1):S23-S30, 2000.

Ancoli-Israel S: Sleep problems in older adults: putting myths to bed, *Geriatrics* 52(1):20-30, 1997.

Barthlen GM: Sleep disorders, obstructive sleep apnea syndrome, restless legs syndrome and insomnia in geriatric patients, *Geriatrics* 57(11):34-39, 2002.

Brostrom A et al: Patients with congestive heart failure and their conceptions of their sleep situation, *J Adv Nurs* 34(4):520-529, 2001.

Brown LK: Sleep and sleep disorders in the elderly, *Nurs Home Med* 5(10):346-353, 1997.

Butler JV et al: Nocturnal leg cramps in older people, *Postgrad Med J* 78:(924):596-598, 2002.

Community Internal Medicine Division, Mayo Clinic: *Geriatric medicine*, Rochester, Minn, 2001, Mayo Foundation for Medical Education and Research.

Dobbin K, Strollo PJ: Obstructive sleep apnea: recognition and management considerations for the aged patient, AACN Clinical Issues: *Advanced Practice in Acute and Critical Care* 13:103-113, 2002.

Eisendrath SJ: Psychiatric disorders. In LM Tierney et al, editors: *Current medical diagnosis and treatment*, ed 26, New York, 2002, Lange Medical Books/McGraw-Hill.

Lee KA: An overview of sleep and common sleep problems, *ANNA J* 24(6):614-623, 1997.

Martin J, Shochat T, Ancoli-Israel S: Assessment and treatment of sleep disturbances in older adults, *Clin Psychol Rev* 20(6):783-805, 2000.

Mendelson WB, Aikens JE: Insomnia: exploring underlying processes and treatment, *Med Behav* October:1-11, 1998.

Montgomery P, Dennis J: Cognitive behavioural interventions for sleep problems in adults aged 60+, *Cochrane Database Syst Rev* 2:CD003161, 2002.

Morgan K: Sleep, aging, and late-life insomnia. In Tallis RC, Fillit HM, editors: *Brocklehurst's textbook of geriatric medicine and gerontology*, ed 6, London, 2003, Churchill Livingstone.

National Center on Sleep Disorders Research: *Insomnia*. NIH Publication no. 95-3801, October 1995.

Neubauer D, Smith P, Earley C: Sleep disorders. In Barker LR et al, editors: *Principles of ambulatory medicine*, ed 6, Philadelphia, 2003, Lippincott Williams & Wilkins.

Nokes KM, Kendrew J: Correlates of sleep quality in persons with HIV, *J Assoc Nurses AIDS Care* 12(1):17-22, 2001.

Simon GE, VonKorff M: Prevalence, burden and treatment of insomnia in primary care, *Am J Psychiatry* 154(10):45-56, 1997.

Vitiello MV, Borson S: Sleep disturbances in patients with Alzheimer's disease: epidemiology, pathophysiology and treatment, *CNS Drugs* 15(10):777-796, 2001.

Young T et al: Epidemiology of obstructive sleep apnea: a population health perspective, *Am J Respir Crit Care Med* 165:1217-1239, 2002.

27

Driving

The health and longevity of the older population in the United States are at unprecedented levels, and many older persons continue to drive throughout their eighth and ninth decades of life. Both the aging of the post-World War II "baby boom" generation and an increasing proportion of women who drive among those turning 65 years of age will contribute to a rapidly growing number of older drivers in the U.S. population in years ahead. One study found that drivers 70 to 74 years of age had a driving life expectancy of about 11 years (Foley et al, 2002).

Like people of all ages, older people prefer to travel by car, reserving public transportation for only about 3% of their trips. Persons over 65 years of age account for about 13% of both the population (33 million older people) and the number of licensed drivers (22 million older drivers). By 2020 about 22 million people over 75 years of age will be eligible for a driver's license, and seven million of these will be 85 years of age or older (American Association of Motor Vehicle Administrators website, www.aamva.org).

Male drivers 65 years of age and older average about 10,000 miles of driving per year, which reflects an increase of 74% over the last three decades. Older female drivers average 5000 miles per year, a 31% increase over the same period (Foley et al, 2002). Compared with middle-aged drivers, older drivers have about a threefold increased risk of crashing per mile driven; however, older persons drive markedly fewer miles annually than middle-aged drivers, resulting in an equivalent annualized risk for crashing (Foley et al, 2002). The roadways most often used by older drivers involve lower speeds but have more intersections and more opportunities for vehicle-to-vehicle conflict.

The greater threat to an older driver is the risk of fatality from an automobile crash. Although the annual risk of crashing remains fairly stable over the years of driving, the risk of dying after involvement in an automobile crash increases significantly with age (Margolis et al, 2002). Compared with middle-aged drivers of the same sex and involved in the same severity of crash, older drivers are three times more likely to die as a result of the crash (Foley et al, 2002).

The reasons for deterioration in driving performance in older adults are multifactorial (Wood, 2002); however, in the absence of certain medical conditions, age alone has not been correlated with poor driving performance (McGregor, 2002). There is evidence to suggest, however, that the skills needed for safe driving begin to deteriorate in later years. Whereas certain adaptations may improve safe and successful driving for older persons, some persons have cognitive problems and driving disabilities that cannot be compensated by more careful behavior on the road (Daigneault, Joly, and Frigon, 2002).

Nationwide, many older drivers quit driving each year and must seek alternative sources of transportation. In general, older drivers decide for themselves when to quit, a decision that often stems from the onset and progression of medical conditions that affect visual, physical, and cognitive functioning and consequently driving skills. Cessation is not an easy decision and may have consequences such as depressed mood and less social engagement because of the loss of mobility. Of paramount concern to the older driver who is pondering cessation is the availability and cost of alternative sources of transportation. Such sources may include formal services such as public transportation systems, taxis, and community-sponsored and church-sponsored van services. More informal support typically comes from family and friends who live nearby and can drive (Foley et al, 2002). Because of differences in life expectancy, women require more years of support for transportation, on average, than men after 70 years of age (Foley et al, 2002).

Although several states and the District of Columbia have established legal restrictions or policies for drivers once they have reached a certain age, the standard licensing and renewal procedures in most states do not adequately assess the ability of an older person to operate a motor vehicle safely. Unless a person has been involved in an at-fault accident, the Department of Motor Vehicles (DMV) in most states will probably never be prompted to investigate an older person's capabilities behind the wheel. At that point (if not before), the primary care provider may be asked by the state's DMV or even family members to perform an assessment and make recommendations regarding the patient's ability to drive. Most providers have never received training in how best to assess a patient's ability to perform this complicated task. No standardized testing procedures have been established, and few resources provide helpful information. The practitioner needs to be aware of the required skills and the potential impact of various factors on a person's ability to operate a motor vehicle safely. It is important to know who should be assessed, how to assess them, and how to proceed appropriately on the basis of findings. Many people at risk can benefit from interventions to improve their driving safety and thus maintain their driving privileges. Others may be deemed unsafe behind the wheel. Just as a young person views a driver's license as a rite of passage into the adult world of independence, when older drivers are deprived of their license, it is viewed as a loss of independence and even identity.

Age-related Risk Factors

A complex interaction of both human (personal) and situational (contextual) factors may affect safety. Studies of crashes and driving cessation among older drivers have shown stronger associations with measures of visual, physical, and cognitive functioning than with diagnoses of specific medical conditions and diseases. Independent risk factors for driving cessation include poor vision, limitations in activities of daily living, poor memory, and depressed mood (Foley et al, 2002). When examining the risk of adverse outcomes from the operation of a motor vehicle, an epidemiologic approach should be considered. Epidemiologists consider three "players" in the evaluation of the risk of any accident or injury: the agent, the host, and the environment.

In this case, the agent is the car: its motion and maneuverability, its mechanical reliability, and all the skills required for its successful operation. The host is the older driver, with all of his or her capabilities and limitations in mastering and maintaining the necessary skills, both in a general sense and at any given moment while driving the car. The environment includes such factors as weather and road conditions. Less than ideal circumstances in any one of these players make the operation of the vehicle more difficult, with less chance of a desirable outcome (i.e., the driver arriving at the chosen destination safely and without incident). Complications in any combination of these factors will cumulatively increase the risk of an adverse outcome (e.g., a crash).

Studies of older drivers have focused on the host (the older driver) and the environment and have found that several factors affect the outcomes within these areas.

THE HOST

A driver must possess a variety of physical and cognitive functions to perform successfully the complicated task of operating a motor vehicle. Motor difficulties such as a loss of strength, coordination, and reaction speed can have serious effects on a person's ability to operate a motor vehicle. Steering, braking, shifting, and monitoring surrounding traffic require certain physical skills such as mobility and strength in the neck, torso, and extremities. Brisk reaction is required to brake urgently or to swerve to avoid an obstacle or collision. Recent and recurrent falls have proven to be a reliable predictor of driving difficulty. Table 27-1 lists the common physical limitations of older drivers and some intervention options.

In many studies sensory deficits, such as those of visual or auditory acuity, have been demonstrated to be a factor in driving performance. Besides near and distance vision, other aspects of vision, such as glare and contrast sensitivity, motion perception, and visual-field perception play important roles. The problem of night and tunnel driving is the most urgent in relation to the effects of glare from vehicle headlights on motion perception of drivers. The reduced mesopic vision and

| **TABLE 27-1** | **Common Physical Limitations of Elderly Drivers** |

Problem	*Impact on Driving*	*Options*
Limited neck ROM	Decreased ability to turn head for visual checks; impairments in seeing cars, traffic signs, and pedestrians	OTR/RPT to increase ROM and strength; driving program or vendor for special mirrors
Limited shoulder ROM	Difficulty or inability to fasten seat belt; difficulty turning the steering wheel	OTR/RPT to increase ROM and strength; OTR to modify seat belt for independent use
Arthritic changes in hand	Difficulty opening car door and grasping/turning keys	OTR key holder, door opener devices; driving program or vendor for steering device, built-up steering wheel, modified dashboard knobs
Impaired or nonfunctional upper limb	Unsafe steering with one hand, especially in turns or emergencies; unsafe operation of transmission shift lever or turn signals	Driving program or vendor for steering device, cross-over transmission, or turn signal lever
Lower back syndrome or orthopedic changes	Impaired visual checks; limited driving; decreased concentration	OTR/RPT to increase strength, flexibility, and positioning; driving program or vendor for lumbar supports, rearview mirror
Lower-extremity impairment	Difficulty lifting legs in and out of car; difficulty lifting foot up from low accelerator pedal to high brake pedal	OTR/RPT to increase ROM and strength, modify transfer technique; driving program or vendor for foot pedal extensions, left foot accelerator
Cognitive	Slow information processing and delayed or impaired judgments; impaired recognition of unsafe driving practices	OTR for cognitive evaluation and training; driving program or motor vehicles department to road test for a minimum of 30 min

From Yoshikawa TT, Cobbs EL, Brummel-Smith K: *Ambulatory geriatric care*, St Louis, 1997, Mosby.
OTR, Occupational therapist, registered; *ROM,* range of motion; *RPT,* registered physical therapist.

increased sensitivity to glare are accompanied by an increased risk of nighttime accidents. Older drivers and patients with early cataract often cannot sufficiently fulfill the criteria for night driving ability because of contrast and glare sensitivity (Babizhayev, 2003). Drivers with greater than 40% reduction in the visual field are five times more likely to have an accident. Hearing loss impairs the driver's awareness of surrounding traffic and ability to respond to the horns of other cars that are sounded in warning.

Driving is a demanding task that requires a person to possess and use many cognitive–perceptual skills and abilities at generally higher levels of intensity in all conditions. Cognitive impairments—for example, problems with attention, scanning, speed in information processing, visuospatial perception, and decision making—have an impact on a person's ability to recognize and react appropriately to the many stimuli received at each moment when driving.

Personality and behavioral disturbances that may cause anxiety or impulsivity can also affect a person's ability to make safe and accurate judgments when driving a car. Boxes 27-1 and 27-2 outline the medical conditions and medications that can affect driving ability.

THE ENVIRONMENT

Driving is regarded as more demanding in some situations than in others, depending on contextual determinants, such as type of driving (e.g., highway, city, residential), density of traffic, weather, and road conditions. Research has centered on the situational determinants of accidents, such as the effects of road designs and highway surfaces (i.e., the environment). Results of this research have shown that accidents in all populations of drivers tend to occur in specific locations (e.g., intersections) and under specific conditions (e.g., glare). In addition, certain operations such as turning left and making right-of-way decisions tend to lead to more accidents. These findings, especially in regard to the negotiation of intersections, have also proven true in studies of older drivers.

When assessing a patient's ability to drive, the provider should determine the type of driving the patient does most often. Driving on the highway demands significantly greater speed and accuracy

---

Box 27-1

Medical Conditions that May Affect Driving Ability

Cardiac disease	Seizure disorder
Memory loss or dementia	Stroke
Diabetes	Glaucoma and macular degeneration
Parkinson's disease	Sleep apnea

From Marottoli RA et al: Development of a test battery to identify older drivers at risk for self-reported adverse driving events, *J Am Geriatr Soc* 46:562-568, 1998; Eberhard JW: Driving is transportation for most older adults, *Geriatrics* 53 (suppl 1):S53-S55, 1998.

Box 27-2

Drugs that May Affect Driving Ability

Antidepressants	Alcohol
Benzodiazepines	Any drug that can cause sedation or drowsiness
Antihistamines	

in information processing and passing skills, whereas city driving demands greater stopping and braking skills. This information helps to guide the assessment of the patient's ability to drive. Box 27-3 lists the errors commonly made by older drivers.

An awareness of the type of behavior that prompted an evaluation will enable the practitioner to evaluate the situation appropriately. Referrals are often prompted by a police officer who has observed the older driver in behaviors or situations that cause concern, such as the following:

- Driving the wrong way or on the wrong side of the road
- Driving off the road
- Rear-ending another vehicle
- Failing to yield the right of way or come to a complete stop at a stop sign
- Infringing on the rights of a pedestrian or cyclist
- Turning across the path of oncoming vehicles
- Crossing lane markings
- Operating at a low speed
- Backing improperly

Once the police officer has made contact with the driver, the following behaviors suggest the need for further evaluation:

- Aberrant behavior (e.g., taking too long to pull over or difficulty in producing identification)
- Attention deficit (unawareness of what he or she did that resulted in a violation or crash)
- Cognitive deficit (lack of recall, inability to comprehend or to follow the rules of the road)
- Medical problems (e.g., blackouts, diabetes, Parkinson's disease, seizure, stroke)
- Mental problems (e.g., slow reflexes, inappropriate manipulation of controls, such as brake and accelerator)
- Sensory deficits (impaired vision or hearing, poor depth perception, degraded night vision, recent eye surgery, cataracts)

Assessment
HISTORY

A thorough medical history is important to ascertain risk factors as well as any medical conditions or medications that could affect a driver's capabilities behind the wheel. Functional status provides important information regarding the patient's general abilities. Information regarding recent or recurrent falls is significant.

Box 27-3

Common Driving Errors in Older Drivers

Difficulty backing up and making turns
Not seeing traffic signs or other cars quickly enough
Difficulty in locating and retrieving information from dashboard displays and traffic signs
Delayed glare recovery when driving at night
Not checking rearview mirrors and blind spots
Bumping into curbs and objects
Not yielding to oncoming traffic or right-of-way vehicles
Irregular or slow vehicle speeds
Difficulty with situations requiring quick decision making

From Yoshikawa TT, Cobbs EL, Brummel-Smith K: *Ambulatory geriatric care*, St Louis, 1997, Mosby.

A driving history inquires about driving habits and problems. Driving habits may include frequency, distance, and circumstances of travel; the use of a copilot; and familiarity with roadways used. Problems may include getting lost, becoming angry or confused while driving, or a history of accidents, traffic violations, and near misses. The observations and concerns of family members may provide additional information, especially if the patient is unaware of or denying the deficits. It is also helpful to elicit details about any prior accidents in which the patient was involved (if he or she is forthcoming with this information). This background may reveal impairments in physical function or judgment that were previously undetected (e.g., a failure to see traffic approaching from the side or to recognize road signs).

PHYSICAL EXAMINATION

The physical examination should assess overall function as well as the presence of any medical conditions that may affect driving abilities. In one study by Marottoli and colleagues (1998), three factors were associated with the occurrence of an adverse event: an inability to copy a design from a brief mental status test, walking fewer blocks, and the presence of foot abnormalities. The study also showed that the factors most closely associated with a self-reported history of adverse driving events were poor near-visual acuity, poor visual attention, and limited neck rotation. Neck rotation is important in detecting cars or objects to the side of or behind a vehicle, particularly at intersections or when merging, areas in which older people typically have problems. Box 27-4 shows elements of the physical examination, including tools used in the assessment of driving ability.

ASSESSMENT TOOLS

One helpful screening tool is the number cancellation test to measure visual attention, an important skill for scanning the visual field for road hazards while driving (Marottoli et al, 1998). The Mini-Mental State Examination is an excellent screening tool for memory and attention. The clock-drawing test elicits information regarding executive functioning. The geriatric depression scale helps to determine the presence of a mood disorder, which may affect judgment and cognitive function.

Some occupational therapists are skilled in performing driving assessments and can provide additional information. Where available, a driving evaluator (e.g., veteran's association, private, or DMV) can also make recommendations.

Box 27-4
Elements of Physical Examination in Assessing Driving Ability

General

Appearance
Affect (Geriatric Depression Scale)
Thought content

Sensory

Hearing
Vision
Near and far vision
Field of vision

Cardiac

Murmurs, carotid bruits, etc.

Musculoskeletal

Range of motion (neck, torso, extremities)
Strength
Gait
Timed distance walking test

Neurologic

Including the number cancellation test, Mini-Mental
State Exam, and the clock drawing test

Interventions

Often an assessment of driving skills does not lead to a clear-cut decision about a person's ability to operate a motor vehicle. Appropriate "in-between ground" of unrestricted driving versus no driving at all may be found. The practitioner's evaluation may be used to determine that a person has ubiquitous driving capacity (i.e., fit to drive in any situation) or only situation-specific driving capacity (i.e., fit to drive in certain situations). Recommendations may range from unconditional motor vehicle operation, to stipulated driving, to complete abstinence from driving. In stipulated driving, a person is restricted to situations for which he or she has the requisite abilities: within his or her familiar community, in good weather, during daytime only, and in areas with no four-way intersections. Whether the provider's findings must be reported to motor vehicle authorities depends on state-determined reporting guidelines.

Licensing procedures vary by state. Renewal procedures for older drivers include accelerated renewal cycles that provide for shorter renewal intervals for drivers older than a specified age, typically 65 or 70, a requirement that they renew their licenses in person rather than electronically or by mail where remote renewal is permitted, and testing that is not routinely required of younger drivers (vision and road tests, for example). If a person's continued fitness to drive is in doubt because of the person's appearance or demeanor at renewal or because of a history of crashes or violations, reports by medical providers, police, and others, state licensing agencies may require renewal applicants to undergo physical or mental examinations or retake the standard licensing tests. States typically have medical review boards comprising health care professionals who advise on licensing standards and on individual cases in which a person's driving ability is in doubt (Insurance Institute for Highway Safety website, www.hwysafety.org). Table 27-2 indicates for the 50 United States and the District of Columbia the periods for which licenses can be renewed and any special provisions for older drivers (www.hwysafety.org).

Specific interventions may be instituted on the basis of the patient's needs. For example, drivers with a field of view in the range of 45 to 70 degrees to either side can install special mirrors to compensate in part for the loss of peripheral vision. Referral to physical and occupational therapy often helps to improve strength, mobility, and motor functioning, thereby preserving driving ability. A few programs are available to assist older drivers to stay on the road safely for as long as possible. One of these is the AARP "55 Alive" program, which provides education that attempts to refine existing skills and to develop defensive techniques for the older driver. This 8-hour course is taught in two 4-hour sessions spanning 2 days; the cost is $10. Drivers completing the course may be eligible for discounts on their automobile insurance premiums. Since 1979 more than 7.5 million people have completed this course (American Association for Retired Persons website, www.aarp.org).

Recommendations should be reviewed with patients and family members. The older person who is still able to drive should be educated about risky driving times and patterns to be avoided. The evaluation should be repeated periodically. A person with advanced cognitive impairment who has been judged to be incapable of driving safely and who continues to have access to an automobile may require creative interventions to maintain this person's safety and dignity. The primary provider needs to work with family members to reach a successful solution to this dilemma.

The loss of a driver's license can seriously affect an older person's ability to take care of day-to-day needs. It can lead to social isolation and depression. Information about public or private transportation may help the higher-risk driver find acceptable alternatives. The involvement of available family members and friends may also provide an alternative transportation system for the older person. A consultation with an experienced social worker may help to address the objections and frustrations associated with the loss of a driver's license and locate alternative transportation resources. Table 27-3 lists resources for older drivers.

TABLE 27-2	U.S. Driver Licensing Renewal Procedures for Older Drivers as of January 2003		
		Special Provisions for Older Drivers	
State	**Length of Renewal Cycle**	**Accelerated Renewal**	**Other Provisions**
Alabama	4 yr	None	None
Alaska	5 yr	None	Mail renewal not available to people 69 and older and to people whose prior renewal was by mail.
Arizona[1]	Until age 65[1]	5 yr for people 65 and older	People 70 and older may not renew by mail.
Arkansas	4 yr	None	None
California	5 yr	None	At age 70, mail renewal is prohibited. No more than two sequential mail renewals are permitted, regardless of age.
Colorado	10 yr (eff. 7/1/01)	5 yr for people 61 and older (eff. 7/1/01)	Mail renewal not available to people 66 and older and to people whose prior renewal was by mail.
Connecticut	4 or 6 yr	None that are safety related[2]	None that are safety related[2]
Delaware	5 yr	None	None
District of Columbia	5 yr	None	None
Florida	6 yr with clean record; 4 yr otherwise	None	None[3]
Georgia	4 yr	None	None
Hawaii	6 yr	2 yr for people 72 and older	None
Idaho	4 yr	Drivers ages 21-62 have the choice of a 4- or 8-yr license; drivers 63 and older will receive a 4-yr license	None
Illinois	4 yr	2 yr for drivers ages 81-86; 1 yr for drivers 87 and older	Renewal applicants 75 and older must take a road test.
Indiana	4 yr	3 yr for drivers 75 and older	None
Iowa	2 or 4 yr at driver's option	2 yr for drivers 70 and older	None
Kansas	6 yr	4 yr for drivers 65 and older	None

TABLE 27-2	U.S. Driver Licensing Renewal Procedures for Older Drivers as of January 2003—cont'd

		Special Provisions for Older Drivers	
State	Length of Renewal Cycle	Accelerated Renewal	Other Provisions
Kentucky	4 yr	None	None
Louisiana	4 yr	None	Mail renewal not available to people 70 and older and to people whose prior renewal was by mail.
Maine	6 yr	4 yr for drivers 65 and older	Vision test required at first renewal after driver's 40th birthday and at every second renewal until age 62; thereafter, at every renewal.
Maryland	5 yr	None	None that are safety related[4]
Massachusetts	5 yr	None	None that are safety related[4]
Michigan	4 yr	None	None
Mississippi	4 yr	None	None
Missouri	6 yr	3 yr for drivers 69 and older and 21 and younger	None
Montana	8 yr, 4 yr if by mail, or on 75th birthday, whichever occurs first	4 yr for drivers 75 and older	None
Nebraska	5 yr	None	None
Nevada	4 yr	None	None that are safety related[4]
New Hampshire	5 yr	None	Renewal applicants age 75 and older must take a road test.
New Jersey	4 yr	None	None
New Mexico	4 or 8 yr at driver's option	4 yrs for drivers who would turn 75 in the last half of an 8-yr renewal cycle	None
New York	5 yr	None	None
North Carolina	5 yr	None	People 60 and older are not required to parallel park in the road test.
North Dakota	4 yr	None	None
Ohio	4 yr	None	None
Oklahoma	4 yr	None	None that are safety related[5]
Oregon	8 yr	None	Vision screening is required every 8 yr for drivers 50 and older.

Continued

TABLE 27-2	U.S. Driver Licensing Renewal Procedures for Older Drivers as of January 2003—cont'd		
		Special Provisions for Older Drivers	
State	**Length of Renewal Cycle**	**Accelerated Renewal**	**Other Provisions**
Pennsylvania	4 yr	None	None
Rhode Island	5 yr	2 yr for drivers 70 and older	None
South Carolina	5 yr	None	None
South Dakota	5 yr	None	None
Tennessee	5 yr	None	Licenses issued to people 65 and older do not expire[5]
Texas	6 yr	None	None
Utah	5 yr	None	Vision test required for people 65 and older
Vermont	4 yr	None	None
Virginia	5 yr	None	None
Washington	5 yr	None	None
West Virginia	5 yr	None	None
Wisconsin	8 yr	None	None
Wyoming	4 yr	None	None

©1996-2003, Insurance Institute for Highway Safety, Highway Loss Data Institute U.S. driver licensing renewal procedures for older drivers as of January 2003.

[1]In Arizona, the license is valid until age 65. Any person 65 years and older who is renewing by mail must submit a vision test verification form, provided by the department, or verification of an examination of the applicant's eyesight. The vision test or examination must be conducted not more than 3 months before.

[2]In Connecticut, people 65 and older may choose a 2-year or 6-year renewal cycle. A personal appearance at renewal generally is required. Upon a showing of hardship, people 65 and older may renew by mail.

[3]In Florida, only two successive renewals may be made electronically or by mail, regardless of age.

[4]Some states' licensing laws specifically prohibit licensing administrators from treating people differently solely by virtue of advanced age. Maryland law specifies that age alone is not a grounds for reexamination of drivers; applicants for an initial license age 70 and older must provide proof of previous satisfactory operation of a vehicle or physician's certificate of fitness. Massachusetts law prohibits discrimination by reason of age with regard to licensing. Minnesota and Nevada law specify that age alone is not a justification for reexamination. In Nevada, applicants for mail renewal age 70 and older must include a medical report.

[5]License fee reduced for drivers 62-64 and are waived for drivers 65 and older in Oklahoma; fees are reduced for drivers 60 and older in Tennessee.

Summary

Each year, hundreds of thousands of older drivers across the country must face the reality of driving cessation and of becoming transportation dependent. Evaluation of the older person's ability to drive a car safely is a skill for which most providers have not received adequate training. The decision to limit or revoke a license to drive can be devastating to the older person who relies on a car for social, professional, and medical contact as well as for routine functioning. It is important to appreciate that it has both emotional and pragmatic consequences (McGregor, 2002). It is crucial to

| TABLE 27-3 | Resources for Older Drivers |

Resource	Service
The Handicapped Driver's Mobility Guide American Automobile Association Traffic Safety Department 1000 AAA Drive Heathrow, FL 32746 Approximately $5.95	Provides state-by-state listing of driver evaluation programs, including those with an occupational therapist, driver instructors, vehicle modification vendors, and basic guidelines for vehicle modification
A Flexibility Fitness Training Package for Improving Older Driver Performance (pamphlet) American Automobile Association Foundation for Traffic Safety 1730 M Street, N.W., Suite 401 Washington, DC 20036	Provides written directions and diagrams for flexibility exercises for the neck, shoulder, trunk, and back specific to driving
Reporting Alzheimer's Disease and Related Disorders: Guidelines for Physicians State of California Health and Welfare Agency Department of Health Services PO Box 942732 Sacramento, CA 94234	Provides reporting guidelines and legal information for patients with dementia; although specific to California law, it is generally useful for determining interventions
Perceptual Motor Evaluation for Head Injured and Other Neurologically Impaired Adults Santa Clara Valley Medical Center Occupational Therapy Department 751 South Bascom Avenue San Jose, CA 95128 Approximately $15.00	Provides directions for administering gross visual screenings and other perceptual motor tests and includes an established scoring system
Drivers 55 Plus: Test Your Own Performance (booklet) *55 Alive/Mature Driving* (pamphlet) Publication No. PF3798(791). D934 American Association of Retired Persons 601 E Street, N.W. Washington, DC 20049	Provides self-test booklet for older drivers, materials on the 55 Alive/Mature Driving Program for both participants and prospective instructors, and other miscellaneous materials
U.S. Department of Transportation National Highway Traffic Safety Administration 400 Seventh Street, N.W. Washington, DC 20590	Provides consumer information in brochures or newsletters about traffic safety for older drivers; gathers data; conducts research; institutes plans for national highway traffic safety of older drivers
Older Driver Resource Directory Circular #385 National Research Council 2101 Constitution Ave., N.W. Washington, DC 20418	Provides domestic and international listing of persons and agencies involved with older drivers

From Yoshikawa TT, Cobbs EL, Brummel-Smith K: Resources for older drivers. In Yoshikawa TT, Cobbs EL, editors: *Ambulatory geriatric care*, St Louis, 1997, Mosby.

the health and well-being of the patient, family, and other drivers on the road to prevent unsafe drivers from placing themselves and others in hazardous situations. Several specific aspects of function have been shown to play a role in the ability to drive safely. Most of these can be assessed effectively in the office of the primary care provider so that appropriate recommendations can be made regarding the person's ability to continue driving.

Resources

American Association of Motor Vehicle Administrators
4301 Wilson Blvd., Suite 400
Arlington, VA 22203
(703) 522-4200
www.aamva.org

American Association of Retired Persons
AARP 55 Alive
601 E Street NW
Washington, DC 20049
(202) 434-2277
www.aarp.org

Insurance Institute for Highway Safety
www.hwysafety.org
National Safety Council
1121 Spring Lake Drive
Itasca, IL 60143-3201
(630) 285-1121
Fax: (630) 285-1315
www.nsc.org

References

Babizhayev MA: Glare disability and driving safety, *Ophthalmic Res* 35(1):19-25, 2003.
Daigneault G, Joly P, Frigon JY: Executive functions in the evaluation of accident risk of older drivers, *J Clin Exp Neuropsychol* 24(2):221-238, 2002.
Foley DJ et al: Driving life expectancy of persons aged 70 years and older in the United States, *Am J Public Health* 92(8):1284-1289, 2002.
Margolis KL et al: Risk factors for motor vehicle crashes in older women, *J Gerontol A Biol Sci Med Sci* 57(3):M186-M191, 2002.
Marottoli RA et al: Development of a test battery to identify older drivers at risk for self-reported adverse driving events, *J Am Geriatr Soc* 46:562-568, 1998.
McGregor D: Driving over 65: proceed with caution, *J Gerontol Nurs* 28(8):22-26, 2002.
Wood JM: Aging, driving and vision, *Clin Exp Optom* 85(4):214-220, 2002.

28

Alcohol Abuse

Substance-related disorders in older adults remain overlooked and undertreated. Up to 16% of older adults have alcohol-use disorders (Menninger, 2002). Alcoholism is the third most prevalent psychiatric disorder among older men, following dementia and anxiety disorders. Evidence exists that light to moderate drinking is associated with a reduced risk of coronary heart disease, total ischemic stroke, and total mortality in middle-aged and older men and women; however, the apparent benefits of moderate drinking on mortality rates from congestive heart disease are offset at higher drinking levels by increasing the risk of death from other types of heart disease (e.g., cardiomyopathy, arrhythmia), neurologic disorders, cancer, liver cirrhosis, and traffic accidents (Agarwal, 2002). Falls have also been found to be a more common cause of injury in older patients who use alcohol than in those who do not use alcohol (Zautcke et al, 2002).

Health-related consequences of alcohol abuse include functional decline, dependency, and cognitive impairments that lead to excessive emergency department visits and hospitalization. Alcohol intake has been associated with an increased risk of adverse drug reactions, including gastrointestinal complications, metabolic and endocrine complications, dermatologic and allergic complications, and arrhythmias (Onder et al, 2002). Studies demonstrate that medical staff make the diagnosis of alcohol abuse in fewer than 25% of older patients who are abusing alcohol and refer to treatment fewer than half of those who are diagnosed (McInnes and Powell, 1994). Other factors that contribute to low reporting rates are listed in Box 28-1.

The underdiagnosis of alcohol abuse is due in part to the facts that the effects of alcohol use among older adults tend to be less clearly visible than among other age groups and that older adults are less likely to seek treatment than are younger age groups. An additional challenge to diagnosis may be a lack of previous alcohol abuse by the patient because about one third of older adults with alcohol-use problems first develop their drinking problem after the age of 60 years. With a demographic shift that is expected to increase the number of older adults with alcohol problems, awareness and understanding of this problem become increasingly important (Barrick and Connors, 2002).

Metabolism of Ethanol

Ethanol (the chemical component of consumable alcohol) has direct toxic effects on the gastrointestinal system, heart, kidney, brain, and liver. Oxidation of ethanol through the alcohol dehydrogenase pathway produces acetaldehyde, which is converted to acetate. Hydrogen is transferred from ethanol to a cofactor, nicotinamide adenine dinucleotide (NAD), which in turn is reduced to NADH.

Box 28-1

Factors Leading to Low Reporting of Alcohol Abuse in Older Adults

Underdiagnosis by health care providers	Increased biologic sensitivity
Denial of condition by patient	Less interaction with social institutions
Unwillingness of family to report	Less pressure to initiate treatment

---

NADH is responsible for many of the metabolic problems associated with alcohol abuse: hyperlactacidemia, hyperuricemia, hypoglycemia, and hyperlipidemia. Advanced age results in a decreased first-pass metabolism of ethanol with elevated serum ethanol concentrations. It is still unknown whether this is due to age alone or to other factors like, for example, atrophic gastritis with decreased activity of alcohol dehydrogenase (Oneta et al, 2001). Ethnic differences are an important consideration; 40% of Japanese for example, have aldehyde dehydrogenase deficiency and thereby are more susceptible to the effects of alcohol.

Age-related Changes and Relationship to Alcohol Consumption

GASTROINTESTINAL SYSTEM

1. Atrophy of the gastric mucosa
2. Alteration of prostaglandin synthesis (which increases the risk for gastritis)
3. Decreased absorption of calcium, iron, lactose, and vitamin D
4. Increased absorption of fat-soluble compounds such as vitamins A and K and cholesterol
5. Decreasing liver mass
6. Decreased blood flow to the liver (about 10% per decade)
7. Blood concentration of alcohol that is increased disproportionately to the amount consumed because *the volume of distribution for alcohol is decreased* in older adults

CARDIOVASCULAR SYSTEM

1. Left ventricular muscle mass increases, and maximum heart rate declines.
2. Systolic and diastolic blood pressures increase with age.
3. The incidence of atherosclerosis and atherosclerotic heart disease increases.
4. Alcohol consumption increases plasma triglyceride levels and elevates blood pressure.

NERVOUS SYSTEM

1. Weight of the brain decreases.
2. Blood supply to the brain decreases.
3. The blood–brain barrier becomes more penetrable, increasing the sensitivity of older adults to the central effects of alcohol.
4. The incidence of short-term memory loss and dementia increases with age.
5. Long-term alcoholism can produce dementia secondary to the nutritional deficit resulting from alcoholism. Estimates are that 10% of dementia cases in older adults are alcohol related (Campbell, 1997). Increasing blood alcohol levels have been associated with progressively decreasing perception, and older subjects perform less well at all blood alcohol levels.

MUSCULAR AND SKELETAL SYSTEMS

1. Gait and balance impairments increase.
2. The incidence of falls in older adults is high. Accidents are the sixth leading cause of death in older adults, and two thirds of these deaths are related to falls.

3. In all age groups alcohol plays a significant role in accidents, especially falls. Alcohol-related cognitive and physical effects contribute to gait and balance impairments and increase the risk of falls.
4. Alcohol is identified as a significant risk factor for the development of osteoporosis.

Diagnostic Criteria

Substance dependence is defined as a maladaptive pattern of use in the presence of three of the seven elements of dependence within a 12-month period. The seven elements of dependence are tolerance, withdrawal, use of the substance in larger amounts and for a longer time than intended, a persistent desire to use and unsuccessful efforts to cut down, spending a great deal of time in obtaining the substance, giving up or reducing activities because of use, and continued use despite recurrent physical or psychological problems caused by use (American Psychiatric Association, 1994).

CRITERIA FOR ALCOHOL ABUSE

According to the *Diagnostic and Statistical Manual of Mental Disorders*, fourth edition (DSM-IV) (American Psychiatric Association, 1994), the following are the criteria for alcohol abuse:
A. A maladaptive pattern of substance use leading to clinically significant impairment or distress, as manifested by one (or more) of the following, occurring within a 12-month period:
   1. Recurrent alcohol use resulting in a failure to fulfill major role obligations at work, school, or home
   2. Recurrent alcohol use in situations in which it is physically hazardous
   3. Recurrent alcohol-related legal problems
   4. Continued alcohol use despite having persistent or recurrent social or interpersonal problems caused or exacerbated by the effects of alcohol
B. The symptoms have never met the criteria for alcohol dependence for this class of substance.

Older adults who abuse alcohol do not always meet the preceding criteria for alcohol abuse. It is difficult to apply these criteria to this group of patients because most are no longer working or in school settings. A decline in social interactions because of retirement and the loss of friends and family to death may make many older adults prone to social isolation. Social isolation, grief, and boredom are often precursors for alcohol abuse and subsequent dependency.

According to the DSM-IV, the criteria for alcohol dependency include a definition of *tolerance:* a need for markedly increased amounts of alcohol to achieve intoxication or markedly diminished effects with continued use of the same amount of alcohol (American Psychiatric Association, 1994). As a person ages, the quantity of alcohol consumed generally decreases; however, as mentioned previously, an older person is more sensitive to the effects of alcohol. The decrease in the amount of alcohol consumed may cause the patient and practitioner to minimize the problem.

Alcohol-use disorders can be categorized into six groupings that are not mutually exclusive: dependence, abuse, harmful, hazardous, heavy drinking, and binge drinking (see Box 28-2 for definitions).

A helpful distinction for older drinkers may be early onset versus late-onset drinkers. Despite the widely held view by clinicians that alcoholics die at a young age, two thirds of older drinkers began drinking in their youth. Those who have survived to old age have multiple medical and psychological problems related to their long pattern of alcohol ingestion. By contrast, late-onset use of alcohol is usually related to the stress associated with age, such as death of a spouse, retirement, and financial strains. This group of older adults has fewer health problems and contains more women than men.

"Ageism" can interfere with the diagnosis and treatment of alcohol abuse: "*He is 85 years old. His wife is dead. He suffers from cataracts, arthritis, hypertension, and diabetes. It is no wonder that he is depressed. Let him drink!*" In this situation, alternatives to alcohol are available. Many patients use alcohol as self-medication for emotional and physical pain and for insomnia because of myths about the effects of alcohol.

Box 28-2

Definitions of Terms

Dependence

Maladaptive pattern of use to include three of the following seven elements of dependence within a 12-mo period (American Psychiatric Association, 1994):

Tolerance

Withdrawal

Use of larger amounts and for longer time periods than intended

Persistent desire to use and unsuccessful efforts to cut down

Giving up activities because of use

Spending a great deal of time in obtaining the substance

Continued use despite adverse problems related to use (DSM-IV)

Abuse

Maladaptive pattern of use to include one or more of the following four elements of abuse within a 12-mo period (American Psychiatric Association, 1994):

Failure to fulfill obligations because of use

Use in situations that are physically hazardous

Legal problems related to use

Persistent use despite social and interpersonal problems

Harmful Drinking

Evidence of adverse physical and psychologic problems related to use

Hazardous Drinking

Use that places user at risk for adverse consequences

Heavy Drinking

Consuming 5 or more drinks* on the same occasion on at least 5 different days in the past month

Binge Drinking

Ingesting 5 or more drinks* on the same occasion once in the past month

_____

*A drink is 12 oz of beer, 5 oz of wine, or 1.5 oz of 80-proof distilled spirits (U.S. Department of Health and Human Services, 1995).

HISTORY

Diagnosing alcohol abuse in older patients requires a high index of suspicion. Clinicians need to be aware of their tendency to overlook many of the presenting symptoms of alcohol abuse in the older person because of *the typical atypical presentation* and because of the stigma attached to the older alcoholic. Clues may include missed appointments, personality changes, irritability, uncontrolled hypertension, uncontrolled diabetes, poor personal hygiene, sleep disturbances, recurrent falls, weight loss, and memory loss (immediate, recent, or remote) (Box 28-3). The concurrent use of cigarettes and a family history of alcohol problems are associated with an increased risk of alcohol abuse. Often family members or friends will bring these problems to the attention of the practitioner. Most patients generally deny that there is a problem, whereas others may defend their drinking and become angry when confronted.

Box 28-3

Symptoms of Alcohol Abuse Missed by Many Health Care Providers and Ascribed to the Aging Process

New symptoms of confusion	Sleep disturbance
Increased short-term memory loss	Functional decline
Weight loss	Self-neglect
Apathy	Chronic fatigue
Falls	Poorly managed disease (diabetes, hypertension)
Bruises	Solution: Maintain a high degree of suspicion and
Polypharmacy	assess for the problem.

At times enabling behavior by the patient's spouse, adult children, or formal caregivers may make the differential diagnosis extremely difficult. For whatever reason, many caregivers use denial to deal with an older person's alcoholism. The primary care provider needs the assistance of caregivers to treat older people who are abusing alcohol successfully.

A review of prescription and over-the-counter medications is normal procedure in the history taking for any older adult, but it is especially critical if there is a suspicion of alcohol abuse. Alcohol is a drug that places the older person at unrecognized risk for adverse drug interactions. Alcohol has the potential to affect adversely medications and can lead to injury, acute illness, or at times even death. A referral to current drug manuals is necessary to check the potential risk for interactions with the patient's prescription and over-the-counter drugs.

Many older women are at risk for the development of late-onset alcohol problems. The practitioner needs to maintain an awareness of the person's individual risk and consider that women tend to outlive their partners and have higher poverty rates and different patterns of intake than men. Women are more likely to drink at home and alone, which makes detection by friends, family, and neighbors quite difficult.

Many tests are available to screen for alcohol abuse. The CAGE (need to *c*ut down on drinking, *a*nnoyance, *g*uilt about drinking, need for *e*ye-opener) questionnaire and the MAST-G (Michigan Alcoholism Screening Test–Geriatric Version) have been studied in older people. The advantages of the four-question CAGE questionnaire are that it is brief and inoffensive and can be given in written or oral form. The CAGE questionnaire does not make a distinction between current and past problems, but the sensitivity and specificity are 70% and 91%, respectively (cutoff two or more yes responses). The MAST-G, a 24-item tool, is age appropriate and quite useful (Box 28-4 and Figure 28-1). It has been suggested that using both brief measures may identify more alcohol-use disorders among older persons because each instrument seems to capture different aspects of unsafe drinking (Moore et al, 2002).

PHYSICAL EXAMINATION

A physical examination of the patient can be helpful in diagnosing alcoholism. Signs to look for include a disheveled appearance, a smell of alcohol or urine, pale conjunctivae, icteric sclerae, a coated tongue, multiple caries, a hyperactive gag reflex, epigastric tenderness, a palpable liver, tremors, and ataxia. Although these signs are inconclusive by themselves, a positive diagnosis can be made in conjunction with a good history and supportive laboratory data.

DIAGNOSTIC TESTS

Diagnostic tests may include blood tests and radiologic evaluation of the liver, pancreas, and heart. Abnormal laboratory results suggestive of alcohol abuse include elevated mean corpuscular cell volume; decreased vitamin B_{12}, folate, and albumin; elevated gamma-glutamyl transferase; and an

		Yes (1)	No (0)

1. After drinking have you ever noticed an increase in your heart rate or beating in your chest?   1. ____ ____
2. When talking with others do you ever underestimate how much you actually drink?   2. ____ ____
3. Does alcohol make you sleepy so that you often fall asleep in your chair?   3. ____ ____
4. After a few drinks have you sometimes not eaten or been able to skip a meal because you didn't feel hungry?   4. ____ ____
5. Does having a few drinks help decrease your shakiness or tremors?   5. ____ ____
6. Does alcohol sometimes make it hard for you to remember parts of the day or night?   6. ____ ____
7. Do you have rules for yourself that you won't drink before a certain time of the day?   7. ____ ____
8. Have you lost interest in hobbies or activities you used to enjoy?   8. ____ ____
9. When you wake up in the morning do you ever have trouble remembering part of the night before?   9. ____ ____
10. Does having a drink help you sleep?   10. ____ ____
11. Do you hide your alcohol bottles from family members?   11. ____ ____
12. After a social gathering have you ever felt embarrassed because you drank too much?   12. ____ ____
13. Have you ever been concerned that drinking might be harmful to your health?   13. ____ ____
14. Do you like to end an evening with a night cap?   14. ____ ____
15. Did you find your drinking increased after someone close to you died?   15. ____ ____
16. In general, would you prefer to have a few drinks at home rather than go out to social events?   16. ____ ____
17. Are you drinking more now than in the past?   17. ____ ____
18. Do you usually take a drink to relax or calm your nerves?   18. ____ ____
19. Do you drink to take your mind off your problems?   19. ____ ____
20. Have you ever increased your drinking after experiencing a loss in your life?   20. ____ ____
21. Do you sometimes drive when you have had too much to drink?   21. ____ ____
22. Has a doctor or nurse ever said they were worried or concerned about your drinking?   22. ____ ____
23. Have you ever made rules to manage your drinking?   23. ____ ____
24. When you feel lonely does having a drink help?   24. ____ ____

Scoring: 5 or more "yes" responses is indicative of alcohol problem.

Figure 28-1   Michigan Alcoholism Screening Test-Geriatric Version (MAST-G). (From Blow FC et al: The Michigan Alcoholism Test-Geriatric Version (MAST-G): a new elderly-specific screening instrument, *Alcohol Clin Exp Res* 16(2):372, 1991. Copyright of The Regents of the University of Michigan.)

Box 28-4
The CAGE Questionnaire

1. Have you ever felt you ought to Cut down?
2. Have you ever been Annoyed by criticism of your drinking?
3. Have you ever felt Guilty about your drinking?
4. Have you ever felt the need for an Eye opener?

aspartate aminotransferase and alanine aminotransferase ratio greater than 2:1. A normal blood alcohol level does not rule out a diagnosis of chronic alcohol abuse. Radiographic studies demonstrating cardiomegaly, hepatomegaly, or pancreatitis also warrant consideration of a diagnosis of alcohol abuse.

Management and Treatment

The general principles of treatment of alcohol abuse emphasize things that can be done and also emphasize building a relationship that allows the patient and caregivers to realize that there is a caring environment and that recovery is a strong possibility. For many older patients the inclusion of family or the caregiver becomes essential to the ability to participate successfully in treatment and recovery.

Care needs to be individualized on the basis of the extent and type of alcohol disorder. Patients with more acute dependence are referred, and hospitalization should be considered for the withdrawal period. Therapy for less acute patients needs to deal with their particular age-related stresses and how their coping mechanism of alcohol use is harmful. When discussing treatment options, the practitioner must be knowledgeable about local programs and community resources available to the patient. Alcoholics Anonymous (AA) members are excellent resources, and the older patient should be informed that AA is certainly appropriate for older adults; more than one third of its members are over 50 years of age. The treatment plan should begin the day the patient is confronted with the diagnosis.

Relapse, or the return to drinking following abstinence, may follow situations that are of particularly high risk for older adults. These include situations related to anxiety, interpersonal conflict, depression, loneliness, loss, or social isolation (Barrick and Connors, 2002).

Treatments such as cognitive–behavioral therapy, group and family therapies, and self-help groups are just as effective for older adults as they are for other age groups. In fact, group and family therapies and self-help groups may be of particular benefit to older adults because of the emphasis on social support (Barrick and Connors, 2002).

One way to approach the treatment of alcohol abuse in older adults is to use a staging process and relate the treatment to the stage that applies to the patient (Table 28-1).

The following paragraphs provide an example of the progression of the staging process: Mr. Recent Widower is an older man who usually has one drink a day after dinner. Since his wife died 3 months ago, he spends his evenings drinking beer while watching television. He has passed out on the couch three times in the last month. This is stage I: nonsocial drinking pattern, and a nonconfrontational approach is recommended. It is important for the patient to hear from the practitioner that his *pattern* of drinking is *problematic*. Appropriate evaluation and treatment for grief and depression are necessary. A 90-day abstinence trial may be effective with weekly AA meetings. Patients should be encouraged to schedule group activities to avoid social isolation. Suggestions may include weekly meals with family members and friends and participation in senior or recreational center activities.

As Mr. Recent Widower enters stage II, his drinking takes precedence over his eating. His daughter finds his home in disarray. The patient is unshaven, and his clothes are dirty. When confronted by his daughter, the patient states, "Stop nagging and leave me alone." The daughter reluctantly complies. The psychological dependency and social problems begin. Temporary inpatient treatment may be necessary; Medicare will cover some of the inpatient days. AA can offer support and guidance to the patient and family members.

Without treatment the patient progresses to stage III. The physiologic dependency begins, and health problems become evident. Emergency department visits become frequent, and hospitalizations for trauma, loss of consciousness, and recurrent infections occur. Diagnoses include peripheral

TABLE 28-1	**Staging of Problem Drinking in Older Patients**			
Stage	*Features*	*Dependency*	*Prognosis*	*Intervention*
I	Nonsocial drinking pattern	Minimal	Good	Nonconfrontational
II	Social problem	Psychologic	Good	Confrontational
III	Health problems	Physiologic	Fair	Group intervention
IV	Laboratory evidence	Severe	Poor	Multidisciplinary intervention
V	Minimal social functioning	Terminal	Poor	Involuntary

neuropathy, pneumonia, urinary tract infections, gastrointestinal bleeding, seizure disorders, cardiomyopathy, and congestive heart failure. Treatment at this stage generally requires benzodiazepines to prevent withdrawal seizures; therefore hospitalization is normally advised. Follow-up should include an outpatient program, AA, and 1 to 2 years of continuing care.

Older patients in stages IV and V are easy to identify. Treatment includes an inpatient program followed by a lifelong outpatient program. Outpatient programs are most effective when tailored to the individual patient. Treatment with individuals in the same age group as the patient also yields a better response.

GUIDELINES FOR INTERVENTION

1. Avoid being judgmental.
2. Persuade the patient to have an evaluation for possible treatment.
3. Do something today.
4. Have the telephone number of an AA person who can talk to the patient.
5. Have a plan.
6. Make use of family and friends.
7. If all else fails, consider legal commitment.

Prevention

Older adults should be counseled about the risks and the age-related changes that increase the dangers of alcohol-related problems. The harmful interactions of alcohol and many medications, both prescription and over the counter, need to be clarified. Information regarding the physical changes that accompany aging and the effects on alcohol metabolism needs to be readily available in all forms: verbal, visual, and written. Abstinence or at least moderation of intake should be strongly encouraged for all older patients.

Summary

Alcohol abuse is a prevalent but commonly overlooked problem in older patients. The economic, social, psychological, and medical consequences of alcohol abuse lead to increased functional impairment and increased risk for dependency in older persons. Alcohol abuse in older adults should be diagnosed and effectively treated to decrease mortality and morbidity. Overall medical costs will be reduced by the decreased need for hospitalization and treatment for alcohol-related medical conditions.

Resources

Alcohol Abuse USA Information Page
www.drug-abuse.com

Alcoholism Net
www.alcoholism.net

National Institute on Alcohol Abuse and Alcoholism
www.niaaa.nih.gov

References

Agarwal DP: Cardioprotective effects of light-moderate consumption of alcohol: a review of putative mechanisms, *Alcohol Alcohol* 37(5):409-415, 2002.
American Psychiatric Association: *Diagnostic and statistical manual of mental disorders*, ed 4, Washington, DC, 1994, American Psychiatric Association.

Barrick C, Connors GJ: Relapse prevention and maintaining abstinence in older adults with alcohol-use disorders, *Drugs Aging* 19(8):583-594, 2002.

Campbell JW: Alcoholism. In Ham R, Sloane P, editors: *Primary care geriatrics: a case-based approach*, ed 3, St Louis, 1997, Mosby.

McInnes E, Powell J: Drug and alcohol referrals: are elderly substance abuse diagnoses and referrals being missed? *BMJ* 308:444-446, 1994.

Menninger JA: Assessment and treatment of alcoholism and substance-related disorders in the elderly, *Bull Menninger Clin* 66(2):166-183, 2002.

Moore AA et al: Are there differences between older persons who screen positive on the CAGE questionnaire and the Short Michigan Alcoholism Screening Test-Geriatric Version? *J Am Geriatr Soc* 50(5):858-862, 2002.

Onder G et al: Moderate alcohol consumption and adverse drug reactions among older adults, *Pharmacoepidemiol Drug Safety* 11(5):385-392, 2002.

Oneta CM et al: Age and bioavailability of alcohol, *Z Gastroenterol* 39(9):783-788, 2001.

Zautcke JL et al: Geriatric trauma in the state of Illinois: substance use and injury patterns, *Am J Emerg Med* 20(1):14-17, 2002.

29

Abuse and Neglect

Mistreatment of older persons in the United States occurs across all social, racial, and class strata. Up to two million older persons are abused or neglected in the United States each year (Harrell et al, 2002). Most cases of elder abuse occur at home rather than in institutions, and evidence suggests that only one in five cases are recognized (Brandl and Horan, 2002). It is estimated that only 1 in 14 incidents of domestic elder abuse is ever reported or detected. Whatever the estimate, it is generally agreed that the number of incidents of older adults will increase over the next 30 years. The projected increase in abuse cases is the result of the following factors: (1) people are living longer, which increases the need for more long-term care; (2) increased demands on family caregivers; and (3) increased legal obligations to report suspected elder abuse.

To determine the boundaries of elder abuse or neglect, the California penal code is an excellent standard; however, providers need to be cognizant of the legal standards of their particular state. *Abuse* is defined in the California Welfare and Institution code as "physical abuse, neglect, intimidation, cruel punishment, financial abuse, abandonment, isolation, abduction or other treatment with resulting physical harm, pain, or mental suffering, or the deprivation by a care custodian of goods or services which are necessary to avoid physical harm or mental suffering" (California Welfare and Institution Code).

Types of Abuse and Neglect

Box 29-1 provides definitions of abuse with examples of behaviors and effects. Physical abuse and neglect produce a wide range of bodily injuries, such as bruising, scratches, broken areas on the skin, undetected and untreated pressure ulcers, and neglected personal grooming. Physical abuse may take the form of striking, shoving, shaking, restraining, or physical coercion. Sexual assault refers to any form of sexual intimacy that occurs without consent or by force or threat of force.

Psychological abuse and neglect encompass behaviors that cause emotional anguish to the older person. This type of abuse includes verbal mistreatment such as threats, insults, or harsh commands as well as silence and ignoring the person.

Material or financial abuse is the misuse or exploitation of, or inattention to, an older person's possessions, funds, or resources. It includes irresponsible management of the older person's money, pressuring of the victim to distribute assets, and outright theft.

Active neglect refers to the refusal or failure to undertake a caregiving obligation (including a conscious and intentional attempt to inflict physical or emotional stress on the older person). *Passive*

Box 29-1

Definitions of Types of Abuse, with Examples of Behavior and Effects

Physical abuse: Nonaccidental infliction of physical force that results in bodily injury, pain or impairment
- *Examples of behavior:* hitting, slapping, pushing, burning, physical restraint
- *Examples of effects:* bruises, fractures, burns, broken teeth, sprains, cuts, hair loss, bleeding from scalp, fear, anxiety, depression

Psychological abuse: The persistent use of threats, humiliation, bullying, swearing and other verbal conduct, and/or of any other form of mental cruelty that results in mental or physical distress
- *Examples of behavior:* treating elder as a child, blaming, swearing, intimidating, name-calling, threatening violence, isolating elder
- *Examples of effects:* fear, depression, confusion, loss of sleep, loss of appetite

Financial abuse: Unauthorized and improper use of funds, property or any resources of an older person
- *Examples of behavior:* misappropriating money, valuables, or property; forcing changes to will; denying elder right to access personal funds
- *Examples of effects:* loss of money, etc., inability to pay bills, deterioration in health or standard of living, lack of amenities, unusual activity in bank accounts, signatures on documents uncertain, lack of solid arrangements for financial management, eviction or house sale notices

Sexual abuse: Direct or indirect involvement in sexual activity without consent
- *Examples of behavior*
  - *Noncontact:* looking, photography, indecent exposure, harassment, serious teasing or innuendo, pornography
  - *Contact:* touching breast, genitals, anus, mouth; masturbation of either or both persons; penetration or attempted penetration of vagina, anus, mouth, with or by penis, fingers, other objects
- *Examples of effects:* difficulty in walking or sitting, bruises, bleeding, venereal disease, psychological trauma

Neglect: Repeated deprivation of assistance needed by the older person for important activities of daily living
- *Examples of behavior:* failure to provide food, shelter, clothing, medical care, hygiene, personal care; inappropriate use of medication or overmedication
- *Examples of effects:* malnutrition, pressure sores, oversedation; untreated medical problems, depression, confusion

Source: McCreadie C, Tinker A: Elder abuse. In Tallis RC, Flint HM: *Brocklehurst's Textbook of Geriatric Medicine and Gerontology*, ed 6, London, 2003, Churchill Livingstone.

neglect is a refusal or failure to fulfill a caretaking obligation (excluding a conscious and intentional attempt to inflict physical or emotional distress on the older person). Interestingly, the most commonly reported type of neglect is *self-neglect,* defined as "an adult's inability, due to physical or mental impairments or diminished capacity, to perform self-care tasks ... to maintain physical health, safety, and/or manage financial affairs" (Capezuti, Brush, and Lawson, 1997). Most self-neglecting older adults have functional or mental impairments as well as a poor social network. Interventions in this situation present many practical and ethical challenges.

Undue influence (UI) is the substitution of one person's will for the true desires of another. Unlike common persuasion and sales techniques, such influence often entails fraud, duress, threats, or other deceits and pressures (Quinn, 2002). UI occurs when one person uses his or her role and power to exploit the trust, dependency, or fear of another to gain psychological control over the weaker person's decision making, usually for financial gain. Although UI has long been recognized in the legal system, it is new to the field of elder abuse and neglect; however, undue influence is common in elder-abuse situations, specifically when psychological abuse works in combination with financial abuse. Older adults may be more vulnerable to UI than other age groups because several factors may be occurring at the same time, such as cognitive problems, drastic changes in life circumstances, and physical health problems (Quinn, 2002).

The circumstances that surround an abusive situation are composed of three elements: the abuser, the abused older person, and the context of the social situation that leads to and supports the act of abuse. No typical abusive scenario is valid. In fact, the diversity of situations that lead to abuse makes it crucial that providers assess all three elements of an abusive situation before making a diagnosis.

ABUSER

Factors that may indicate that a caregiver is at risk of becoming an abuser include substance abuse; poor physical health; mental confusion or cognitive impairment; emotional or mental illness; inexperience in caregiving; emotional or financial dependence on the care recipient; having been abused as a child, especially if the older person was the abuser; social isolation and lack of a support system; and being involved in conflict either with the older person or with an outside relationship, which may increase stress. Caregivers who have a history of alcoholism, drug use, or gambling addiction may resort to financial abuse of an older adult to support these habits or to escape financial crisis. Many caregivers are older themselves and may have physical or medical problems. The behavior traits of the older person, the daily tasks to be performed, and isolation and frustration can lead to stress. Unintentional abuse, or *neglect,* can be the result of ignorance, inexperience, overburdened caregivers, or a lack of desire or ability to provide proper care.

ABUSED OLDER PERSON

Common characteristics of abused older persons include being older, female, dependent, of low socioeconomic status, alcoholic, isolated, or impaired; having a history of abuse; engaging in provocative (e.g., overly demanding, unappreciative) or aggressive and combative behavior; and having unrealistic expectations (Harrell et al, 2002). Although victims of elder abuse have long been characterized as being frail, dependent women, it is important to remember that any older person, male or female, cognitively impaired or intact, can be a victim.

SOCIAL CONTEXT

The history of the relationship between the caregiver and the care recipient must also be considered. A parent–child (or other) relationship that was always strained or abusive cannot be expected to improve when the stresses of caregiving and dependence are added. Dependence of the caregiver on the older person for financial support or housing can also lead to or sustain an abusive relationship.

ABUSE OF AGING CAREGIVERS

Whereas the study of abuse of aging persons in family caregiving situations has traditionally focused on abuse of the dependent care receiver, evidence supports the health risks related to abuse of aging caregivers as well. Women, usually spouses, daughters, or daughters-in-law, most frequently assume the caregiver role. Aging caregivers can be placed at risk by verbally and physically abusive behaviors of older persons for whom they provide care. Caregivers use metaphors, substituted terms, alternative words, analogies, and interpretive phrases in place of the word "abuse." For example, caregivers may refer to verbal abuse by describing the abusive older person as "unkind," "nasty," or "manipulative." Use of terms such as "tyrant," "explosive," and "verbal knives" reflect the strategies caregivers use of avoidance, denial, explanations, and descriptions to characterize the hurtful behavior in ways that normalize the abusive actions (Ayres and Woodtli, 2001). It is important that primary care providers be alert to these signals from caregivers and be prepared to provide counseling and assistance.

Subjective Findings

As mentioned, elder abuse can be physical, emotional, or financial. It is a serious and often overlooked problem. Many patients may be too cognitively impaired to explain the situation adequately. Others may be afraid of caregivers, on whom they are dependent. It is important to screen patients by asking whether anyone has ever hurt them or abused them emotionally or financially (Devons, 2002).

The abuse or neglect of older adults by their caregivers is not always readily visible or obvious to providers. Unfortunately, few validated screening measures exist to assist providers in identifying cases of abuse. One tool that is based on abuse indicators and is designed to be completed by the practitioner is the Indicators of Abuse Screen in Box 29-2. A score of 16 or greater, the "abuse alert" score, is considered indicative of abuse; however, the need for more research into the use of this tool has been recognized (Reis and Nahmiash, 1998).

The practitioner cannot rely solely on interviews with, or reports from, abusers or victims. Communication barriers such as dementia, aphasia, or delusions may render a victim incapable of alerting a practitioner to an abusive situation. In rare cases a victim who is able will talk openly about ongoing abuse. More often, however, victims do not want to report abuse because of embar-

---

Box 29-2

Indicators of Abuse (IOA) Screen

Indicators of abuse are listed below, numbered in order of importance.* After a two- to three-hour home assessment (or other intensive assessment) please rate each of the following items on a scale of 0 to 4. Do not omit any items. Rate according to your *current opinion*.

Scale: Estimated extent of problem:
- 0 = nonexistent
- 1 = slight
- 2 = moderate
- 3 = probable/moderately severe
- 4 = yes/severe
- 00 = not applicable
- 000 = don't know

Caregiver Age _____ years
Caregiver and Care Receiver Kinship ___ spouse
_____ nonspouse

Caregiver
- ___ 1. Has behavior problems
- ___ 2. Is financially dependent
- ___ 3. Has mental/emotional difficulties
- ___ 6. Has alcohol/substance abuse problem
- ___ 7. Has unrealistic expectations
- ___ 9. Lacks understanding of medical condition
- ___ 10. Caregiving reluctancy
- ___ 12. Has marital/family conflict
- ___ 13. Has poor current relationship
- ___ 14. Caregiving inexperience
- ___ 17. Is a blamer
- ___ 24. Had poor past relationship

Care Receiver
- ___ 4. Has been abused in the past
- ___ 5. Has marital/family conflict
- ___ 8. Lacks understanding of medical condition
- ___ 11. Is socially isolated
- ___ 15. Lacks social support
- ___ 16. Has behavior problems
- ___ 18. Is financially dependent
- ___ 19. Has unrealistic expectations
- ___ 20. Has alcohol/medication problem
- ___ 21. Has poor current relationship
- ___ 22. Has suspicious falls/injuries
- ___ 23. Has mental/emotional difficulties
- ___ 25. Is a blamer
- ___ 26. Is emotionally dependent
- ___ 27. No regular doctor

From Reis M, Nahmiash D: Validation of the indicators of abuse screen, *Gerontologist* 38(4):471-480, 1998.
* The majority of the most important indicators are the caregiver ones.

rassment, shame, intimidation, or fear. Some victims even blame themselves for the abuse and believe it is somehow deserved. They may be unwilling to talk openly and may respond to questions with implausible stories, anger, or denial.

Despite the importance of avoiding confrontation with the victim and the caregiver, it is possible to elicit reports of abuse with direct questions: Do you feel safe where you live? Do you ever have disagreements with your caregiver? Have you ever been treated roughly or intimidated? The responses to such questions are often revealing. Conversations with the caregiver usually rely on opened-ended types of questions worded in a nonthreatening, nonjudgmental way: Can you tell me what a normal day providing care for [the patient] is like for you? It must be difficult. Do you ever lose control?

These types of questions allow the abuser to perceive the practitioner as empathic and create a nonjudgmental environment that is helpful in obtaining necessary information. Victims fear reporting abuse for a number of reasons. They may want to protect their loved one from criminal action. The older person may have a long history of "saving" the abuser, who is often an alcoholic, drug-dependent, or mentally ill adult child. It is important to interview the patient and suspected abuser both together *and* individually and to observe the interactions between them, making note of disparities in their accounts regarding care routines, history, and especially injuries. Behavioral indications of an abusive relationship are identified in Box 29-3.

Objective Findings

Most cases, whether in domestic or institutional settings, are likely to arise in primary or secondary care as part of some other presenting problem. Identification relies on a high index of suspicion (McCreadie and Tinker, 2003). Issues in the patient history that may indicate abuse include delay in time between onset of illness and presentation to a health care provider, repeated injuries, missed appointments or frequent changes in doctors, inconsistencies between the history given by patient and caregiver, strain in the relationship between the caregiver and the patient, and fearfulness of the patient (Harrell et al, 2002).

Physical examination of the abused or neglected older adult may reveal the following findings:
- *General appearance:* poor hygiene, inappropriate dress
- *Skin:* poor turgor, skin lesions, bruises, pressure ulcers, burns
- *Head and neck:* trauma (hematomas, lacerations, abrasions), alopecia
- *Trunk:* bruises, welts
- *Genitourinary tract:* rectal or vaginal bleeding, infestations
- *Extremities:* wrist or ankle bruising, immersion (or other) burns

---

Box 29-3

Behavioral Clues to an Abusive Relationship

- The patient is not given the opportunity to speak for himself or herself or to see others except in the presence of the caregiver.
- The caregiver exhibits an attitude of indifference or anger toward the dependent person.
- The caregiver blames the patient for his or her condition, for example, by claiming that the patient's incontinence is a deliberate act.
- The caregiver exhibits aggressive behavior toward the patient or toward health care providers, including threats, insults, or harassment.
- The caregiver and the patient present conflicting accounts of incidents.
- The caregiver shows an unwillingness or reluctance to comply with planning for care.

Data from Murray L, DeVos D: The escalating problem of elder abuse, *Radiol Technol* 68(4):351-353, 1997.

- *Musculoskeletal:* fractures, pain (observe gait)
- *Neurologic:* cognitive deficits
  Signs that indicate abuse or neglect are listed in Box 29-4.

Discernment Before Intervention

Once a diagnosis is made, a review of the data obtained during the assessment phase is essential before any intervention can be implemented. Interventions must be based on the identified underlying causes; and a comprehensive, multidisciplinary long-term care plan must be formulated to ensure patient safety while respecting the autonomy of a competent individual (Chen and Koval, 2002). Figure 29-1 suggests steps for the management of abuse.

The review of data includes the following:

1. Is access to the victim a problem? Victims and abusers are often reluctant to allow contact by health care professionals. Practitioners may need to be creative in their approach to the situation and must always be aware of safety and other risks to themselves.
2. How serious is the abuse? If the pattern of abuse has escalated, the victim may be in serious danger, which may increase the urgency for intervention.
3. Is the victim aware of the problem? The victim's awareness of and reaction to the abuse will affect the practitioner's options in the situation.
4. Who is inflicting the abuse? Is it a family member or an outside caregiver? Does the victim have access to other family or friends? It is also important to remember that more than one person may be involved.
5. What is the victim's cognitive status? Does the victim have the capacity to make decisions regarding her or his care? Is the victim capable of following a plan of action if the situation becomes dangerous? It is important to determine whether any apparent cognitive deficits are actually pseudodementia caused by dehydration, improper medication management, or other acute disease that has been neglected or caused by the abuse itself.

Box 29-4

Indications of an Abusive Relationship

- Pattern of physician or hospital "hopping"
- An injury that has not been properly treated
- Any injury that is not compatible with the given history
- Recurrent injuries due to "accidents"
- Frequent trips to the emergency department for injuries
- Pain on touching (requires further assessment)
- Cuts, lacerations, or puncture wounds
- Bruises, welts, and discolorations (especially those in a suspicious pattern)
- The presence of new and old bruises together
- Dehydration or malnutrition without illness or related cause
- Sunken eyes or cheeks
- Evidence of inadequate care, such as pressure ulcers, weight loss, unfilled prescriptions, unscheduled or unkept appointments
- Poor hygiene or soiled clothing or bed linens
- Burns (especially those that appear due to cigarettes, ropes, etc.)
- Signs of confinement
- Lack of bandages on injuries, unset fractures, lack of sutures if needed
- Signs of sleep disruption (e.g., complaints of insomnia, excessive sleepiness)
- Absence of assistive devices (e.g., cane, hearing aids, dentures)

6. What is the victim's health and functional status? Does the victim have a medical condition or mobility problem that will modify management?
7. What are the victim's resources? What are the financial resources? Are there supportive family members, concerned neighbors, and friends?
8. What community resources are available? Are respite care options available (e.g., temporary shelters, day care, or foster care)?
9. Has any intervention been made in the past? Information about previous interventions (e.g., court orders of protection) and why they failed should be obtained to avoid embarking on the same approach.

Intervention
ABUSER

The counseling of abusers must start with an assessment of their abilities and knowledge level so that deficits can be corrected. This step is especially important in attempting to discern between intentional and unintentional neglect.

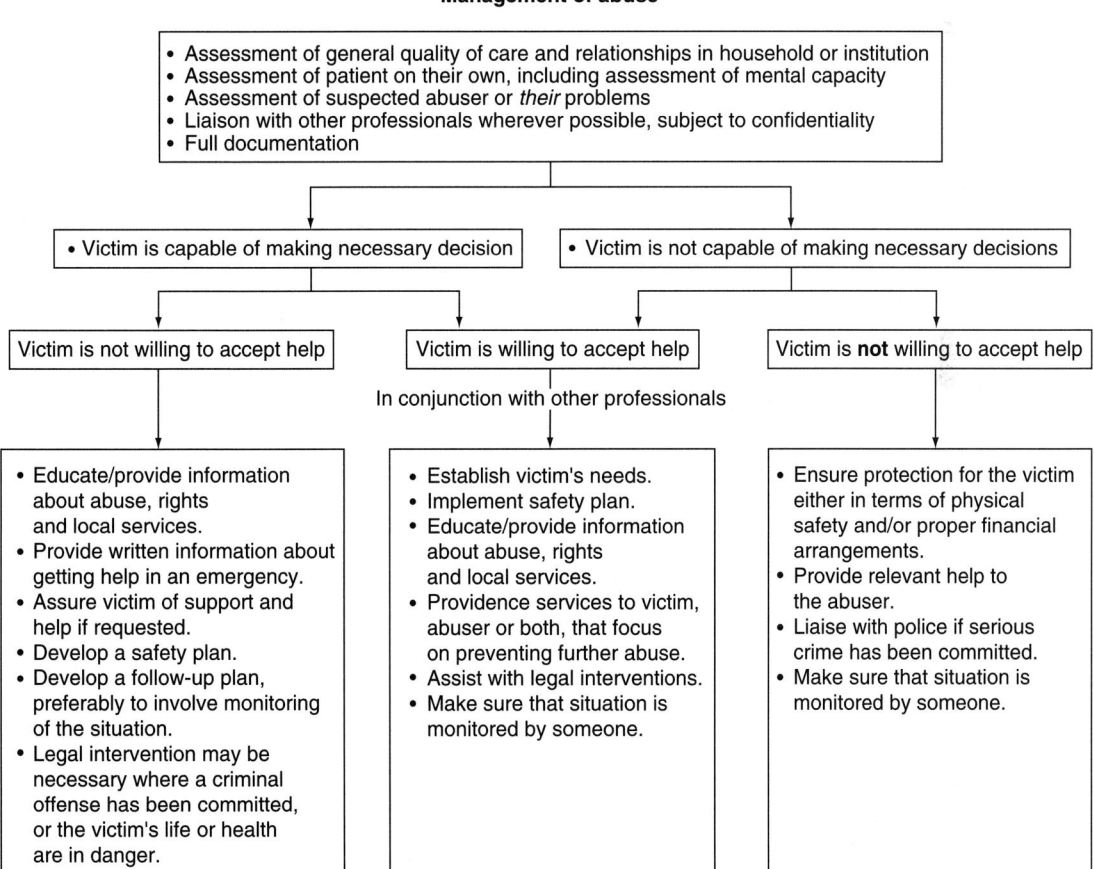

Management of abuse

- Assessment of general quality of care and relationships in household or institution
- Assessment of patient on their own, including assessment of mental capacity
- Assessment of suspected abuser or *their* problems
- Liaison with other professionals wherever possible, subject to confidentiality
- Full documentation

| • Victim is capable of making necessary decision | • Victim is not capable of making necessary decisions |

| Victim is not willing to accept help | Victim is willing to accept help | Victim is **not** willing to accept help |

In conjunction with other professionals

- Educate/provide information about abuse, rights and local services.
- Provide written information about getting help in an emergency.
- Assure victim of support and help if requested.
- Develop a safety plan.
- Develop a follow-up plan, preferably to involve monitoring of the situation.
- Legal intervention may be necessary where a criminal offense has been committed, or the victim's life or health are in danger.

- Establish victim's needs.
- Implement safety plan.
- Educate/provide information about abuse, rights and local services.
- Providence services to victim, abuser or both, that focus on preventing further abuse.
- Assist with legal interventions.
- Make sure that situation is monitored by someone.

- Ensure protection for the victim either in terms of physical safety and/or proper financial arrangements.
- Provide relevant help to the abuser.
- Liaise with police if serious crime has been committed.
- Make sure that situation is monitored by someone.

Figure 29-1 Management of abuse. (From McCreadie C, Tinker A: Elder abuse in Tallis RC, Flint HM, editors: *Brocklehurst's textbook of geriatric medicine and gerontology,* ed 6, London, 2003, Churchill Livingstone.)

Counseling can include the following:

1. Assess the caregiver's understanding of the illness and knowledge of the patient's care needs (e.g., medication schedules, tube-feeding administration, pressure relief).
2. Assess the caregiver's physical capabilities in caring for a dependent older person. The caregiver's physical health, emotional stability, social support system, and other responsibilities must also be taken into consideration.
3. Educate the caregiver regarding the patient's illness, follow-up care, medications, behavior management, and hands-on caregiving; this can reduce confusion and alleviate stress.
4. Explore insurance benefits, financial relief programs, free medication programs offered by some pharmaceutical companies, and other resources that could help ease the burden of paying for medication and supplies. A social work consultation may help to provide this information.
5. Arrange respite time for the caregiver to provide a "break" from responsibilities.
6. Seek alternative or assistant caregivers if a caregiver is thought to have mental or psychologic impairments that affect his or her ability to provide care. If the impairment is related to substance abuse, the provider can attempt to assist the caregiver in seeking treatment, including provision of care for the older person while the caregiver is undergoing rehabilitation.

ABUSED OLDER PERSON

Victims often require education and time before the decision is made to change the situation. The provider must develop a trusting and therapeutic alliance with the abused older person. Allowing the victim the opportunity to recognize the danger inherent in the situation and the benefits of alternatives can take time.

Counseling of the victim should consist of the following:

1. Educating the victim regarding options (e.g., making other living arrangements, obtaining an order of protection, having the abuser evicted, having the locks changed, or pressing formal charges). Legal options can be discussed with the office of the local district attorney.
2. Examining the positive and negative aspects of each option
3. Allowing the victim to talk about feelings in a nonjudgmental atmosphere
4. Enabling the victim to express his or her angers or fears
5. Assuring the victim that these feelings are normal
6. Helping the victim understand that choosing an option different from the caregiver's wishes would not necessarily sever the relationship if the patient wants to retain it

SOCIAL CONTEXT

Elder abuse reporting laws exist in every state to protect older persons from being abused physically or emotionally, suffering from neglect, or experiencing financial exploitation. Support groups for caregivers of older persons may help prevent elder abuse by reducing caregiver stress and linking caregivers to community services (Bergeron and Gray, 2003).

If possible, every effort should be made to correct situations so that the older person can remain in as independent a setting as possible. Occasionally the abused older person will not allow intervention. Although victims who have been determined to have capacity may refuse help, they cannot prevent the practitioner from reporting the problem as required by law. Most states require health care professionals to report suspected cases of abuse or neglect to the state's adult protective services (APS) agency. These mandatory reporting laws require the disclosure of suspected abuse or mistreatment regardless of the wishes of the adult victim. The APS agencies must then investigate reports by interviewing victims and others who may be knowledgeable about the situation. According the *APS Handbook*, all patients receive voluntary protective services with consent, they participate in decisions as they are able, the least restrictive alternative is chosen, and patients may refuse or withdraw from protective services. Up to 70% of confirmed cases receive no intervention because of refusal by patients who are deemed competent (Harrell et al, 2002). "At-risk" older persons who refuse the needed help are of great concern to health care providers, who often must grapple with difficult ethical and legal issues concerning when to intervene against a person's will and when to respect his or her right to self-determination.

Older adults for whom self-neglect is an issue present a variety of practical and ethical challenges. The person's capacity to make decisions must often be assessed to determine that he or she understands the potential risks in deciding to decline intervention. A surrogate or guardian is often assigned until an evaluation and determination can be completed. When working with a judgmentally impaired person, it is necessary to consider that person's lifestyle choices and try to make decisions consistent with those choices. Persons must not be judged incapable if their choices are consistent with those made over the course of their lives, even if they seem eccentric or outlandish to others. Regardless of the individual aspects of a situation, the least restrictive choice should be made, so long as it ensures safe and appropriate care for the older person.

Summary

Health professionals have been found to lack knowledge regarding assessment, diagnosis, intervention, and reporting criteria of elder mistreatment (Cowen and Cowen, 2002). The diagnosis of elder abuse is seldom straightforward because of social issues, cognitive impairment, and comorbid conditions, and requires careful correlation of historical and clinical findings. Comprehensive evaluation, including a detailed history, systematic physical examination, and appropriate laboratory and radiographic assessment, is essential (Chen and Koval, 2002).

Resources

California Law Website
www.leginfo.ca.gov

National Center on Elder Abuse
www.elderabusecenter.org

Web Resources on Elder Abuse
www.seniorlaw.com/elderabuse.htm

References

Abrams WB, Berkow R: *The Merck manual of geriatrics*, Rahway, NJ, 1990, Merck Sharp & Dohme Research Laboratories.

Ayres MM, Woodtli A: Concept analysis: abuse of ageing caregivers by elderly care recipients, *J Adv Nurs* 35(3):326-334, 2001.

Bergeron LR, Gray B: Ethical dilemmas of reporting suspected elder abuse, *Social Work* 48(1):96-105, 2003.

Brandl B, Horan DL: Domestic violence in later life: an overview for health care providers, *Women & Health* 35(2-3):41-54, 2002.

California Welfare and Institution Code: Section 15610.07.

Capezuti E, Brush BL, Lawson WT: Reporting elder mistreatment, *J Gerontol Nurs* 23(7):24-32, 1997.

Chen AL, Koval K: Elder abuse: the role of the orthopaedic surgeon in diagnosis and management, *J Am Acad Orthop Surg* 10(1):25-31, 2002.

Cowen HJ, Cowen PS: Elder mistreatment: dental assessment and intervention, *Special Care in Dentistry* 22(1):23-32, 2002.

Devons C: Comprehensive geriatric assessment: making the most of the aging years, *Curr Opin Clin Nutr Metabolic Care* 5(1):19-24, 2002.

Harrell R et al: How geriatricians identify elder abuse and neglect, *Am J Med Sci* 323(1):34-38, 2002.

McCreadie C, Tinker A: Elder abuse. In Tallis RC, Flint HM, editors: *Brocklehurst's textbook of geriatric medicine and gerontology*, ed 6, London, 2003, Churchill Livingstone.

Reis M, Nahmiash D: Validation of the indicators of abuse screen, *Gerontologist* 38(4):471-480, 1998.

Quinn MJ: Undue influence and elder abuse: recognition and intervention strategies, *Geriatr Nurs* 2(1):11-17, 2002.

30

Grief

Role of Spirituality in Coping with Loss

One of the essential elements of the grieving process is finding meaning in the loss and suffering. Most people have something in their life that gives them meaning. To many this meaning is defined in terms of their careers, their relationships, or their social status; but once a person experiences a loss such as a death of a loved one or the loss of health or previous level of functioning, the previous way of looking at the world and at defining meaning may not suffice. Illness or death of a loved one is a major life event that causes people to question themselves, their purpose, and the meaning in life (Van Ness and Larson, 2002). Grief and loss disrupt career, family life, and ability to enjoy life, three areas essential to a healthy mind. These losses inevitably raise profound questions as to who we are and the purpose of our lives. The process of dealing with these questions is really one of finding new meaning in life. This is the essence of a spiritual journey. Frankl (1993) wrote, "Man is not destroyed by suffering; he is destroyed by suffering without meaning." When he wrote about concentration camp victims, he noted that survival itself may depend on seeking and finding meaning. People can cope with their suffering by seeking and finding meaning in it. Thus spirituality can play such a critical role.

Spirituality can be defined as the transcendent relationship that gives meaning and purpose to people's lives, joys, and sufferings. Downey (1997) defines spirituality as "an awareness that there are levels of reality not immediately apparent and that there is a quest for personal integration in the face of forces of fragmentation and depersonalization." It is the aspect of human beings that seeks to heal. The healing of grief involves an acceptance of the loss, be it of a loved one or of one's health. Spirituality offers people hope and helps them understand their grief in the context of a deeper reality.

SPIRITUALITY AND RELIGION

Confusion about the differences between spirituality and religion is common. As we work with patients, it is important to recognize that spirituality is universal. Individual patients may or may not be religious, but spirituality is inherent in everyone. *Religion* is the expression of one's spirituality in a particular, organized community with a set of doctrines accepted by the community. In a study of community-dwelling older adults, 96% used prayer as a spiritual modality adopted to cope with stress (Dun and Horgas, 2000).

Historically, spirituality was referenced only in the context of religion. The current use of the term *spirituality* as separate from religion is thought to originate from the rise of secularism in the late twentieth century and from a growing disillusionment with religious institutions in Western society. In the 1960s and 1970s, *spirituality* began to acquire distinct meanings separate from *religion*. As spirituality has become differentiated from religion, spirituality has become the broader, more inclusive term (Pargament, 1997). Nonetheless, it is important to recognize that, according to a Gallop survey, Americans are religious, with more than 90% of the population believing in God and a large segment of the population attending religious services regularly (Gallop, 1990). *Spirituality*, defined as a universal concept of search for meaning, can appeal and provide solace to a large segment of the population served by the health care system. This definition allows for the diversity in beliefs and backgrounds. The search for meaning through a relationship with the transcendent or divine can be expressed in many ways: religion, nature, music, art, and relationship with others. There is no one expression of spirituality: everyone has a personal understanding and expression of his or her beliefs. What is uniform is that these beliefs help people cope with their grief, loss, and suffering.

PATIENT NEED

Several national surveys have documented patients' desire to have spiritual concerns addressed by health care professionals who are providing their care. When asked, 95% of Americans surveyed espouse a belief in God, 57% report praying daily, and 42% report attending a worship service in the prior week (Gallop, 1990). The need for attentiveness to the spiritual concerns of seriously ill patients has been well recognized by many. Researchers at Johns Hopkins University Medical Center talked to 22 patients who had experienced life-threatening illness for the purpose of identifying their concerns about discussing religious and spiritual beliefs with physicians. God, prayer, and spiritual beliefs were frequently mentioned as sources of comfort, support, and healing. All 22 subjects, when discussing physician–patient relationships, stressed the importance of empathy and strong interpersonal skills (Hebert et al, 2001). In a survey by Gallop, people overwhelmingly want their spiritual needs addressed when they are close to death. Gallop (1997) writes, "The overarching message that emerges from this study is that the American people want to reclaim and reassert the spiritual dimensions in dying." Other surveys found that 75% of Americans say that religion is central to their lives; most believe that their spiritual faith can help them recover from their illness. To prepare physicians to respond to this growing need, spirituality and medicine courses are being incorporated into medical school curricula (Puchalski and Larson, 1998; Levin, Larson, and Puchalski, 1997). Historically, nursing schools have always emphasized the role of spirituality in health care.

Putting Spirituality in the Practice of Medicine and the Art of Healing

Cassell (1991) writes, "Since in suffering, disruption of the whole person is the dominant theme, we know the losses and their losses and their meaning by what we know of others out of compassion for their suffering." It should be the obligation of all health care providers to respond to all types of suffering as well as to relieve all physical suffering. We have seen from the survey data that patients would like to discuss their spiritual beliefs with health care providers and incorporate those beliefs into the therapeutic plan. Data also demonstrate the beneficial effects of spirituality in health, particularly in chronic and serious illness and bereavement. Therefore health care providers should be able to communicate with patients about spirituality as integral to health and as an aid in coping with suffering.

Spiritual issues can be explored effectively with patients of all ages, including children and older demented adults (Frankel, 1993; Maugins, 1996). The depth and focus of the discussion will vary, depending on the cognitive and developmental ability of the patient. The goals of a spiritual history are to recognize the spiritual belief of the patient and to make the appropriate referral if necessary. One way to obtain a patient's spiritual history is to talk with a patient and listen to that patient's story about what is central and important to him or her (i.e., who the patient is at his or her deepest core). Kuhn (1988) identified 14 items one might ask in a spiritual history: questions about what a person believes in, whom a person loves, whether patients pray or enjoy being alone, and whether patients can forgive. Another approach to a spiritual history is suggested by Maugins (1996), who describes an assessment using the mnemonic SPIRIT, which lists several questions for each of six categories: (1) spiritual belief system, (2) personal spirituality, (3) integration in a spiritual community, (4) ritualized practices and restriction, (5) implications for medical care, and (6) terminal events planning.

Yet another effective spiritual assessment tool is "FICA" (Puchalski et al, 1999), which is currently being used in both academic and practice settings. The use of this tool, like all such tools, must be used with a deep respect for each patient's beliefs, strengths, and needs. FICA is outlined briefly below.

F: FAITH AND BELIEFS

The provider asks the patient about the faith or beliefs that are important to the patient. It seeks to understand what gives meaning to the person's life. The provider should use language that is familiar and comfortable for the provider. The following are some open-ended questions that can be used:

- Do you consider yourself spiritual or religious?
- What gives your life meaning and purpose?
- What types of beliefs help you cope?

I: IMPORTANCE AND INFLUENCE

One needs to know what role these beliefs play in the person's life. Are they important, and what role do they play in how the patient takes care of his or her health? For example, a patient may be very religious, attending services regularly and seeing God as central in his or her life. For that person, any "bad news" may eventually be viewed as God's will, and such views may enable a person to cope better with illness. On the other hand, patients may have left their church and are searching for something broader. Patients may want the provider to give them referrals to chaplains or other spiritual resources. How a provider responds to patients regarding their spirituality varies, depending on the role spiritual belief has in that patient's life.

It is important to recognize that not all spiritual beliefs are helpful. In fact, some may interfere with the patient's ability to heal. For example, in many cases a patient's relationship with God is positive and supportive, but patients may see God in ways that can interfere with care. For example, patients may view God as punitive and refuse medical treatment because they believe the illness is deserved. Others may refuse to take any tests or medication because they believe that any outcome is in God's hands. Therefore it is important for providers to refer to professionals such as chaplains trained as clinical pastoral educators, spiritual directors, and pastoral counselors to help patients differentiate between healthy and unhealthy beliefs.

C: COMMUNITY

It is important to know whether the patient expresses his or her spiritual beliefs in the context of a religious or spiritual community. This could be a church, temple, or mosque, or it could be a group of like-minded friends who could provide social support and assistance when the patient is facing serious or chronic illness. Many people, particularly older patients who are often alone, may be supported by and even brought to their provider's offices by their faith's community members.

A: ADDRESS AND APPLICATION

The provider needs to know how the patient would like the provider to address the patient's beliefs in the context of the patient–provider relationship. Some patients may want to discuss their spiritual issues briefly and routinely at each visit. Some may simply want them noted in the event of some serious life-threatening event in the future. In addition, it is important to know what actions the patient would like the provider to take with respect to the patient's responses stemming from the initial spiritual history-taking discussion. For example, patients may need or want a referral to a chaplain, they may want clergy involved, or they may want advice regarding community resources, such as meditation classes. Most patients want their beliefs to be respected and advocated by their provider.

With the ever-increasing diversity of the American population, health care organizations, providers, and government policy makers are becoming increasingly aware of the troubling disparities in access to care, utilization, and health outcomes of minority older adults. Recent federal requirements for health care systems ensure that all persons receive equitable and effective treatment in a culturally sensitive manner (*Federal Register*, 2000). In developing a clinical tool for ethnogeriatric education, Kobylarz and associates (2002) revised the mnemonic teaching tool ETHNIC to include spirituality ETHNICS. The realization of the universality of spirituality as a component of all cultures prompted the inclusion of spirituality in multicultural curricula. For the health professional the influence of spirituality becomes apparent when the patient or the patient's family is dealing with severity of illness, advanced directives, and end-of-life care. Prayer in all its forms and accompanying rituals as a personal intervention is an example of the relevance of spirituality and the need for sensitivity to diverse beliefs and practices. See Box 30-1 for an explanation of ETHNIC.

The health care provider should use FICA as a guide, not as a checklist. Many times a patient is so pleased to have the issue of spirituality addressed that the conversation flows naturally after the first question regarding the patient's beliefs. Others may not be willing to discuss spirituality. If a patient is not interested in talking about his or her beliefs, the conversation should not be pursued

---

Box 30-1

ETHNIC(S): A Clinical Tool

(E) Explanation
To increase awareness of health professionals to the problem that many older people may be reluctant to ask questions or seek explanations of care. This can negatively impact their compliance with treatment.

(T) Treatment
Older patients from varying cultures many times seek parallel care from alternative medical providers. Herbal supplements and vitamins also fall into this category, and therefore all persons should be asked, "What have you done to alleviate your suffering before you came to see me?" Or some other appropriate open-ended question can be asked.

(H) Healers
Again the need to understand how the patient is using the alternative healing system is crucial. In many cultures respected, culturally important persons hold the position of healer. Acknowledgement of the patient's beliefs will facilitate further communication.

(N) Negotiate
The ability to establish mutual objectives in regard to the care of the older person with realistic outcomes will require an open, knowledgeable communication that demonstrates respect for all participants.

(I) Intervention
Original treatment decisions may need to be modified and individualized after proceeding through this process.

(C) Collaborate
Collaboration refers to all professional and family members involved in the patient's care. This is an interactive process leading to a therapeutic relationship between the patient and the health professional and that takes time to build a trusting and mutually beneficial relationship.

(S) Spirituality
Acknowledging patient's spiritual beliefs when appropriate enhances the therapeutic relationship.

Adapted from Kobylarz FA et al: The ETHNIC(S) mnemonic: a clinical tool for ethnogeriatric education, *J Am Geriatr Soc* 50(9):1582-1589, 2002.

further. It is critical that these conversations should never appear to be coercive. No health care provider should let these conversations seem to proselytize or ridicule a patient for his or her beliefs. Respect for the patient's privacy regarding these issues is paramount.

Resources Available in the Community

It is also important to know what spiritual resources are available in the community. Chaplains with training in clinical pastoral education (CPE) are skilled at helping patients resolve spiritual crises or questions. A CPE-certified chaplain is trained to work with patients of any religious denomination or spiritual belief system. Many hospitals have CPE-certified chaplains. In addition, a growing movement is under way to include chaplains in outpatient settings. Referrals to chaplains are as appropriate as referrals to any other specialty. Because the spirituality of patients is so important to patients and to potential outcomes, chaplains should be integral to health care teams.

The patient may also want to discuss issues with a member of the clergy (i.e., his or her own minister, priest, rabbi, or imam). Clergy are not trained in the same way as chaplains and therefore usually do not work with patients of religious beliefs different from their own. Some religious denominations also have spiritual directors who are trained specifically to work with people on spiritual issues. They are not counselors; they work specifically on a person's spiritual journey.

Many other resources are available that may be appropriate for particular patients (e.g., music therapy, art therapy, guided imagery, meditation, and yoga).

Summary

In working with geriatric patients, practitioners will encounter many cases of bereavement, ranging from grief following the loss of a loved one to grief associated with serious illness. Grief associated with depression may need to be treated with medications or psychotherapy. Many people who grieve become stressed and consequently are more susceptible to colds, headaches, and other maladies, which may be stress related. In all cases of grief, however, spirituality plays a central role in how people cope with loss. Substantial data exist from both surveys and other studies to support the beneficial role spirituality plays in health care. Therefore it is important for all health care providers to be able to recognize this important factor in patients' lives and to be able to communicate with patients about their spiritual beliefs and incorporate those beliefs into the patients' therapeutic plan. In patient care spirituality is an ongoing issue and one frequently discussed at subsequent visits, particularly with patients who are experiencing suffering and loss. Health care providers who can speak and listen to patients discuss their beliefs, fears, and concerns in terms of spirituality have an opportunity to bring a form of healing from pain, loss, and suffering into a patient's life.

Resources

Family Caregiving Alliance
www.caregiver.org/factsheets/grief.html

References

Cassell EJ: *The nature of suffering and the goals of medicine*, New York, 1991, Oxford University Press.
Downey M: *Understanding Christian spirituality*, Machwah, NJ, 1997, Paulist Press.
Dunn KS, Horgas AL: The prevalence of prayer as a spiritual self-care modality in elders, *J Holist Nurs* 18(4):337-351, 2000.
Frankl VE: *Man's search for meaning*, Long Island, NY, 1993, Buccaneer Books.
Gallop G: *Religion in America: 1990*, Princeton, NJ, 1990, Princeton Religion and Research Center.
Gallop G: *Spiritual beliefs and the dying process*, 1997, National Survey for the Nathans Cummings Foundation and the Fetzer Institute.

Herbert RS et al: Patient perspectives on spirituality and the patient-physician relationship, *J Gen Intern Med* 16(10):685-692, 2001.

Kobylarz FA et al: The ETHNIC(S) mnemonic: a clinical tool for ethnogeriatric education, *J Am Geriatr Soc* 50(9):1582-1589, 2002.

Kuhn CC: A spiritual inventory of the medically ill patient, *Psychiatr Med* 6(2):87-100, 1988.

Levin JS, Larson DB, Puchalski DM: Religion and spirituality in medicine: research and education, *JAMA* 278(9):792-793, 1997.

Maugins TA: The SPIRITual history, *Arch Fam Med* 5:11-16, 1996.

Office of Minority Health: National standards on culturally and linguistically appropriate services in health care, *Federal Register* 65:80865-80879, December 20, 2000.

Pargament KI: The psychology of religion and spirituality? yes and no. Paper presented at the American Psychological Association Annual Conference, Chicago, 1997.

Puchalski CM, Larson DB. Developing curricula in spirituality and medicine, *Acad Med* 73(9):970-974, 1998.

Puchalski CM et al: *FICA: a guide to spiritual assessment in the clinical setting*, in press.

Van Ness PH, Larson DB: Religion, senescence, and mental health: the end of life is not the end of hope, *Am J Geriatr Psychiatry* 10(4):386-397, 2002.

31

Caregivers

As society ages and people are living longer, issues that were never considered in another time emerge as societal problems. One risk of an extended life is the possibility of becoming unable to provide for oneself in the normal activities of daily living, thereby becoming dependent on others, often female family members. Since the middle of the twentieth century, the roles and composition of American families have changed in ways that limit the number of caregivers for older, frail family members. As a result of there being fewer members per family, dual-income families, and shifting of roles, fewer women are available to provide full-time care for older people. Despite these changes, women continue to be 80% of the caregivers (Yin et al, 2002).

Health care providers are in a unique position to influence the health and well-being of family caregivers. Usually the issues associated with caring are not presented as a primary reason for seeking medical intervention, and yet these issues may lie at the heart of medical problems for which the patient or caregiver is seeking treatment. When the functionally dependent family member is the patient, a prudent health care provider knows to inquire about the health of his or her caregiver(s). Nurse practitioners, with their health-promotion and family-based approach, are trained to identify and intervene in the spiral of interconnected medical, psychological, and emotional issues that surround family caregiving. This chapter provides the background necessary to form health-promoting partnerships with family caregivers—including caregiver characteristics, role responsibilities, and needs—in relationship to their implications for assessment and intervention by health care providers.

Caregivers

Family caregiving is a recognized strain or burden that has become a living reality for a large number of middle-aged Americans. Caregivers have long been recognized as a group characterized by high levels of poor health, depression, burden, and stress (Chappell and Reid, 2002). Caregiver burden is recognized to include physical, psychological, social, and financial problems experienced by family members caring for an impaired older adult.

Despite these obstacles, family caring is widespread and accounts for most long-term care provided in the United States. Unpaid family caregivers provide the bulk of care required by a dependent older person who lives at home, and as a group these caregivers perform tasks that range from buying groceries to physically caring for a bed-bound person. At times they are called on to perform tasks that once were done by registered nurses (Hoffman and Mitchell, 1998). Caregiving by family or friends is the primary resource preventing or forestalling institutionalization of a great number of older people. Nearly one in four households in the United States is involved in providing some type of care for an older family member (Coleman, 2000). This proportion is expected to grow as diseases that are strongly associated with aging, such as Alzheimer's disease, drive the demand for both family and formal supports.

Traditionally, when the need for direct care arises, families turn to the spouse, then a daughter, and finally a daughter-in-law. Caregiving is widely regarded as a female issue, largely because of the fact that the average caregiver is a middle-aged female relative of the person needing care. More recently and in response to lack of available caregivers, a greater number of older men and sons have become involved in their aging parents' care (Houde, 2001; Jansson et al, 2001). The role of caregiver is often compounded by conflicting responsibilities, including job, children, family, and friends. Such conflicts are easy to understand when considered in light of the fact that some caregivers spend up to 35 hours per week providing care in addition to working at full-time jobs outside the home.

Family caregiving problems are complicated by a widespread lack of affordable services that could potentially ease these problems. State-supported services for family caregivers are widely divergent, with some states offering a comprehensive program with respite-care support groups, specialized information and referral, and family consultation; other states have a much smaller range of services. Although most states offer respite care, eligibility requirements differ considerably (Coleman, 2000). Out-of-pocket expenses for caring for an older, frail adult can be a great financial strain, with costs in some parts of the country being beyond the means of an average family. Adult day-care rates can easily exceed $60 per day, and it is typical for personal-care aides to cost $15 to $20 per hour. When the family is facing a devastating and progressive disease such as Alzheimer's, the economic toll is even greater. At times, it may be less expensive to stop working to care for an older relative than to hire formal supports.

Dementia and Caregiver's Burden

A special note is in order regarding care for an individual with Alzheimer's disease or a related dementia. Despite scientific advances in understanding the etiology and progression of Alzheimer's disease, concern continues that dementia care will place a tremendous burden on our health care system and the informal network of family caregivers who provide the bulk of care. It is projected that the incidence of Alzheimer's disease in the United States will exceed five million by 2030 (Brookmeyer, Gray, and Kawas, 1998). Most persons with Alzheimer's disease will continue to be females without a living spouse, meaning that adult daughters will constitute the largest group of caregivers. One major effort in response to these projections is an attempt to delay onset of symptoms with medication; however, the effectiveness of medications introduced up to this point is marginal. Thus it is clear that health care providers must expect to encounter in their daily practice a significant number of middle-aged women who are fatigued, depressed, and overwhelmed as a result of caregiving.

Caregivers face a daunting task when providing care for a loved one with dementia, especially when the disease has progressed to the moderate and severe stages of impairment. In a study with a national population-based sample of community-dwelling older adults 70 years of age and older (n = 7443), Langa and associates reported caregiver time and cost relative to the severity of dementia compared with older adults with normal cognition. Those with normal cognition received an average of 4.6 hours a week of informal care; those with mild dementia received an average of 8.5 hours per week of informal care; and those with moderate and severe dementia received an additional 17.4 and 41.5 hours a week, respectively. The annual associated additional costs of informal care per case were $3630 for mild dementia, $7420 for moderate dementia, and $17,700 for severe dementia (Langa et al 2001).

Another study investigated the informal costs of caring for community-dwelling male veterans with dementia and female caregivers. The study comprised 2043 female caregivers. Cost measures included the value of caregivers' time, caregivers' lost income, out-of-pocket expenses for formal caregiving, and caregivers' excess health costs. The results found annual cost of providing informal care to older community-dwelling veterans with dementia to be $18,385, and this cost increased with the severity of the dementia; the largest costs were caregiver time and loss of income (Moore et al, 2001).

Loneliness and depression among caregiving wives and daughters have been widely reported (Besson et al, 2000; Marwit and Meuser, 2002). The grief that surrounds this type of loss is characterized as heartfelt sorrow and longing for the person who once was. It is not uncommon for these overworked caregivers to be isolated from family and friends who are uncomfortable with the disease and have no understanding of how to help. Of all caregiving groups, persons who live with and care for a loved one with dementia pay the highest toll in terms of emotional and physical well-being and should be the concern of health care providers in every clinical arena.

Caregiver Needs and Issues

It is crucial for anyone interacting with older adults to understand the network of aging services in their community. Also, because of the recent state budgetary problems, providers must keep themselves informed of any new requirements for or limitations of services that have been available in the recent past.

States and local communities for the most part decide which type of projects will be funded. For instance, in Philadelphia County a home-modification program is available through the local Area Agency on Aging (Philadelphia Corporation for Aging). This unique program provides adaptive equipment (e.g., bath benches, raised toilet seats) and home modifications (e.g., ramps, banisters) for older persons who qualify. Other possibilities include professional programs at local universities who may wish to find unique clinical placements for their students. The best place to start may be a presentation by a social worker specializing in community resources for adults in a specific area.

Programs may be available on either a county or regional basis. The Office on Aging in all counties is a valuable resource of information about county-wide services. Often the Office on Aging has programs that provide adult day care and transportation on a sliding-fee basis. Also locally, many services are provided by the Area Agency on Aging (AAA), which is legislated by the Older Americans Act. The range of services among AAAs is broad, but each agency serves the primary function of coordinating aging services and providing case management. The vast majority of AAAs also provide the opportunity for meals (Meals on Wheels), recreation (Senior Citizens Centers), and personal-care assistance. Finally, for persons caring for an older adult with memory loss, the local chapter of the Alzheimer's Association is an invaluable resource. This nonprofit organization serves the public through support groups, educational programs, a lending library, telephone information and referral, and programs to assist the safe return of individuals who wander away from home. Recently a survey conducted by the Northern Virginia Chapter of the Alzheimer's Association indicated that caregivers are primarily concerned with accessing information about the disease process and management.

A metaanalysis of studies to assess effectiveness of intervention studies to reduce the perception of burden for caregivers of frail older adults was undertaken by Yin and associates. Eighteen group intervention studies and eight individual intervention studies were included in the analysis.

The total number of subjects in the 18 group intervention studies was 1970; the mean age of the caregivers was 60.1 years of age, and 78.8% were women, 86% were white, and 80% lived in the same house as the care receiver. The mean age of the care receiver was 78.8 years, and 55% had dementia.

Group interventions in 93% of the studies contained an educational component in combination with peer support, 33% specialized group counseling, and 27% respite care and stress management. The duration of the intervention varied from 2 weeks to 1 year. Sample size for the eight individual intervention studies was 272 subjects. Table 31-1 summaries characteristics of the eight studies with explanation of the intervention.

| TABLE 31-1 | Summary of Eight Intervention Studies |

Study	N	Caregiver Characteristic	Assignment	Intervention
Archbold et al, 1995	9T 10C	100% primary 23% male 82% spouse 14% minority	Nonrandom	Family focused, individualized interventions PREP system of intervention, including expanded in-home services, the advice line, and the keep-in-touch system, provided by trained nurses
Chang, 1999	34T 31C	No info. on primary 100% female 89% spouse 21% minority (including 16% African American)	Random	8-wk cognitive-behavioral intervention Videotapes and Nurseline support program to assist caregivers individually
Montgomery and Borgatta, 1989*	83T 85C	100% primary 21% male 31% spouse No info. on ethnicity	Random	Family consultation (group 4 only) to provide individualized training and assistance Social worker home visit One session only
Quayhagen and Quayhagen, 1989*	14T 6C	100% primary 62.5% male No info. on spouse No info. on ethnicity	Nonrandom	Clinic and home cognitive stimulation training sessions Caregiver worked 6 hr per week Booster contact maintained on a monthly basis for 8 mo
Scharlach, 1987*	14T 10C	No info. on primary All daughters All white	Nonrandom	Cognitive-behavioral intervention (condition A only) Two 90-minutes sessions 10-min phone contact each week for 6 wk
Toseland et al, 1990*	51T 33C	100% primary All daughters or daughter-in-laws 5% minority	Random	Individual professional and peer counseling Eight weekly 1-hr sessions
Wishart et al, 2000	11T 10C	No info. on primary 14% male 33% spouse No info. on ethnicity	Random	In-home care and supervision by a trained volunteer on a regular basis Used walking as physical and psychological stimulation 2.5 hr visitation each week for 6 wk

TABLE 31-1	Summary of Eight Intervention Studies—cont'd			
Study	**N**	**Caregiver Characteristic**	**Assignment**	**Intervention**
Zarit et al, 1987[*]	36T 39C	100% primary 30% male 52% spouse 13% minority	Random	Individual and family counseling Stress management and problem solving Eight weekly sessions

From Yin T et al: Burden on family members: caring for frail elderly: a meta-analysis of interventions, *Nurs Res* 51(3):199-208, 2002.

Note. *Included in Knont et al (1993) meta-analysis.

Results of the metanalyses showed a consistent positive impact on the caregiver's sense of burden in all types of interventions. Generally, interventions were psychosocial counseling, support-group therapy and counseling, psychoeducational programs, or combinations of behavior and cognitive educational programs. Women had a higher level of pretreatment burden and also showed a higher level of stress reduction after the intervention (Yin et al, 2002). One assumption that could be made in regard to this study is that any intervention that recognizes the difficulty of caregiving and tries to address caregiver concerns will have a positive impact.

Caregivers have a need for specific information concerning diagnosis and treatment and most importantly, information regarding financial and legal issues related to their health plan coverage (Wackerbarth and Johnson, 2002). At times this type of information is difficult to access, but practitioners at the very least need to refer patients to appropriate resources that can assist them with this issue.

The stressors that impinge on caregivers can be summarized as the cognitive, physical, and behavioral functioning of the care recipient and the tasks and amount of hours per day spent in the caregiver role. Aspects of formal and informal assistance that mitigate the burden are frequency of getting a break, social support, hours of formal services, personal attributes of high self-esteem, and a close relationship with the recipient of care (Chappell and Reid, 2002).

PROVIDING HEALTH CARE TO CAREGIVERS

Working with caregivers, who are often stressed and isolated, requires careful listening to understand the individual's mix of emotions. Caregivers can simultaneously experience a vast range of responses, including guilt, remorse, grief, resentment, and embarrassment. For instance, a wife caring for her husband may feel guilty at anything less than perfection in her own performance while resentful that she has to provide care during her "golden years." It is important to listen and acknowledge caregivers' feelings without judgment while focusing on the disease as the culprit responsible for the family member's dependency or difficult behaviors. At times wives in particular are embarrassed to disclose all their caregiving issues for fear that some situations will reflect badly on the caregiver herself. When a caregiver seems reticent to discuss the issues fully, it is important to listen and acknowledge the caregiver's feelings while assuring him or her that the disease has caused the family member to behave irrationally rather than the cause being a bad choice in a marriage partner.

Unfortunately, in today's health care industry, some encounters with caregivers are brief, infrequent, or one time only. Caregivers require a level of sustained availability to identify care problems and develop potential solutions. An effective schedule involves regular visits with the same health care provider over time and the opportunity for telephone contact if a serious issue arises or worsens. These visits and contacts do not have to be lengthy or frequent; often only a few minutes are needed for the caregiver to discuss how things are going. If this type of encounter is not possible in the clinical arena, the caregiver can be referred to a professional who will be available to address the care issues specifically.

If the health care provider is in a position to sustain availability with the caregiver, the next set of personal characteristics that caregivers request is a creative and flexible approach to problem solving. Caregiving problems are naturally complex, involving interactions among several family members, environmental demands, sociocultural constraints, financial resources, and functional abilities. Solutions rarely come easily or quickly and often involve several refinements to find a workable approach.

Health care providers should be willing to familiarize themselves with the family's idiosyncrasies. Caregiving is a cultural activity, and no two families are alike. Rich sources of information about the family are found in responses to questions about caregiving goals and methods as well as daily routines. Particular attention should be paid to how the caregiver describes acceptable uses of time. Conflicts often arise when a resting or fatigued family member is regarded by the caregiver as lazy, unwilling to help, or unconcerned with the caregiver's needs. In this case, education about the typical effects of the disease on activity levels may reduce this source of conflict. Education may be followed up with suggestions about how the caregiver can prioritize care tasks, simplify them, and pace their presentation to optimize participation by the care recipient. This process, known as *task breakdown*, is also available from occupational therapists (OTs), who are uniquely trained in these procedures.

ASSESSMENT

As with any clinical issue, the success of interactions with caregivers depends on a comprehensive assessment; however, it is difficult to know where to start the assessment process when confronted with an overwhelmed, stressed, and fatigued caregiver reciting a litany of complaints about the dependent family member. Experienced clinicians recognize the issues in such a litany and consider four overlapping areas to include in the assessment process: (1) the care context, (2) the caregiver's emotional and physical health, (3) the care recipient's level of *excess disability*, and (4) the caregiver's knowledge and skills. Each is discussed in more detail in the following paragraphs.

CONTEXT OF CARE

The context of care is described as consisting of three dimensions: objects, tasks, and supports. *Object* evaluation includes all physical items and structural attributes. The home should be observed to determine whether necessary objects are present, easily accessible when needed, and yet not so cluttered as to cause a home accident or confusion. In addition, the physical structure should support easy and safe access and ideally allow a balance of privacy, comfort, and utility. *Tasks* can be assessed through detailed interview, simulation, and observation. In particular, tasks should be evaluated for their complexity, efficiency, and timing. For instance, is the caregiver spreading care tasks over time or rushing to fit them all in a few hours? *Support* evaluation primarily involves understanding the effectiveness of the caregiving network. Health care providers should evaluate the family in terms of who is available to help with caregiving, how care is coordinated, and how each family member interacts with the disabled older person.

CAREGIVER'S EMOTIONAL AND PHYSICAL HEALTH

In a comprehensive assessment of any frail community-dwelling older person, it is essential to include a caregiver assessment. Caregiver assessments should focus on the person's physical and emotional health and the social support system available with intent to assess the capacity to provide care.

CARE RECIPIENT'S LEVEL OF EXCESS DISABILITY

To develop effective health care, it is useful to understand the range of disabilities addressed by caregivers. The most common physical ailments are arthritis (50%), hypertension and heart disease (33%), and diabetes (11%). Dementia is the most common source of disability related to psychiatric problems and may be attributed to a range of pathologies, including Alzheimer's disease, multiinfarct dementia, and Parkinson's disease. It is not uncommon for caregivers to be caring for a person who has several physical and psychiatric disorders, which can make care tasks time consuming and nearly constant.

CAREGIVER'S KNOWLEDGE AND SKILLS

As part of the comprehensive assessment, the health care providers should interview the caregiver to gain information about his or her knowledge and skills for managing the care recipient's condition. If needed, the caregiver can be asked directly to define the condition ("How would you explain this condition to a neighbor or friend?") and to describe his or her care techniques. As a result, the health care provider will gain important assessment information about the strengths and weaknesses of the caregiver that could be the basis for referral or intervention. See Table 31-2 for the key elements of a caregiver assessment.

Caregiving Interventions

Typically the short-term services of a team of health care professionals are required for implementing the caregiver care plan. For instance, a physical therapist may use one session with the caregiver to teach proper body mechanics, in addition to any therapy or use of mobility equipment required for the care recipient. OTs help with task breakdown and use a range of methods to restore maximal functional independence (including adaptive equipment), make caregiving easier, and establish an energy-conserving routine. An OT may be indicated for the caregiver (to assist with dementia management strategies), the dependent family member (to improve function), or both. Social work is essential when financial or community resource needs are identified, especially a seasoned social worker who has an in-depth understanding of the local aging network.

A comprehensive intervention program dealing with the issue of caregiving can include treatments both for the person receiving the care and the family caregiver. One type of intervention is aimed at the behavior of the family member who is the care recipient. This type of intervention may serve to lessen the caregiver's problems indirectly.

The caregiver may benefit from education concerning the particular illness that is afflicting his or her family member. Effective management techniques such as communication skills can be taught, which may prove to be a substantial benefit. Interventions aimed at reducing isolation and stress include support groups, respite care, and family therapy.

The need for information is a major issue for caregivers. The following list provides a framework by which health practitioners can meet the caregiver's needs:

- Health care plans
- Information about the pathology
    Disease course
    Etiology
    Prognosis
    Genetic disposition (when relevant)
    Treatments
    Research findings
- Skills to manage symptoms related to the pathology
    Effect of the environment on functional ability
    How to promote independence in self care
    Maintaining health
    Adaptive equipment
    Transfer and handling techniques
    Methods for interacting with professionals and para-professionals
- Supports
    Support groups

| TABLE 31-2 | Assessment of Caregivers |

Domain	Key Elements
Ethnic and cultural issues	Primary language
	Level of acculturation of caregiver versus majority culture
	Level of acculturation of caregiver versus other family members
	Values regarding elder care
	Values regarding help-seeking
Knowledge base	Expected signs, symptoms, and course
	Causal attributions for difficult behaviors
	Communication skills
	Behavioral management techniques
	Local services
Social support	Extent of social network
	Local presence of extended family
	Availability of support and instrumental aid
	Satisfaction with support
Psychiatric symptomatology and burden	Depression, including vegetative signs
	Anxiety and stress-related symptoms
	Caregiver's perception of adverse impact
Family conflict	Quality of past relationship
	Degree of unresolved family issues
	Hostility and criticism toward patient
	Elder abuse

From Dunkin J, Cay A: Dementia caregiver burden: a review of the literature and guidelines for assessment and intervention, *Neurology* 51 (Suppl 1):S53-S60, 1998.

       Educational programs
       Social service organizations
       Self-help programs
       Demonstration
- Services
       Financial and legal advice
       Chore services
       Respite
       Adult day care
       Transportation support groups
       Educational programs
       Social service organizations
       Self-help programs

Summary

The complexity of family caregiving requires a comprehensive approach to health care. As with any dynamic system that has multiple components, change in any one component will potentially resonate to the rest of the system. Therefore problems experienced by an older adult may have implications for the health and well-being of the rest of the family. In turn, an ineffective family care network is likely to promote further dependence and health issues for the older person. The unique challenge in partnering with family caregivers to promote health is initially identifying who is experiencing negative consequences from caregiving. Because these negative consequences may not be the primary reason for contact with a health provider, their presence may go undetected. One solution for effectively identifying family members who need additional knowledge and skills is for all health professionals to be vigilant about examining the status not only of an individual patient but also the family system that supports that individual.

Resources

Administration on Aging
www.aoa.gov

AGENET
www.caregivers.com

Alzheimer's Caregiving Page
www.alzwell.com

Caregiving Online Newsletter
www.caregiving.com

Elderweb Online Eldercare Sourcebook
www.elderweb.com

References

Beeson R et al: Loneliness and depression in caregivers of persons with Alzheimer's disease or related disorders, *Issues Ment Health Nurs* 21(8):779-806, 2000.

Brookmeyer R, Gray S, Kawas C: Projections of Alzheimer's disease in the United States and the public health impact of delaying disease onset, *Am J Public Health* 88(9):1337-1341, 1998.

Chappell NL, Reid RC: Burden and well-being among caregivers: examining the distinction, *Gerontologist* 42:772-780, 2002.

Coleman B: *Helping the helpers: state-supported services for family caregivers—executive summary*, Publication ID 2000-2007, Washington DC, 2000, AARP Research.

Hoffmann RL, Mitchell AM: Caregiver burden: historical development, *Nurs Forum* 33(4) 5-11, 1998.

Houde SC: Men providing care for older adults in the home, *J Gerontol Nurs* 34(60):804-812, 2001.

Jansson W et al: Patterns of elderly spousal caregiving in dementia care: an observational study, *J Adv Nurs* 34(6):804-812, 2001.

Langa KM et al: National estimates of the quantity and cost of informal caregiving for the elderly with dementia, *J Gen Intern Med* 16(110):770-778, 2001.

Marwit SJ, Meuser T: Development and initial validation of an inventory to assess grief in caregivers of a person with Alzheimer's disease, *Gerontologist* 42:751-765, 2002.

Moore MJ et al: Informal costs of dementia care: estimates from the National Longitudinal Caregiver Study, *J Gerontol B Psychol Sci Soc Sci* 56(4):S219-S228, 2001.

Wackerbarth SB, Johnson MM: Essential information and support needs of family caregivers, *Patient Educ Couns* 47(2):95-100, 2002.

Yin T et al: Burden on family members: caring for frail elderly: a meta-analysis intervention, *Nurs Res* 51:199-2080, 2002.

32

Epidemiology of Aging: The Older Population in the United States

Chronological age is an unreliable predictor of a person's performance or health, but at the population level, it is a sensitive discriminator among groups. This distinction is important because a general inventory of the health status of older people is essential for public health planning and can provide insights into future needs of the health care system. The information gleaned from population studies, however, may be irrelevant in regard to a specific older patient. The epidemiology of aging can demonstrate the effectiveness of health-promoting behaviors and outcomes from government intervention programs. Therefore it is appropriate that health care professionals have global, national, and local population-based information concerning the aging population.

Growth of the Aging Population
GLOBAL AGING

The rapid pace of global aging is startling. The net balance of the world's older population grew at a rate of 795,00 each month of the year 2000. Global figures of persons 65 years of age and older in 2000 were estimated to be 450 million. In 1990, 26 nations had older adult populations of at least two million; in 2000, 31 countries had reached that mark; with projections that by the year 2030, 60 countries will reach that figure (Kinsella and Velkoff, 2001). See Table 32-1 for a list of countries in the year 2000 with more than 12% of their total population over 65 years of age.

In 2000, persons 80 years of age and older constituted 17% of the world's older population, with more than half (53%) living in six countries: China, United States, India, Japan, Germany, and Russia. One historical factor in population aging has been the fertility decline throughout the developed world (Figure 32-1). Rapidly expanding numbers of older persons will call for redefining public policies to meet individual needs as World War II baby-boom cohorts join the ranks of the older population in the year 2010. The coming growth of the oldest old population will bring new challenges, and the effects of this new cohort will be felt throughout the global economy. See Figure 32-2 for the global distribution of population over 80 years of age.

TABLE 32-1	Percentage of the Population 65 Years of Age and Older, by Country, 2000		
Austria	15.6	Italy	18.2
Belarus	13.6	Japan	17.0
Belgium	17.1	Latvia	15.3
Bulgaria	16.5	Lithuania	13.4
Canada	12.6	Netherlands	13.7
Croatia	15.4	Norway	15.3
Czech Republic	13.8	Poland	12.2
Denmark	14.9	Portugal	15.5
Estonia	14.7	Romania	13.5
Finland	14.9	Russia	12.6
France	16.1	Spain	16.8
Germany	16.5	Sweden	17.2
Greece	17.2	Switzerland	15.2
Hungary	14.6	Ukraine	13.9
Iceland	11.9	United Kingdom	15.7
Ireland	11.3	United States	12.7

From Kinsella K, Velkoff V: *An aging world, 2001*, U.S. Census Bureau Series, pp 95/01-1, Washington DC, 2001, U.S. Government Printing Office.

One important factor to consider when attempting to understand the impact of aging on a country's economy is to consider the median age of its citizens. Significant differences exist between developed and developing countries, but large differences also exist between countries that share the same type of economy. The impact of low fertility rates, which influence the numbers and actual percentage of the older population within a country, and the reverse with high fertility rates and low percentage of older population, is exemplified by the figures for by Germany and Mexico. See Figure 32-3 for median age projections for developed and developing countries.

AGING IN THE UNITED STATES

The growth in life expectancy is one of the great accomplishments of the twentieth century. In 1900, adults over 65 years of age accounted for 4% of the total U.S. population, and the life expectancy of an American child born in that year was 46.4 years for boys and 49.0 years for girls. Advances in medical technology in combination with public health measures such as clean water, sanitation, work safety laws, and better nutrition have contributed to the increased life expectancy. In the year 2000 older adults accounted for 12.7% of the total U.S. population, and life expectancy at birth in the year 2000 was 73.6 years for males and 79.5 years for females (Table 32-2). Within the U.S. population, however, significant differences in life expectancy at birth can be found in relationship to race (Table 32-3).

The proportion of older adults will remain constant until around 2010, when the first wave of baby-boom cohort turns 65 years of age. This event will trigger large increases in the number and proportion of older people. In recent years the many articles discussing the impact of baby boomers on social services, pensions, the economy, the health care industry, and even national production have illustrated the concern and attention this population shift has been receiving. The growth rate in the older population has implications for the sheer number of people requiring services (e.g., housing, health, nutrition, information, and entitlement programs).

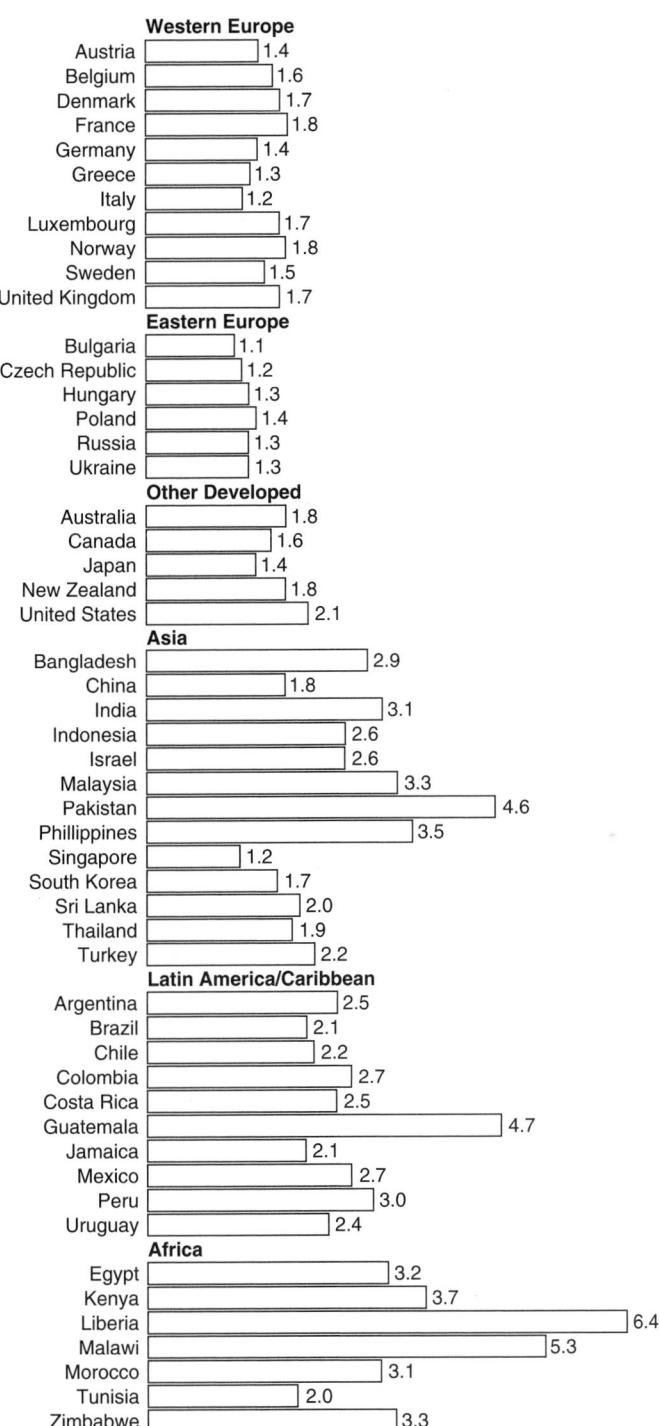

Figure 32-1 Fertility rate: births per woman. (From Kinsella K, Velkoff V: *An aging world, 2001*, U.S. Census Bureau Series, pp 95/01-1, Washington, DC, 2001, U.S. Government Printing Office.)

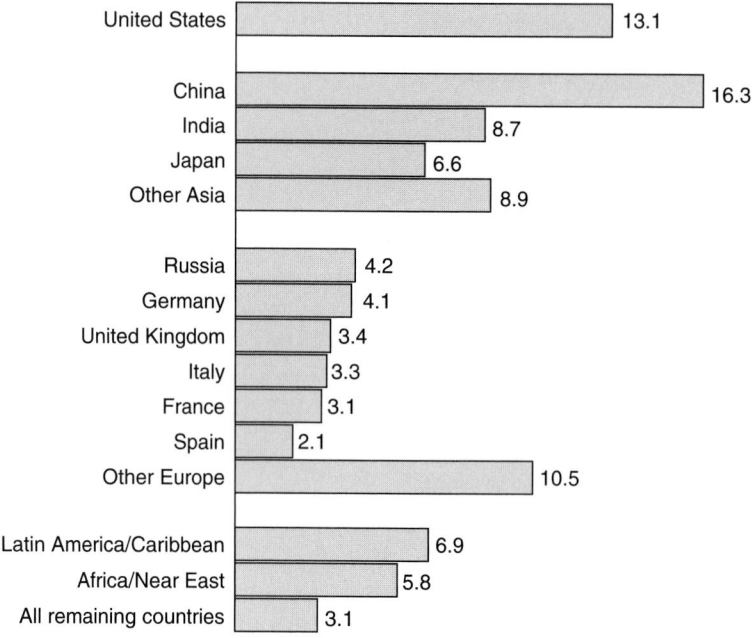

Figure 32-2   Percent distribution of worldwide population 80 years of age and older: 2000. (From Kinsella K, Velkoff V: *An aging world,* 2001, U.S. Census Bureau Series, pp 95/01-1, Washington, DC, 2001, U.S. Government Printing Office.)

The projections of a high and increasing proportion of older adults from 2010 to 2030 are attributed to three factors: (1) declining and low fertility, (2) maturing of the baby-boom cohort, and (3) sharp declines in mortality at older ages.

Socioeconomic Factors

The socioeconomic characteristics of the older population include elements such as income, gender, and race. An understanding of how various socioeconomic factors are interwoven and impact primary health care is more important than simply defining individual socioeconomic factors.

INCOME

Because of government social programs such as Social Security and Medicare, combined with a corporate culture that provided defined pension benefits plans to workers and a growing economy that provided jobs for most able Americans, the poverty rate improved markedly over the last 50 years. The percentage of older people living in poverty declined from 35% in 1959 to 10.5% in 1998. Social Security accounts for 82% of the income for older Americans with the lowest level of income. In 1998 Social Security provided about 40% of the income of older Americans.

Pensions expanded for at least 20 to 30 years after the Second World War, but recent changes have encouraged corporations to revise their pension programs from defined benefits to defined contribution for their employee-sponsored pension. The future benefits of this type of plan depend on investment earnings and the amount of money the employee is allowed to invest along with (for some but not all) a contribution from the employer. Surveys have found that a large percentage of workers are not maximizing their contribution to these plans, known as 401K or 401b plans. Recent scandals (e.g., Enron, World Com) and a decline in the stock market have shown the inherent risk for workers in this type of pension program. Little regulation has been enacted to reform the investment culture or to protect workers from losses that result from corporate malfeasance. In fact, a

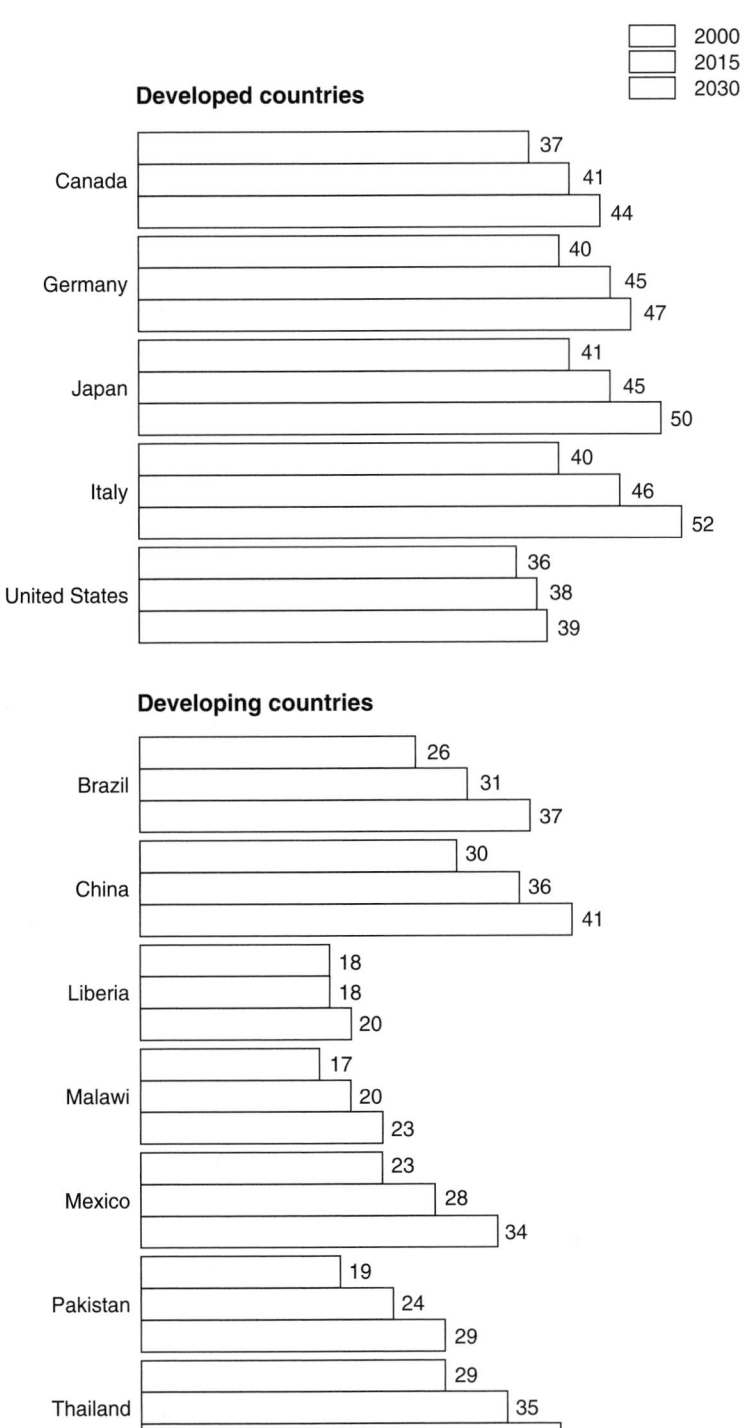

Figure 32-3   Median age: 12 countries, 2000, 2015, and 2030. (From Kinsella K, Velkoff V: *An aging world, 2001,* U.S. Census Bureau Series, pp 95/01-1, Washington, DC, 2001, U.S. Government Printing Office.)

TABLE 32-2	Life Expectancy by Age Group and Sex, in Years, 1900 to 1997

	1900	1910	1920	1930	1940	1950	1960	1970	1980	1990	1997
Total	49.2	51.5	56.4	59.2	63.6	68.1	69.9	70.8	73.9	75.4	76.5
Men	47.9	49.9	55.5	57.7	61.6	65.5	66.8	67.0	70.1	71.8	73.6
Women	50.7	53.2	57.4	60.9	65.9	71.0	73.2	74.6	77.6	78.8	79.4
Life Expectancy at Age 65											
Total	11.9	11.6	12.5	12.2	12.8	13.8	14.4	15.0	16.5	17.3	17.7
Men	11.5	11.2	12.2	11.7	12.1	12.7	13.0	13.0	14.2	15.1	15.9
Women	12.2	12.0	12.7	12.8	13.6	15.0	15.8	16.8	18.4	19.0	19.2
Life Expectancy at Age 85											
Total	4.0	4.0	4.2	4.2	4.3	4.7	4.6	5.3	6.0	6.2	6.3
Men	3.8	3.9	4.1	4.0	4.1	4.4	4.4	4.7	5.1	5.3	5.5
Women	4.1	4.1	4.3	4.3	4.5	4.9	4.7	5.6	6.4	6.7	6.6

From Federal Interagency Forum on Aging-Related Statistics: *Older Americans 2000: key indicators of well-being*, Washington, DC, 2000, U.S. Government Printing Office.

large media campaign constantly reminds workers to increase their savings and that "you are responsible for your retirement." It is too early to tell whether poverty rates will increase in the older population as a result of changes in government programs and changes in the pension system. Nonetheless, primary care providers are dealing every day with older adults who are being forced to make health care decisions based on cost.

More than 10% of persons 65 years of age and older living in the United States are living at the poverty level or below, and 2.3% are living in extreme poverty ($3909 yearly income for one person). Poverty is considered to be yearly income in a range of $3909 to $7817 for one person. Significant differences in income and poverty can be found within the older population based on gender and race (Table 32-4). On the other hand, since 1974 a decline has occurred in the number of older adults living in poverty and an increase in the number of older persons enjoying higher incomes. An interesting fact concerns the difference between sources of income for the highest and lowest income levels. The highest income group receives only 18.3% of its income from Social Security and 31.1% from earnings, whereas the lowest group receives 82.1% from Social Security and only 0.7% from earnings. See Table 32-5 for income distribution among income groups.

TABLE 32-3	Life Expectancy by Age Group and Race, in Years, 1997

	White	Black
Life expectancy at birth	77.1	71.1
Life expectancy at age 65	17.8	16.1
Life expectancy at age 85	6.2	6.4

From Federal Interagency Forum on Aging-Related Statistics: *Older Americans 2000: key indicators of well-being*, Washington, DC, 2000, U.S. Government Printing Office.

TABLE 32-4	Percentage of Persons 65 Years of Age or Older Living in Poverty, by Selected Characteristics, 1998
Total	10.5
Men	7.2
Women	12.8
Married	4.9
Nonmarried	17.4
Non-Hispanic white	8.2
Non-Hispanic black	26.4
Non-Hispanic Asian and Pacific Islander	16.0
Hispanic	21.0

From Federal Interagency Forum on Aging-Related Statistics: *Older Americans 2000: key indicators of well-being*, Washington, DC, 2000, U.S. Government Printing Office.
Note: The poverty level is based on money income and does not include noncash benefits, such as food stamps. Poverty thresholds reflect family size and composition and are adjusted each year using the annual average Consumer Price Index level.

EMPLOYMENT

Although older adults represent a growing proportion of the total population and life expectancy has increased, the older population represents a smaller share of the nation's labor force today than they did in 1963. Between 1963 and 1999, labor force participation declined from 90% to 75% among men 55 to 61 years of age and declined from 76% to 47% among men 62 to 64 years of age. For men 70 years and older the 1963 participation rate was 21%, and 1999 brought a decline to less than 12%. The Bureau of Labor Statistics predicts that the percentage of men 55 to 59 years of age in the labor force will continue to decline through 2005 but at a slower rate. The change in labor force participation has not been as striking for older women; participation actually increased in the 55 to 61 age group, from 43.7% in 1963 to 57.9%; in the 62 to 64 age group, from 28.8% to 33.7%; and in the 65 to 69 age group, from 16.5% to 18.4%. A labor force participation of more than 5% of women over 70 years of age has been a constant over the span of years since 1963 to 1999.

TABLE 32-5	Sources of Income Among Persons 65 Years of Age or Older, by Income Level, 1998				
	Lowest Fifth	*Second Fifth*	*Third Fifth*	*Fourth Fifth*	*Highest Fifth*
Total	100	100	100	100	100
Social Security	82.1	80.5	63.8	45.2	18.3
Asset Income	2.4	6.1	10.5	13.7	27.9
Pensions	3.3	6.6	14.9	24.4	20.5
Earnings	0.7	3.2	7.3	13.1	31.1
Public Assistance	9.8	1.8	0.7	0.2	0.0
Other	1.8	1.8	2.8	3.3	2.1

From Federal Interagency Forum on Aging-Related Statistics: *Older Americans 2000: key indicators of well-being*, Washington, DC, 2000, U.S. Government Printing Office.

ASSETS

Because financial soundness includes a person's lifetime accrual of assets in addition to net income, it is not surprising that the median net worth of older adults is much higher than that of households headed by the under-35 age group. Huge income and asset disparities are found within the population of the United States, and the older population reflects this fact. The three most significant factors that affect income and asset achievement are race, marital status, and education level (Table 32-6).

Despite the optimistic picture that their high median net worth presents, a large number of people are reaching retirement age with little or no savings. This fact can have considerable implications for their ability to finance potential long-term care services and to assume the burden of other health care expenditures because older adults face an increased risk for more serious and expensive health care problems.

GENDER

The percent of women in the older population is 58% of the total of those over 65 years of age. Furthermore, women make up 70% of the population of those over 85 years of age and older. Older women are more likely to be unmarried than older men and more likely to be living alone. In 1998 41% of older women were living alone compared with only 17% of older men. The imbalance between genders in older adults has implications for the types of integrated primary health care delivery systems that will be developed over the next decades. Planning and policy efforts regarding primary health care should reflect gender proportions within the population cohort. Although the projected gender imbalance in the 65+ age group will decrease because of converging mortality rates, women are projected to continue to outnumber men, especially in the over-85 age group.

TABLE 32-6 Median Household Net Worth, by Selected Characteristics, in Thousands of 1999 Dollars, 1984 to 1999				
	1984	*1989*	*1994*	*1999*
Age of Head Household				
45 to 54	$ 110.6	$ 98.5	$ 107.3	$ 85.0
55 to 64	118.6	149.8	157.4	145.0
65 to 74	109.2	126.3	130.4	190.0
65 or older	93.0	101.5	112.4	157.6
75 or older	80.2	84.0	93.9	132.9
Marital Status, Head of Household Age 65 or Older				
Married	$ 145.9	$ 184.8	$ 204.6	$ 234.0
Unmarried	65.7	61.8	70.8	83.7
Race, Head of Household Age 65 or Older				
BLACK	$ 24.0	$ 30.2	$ 41.6	$ 13.0
WHITE	105.3	115.6	125.9	181.0
Education, Head of Household Age 65 or Older				
No high school diploma	$ 52.0	$ 53.1	$ 61.8	$ 63.1
High school diploma only	128.7	137.0	120.3	157.4
Some college or more	203.6	235.2	265.3	301.0

From Federal Interagency Forum on Aging-Related Statistics: *Older Americans 2000: key indicators of well-being,* Washington, DC, 2000, U.S. Government Printing Office.

MIGRATION

In general, the older population remains geographically stationary. Older adults represent only about 4% of all persons who move in the United States; only 3% of all older persons who moved actually changed their county of residence, only 1% moved as far as another state, and 8% moved from a metropolitan area to a nonmetropolitan area. In addition, of all people 65 years of age and older, about 6% moved within the county compared with about 18% of all younger people. Older people moving from warmer to colder states tend to be disproportionately disabled and widowed compared with those moving from colder to warmer states. This phenomenon probably occurs after the death of a spouse and in combination with other illness, which causes an older person to move closer to children or other family members in their original home communities, presumably to receive support. The most salient fact to be drawn from these data, however, is that most older adults remain either in their primary residence or in the same geographic location where they have spent their adult lives, and this fact remains constant.

LIVING ARRANGEMENTS

Because women live longer than men, it is not surprising that 41% of women and 73% of men 65 years of age and older live with their spouses. Living arrangements of older women vary by race, with about 41% of black and white older women living alone compared with only 27% of Hispanic older women and 21% of older Asian and Pacific Islanders. Living with other relatives demonstrated a reverse, with only 15% of older white women but up to one third of black, Hispanic, and Asian and Pacific islanders having this living arrangement (Federal Interagency Forum on Age-Related Statistics, 2000).

Not surprisingly, older adults with declining health and economic resources are more likely to form a household with one of their children (Burr and Mutchler, 1995). On the other extreme, one in 10 grandparents raises a grandchild for at least 6 months, often longer (Gerontological Society of America, 1997).

RACE

The racial and ethnic composition of the United States is changing, a reflection of the demographic shifts of the total population. A more diverse older population than that of a decade ago will call for flexibility in programs and services. In the year 2000, 84% of the over-65 population were non-Hispanic whites; by the year 2050 projections are that the percentage of non-Hispanic whites will decline to 64% (Figure 32-4) (Federal Interagency Forum on Aging-Related Statistics, 2000).

The Hispanic proportion of the over-65 age group is projected to increase from 4.5% in 1995 to more than 16% in 2050. The proportion of blacks in the 65+ age group is also projected to increase, but not so dramatically: from 8% in 1995 to almost 11% in 2050. The proportion of other races (mainly Asian and Pacific Islanders) is projected to increase significantly during this same period: from 2.3% to 7.4%. These projections are estimates of future changes, and the proportion may vary; however, the undeniable fact is that the composition of the population in 2050 will differ from that in 2000.

Racial differences are important factors for primary care health policy. For example, black Americans report higher rates of hypertension, diabetes, and arthritis than other races. People of Hispanic descent report higher rates of hypertension and diabetes and lower rates of heart conditions than other races. Although socioeconomic status accounts for much of the difference in functional status associated with these chronic diseases, it does not explain the differences in the prevalence of these diseases among the different groups. These differences suggest varying causal pathways among racial and ethnic groups (Kington and Smith, 1997).

Race alone is not necessarily the causative biologic factor determining health status and utilization of health services, however. Race and ethnicity are fluid categories defined as much by social and historical context as by how a person responds to race questions on a survey. Intermarriage, socioeconomic integration, and cultural exchange will continue to contribute to significant changes in "standard" race definitions and the association between race and health or race and primary health care utilization (Muller, 2002).

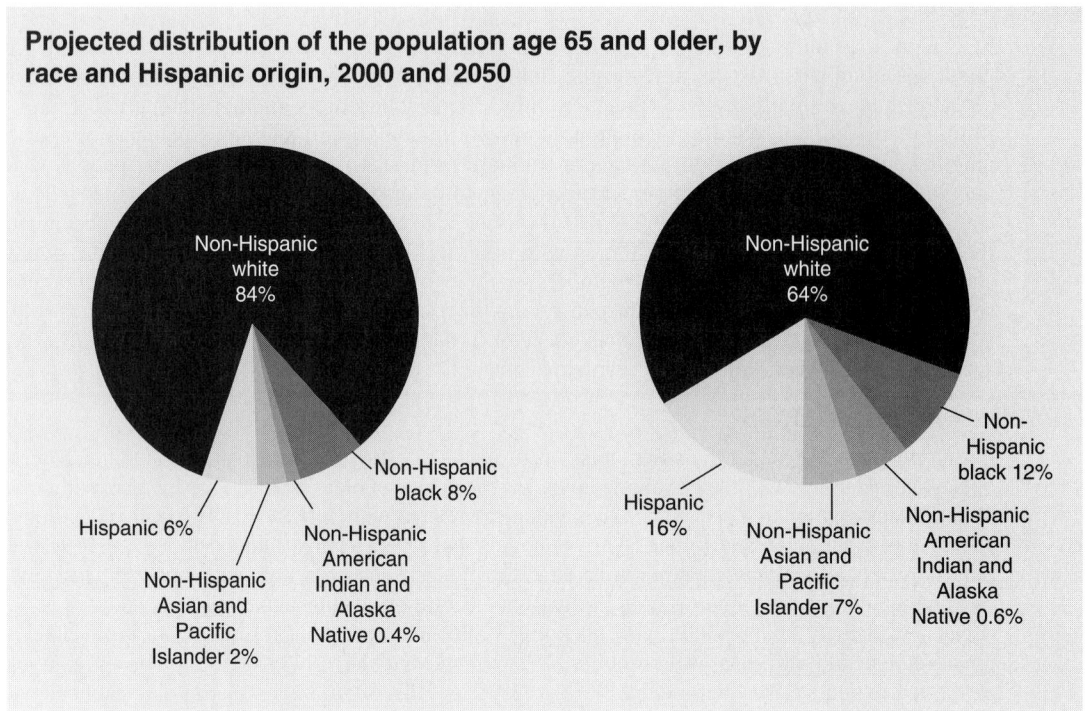

Figure 32-4   Projected distribution of the population 65 years of age and older, by race and Hispanic origin, 2000 and 2050. (From Federal Interagency Forum on Aging-Related Statistics: *Older Americans 2000: key indicators of well-being,* Washington, DC, 2000, U.S. Government Printing Office.)

EDUCATION

A person's educational level is often used as a gauge for both economic well-being and health status. Indeed, research has shown that mortality more than doubles for those who did not finish high school compared with those who did graduate from high school. The death rate among high school graduates is 79% higher than for those whose education continued beyond high school. In addition, those without a high school education were more likely to have a disability than better-educated people (U.S. Bureau of the Census, 1996).

In a study analysis of census data, Muller tested the relationship between income inequality and mortality and different levels of formal education (Muller, 2002). Higher education degrees are usually prerequisites for work that is highly compensated. The median earnings of workers with professional degrees are about four times higher than those who have not completed high school. Lack of high school education results in income inequality and indicates low status, adverse life circumstances, lack of health insurance, high risk of injury, and smoking, which lead to poorer health and greater mortality. The conclusion of the study was that a lack of high school education accounts for income inequality and is a powerful predictor of mortality variation within the United States (Muller, 2002).

In 1950, 18% of the older population had finished high school, but by 1980, 67% of Americans 65 years of age and older had completed their high school education. Furthermore, in 1950 only 4% of the older population had attained a bachelor's degree; this number increased to almost 15% by 1998, with 20% of older men and 11% of older women holding a bachelor's degree (Federal Interagency Forum on Aging-Related Statistics, 2000).

The educational level of the older population is rising, and the proportion of the older population with at least a high school education will notably increase. Therefore older adults of the future will be better educated. This significant progression in educational attainments presumably will have a positive impact on the overall well-being of older adults. Despite the increase in educational attainment of the older population, substantial disparities exist among racial and ethnic groups; the lowest educational attainment is in the Hispanic older population (see Figure 32-5 for educational attainment for racial and ethnic older American populations).

Health Status

Various life-expectancy projections have shown that older adults can expect a longer average life by the year 2050. In fact, by the year 2050 the average 65-year-old white woman can expect to live to almost age 90. These projections are based in part on the estimates of decreasing mortality rates, particularly among the older age groups. Although this projection indicates that older persons are living longer, the question of quality of life is not addressed solely by number of years. The issue of a healthy life during the last years is an important consideration for all primary care providers.

When older adults were asked to assess their own health, almost three of four noninstitutionalized persons 65 to 74 years of age indicated that they thought their health was good, very good, or excellent (Federal Interagency Forum on Aging-Related Statistics, 2000). Positive health evaluations declined somewhat with advanced age in all racial groups. These data seem to indicate that, at least in their viewpoint, older Americans are generally in good health. Although there was no significant gender difference in this self-assessment of health, there was a significant ethnic difference (Figure 32-6).

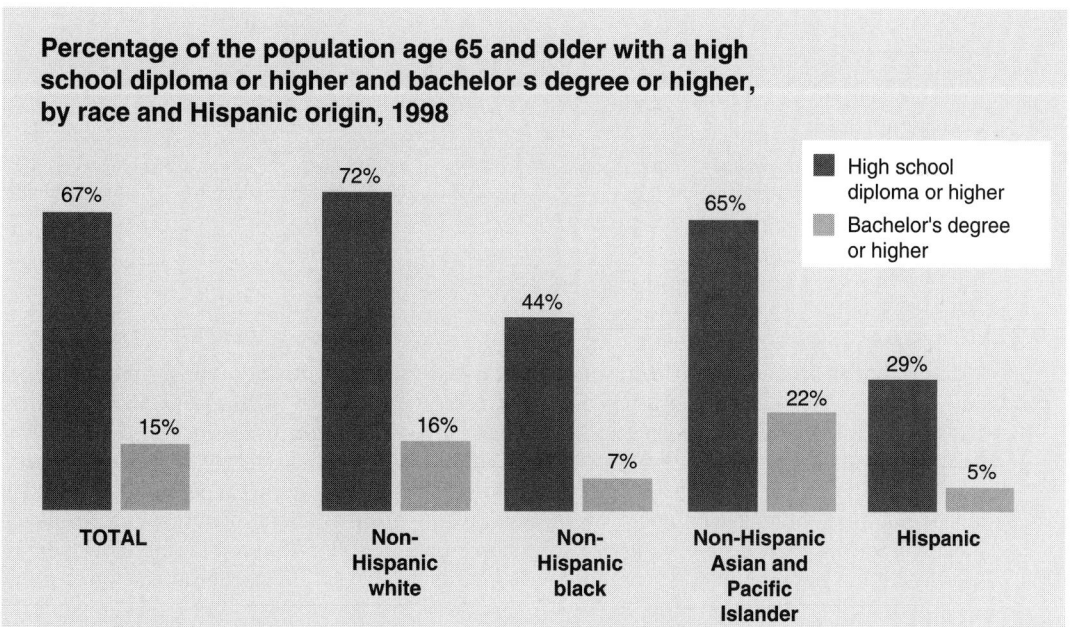

Figure 32-5   Percentage of the population 65 years of age and older with a high school diploma or higher and bachelor's degree or higher by race and Hispanic origin, 1998. (From Federal Interagency Forum on Aging-Related Statistics: *Older Americans 2000: key indicators of well-being*, Washington, DC, 2000, U.S. Government Printing Office.

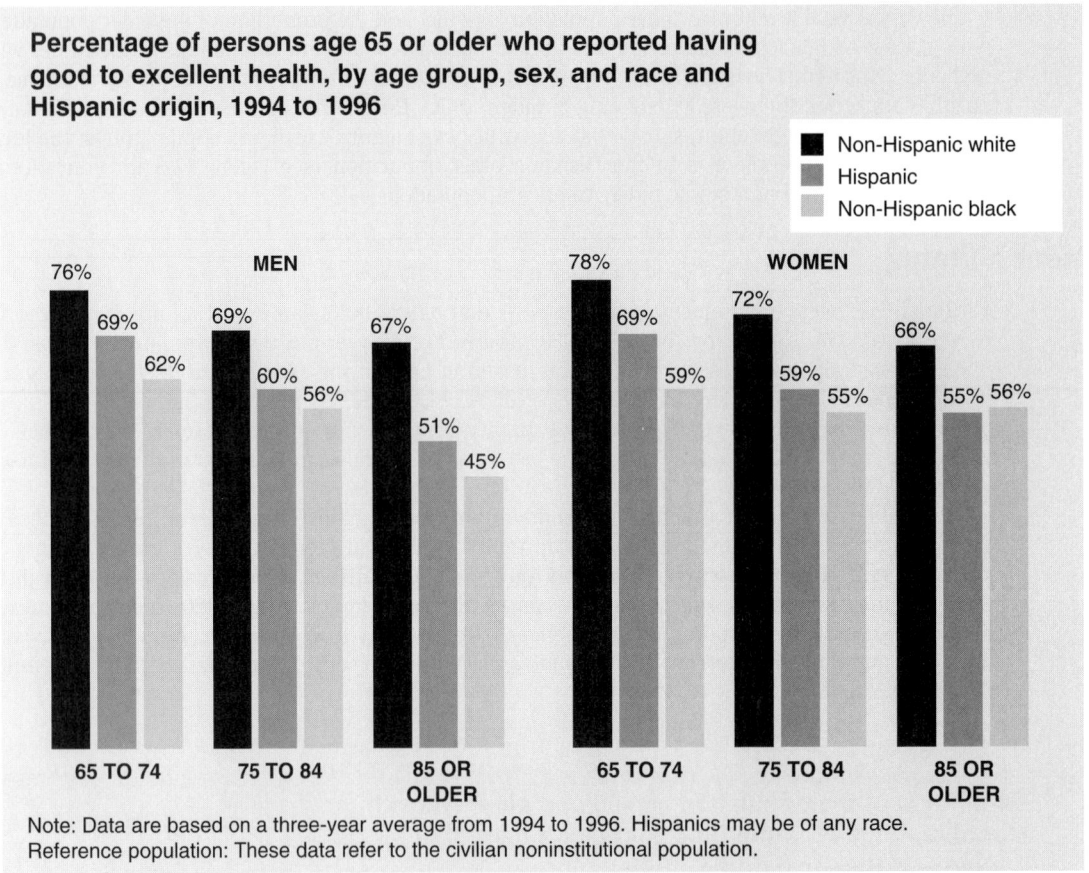

Percentage of persons age 65 or older who reported having good to excellent health, by age group, sex, and race and Hispanic origin, 1994 to 1996

Note: Data are based on a three-year average from 1994 to 1996. Hispanics may be of any race.
Reference population: These data refer to the civilian noninstitutional population.

Figure 32-6 Percentage of persons 65 years of age or older who reported having good to excellent health, by age group, sex, race, and Hispanic origin, 1994 to 1996. (From Federal Interagency Forum on Aging-Related Statistics: *Older Americans 2000: key indicators of well-being*, Washington, DC, 2000, U.S. Government Printing Office.

CHRONIC CONDITIONS

Chronic conditions such as arthritis and heart disease have become increasingly important public health concerns. The interesting aspect of these two disease processes is that arthritis is rarely the cause of death; in contrast, heart disease is a leading cause of death. Cause-specific mortality statistics project that more than half of older Americans will die of heart disease. On the other hand, disability caused by arthritis varies greatly even among older adults with a similar degree of arthritis (Grundy, 2003). Acknowledgment of differences in response to disease processes rather than accepting a view of disease as a sole determinant of the older person's health state is paramount for a practitioner's ability to assess the strengths and limitation of each patient.

Most older adults have at least one chronic disease, and many have multiple chronic diseases. Figure 32-7 lists the percentage of those over 70 years of age that report selected chronic diseases. Well-being of older people is greatly influenced by their mental state and cognitive

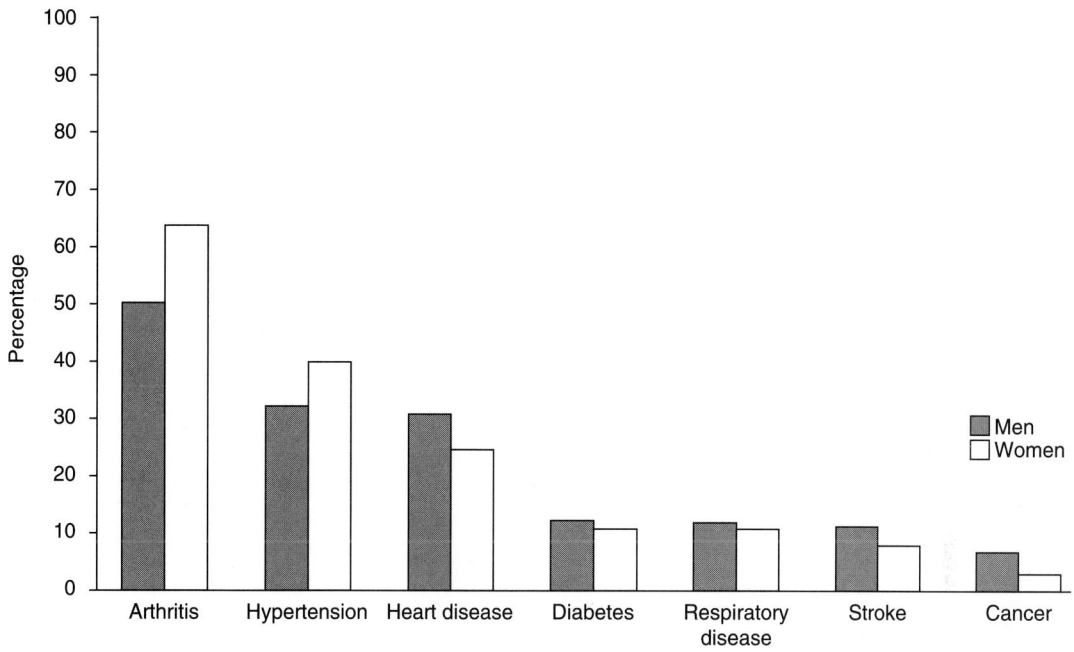

Figure 32-7   Percentage of people in the United States 70 years of age and older reporting selected chronic disease. (From Grundy E: The epidemiology of aging. In Tallis RC and Fillit HM, editors: *Brocklehurst's textbook of geriatric medicine and gerontology*, ed 6, London, 2003, Churchill Livingstone.)

abilities. Memory skills are important to general cognitive functioning, and many older adults fear the loss of memory. In 1998 the percentage of older persons with moderate or severe memory loss ranged from 4% of those 65 to 69 years of age up to 36% of those over 85 years of age. Depressive symptoms are associated with higher rates of physical illness, greater functional disability, and higher utilization of health care resources. Older women are more likely than older men to have severe depressive symptoms until the age of 85, when a similar prevalence between men and women occurs (Federal Interagency Forum on Aging-Related Statistics, 2000). See Figure 32-8.

FUNCTIONAL HEALTH

There is an ongoing debate in the field of aging concerning the extent and length of time older persons experience the loss of many functional abilities and thereby lose degrees of independence. Data on the disability and limitations status of the noninstitutionalized older person are of importance to policymakers, researchers, and service planners to assess service needs. The statistics and information presented in this discussion of disability indicate that older persons are vulnerable to the onset of disability and activities of daily living (ADL) dependencies and that the number of disabled older adults may increase in the future. Recent research, however, demonstrates that disability rates among older adults in the United States are actually declining dramatically and that this rate of reduction is increasing. Researchers found that the actual number of older people with disability in 1994 was 7.1 million, and not the expected 8.3 million, an estimate based on the assumption that the 1982 disability rates would remain unchanged (Manton and XiLiang, 2001). Significant declines in the prevalence of chronic disability in the older population have been observed from 1982 to 1999

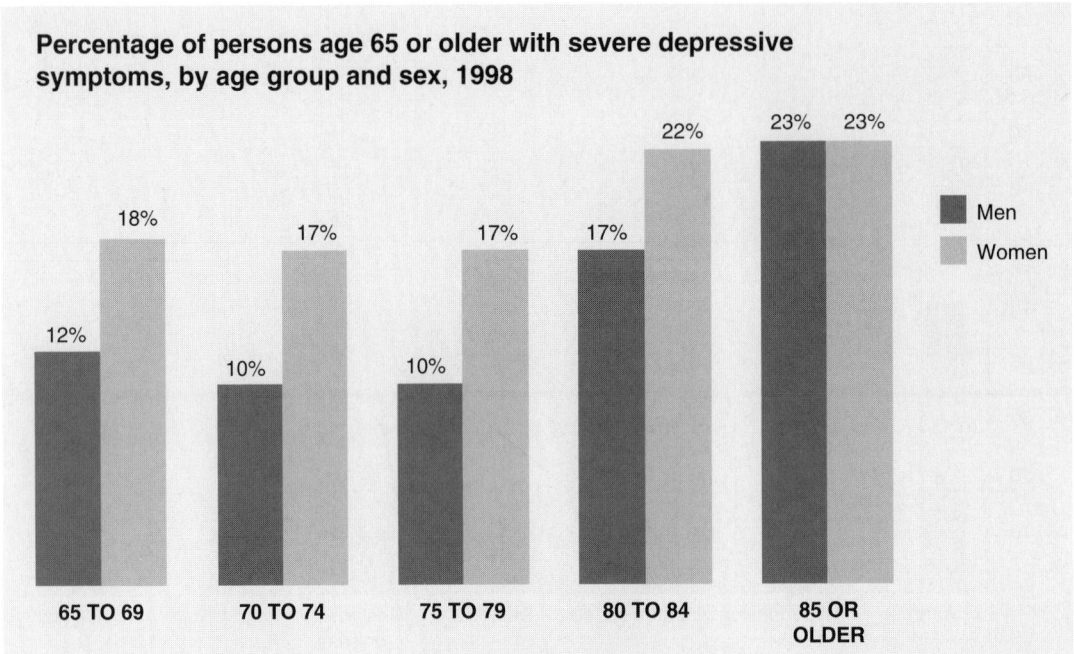

Figure 32-8   Percentage of persons age 65 or older with severe depressive symptoms, by age group and sex, 1998. (From Federal Interagency Forum on Aging-Related Statistics: Older *Americans 2000: key indicators of well-being,* Washington, DC, 2000, U.S. Government Printing Office.)

(Manton and XiLiang, 2001). This trend of declining disability among older adults (if it continues) will have a profound effect on health care delivery systems and government programs that serve the older population.

Not surprisingly, the likelihood of having a disability increases with age. Disability can be measured by certain indicators, such as limitations in ADLs; instrumental activities of daily living (IADLs); and measures of physical, cognitive, and social functioning. The proportion of people 65 years of age and older with a chronic disability declined from 24% in 1982 to 21% in 1994. The decline rates slowed the growth of the actual numbers of older adults with disabilities, although because of the growth in the older population the numbers of disabled older adults increased by about 600,000 in the period; however, if the disability rates had not declined, the disabled population would have increased by 1.5 million older adults. It is well to remember that there is a wide variation in the degree of disability (Figure 32-9). Some diseases are considered responsible for a large share of severe disability in older persons: stroke, hip fracture, congestive heart failure, pneumonia, coronary heart disease, diabetes, and dehydration. Targeting these conditions could help to decrease severe disability among older adults and improve their independent functioning (Ferrucci et al, 1997).

Functional health is often measured in terms of a person's ability to perform ADLs and IADLs. ADLs include bathing, dressing, toileting, walking, eating, and getting in and out of a bed or chair. IADLs include housekeeping tasks such as preparing meals, shopping, managing money, using the telephone, doing light housework, and doing heavy housework. Table 32-7 shows the percentage of people 70 years of age and older who require assistance with one or more ADLs and IADLs. Women more than men need assistance, and for those over 80 years of age, both men and women, the need

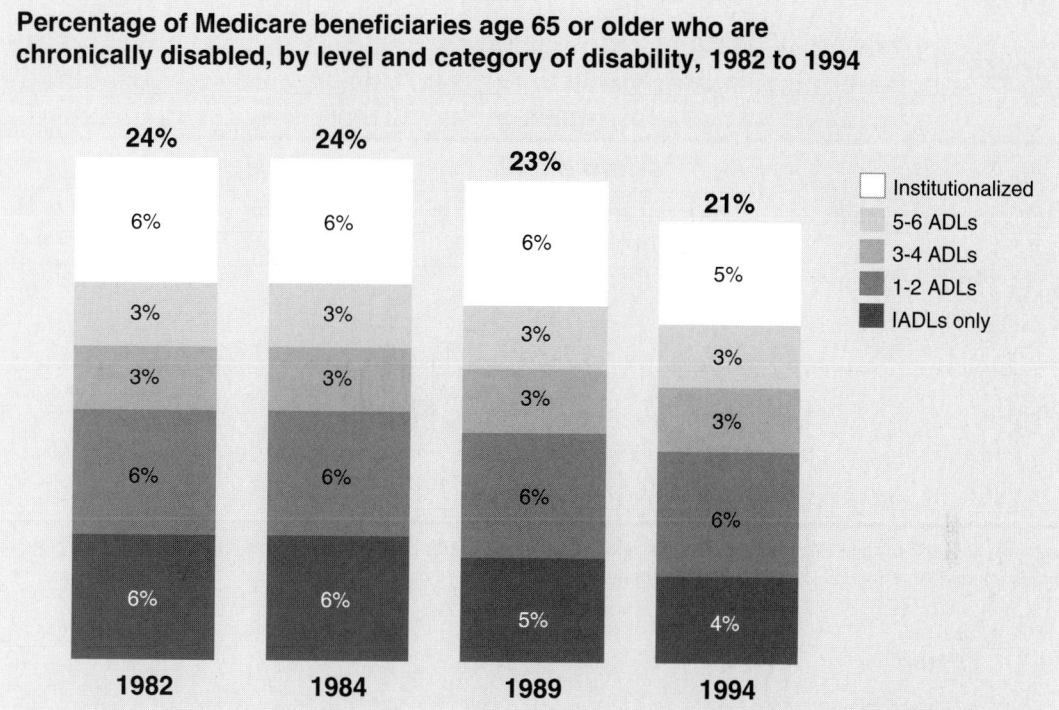

Figure 32-9 Percentage of Medicare beneficiaries 65 years of age or older who are chronically disabled, by level and category of disability, 1982 to 1994. (From Federal Interagency Forum on Aging-Related Statistics: *Older Americans 2000: key indicators of well-being*, Washington, DC, 2000, U.S. Government Printing Office.)

for assistance increases. It is important to realize that if 21% of persons in the over-65 age group have some type of disability, then 79% are able to function independently. Many projections have been made concerning this group of older independent people, but it behooves all health professionals to recognize and affirm the strengths of older people and support them and their network of informal support.

Summary

This chapter provides an overview of the nation's older population, with an emphasis on the importance of the relationship between demographic data and health care delivery. Primary care providers need to be able to access this information for their community to advocate health policy developments that will meet the needs of the older population they serve.

| TABLE 32-7 | Percentage of People 70 Years of Age and Older Who Have Difficulty Performing, or are Unable to Perform, One or More Activities of Daily Living (ADLs) and Instrumental Activities of Daily Living (IADLs) |

		At least one ADL		At least one IADL	
Age group	Gender	Performs with difficulty	Unable to perform	Performs with difficulty	Unable to perform
70-74	M	14	4	6	8
	F	20	5	13	16
75-79	M	17	6	8	11
	F	19	9	12	21
80-84	M	20	10	8	20
	F	24	12	14	27
85+	M	23	19	8	27
	F	33	23	13	44

Adapted from Grundy E: The epidemiology of aging. In Tallis RC, Fillit HM, editors: *Brocklehurst's textbook of geriatric medicine and gerontology*, London, 2003, Churchill Livingstone.

Resources

Administration on Aging
www.aoa.dhhs.gov

American Association of Retired Persons
www.aarp.org

American Public Health Association (APHA)
www.apha.org

Bureau of Labor Statistics
stats.bls.gov

National Center for Health Statistics
www.cdc.gov/nchs

National Institute on Aging
www.nih.gov/nia

National Library of Medicine (includes free MEDLINE service)
www.nlm.nih.gov

References

Burr J, Mutchler J: *Intergenerational living arrangements: new evidence from the national survey of families and households*, Paper presented at the American Sociological Association, Amherst, NY, 1995.

Federal Interagency Forum on Aging-Related Statistics: *Older Americans 2000: key indicators of well-being*, Washington DC, 2000, U.S. Government Printing Office.

Ferrucci L et al: Hospital diagnoses, Medicare charges, and nursing home admissions in the year when older persons become severely disabled, *JAMA* 277:728-734, 1997.

Gerontological Society of America: *One in ten grandparents raises a grandchild*, news release, May 29, 1997. Available at gsa.iog.wayne.edu/press.html.

Grundy EM: The epidemiology of aging. In Tallis RC and Fillit FM, editors: *Brocklehurst's textbook of geriatric medicine and gerontology*, ed 6, London, 2003, Churchill Livingstone.

Kington R, Smith J: Socioeconomic status and racial and ethnic differences in functional status associated with chronic diseases, *Am J Public Health* 87(5):805-810, 1997.

Kinsella K, Velkoff V: *An aging world, 2001*, U.S. Census Bureau Series pp 95/01-1, Washington DC, 2001, U.S. Government Printing Office.

Manton KG, XiLiang GU: Changes in the prevalence of chronic disability in the United States black and nonblack population above the age of 65 from 1982 to 1999, *Proc Natl Acad Sci USA* 98:6354-6359, 2001.

Manton KG et al: Estimates of change in chronic disability and institutional incidence and prevalence rates in the U.S. elderly population from the 1982, 1984, and 1989 National Long Term Care Survey, *J Gerontol* 48(4):S153-S166, 1993.

Muller A: Education, income inequality, and mortality: a multiple regression analysis, *BMJ* 324(7328):23, 2002.

U.S. Bureau of the Census: *Population projection of the United States by age, sex, race, and Hispanic origin: 1992-2050* (Current Population Report, pp 25-1092), Washington, DC, 1990, U.S. Government Printing Office.

U.S. Bureau of the Census: *Educational attainment in the United States: March 1992 and 1993* (Current Population Report, pp 20-476), Washington, DC, 1993, U.S. Government Printing Office.

U.S. Bureau of the Census: *Americans with disabilities: statistical brief*, Washington, DC, 1996, U.S. Department of Commerce, Economics and Statistics Administration.

33

Health Care Delivery System

Demographic shifts, which have shown significant increases in longevity and thereby increased total numbers of older people, are a cause of economic and political concern within the U.S. government. Health care for older citizens is funded by either one or a combination of (1) private insurance, (2) Medicare, (3) Medicaid, or (4) out-of-pocket expenditures. Medicare, the federal program that provides health care payment for older adults, has been and continues to be a political issue. How and when any resolution of the issue will be forthcoming is uncertain. This chapter reviews the federal programs that provide for older adults' health care, discusses the current state of health care delivery to the nation's older adults, and discusses some of the current controversies concerning Medicare services, with a look to the future.

Federal Health Care Insurance Programs: Medicare and Medicaid

In 1965 Congress passed the Title 18 and 19 amendments to the Social Security Act, which enacted the Medicare and Medicaid programs. Medicare is a federal government entitlement program, and Medicaid is a joint federal and state need-based program.

Medicare covers 40 million Americans. People over age 65 who are eligible (by virtue of their contributions made during their working years) for Social Security, people who have been disabled for at least 2 years, people with end-stage renal disease, and all people over 80 years of age are eligible for Medicare. Medicare part A includes coverage of inpatient hospital services, skilled nursing facilities, home health, and hospice benefits. There are co-payments and caps on most part A benefits. Optional Medicare part B covers partial physician services, outpatient hospital services, medical equipment and supplies, and other health services and supplies (Health Care Financing Administration, 1997). Beneficiaries must pay a monthly fee for part B coverage. A beneficiary who is enrolled in a managed care system must carry part B. Not all primary care costs and services are covered by Medicare (e.g., prescription drugs, vision, and hearing aids).

Medicaid, the federal–state matching entitlement program (administered by the state) provides health care services for the poor and near poor. Medicaid is the health care safety net for older adults. Many of the expenditures are for nursing home care, after older people have spent their life savings for nursing home care and become destitute, thereby becoming eligible for Medicaid. The Center for Medicare and Medicaid Services (CMS [formerly Health Care Financing Administration]) within the Health and Human Services Department regulates and provides national standards for both the Medicaid and Medicare programs. Medicare or Medicaid coverage usually determines where older adults will seek primary care.

Medicare coverage includes primary health care services. Typical Medicare coverage allows the Medicare beneficiary to select a physician of choice. Since the decade of the 1990s focus has been increasingly on persuading beneficiaries to enroll in managed care programs.

Sources of Primary Health Care for the Older Patient

Primary health care is delivered in a myriad of settings: physician offices, health maintenance organizations (HMOs), other managed care systems, outpatient departments, emergency departments, community health centers, and nursing homes.

PHYSICIAN'S OFFICE

The numbers of visits to physicians' offices have risen steadily over the past decade (Federal Agency Forum on Age-Related Statistics, 2000). Physician visits and consultations increased from 10,800 per 1000 beneficiaries in 1990 to 13,100 per 1000 in 1998 (Table 33-1). On average, older adults made between five (by the 65 to 74 age group) and 6.5 visits (75+ age group) to a physician's office per year (National Center for Health Statistics, 1998). Of these, more than 70% were covered by Medicare, about 15% were self-pay, and about 5% were covered by Medicaid. Medicare reimburses the physician up to a certain amount. Unless otherwise specified, the physician may "balance bill" the patient for the amount Medicare does not reimburse. Physicians may or may not choose to participate in the Medicare program. The usual incentive not to participate is remuneration: often the physician is unable to recoup costs incurred for delivering primary care services to older adults. In

TABLE 33-1	Rates of Health Care Service Usage by Medicare Beneficiaries Age 65 or Older, 1990 to 1998 (PER 1000)								
Type of Service	*1990*	*1991*	*1992*	*1993*	*1994*	*1995*	*1996*	*1997*	*1998*
Hospitalization	307	311	311	306	337	344	352	364	365
Home health visits	2141	—	3822	4648	6352	7608	8376	8227	5058
Skilled nursing facility admissions	23	—	28	33	43	50	59	67	69
Physician visits and consultations	10,800	11,800	11,800	12,100	12,500	12,900	13,000	13,000	13,100
Average length of hospital stay (days)	8.8	8.6	8.3	7.9	7.4	6.9	6.5	6.2	6.1

From Federal Interagency Forum on Aging-Related Statistics: *Older Americans 2000: key indicators of well-being*, Washington, DC, 2000, U.S. Government Printing Office.

— = NOT AVAILABLE

Note: Data for 1998 should be considered preliminary. Some data for 1991 are not available (—). For hospitalizations, home health visits, and skilled nursing facility admissions, utilization rates for 1994-1998 exclude HMO enrollees from the numerator and denominator because utilization data are not available for this group. Prior to 1994, HMO enrollees were included in the denominators causing utilization rates to be understated. Prior to 1994, HMO enrollees represented 7 percent or less of the Medicare population; in 1998 they represented about 18 percent. For physician visits, data on HMO enrollees are excluded for all years.

Reference population: These data refer to Medicare beneficiaries in fee-for-service only.

Source: Medicare claims and enrollment data.

2003 Medicare was scheduled to decrease physician payment by 4.4%; instead, after pressure from Congress, Medicare reversed the decision and raised the rates by 1.9% (Center for Medicare and Medicaid Services, 2003).

To protect themselves from the circumstances of "balance billing," Medicare recipients can purchase supplemental health insurance. Medi-gap policies are regulated, and the Medicare beneficiary can choose from different offerings. Like most medical insurance policies, higher cost leads to an increase in benefits. Many older adults have private insurance coverage as an aspect of their retirement pension that supplements Medicare, but for many this benefit is being withdrawn as large corporations cut back on their retirement programs.

HEALTH MAINTENANCE ORGANIZATIONS AND MANAGED GERIATRIC PRIMARY CARE

Policy makers assumed that the enrollment of Medicare beneficiaries in HMOs would generate cost savings. The 1997 Balanced Budget Act (BBA) Medicare+Choice was thought to be a partial solution to the spiraling cost of the program. After the 1997 BBA cost reduction in the payment formula for the Medicare managed care system, 33 managed care contractors (i.e., HMOs) opted not to renew their 1999 contracts, thereby disenrolling 400,000 Medicare beneficiaries. In other words the health care system terminated 400,000 people with no warning and for no health reasons. Luckily these people still have Medicare coverage, but for many significant problems resulted that required them to make multiple, somewhat complex decisions in a short time and designate certain options to ensure health care coverage within the Medicare program. The HMOs raised premiums and reduced benefits to an unprecedented level (Pizer and Frakt, 2002).

In general, members of an HMO pay a set amount each month for complete health care services, regardless of utilization. Conventional HMOs participating in the Medicare program are required to provide a full range of benefits, including post-acute benefits that are especially important for older adults, who themselves must be astute purchasers of health care, even in instances (such as an HMO) in which it appears that all their primary care needs and associated costs will be covered.

These plans receive monthly payments based on risk or cost. Calculations regarding current health care expenditures are made by adding the annual premium and annual co-payment amount. In addition, expenditures beyond the maximum annual benefit (sometimes called the *cap*) are estimated. Finally, an estimated health risk of using other services in the future that are outside the HMO-reimbursed services are made and added to current expenditures.

As part of the health care coverage, Medicare HMOs provide primary care services for older patients. They may pay a specific provider group a set amount each month to provide health care services for a Medicare beneficiary. The beneficiary must use specific providers unless the HMO offers a point-of-service option by which the beneficiary is permitted to use other providers, usually at an increased cost.

Mirvis, Chang, and Morreim (1997) point out the complex and often competing incentives in a managed care delivery system for older adults. They begin by stating that, given multiple health problems, older patients would benefit most from high-quality managed care that coordinates primary care across chronic conditions; however, managed care generally limits enrollment of older patients, inappropriately uses advance directives, and applies selective criteria to limit care. The limited enrollment techniques are often called "cherry picking," a term that refers to the practice of enticing into the managed care programs younger beneficiaries who are less costly and avoiding the more costly oldest old. Under a poor-quality managed care system, older patients are most vulnerable to financial manipulation in that they consume a disproportionate amount of resources, making them a target for cost-containment measures (Lachs et al, 1997).

In March 2003 CMS published a market update that focused on managed care organizations. The report cited the following:

1. The year 2003 marked the third consecutive year of double-digit premium increases.
2. Employers continue to shift more costs onto employees.

3. Profit margins are expanding from an average of 1.9% in 1999 to 4.4% in 2002.
4. Commercial managed care organizations have reduced Medicare managed care (Medicare+Choice) exposure over the last several years.
5. Fifty-eight percent of Medicaid beneficiaries are covered by managed care plans. Growth is expected in this area, but concerns remain about the impact of state deficits (Center for Medicare and Medicaid Services, 2003).

It seems obvious in a free market system that capitation for health care for older adults, some of whom may be sick and frail, is a disincentive to providing optimum care in systems in which one of the primary missions is to achieve a profit margin that satisfies shareholders and other market demands.

SOCIAL HEALTH MAINTENANCE ORGANIZATIONS

A Medicare demonstration project sponsored by the Health Care Financing Administration is the social health maintenance organization (SHMO). The SHMO is a Medicare HMO that includes long-term care benefits. The program seeks to enroll a broad cross-section of older adults in terms of disability and financial status. Another project is the Program for All-Inclusive Care for the Elderly (PACE). This program provides an extensive set of acute and long-term care services on a capitated basis to frail older patients who wish to continue to live at home (avoiding nursing home placement) (Irvin, Massey, and Dorsey, 1997). The program aims to integrate a wide range of primary care services that older patients typically need into one delivery program that coordinates these services. The success of programs that offer an extensive array of services varies. Much depends on the primary care delivery structure in relation to the preferences of the Medicare recipient. For example, the PACE program offers adult day care. This structure is designed to monitor and deliver primary care for a chronically ill older population. The facts remain that many, if not most, older adults prefer the costly route of staying in their homes during the day and that any capitated payment structure creates an incentive for the program to avoid costly individuals.

MEDICAID PROGRAMS

Medicaid is a need-based program, and certain low-income older adults are considered to have dual eligibility for both Medicare and Medicaid programs. Most of the Medicaid outlays for older Americans are for nursing home care, which occurs after the older person has spent his or her life savings on nursing home bills and is left destitute and thereby eligible for the need-based program, Medicaid. At this time few older persons have long-term care (LTC) insurance, although there is a strong impetus from government to influence the population to begin to purchase this type of insurance. The vast majority of funding for LTC comes out of pocket and Medicaid; however, because the private pay rate for nursing home care is in the range of $4000 to $5000 a month, spend-down comes quickly for most families of older adults (Ouslander and Weinberg, 2003). The number of Americans residing in the nation's 16,706 nursing homes at one time is estimated at 1.8 million, although between 1985 to 1997 the total number of residents declined, with more than half of the residents being 85 years of age or older (Federal Interagency Forum on Aging-Related Statistics, 2000; Ouslander and Weinberg, 2003). This decline in the number of LTC residents may be accounted for by the extraordinary rapid growth of assisted-living facilities (ALF), which provide an alternative to LTC. There are 11,472 ALFs, with estimates of the population ranging from 500,000 to 1.1 million residents. ALFs are not eligible for Medicare reimbursement; on the other hand by not being federally regulated they are able to decide the level of professional staff in relation to the acuity of their group of residents. It is not surprising that ALFs have few, if any, professional staff; that most are for profit; and that many are owned by publicly traded corporations listed on the New York Stock Exchange. An in-depth discussion of the issues surrounding LTC in the United States is truly beyond the scope of this chapter, but all Americans need to stay informed and advocate for better and more humane care for the most vulnerable of our older population.

HOSPITALS

For most older adults, the hospital is not the source of primary care; however, about 10% of older patients report the hospital outpatient department as their usual source of care, and fewer than 1% report the hospital emergency department as their usual source of care (Agency for Health Care Policy and Research, 1998). On average these older patients visit either the hospital outpatient department or the emergency department less often than once per year (National Center for Health Statistics, 1998).

The hospital emergency department and the outpatient department are not structured to deliver integrated primary care services for older adults. Primary care services are typically delivered a la carte—on an as-needed, one-time-only basis. Given the structure of the hospital outpatient setting, little attempt may be made to monitor chronic conditions or to incorporate (or even know about) confounding diseases.

Acute care hospitalizations showed a moderate increase from 1990 to 1998, with 307 hospitalizations per 1000 per beneficiary in 1990 to 365 per 1000 in 1998, although the average length of stay declined from 9 days in 1990 to 6 days in 1998 (Federal Interagency Forum on Aging-Related Statistics, 2000). In California, between 1986 and 1995, the hospitalization rates declined; however, the trend was one of increasing total charges (Koziol et al, 2002). With the increased projections of a substantial increase in the older population, concern about the financial burden to the state and its citizens remains.

HOME HEALTH

The recent changes in home health care utilization gives credence to this author's contention that in the United States practice follows funding. In 1989 home health care delivery began a dramatic increase that lasted until the BBA of 1997. In 1989, as part of an agreement reached in a lawsuit, the Health Care Financing Administration expanded eligibility and coverage. The proportion of Medicare enrollees who experienced home health visits doubled between 1988 and 1996, rising from 4.8% to almost 11%, and the average number of visits increased from 24 visits per enrollee to 74 visits. Needless to say, expenditures for home health grew from $83 per enrollee in 1988 to $528 in 1996. The objective of the BBA was to control the price of home health services and to constrain the volume of services. This was done by changing the financial incentives for Home Health Agencies (Kowisar, 2002). Two years after enactment of the 1997 BBA, the average number of visits fell by 54%, the share of enrollees receiving home health declined by 21%, and spending for home health fell from $520 to $249 (Table 33-2).

It is difficult to assess the health consequences of this rationing of services. On the one hand the steep increase may have served only to enrich the owners of the agencies; on the other hand, perhaps for some frail older patients, home care delayed nursing home care. The other aspect of this conundrum is that most older adults wish to remain in their own living arrangement (aging-in-place) rather than face institutionalization.

PRIVATE-PAY COMMUNITY LONG-TERM CARE

The success of community-based care depends on closely monitored service integration and a willingness to invest in clinical caregivers, appropriate equipment, and clinical care planning. Federal and state regulations at present provide little guidance in defining an integrated community-based delivery system. As such, the most successful community-based systems plan and provide care beyond the current minimum legal requirements. Growth in community-based primary health care is due to an increase in the percentage and number of older persons who have the economic resources to purchase community-based health services or alternative community housing arrangements such as continuing care communities. The growth of these services is accentuated by the combination of need for health care and supportive services and the demand or ability to pay for services that allow older adults to remain in the community.

TABLE 33-2   Medicare Home Health Care Use, by Characteristics of Enrollees: Fiscal Years 1997 and 1999

Characteristic	Home Health Users as a Percent of Enrollees			Number of Visits per User			Number of Visits per Enrollee		
	1997	1999	Percent Change	1997	1999	Percent Change	1997	1999	Percent Change
Total	10.1	8.0	−21	79	46	−41	8.0	3.7	−54
Age									
Under 65 yr	5.6	4.5	−20	87	56	−35	4.9	2.5	−48
65-74 yr	5.9	4.8	−20	68	42	−39	4.1	2.0	−51
75-84 yr	13.3	10.2	−23	76	44	−42	10.1	4.5	−55
85 yr or Over	22.2	17.2	−22	91	50	−45	20.3	8.6	−58
Sex									
Female	11.5	9.1	−21	82	47	−43	9.4	4.3	−55
Male	8.2	6.5	−21	74	45	−39	6.0	2.9	−52
Age and Sex									
Under 65 yr, Female	6.6	5.3	−20	89	55	−39	5.9	2.9	−51
Under 65 yr, Male	4.8	3.8	−19	85	58	−32	4.1	2.2	−45
65-74 yr, Female	6.5	5.2	−19	73	43	−41	4.7	2.2	−53
65-74 yr, Male	5.2	4.2	−20	62	40	−35	3.3	1.7	48
75-84 yr, Female	14.4	11.0	−24	79	45	−43	11.3	5.0	−56
75-84 yr, Male	11.5	9.1	−21	71	42	−41	8.1	3.8	−53
85 yr or Over, Female	22.4	17.7	−21	92	50	−46	20.6	8.8	−57
85 yr or Over, Male	21.6	16.2	−25	90	50	−45	19.4	8.0	−59
Medicaid Enrolled									
Yes	15.3	11.4	−25	102	58	−43	15.6	6.7	−57
No	9.2	7.3	−20	72	43	−41	6.6	3.1	−53
Urban/Rural Location									
Rural	10.4	7.7	−26	85	49	−42	8.8	3.8	−57
Urban	10.0	8.1	−19	76	45	−41	7.7	3.7	−52

Spending per Enrollee in 1996								
Lowest One-Third of States	8.2	6.9	−15	51	34	−33	4.2	2.4	−43
Middle One-Third of States	9.9	8.0	−19	59	38	−36	5.8	3.0	−48
Highest One-Third of States	12.0	8.9	−26	114	63	−45	13.8	5.6	−59
Historic Growth in Spending									
Lowest One-Third of States	10.1	8.2	−19	67	42	−36	6.7	3.5	−48
Middle One-Third of States	9.6	7.8	−19	65	40	−39	6.3	3.1	−50
Highest One-Third of States	11.1	8.2	−26	114	62	−46	12.7	5.1	−60
Census Region									
New England	12.9	10.9	−16	90	54	−40	11.7	5.9	−49
Middle Atlantic	9.7	9.0	−8	53	37	−31	5.1	3.3	−36
South Atlantic	10.1	8.1	−20	73	44	−39	7.3	3.6	−51
East North Central	9.1	7.1	−21	58	38	−35	5.3	2.7	−49
East South Central	12.6	8.6	−31	117	69	−41	14.7	6.0	−59
West North Central	8.3	6.4	−23	55	34	−38	4.6	2.2	−52
West South Central	12.4	8.7	−30	147	78	−47	18.2	6.8	−63
Mountain	8.3	6.4	−23	77	40	−48	6.4	2.6	−60
Pacific	9.2	7.3	−21	48	29	−39	4.4	2.1	−52

From Komisar HL: Rolling back Medicare home health, *Health Care Financing Rev* 24(2):33-55, 2002.
Notes: Medicare expenditures used to group states are from Medicare Home Health Agency National State Summary, dated May 26, 2000, and the enrollment data are from the Health Care Financing Administration website http://cms.hhs.gov/statistics/enrollment /stenrtrend95_98.asp. Historic growth is based on the percentage change in spending per enrollee between 1990 and 1994.

Medicare Current Issues

In 1998 older Americans spent a significant proportion of their total household expenditures for health care. Average dollar amount increased with income; families in the lower fifth of the income distribution spent an annual average of $1654 compared with the $3614 spent by the top fifth families. During the past decade the share of out-of-pocket costs ranged from 9% to 16% of total household expenditures, and the dollar amount has shown a slow but steady increase (Federal Interagency Forum on Aging-Related Statistics, 2000) (Table 33-3).

During the stock market decline from 2000 to 2003, many older Americans lost a significant portion of their retirement income from multiple sources. These losses may include a reduction in pension coverage for health care by increasing costs to participants, stock market losses via mutual

TABLE 33-3	Percentage of Total Out-of-pocket Expenditures Allocated to Health Care Costs in Households Headed by Persons 65 Years of Age or Older, by Income Level, 1987 to 1998					
	1987	*1989*	*1992*	*1994*	*1996*	*1998*
Percent of Income						
Lowest fifth	10.4%	11.6%	13.5%	14.8%	12.5%	12.7%
Second fifth	13.5	14.4	15.8	15.4	14.4	13.9
Third fifth	12.7	14.6	14.9	14.7	14.6	15.6
Fourth fifth	12.3	13.2	13.2	12.0	13.3	13.3
Highest fifth	7.9	8.0	9.4	8.9	8.6	9.2
Average Dollar Amount						
Lowest fifth	$ 886	$ 1,029	$ 1,375	$ 1,685	$ 1,488	$ 1,654
Second fifth	1,390	1,670	2,022	2,112	2,064	2,265
Third fifth	1,550	2,185	2,413	2,700	2,828	3,228
Fourth fifth	1,926	2,613	2,911	2,990	3,152	3,398
Highest fifth	2,065	2,566	3,086	3,376	3,483	3,614
Average Total Expenditures						
Lowest fifth	$ 8,502	$ 8,835	$10,172	$11,375	$11,900	$13,032
Second fifth	10,332	11,617	12,784	13,747	14,378	16,252
Third fifth	12,232	14,965	16,189	18,401	19,315	20,696
Fourth fifth	15,676	19,788	22,011	24,894	23,647	25,509
Highest fifth	26,301	32,117	32,659	37,757	40,602	39,170

From Federal Interagency Forum on Aging and Related Statistics: *Older Americans 2000: key indicators of well-being,* Washington, DC, 2000, U.S. Government Printing Office.

Note: Expenditures on health care, for purposes of this report, include out-of-pocket spending on health insurance, medical services and supplies and prescription drugs. Quintiles are used to define the five levels of income. In this analysis, the term "household" is used in place of "consumer unit." A consumer unit is used to describe members of a household related by blood, marriage, adoption, or other legal arrangement; single persons who are living alone or sharing a household with others but who are financially independent; or two or more persons living together who share responsibility for at least two of three major types of expenses—food, housing, and other expenses. The income distribution was determined for the subset of all consumer units where the reference person was age 65 or older. Reference population: These data refer to the resident noninstitutional population.

Source: Consumer Expenditure Survey.

funds and individually owned stocks, loss of income in bonds and money market funds as a result of low interest rates, and for some older adults corporation defaulting or reducing pension benefits. With these increasing financial pressures, older adults and the federal government (with costs of war and large federal deficit) are concerned about the future state of health care services and future levels of coverage available through Medicare. The first Baby Boomers will turn 65 in 2011, and these numbers of new beneficiaries will, over time, tax the Medicare system.

Both political parties have Medicare reform as part of their political agenda, and questions abound, especially the long-standing political issue of a prescription drugs benefit for Medicare beneficiaries. Pharmaceutical costs have risen faster than inflation. Older persons are more likely to have a chronic condition than are younger people, which leads to more prescription drugs adding to the increasing cost to older adults. What type of coverage will be available? What types of health care will be affordable? How will payment for health care services evolve? What type of protection will frail older patients have if Medicare turns to the free market–driven system? Will the actions of the 33 HMOs who disenrolled beneficiaries for no health reason be repeated? Will insurance companies be able to refuse coverage to the frail and sick? Will they be able to drop a beneficiary who becomes an expensive outlier? Will Medicaid be the place of last resort for poor and near-poor older adults, passing a huge fiscal responsibility to the states? Will the numbers of poor and near poor elderly levels rise? The answers to these and many other questions that surround the current Medicare system are not easy or simple.

Summary

The development of an integrated health care system to provide appropriate services across settings for the older population is the challenge of the twenty-first century. An integrated gerontologic primary health care system reflects the dynamic life transitions of the older population, accounts for the changing social and physical conditions of older adults, and results in individual patients and primary care providers focusing on prevention and early recognition of disease and promotion of health and well-being.

Creative concepts regarding organization of primary care services, multidisciplinary practice, and education of primary care providers that support accountability for improving the health of older patients are the hope for the future. Policy makers are challenged by the constraints of a society that is unable or unwilling to accept tax increases to pay for the service increases that appear necessary to protect the health of the aging population. The government continues to mount a wide cost-containment campaign to include the 1997 BBA, accosting fraud and abuse in the Medicare system, and the 2003 President's Framework to Modernize and Improve Medicare by partial privatization of Medicare. The President's plan is available on the CMS.gov website.

The question that remains to be answered over the next decade is whether adequate and affordable health care will be available for all older Americans. Practitioners need to stay current on this issue because, as stated early in this chapter, practice follows funding. If the highest priority is cost containment, with little or no regard for quality of care, the integrity of the health care delivery system will be at risk as will the well-being of patients. Health care professionals have a responsibility to be part of the solution that protects and provides appropriate primary health care for older Americans.

Resources

Center for Medicare and Medicaid Services
www.cms.gov

References

Agency for Health Care Policy and Research: *Medical expenditure panel survey, household component*, 1996, Rockville, Md, 1998, Center for Cost and Financing Studies.

Center for Medicare and Medicaid Services: *Health care market update: managed care*, March 24, 2003. Availabled at www.cms.gov. Accessed April 9, 2003.

Federal Interagency Forum on Aging-Related Statistics: *Older Americans 2000: key indicators of well-being. Forum on Aging-Related Statistics*, Washington DC, 2000, U.S. Government Printing Office.

Health Care Financing Administration: *Highlights of the national expenditure projections 1997-2007*, Baltimore, 1998, Health and Human Services.

Irvin C, Massey S, Dorsey T: Determinants of enrollment among applicants to PACE, *Health Care Finance Rev* 19(2):135-151, 1997.

Kowisar HL: Rolling back Medicare home health, *Health Care Finance Rev* 24(2):33-55, 2002.

Koziel JA et al: Health care consumption among elderly patients in California: a comprehensive 10-year evaluation of trends in hospitalization rates and charges, *Gerontologist* 42(2):207-216, 2002

Lachs MS et al: Is managed care good or bad for geriatric medicine? *J Am Geriatr Soc* 45(9):1123-1127, 1997.

Mirvis D, Chang C, Morreim H: Protecting older people while managing their care, *J Am Geriatr Soc* 45:645-646, 1997.

National Center for Health Statistics: *1996 National Ambulatory Medical Care Survey*, Hyattsville, Md, 1998, Public Health Service.

Ouslander JG, Weinberg AD: Institutional long-term-care in the USA. In Tallis RC and Fillit HM, editors: *Brocklehurst's textbook of geriatric medicine and gerontology*, ed 6, London, 2003, Churchill Livingstone.

Pizer SDS, Frakt AB: Payment policy and competition in the Medicare+Choice program, *Health Care Finance Rev* 24(1):83-94, 2002.

34

Ethics

Ethical Standards

Those responsible for educating today's health care professionals have also taken measures to ensure that graduates possess the ethical competence necessary to execute their public charge faithfully. The American Association of Colleges of Nursing (AACN) identifies the following core values for caring professional nurses: altruism, autonomy, human dignity, integrity, and social justice (AACN, 1998). The AACN report on the essentials of master's education for advanced practice nursing (AACN, 1996) charged master's nursing education to develop an understanding of the principles, personal values, and beliefs that provide a framework for nursing practice.

The graduate educational experience should provide students the opportunity to explore their values, analyze how these values shape their professional practice and influence their decisions, and analyze systems of health care and determine how the values underpinning them influence the interventions and care delivered. Course work should provide graduates with the knowledge and skills to do the following:

1. Identify and analyze common ethical dilemmas and the ways in which these dilemmas impact patient care
2. Evaluate ethical methods of decision making and engage in an ethical decision-making process
3. Evaluate ethical decision making from both personal and organizational perspectives and develop an understanding of how these two perspectives may create conflicts of interest
4. Identify areas in which a personal conflict of interest may arise; propose resolutions or actions to resolve the conflict
5. Understand the role of an ethics committee in health delivery systems; serve on ethics committees
6. Assume accountability for the quality of one's own practice

The Association of American Medical Colleges (AAMC) published a broad set of objectives designed to ensure that physicians possess the attributes necessary in meeting their individual and collective responsibilities to society (AAMC, 1998):

- Physicians must be altruistic.
- Physicians must be knowledgeable.
- Physicians must be skillful.
- Physicians must be dutiful.

Because many primary-care providers are preceptors to advanced-practice nurses and medical students and residents, it is helpful to seize the "teachable moments" that occur in daily practice to explore the ethical dimensions of gerontologic care. This chapter uses practice vignettes to highlight challenges to ethical competence and concludes with a description of strategies to develop ethical competence.

Challenges to Ethical Competence

A primary care provider's ethical competence is the patient's (and the public's) best security that health care needs will be adequately met. Ethically competent primary care providers have the following characteristics (Taylor, 1997):

1. They are clinically competent.
2. They can be trusted to act in ways that advance the best interests of the patients entrusted to their care.
3. They hold themselves and their colleagues accountable for their practice.
4. They work collaboratively to advocate for patients, families, and communities.
5. They mediate ethical conflicts that occur between the patient, significant others, the health care team, and other interested parties.
6. They critique new health care technologies and changes in the way health care is defined, administered, delivered, and financed in light of their potential to influence human well-being.

Clinical Competence

Clinical competence is obviously a prerequisite of ethical competence. Effective practitioners today value evidence-based practice and work hard to develop the interpersonal and therapeutic skills that equate with high-quality care. The Institute of Medicine defines *quality of care* as the degree to which health services for individuals and populations increase the likelihood of desired health outcomes and are consistent with current professional knowledge. It has also identified three fundamental quality-of-care issues: (1) use of unnecessary or inappropriate care; (2) underuse of needed, effective, and appropriate care; and (3) shortcomings in technical and interpersonal aspects of care (Institute of Medicine, 1994).

Deficient Clinical Competence: Case Studies

The following scenarios illustrate one or more types of deficiency in clinical competence. In the first case study, a family nurse practitioner notices that an older oncology patient is becoming more and more depressed, but the practitioner fails to explore or treat the patient's depression. The patient moved in with her daughter 14 months earlier after learning that she most likely had fewer than 6 months to live. When the patient's daughter asks about her mother's growing depression, the nurse practitioner responds, "Well, she certainly has lots to be depressed about" and changes the subject. In the second scenario, a surgical resident explains his practice of undermedicating older patients postoperatively by telling a medical student that older patients do not experience pain to the same degree as younger patients, as evidenced by their lack of complaints. In the third example, the neurology practice responsible for a large population of patients with Alzheimer's disease, Parkinson's disease, and other predictably debilitating neurologic disorders makes no effort to encourage its members to talk with patients about their end-of-life treatment preferences and advance directives and to document these discussions. When questioned, they reply that they have no time for these conversations.

    These scenarios illustrate why it is important to assess whether or not the goals being sought for a particular patient or population aggregate are adequate and whether or not the provider or caregiving team's competence, motivation, and resources are adequate. An oncologist recently confided how "beaten and defeated" he felt after the death of a woman he had cared for over several years. He shared his puzzlement on learning that the chaplain who had cared for this woman in her last days found the experience "transcendent and transforming." A physician unable to accept "helping people die well" as a legitimate goal of medicine may never be able to feel a sense of accomplishment or peace when one of his or her patients dies. More important, he or she will be deficient clinically by being unable to bring his or her otherwise powerful clinical skills to bear in helping patients experience a comfortable and dignified death.

Trustworthiness

Clinical competence in and of itself cannot guarantee that patients and the public will be well served. Most of us can remember hiring a practitioner who "looked good on paper" but whose presence in the clinic was frustrating because the promised skills were rarely or erratically displayed. Trustworthiness is the character criterion. Can patients and their families, the public, count on the clinician to secure their interests? In today's culture, where the overwhelming majority of Americans surveyed believe that the rush to manage costs has sacrificed safety and quality, trustworthiness is paramount. Clinicians are trustworthy to the extent that they habitually display those human qualities or virtues that equate with excellent care. Fletcher, Miller, and Spencer (1995) define *virtues* as "those dispositions of character and conduct which motivate and enable clinicians to provide good care to patients. The clinical virtues function as habits conducive to good practice as well as guides to healing and caring interactions with patients." Their list of clinical virtues includes technical competence, objectivity and detachment, caring, clinical benevolence, subordination of self-interest to patient care, reflective intelligence, humility, practical wisdom, and courage. Imagine that you learned at the end of a clinical day that someone had secretly videotaped each interaction you had with patients, families, and colleagues. Would you greet with pride or horror the announcement that your videotape was to be shown to colleagues as an example of "excellence in practice"? Which of the preceding clinical virtues would be glaring by their preponderance or absence?

The trustworthiness criterion is displayed in the following scenarios. In the first example, a new gerontologic case manager in a Medicare-managed care program becomes convinced that deficient screening and follow-up services for a large cohort of enrolled elderly patients with diabetes are resulting in unnecessary complications and repeat hospitalizations. When she reports this to the medical director, she is thanked for her observation but is told that the health plan simply cannot afford to make routine the benefits she is recommending. Undaunted, she begins to gather data about the costs associated with the repeat hospitalizations to convince senior management by talking in terms they understand. Choosing to remain an advocate for this population illustrates her ability to be trusted. A more mundane example is that of a clinician who is tempted to abbreviate an intake examination on an "ornery" patient because of extreme fatigue, feelings of impatience or natural aversion, or simply time constraints. The clinician's decision to be faithful to the time needed to conduct a thorough examination in the face of personal constraints to do less is a decision to be trustworthy.

Accountability

As the preceding illustrations make clear, it is often difficult to hold ourselves accountable for high-quality practice, let alone our colleagues. Self-regulation is one of the hallmarks of a moral profession. We earn the right to practice by professing to the public that we can be accountable. Because trustworthiness in individuals and health care institutions and systems is not a given, accountability is another criterion of ethical competence. What does it mean to hold health care professionals accountable for safe and good-quality practice? At the very least this entails periodically stepping back from practice to gain enough distance to be critically reflective about what is being done. A helpful practice is to perform a chart review on an individual patient for whom you established a treatment plan to determine the weight each of the following has in determining the interventions selected:

- Maintenance of status quo
- Clear demonstration by research that this is the best option for the condition(s) being treated

- Availability of resources to execute this plan of care
- Willingness of payers to reimburse for all aspects of the proposed treatment plan
- Patient preferences for the plan of care
- Convenience for providers with the plan of care
- Past experience that demonstrates a high level of patient and family satisfaction with this approach
  Obviously the ideal is to give greatest weight to the variables that best serve patients and the public. Another helpful exercise is to think back to the quality-of-care issues identified previously: (1) use of unnecessary or inappropriate care; (2) underuse of needed, effective, and appropriate care; and (3) shortcomings in technical and interpersonal aspects of care. The next step is to identify a recent practice situation where one or more of these problems was noted and to think carefully about how you responded to the initial sense that something was wrong. Which of the following characterizes your typical response to problems of quality (exercises adapted from Taylor and Barnet, 1999)?
- Try to ignore discomfort and pretend there is no problem
- Experience the frustration of knowing that conditions are less than optimal but accept that you are powerless to effect a solution
- Commit your best energies to attempting to resolve the problem
  Reflection on this sort of challenge and your characteristic responses will yield valuable information about your competence, willingness, and confidence to address challenges to quality. Deficient accountability occurs in many forms:
- Unwillingness to challenge a colleague who often prejudices caregivers negatively toward patients and families by the tone and content of his or her report
- Doing nothing to address staff concerns about certain practitioners or departments who routinely do poorly on measures of performance and patient outcome
- Accepting "playing rules" when changes in the reimbursement levels result in a dangerous reduction of services to older adults

Advocacy

The ability to collaborate with others to secure the health care resources and services needed by older adults is essential to ethical competence. Because few providers work independently, advocacy strengths must include strong interpersonal skills to facilitate the coordination of resources needed in any clinical situation. Any attempt to rely solely on oneself to "make up" for deficient resources in the system or the team is bound to result in failure and burnout. Increasingly today this includes being able to work with payers and community-based support groups. Professional barriers to effective advocacy include the following:

- Low value attached to advocacy ("It's not my job!")—the character issue
- Inadequate knowledge or interpersonal skills—the competence issue
- Low morale and the mediocrity-sustaining cycle: initial enthusiasm, frustration when things do not change, and cynicism (e.g., "nothing ever changes for the better around here" syndrome)—the motivation issue
- Fear of reprisal: how much are we willing to risk to secure valued health
- Outcomes for the patients or communities entrusted to our care—the balancing issue
  Chief among the professional barriers to effective advocacy is the degree to which external forces are redefining the nature of professional health care practice (threats to health care professional–patient relationships, policies that compromise clinical judgments, increasing demand to resolve conflicting obligations). System barriers to effective advocacy are unresponsive or ineffective systems and unsafe systems resulting from the increasing tendency to prioritize cost containment over quality, a preference toward underutilization of services, the gradual "deskilling" of the workforce, and financial incentives that reward denying or reducing indicated treatment and care. The many examples of excellence in advocacy that can be found in practice range from the simple confrontation of a colleague whose commitment to excellence seems to be slipping to testi-

fying before the U.S. Congress on the health needs of older Americans. The major changes needed to ensure a "basic decent minimum of care" for all older Americans mandate that we work collectively to advocate for older adults. No one is capable of orchestrating the needed change alone; participation in professional societies and organizations that can lobby for better gerontologic care is needed more now than ever before.

Conflict Mediation

Ethically competent primary-care providers mediate ethical conflict between patients, families, health care professionals, payers, and other interested parties. The first "trick" in mediating ethical conflict is to identify it early and begin to intervene. Although it is easy to identify older adults at risk for skin impairment or falls, the families and caregiving teams at high risk for decisional conflict are often ignored, and intervention does not occur until adversarial camps have developed. At this point, resorting to a legal court often seems to be the only option.

Successful conflict mediation entails recognizing conflict early, developing the trusting relationships and communication skills that facilitate the identification of variables causing or contributing to the conflict, becoming skilled in facilitating the type of dialogue that results in consensus about prudential judgments that best serve the interested parties, and knowing and assessing the resources available to facilitate conflict resolution. Central to its process is the identification of key stakeholders and their interests, values, and beliefs. We often presume to know what other stakeholders value and believe when nothing is further from the truth.

When conflicts develop between patients and providers about treatment decisions, a patient advocate stands in the middle and does the hard work of uncovering exactly what underlies the patient's and surrogate's demands as well as what makes providers uncomfortable with these demands. Providers often dismiss patients and family members as being "unreasonable" or "sick in the head" because what they want is something other than what the provider has decided ought to be done. The objective is to facilitate patient autonomy without compromising the autonomy of individual health care providers or the internal morality of the health professions. At issue is the patient's right to be self-determining, to demand treatment believed to be in his or her best interests, and to refuse treatment not believed to be in his or her best interests as well as the health care professional's right to control practice and to use only those diagnostic and therapeutic measures consistent with the internal morality of the profession. In the case that follows it is easy to predict two very different outcomes on the basis of the ability of the professional caregivers to be a patient advocate and their willingness to get involved.

CASE STUDY

A 74-year-old man develops a mesenteric infarct after a resection for a meningioma that impaired his vision. His wife withholds consent for surgical repair of the bowel, to the consternation of the neurosurgeon and consulting gastroenterologist. They explain to her that this is a reversible problem that must be treated. The wife explains that the patient, who "crashed" after surgery and is now incapacitated, on a ventilator, and receiving vasopressors, would never want anything done to prolong his life in this condition. The patient is a lawyer who has been married for 49 years, has five children, and according to his wife did not want surgery the second time around for the meningioma but allowed himself to be "talked into it" by his children. He places a high value on being active and independent. The wife consults you, the primary care provider who initially referred her husband to a specialist for the meningioma, and asks you to plead their case.

Commitment to Human Well-Being

The ability to critique new health care technologies and changes in the way health care is defined, administered, delivered, and financed in light of their potential to influence human well-being is critical for gerontologic providers. On entry to the health professions, each of us adopts, along with our white coats or uniforms, a particular lens for viewing the world. This lens focuses our attention on certain phenomena and screens out others. We would go crazy if we ever attempted to pay attention to everything that is going on around us at any point in time. The phenomena of concern to health professionals must be health and human well-being. As we sit at decision-making tables, our voices should be raised on behalf of the people we serve and should ask, "What are the human consequences of what we are proposing?" "How will the people we serve be affected by our decisions?" Although this point might seem self-evident, the fact is that often we are not present when decisions that affect health care for older adults are made and that, when present, we fail to articulate concerns about the human consequences of what is being decided. In today's health culture we can be sure that someone is examining the economic and legal implications of our decisions, which affect health care for older adults in both small and major ways. If we think carefully about how our death-denying culture affects end-of-life care for the older adults or how our car-repair-shop model of health care, with its focus of wholeness of body versus wholeness of being influences reimbursable health care priorities, we begin to see problems. When the old family car is no longer deemed "worthy" of an expensive repair, it is likely to be driven or towed to a junkyard. Some find striking parallels with the nursing home industry. We need to be able to think critically about how the explosion of genetic information, Medicare-managed care alternatives, and health care research will affect the daily lives of older adults and their families. Never has so much change occurred in so little time. Ethically competent providers are committed to shaping change to ensure that older patients are well served. This stance is quite different from an after-the-fact accommodation to change dictated by a lust for profit, misguided altruism, or faulty reasoning.

Developing Ethical Competence

A commitment to develop ethical competence requires taking a careful inventory of our knowledge and skills. Once we know our personal strengths and limitations, we can strategize to address the deficits. This chapter concludes with a discussion of practical strategies to develop ethical competence.

KNOWLEDGE

As with clinical reasoning, ethical reasoning and analysis require a knowledge base. Familiarity with major theoretic and practical ways of "doing" clinical ethics may be obtained by reading, taking a formal course in bioethics at a neighboring university, or attending a continuing education workshop or seminar. Although many specialty-practice journals routinely address ethical issues, the most accessible journals devoted exclusively to bioethics and health care ethics are the *Hastings Center Report* and the *Journal of Clinical Ethics*. One of the chief objectives in acquiring some formal knowledge of ethical theory and systems of justification is to provide a language by which to facilitate conversation and dialogue about ethical matters. The ideal would be for us to consult both formally and informally with our colleagues about perplexing ethical matters in the same way that we consult on interesting clinical questions. Just as we confer with a colleague about a drug regimen ("I'm not sure why she isn't responding to this drug, given its pharmacokinetics"), we should be able to confer about our role in working with proxy decision makers to get the best decision for a patient ("I'm not sure why this family is so reluctant to do any sort of advance planning. Clearly the patient is not responding to treatment, and we are very close to that time when aggressive interventions will be futile"). Initiating some regular forum for the discussion of ethical concerns is an important way to "own the language" of ethics and to develop facility in ethical discourse. Structured ways to do this include having ethics as a topic for a regular team meeting, discussing ethical issues in regularly scheduled team meetings as appropriate, having brown-bag lunch conferences on interesting "cases" or issues, or dedicating one grand round a semester to an ethics case or topic.

SKILLS

Ethically competent providers possess a variety of ethical skills that range from the ability to establish trusting professional relationships to sophisticated conflict-mediation skills. Providers working with older patients and their families should be skilled in most of the following:

- Establishing trusting professional relationships with patients, family members, colleagues, payers, and other interested parties
- Communicating respect and promoting dignity
- Identifying and supporting appropriate decision makers
- Using the shared decision-making model to facilitate health care decision making that best advances patient interests
- Patient advocacy
- Advance care planning (advance directives, special orders: do not resuscitate, comfort measures only, do not hospitalize)
- Preventing and resolving conflicts
- Initiating and facilitating an ethics consult
- Distributing scarce resources
- Preparing for comfortable, dignified deaths
- Reporting unethical, illegal, and incompetent practice

Because most educational programs do not guarantee mastery of these skills, it is helpful for providers to determine their competence and confidence level in the skills that equate with excellent care in their practice setting and then strategize to remedy any deficiencies. For example, a provider who has never initiated an ethics consult and who routinely "muddles through" dilemmas that divide patients, families, and caregiving teams would be well advised to explore the ethics resources available within his or her setting and to practice the skill of facilitating an ethics consult or committee meeting. A provider who works in a culture that routinely dehumanizes older adults and their spouses and families may call a group meeting to explore how staff can change the culture of care and can practice developing and monitoring outcomes that reverse the forces of objectification and dehumanization.

Summary

Older adults have much to lose if a practitioner's ethical competence is undeveloped or undervalued. Long presumed to be somehow inherently present in health care professionals ("only good people are attracted to the health professions for all the right reasons, so it is safe to presume that ethical competence is a given"), ethical competence is beginning to get the attention it deserves. Until all health professionals hold themselves and one another accountable for ethical competence, high-quality health care will continue to be at best a fond hope and a sometimes reality.

Resources

The Ability Project
www.ability.org.uk/bioethics.html

Ethics in Aging
www.grants.cohpa.ucf.ed/age-ethics

References

American Association of Colleges of Nursing (AACN): *The essentials of master's education for advanced practice nursing*, Washington, DC, 1996, AACN.
American Association of Colleges of Nursing (AACN): *The essentials of baccalaureate education for professional nursing practice*, Washington, DC, 1998, AACN.

Association of American Medical Colleges (AAMC): *Report 1: learning objectives for medical student education—guidelines for medical schools*, Washington, DC, 1998, AAMC.

Fletcher JC, Miller FG, Spencer EM: Clinical ethics: history, content and resources. In Fletcher JC et al, editors: *Introduction to clinical ethics*, Frederick, Md, 1995, University Publishing Group.

Goldstein A: Medical competency tests proposed, *Washington Post*, p A2, October 24, 1998.

Institute of Medicine: *America's health in transition: protecting and improving quality*, Washington, DC, 1994, National Academy Press.

Taylor C: Ethical issues in case management. In Cohen E, Cesta T, editors: *Nursing case management: from concept to evaluation*, ed 2, St Louis, 1997, Mosby.

Taylor C, Barnet R: The ethics of case management: the quality/cost conundrum. In Cohen E, DeBack V, editors: *The outcomes mandate: case management in health care today*, St Louis, 1999, Mosby.

Minimum Data Set for Nursing Home Resident Assessment and Care Screening—Version 2.0

Numeric Identifier_____

MINIMUM DATA SET (MDS) — *VERSION 2.0*
FOR NURSING HOME RESIDENT ASSESSMENT AND CARE SCREENING

BASIC ASSESSMENT TRACKING FORM

SECTION AA. IDENTIFICATION INFORMATION

1. RESIDENT NAME⊙

a. (First)   b. (Middle Initial)   c. (Last)   d. (Jr/Sr)

2. GENDER⊙ 1. Male   2. Female

3. BIRTHDATE⊙

Month   Day   Year

4. RACE/⊙ ETHNICITY
1. American Indian/Alaskan Native
2. Asian/Pacific Islander
3. Black, not of Hispanic origin
4. Hispanic
5. White, not of Hispanic origin

5. SOCIAL SECURITY⊙ AND MEDICARE NUMBERS⊙ [C in 1st box if non med. no.]

a. Social Security Number

b. Medicare number (or comparable railroad insurance number)

6. FACILITY PROVIDER NO.⊙

a. State No.

b. Federal No.

7. MEDICAID NO. ["+" if pending, "N" if not a Medicaid recipient]⊙

8. REASONS FOR ASSESS-MENT

[Note—Other codes do not apply to this form]

a. Primary reason for assessment
1. Admission assessment (required by day 14)
2. Annual assessment
3. Significant change in status assessment
4. Significant correction of prior full assessment
5. Quarterly review assessment
10. Significant correction of prior quarterly assessment
0. *NONE OF ABOVE*

b. *Codes for assessments required for Medicare PPS or the State*
1. *Medicare 5 day assessment*
2. *Medicare 30 day assessment*
3. *Medicare 60 day assessment*
4. *Medicare 90 day assessment*
5. *Medicare readmission/return assessment*
6. *Other state required assessment*
7. *Medicare 14 day assessment*
8. *Other Medicare required assessment*

9. Signatures of Persons who Completed a Portion of the Accompanying Assessment or Tracking Form

I certify that the accompanying information accurately reflects resident assessment or tracking information for this resident and that I collected or coordinated collection of this information on the dates specified. To the best of my knowledge, this information was collected in accordance with applicable Medicare and Medicaid requirements. I understand that this information is used as a basis for ensuring that residents receive appropriate and quality care, and as a basis for payment from federal funds. I further understand that payment of such federal funds and continued partici-pation in the government-funded health care programs is conditioned on the accuracy and truthful-ness of this information, and that I may be personally subject to or may subject my organization to substantial criminal, civil, and/or administrative penalties for submitting false information. I also certify that I am authorized to submit this information by this facility on its behalf.

Signature and Title	Sections	Date
a.		
b.		
c.		
d.		
e.		
f.		
g.		
h.		
i.		
j.		
k.		
l.		

GENERAL INSTRUCTIONS

Complete this information for submission with all full and quarterly assessments (Admission, Annual, Significant Change, State or Medicare required assessments, or Quarterly Reviews, etc.)

⊙ = Key items for computerized resident tracking

☐ = When box blank, must enter number or letter   a. = When letter in box, check if condition applies

MDS MEDICARE PPS ASSESSMENT FORM
(VERSION JULY 2002)

Numeric Identifier _____

AB5.	**RESIDEN-TIAL HISTORY 5 YEARS PRIOR TO ENTRY**	(*Check all settings resident lived in during 5 years prior to date of entry.*) a. Prior stay at this nursing home b. Stay in other nursing home c. Other residential facility—board and care home, assisted living, group home d. MH/psychiatric setting e. MR/DD setting f. *NONE OF ABOVE*
A1.	**RESIDENT NAME**	a. (First) b. (Middle Initial) c. (Last) d. (Jr/Sr)
A2.	**ROOM NUMBER**	
A3.	**ASSESS-MENT REFERENCE DATE**	a. Last day of MDS observation period Month — Day — Year
A4a	**DATE OF REENTRY**	Date of reentry from most recent temporary discharge to a hospital in last 90 days (or since last assessment or admission if less than 90 days) Month — Day — Year
A5.	**MARITAL STATUS**	1. Never married 3. Widowed 5. Divorced 2. Married 4. Separated
A6.	**MEDICAL RECORD NO.**	
A10.	**ADVANCED DIRECTIVES**	(For those items with supporting **documentation** in the medical record, check all that apply) b. Do not resuscitate ___ c. Do not hospitalize ___
B1.	**COMATOSE**	(*Persistent vegetative state/no discernible consciousness*) 0. No 1. Yes (*If Yes, skip to Section G*)
B2.	**MEMORY**	(*Recall of what was learned or known*) a. Short-term memory OK—seems/appears to recall after 5 minutes 0. Memory OK 1. Memory problem b. Long-term memory OK—seems/appears to recall long past 0. Memory OK 1. Memory problem
B3.	**MEMORY/ RECALL ABILITY**	(*Check all that resident was **normally able to recall** during last 7 days*) a. Current season b. Location of own room c. Staff names/faces d. That he/she is in a nursing home e. *NONE OF ABOVE* are recalled
B4.	**COGNITIVE SKILLS FOR DAILY DECISION-MAKING**	(*Made decisions regarding tasks of daily life*) 0. *INDEPENDENT*—decisions consistent/reasonable 1. *MODIFIED INDEPENDENCE*—some difficulty in new situations only 2. *MODERATELY IMPAIRED*—decisions poor; cues/supervision required 3. *SEVERELY IMPAIRED*—never/rarely made decisions
B5.	**INDICATORS OF DELIRIUM— PERIODIC DISOR-DERED THINKING/ AWARENESS**	(*Code for behavior in the last 7 days.*) **[Note: Accurate assessment requires conversations with staff and family who have direct knowledge of resident's behavior over this time].** 0. Behavior not present 1. Behavior present, not of recent onset 2. Behavior present, over last 7 days appears different from resident's usual functioning (e.g., new onset or worsening) a. EASILY DISTRACTED—(e.g., difficulty paying attention; gets sidetracked) b. PERIODS OF ALTERED PERCEPTION OR AWARENESS OF SURROUNDINGS—(e.g., moves lips or talks to someone not present; believes he/she is somewhere else; confuses night and day) c. EPISODES OF DISORGANIZED SPEECH—(e.g., speech is incoherent, nonsensical, irrelevant, or rambling from subject to subject; loses train of thought) d. PERIODS OF RESTLESSNESS—(e.g., fidgeting or picking at skin, clothing, napkins, etc; frequent position changes; repetitive physical movements or calling out) e. PERIODS OF LETHARGY—(e.g., sluggishness; staring into space; difficult to arouse; little body movement) f. MENTAL FUNCTION VARIES OVER THE COURSE OF THE DAY—(e.g., sometimes better, sometimes worse; behaviors sometimes present, sometimes not)

C4.	**MAKING SELF UNDER-STOOD**	(*Expressing information content—however able*) 0. *UNDERSTOOD* 1. *USUALLY UNDERSTOOD*—difficulty finding words or finishing thoughts 2. *SOMETIMES UNDERSTOOD*—ability is limited to making concrete requests 3. *RARELY/NEVER UNDERSTOOD*
C6.	**ABILITY TO UNDER-STAND OTHERS**	(*Understanding verbal information content—however able*) 0. *UNDERSTANDS* 1. *USUALLY UNDERSTANDS*—may miss some part/intent of message 2. *SOMETIMES UNDERSTANDS*—responds adequately to simple, direct communication 3. *RARELY/NEVER UNDERSTANDS*
D1.	**VISION**	(*Ability to see in adequate light and with glasses if used*) 0. *ADEQUATE*—sees fine detail, including regular print in newspapers/books 1. *IMPAIRED*—sees large print, but not regular print in newspapers/books 2. *MODERATELY IMPAIRED*—limited vision; not able to see newspaper headlines, but can identify objects 3. *HIGHLY IMPAIRED*—object identification in question, but eyes appear to follow objects 4. *SEVERELY IMPAIRED*—no vision or sees only light, colors, or shapes; eyes do not appear to follow objects
E1.	**INDICATORS OF DEPRES-SION, ANXIETY, SAD MOOD**	(*Code for indicators observed in last 30 days, irrespective of the assumed cause*) 0. Indicator not exhibited in last 30 days 1. Indicator of this type exhibited up to five days a week 2. Indicator of this type exhibited daily or almost daily (6, 7 days a week)

VERBAL EXPRESSIONS OF DISTRESS

a. Resident made negative statements—e.g., "Nothing matters; Would rather be dead; What's the use; Regrets having lived so long; Let me die"

b. Repetitive questions—e.g., "Where do I go; What do I do?"

c. Repetitive verbalizations—e.g., calling out for help, ("God help me")

d. Persistent anger with self or others—e.g., easily annoyed, anger at placement in nursing home; anger at care received

e. Self deprecation—e.g., "I am nothing; I am of no use to anyone"

f. Expressions of what appear to be unrealistic fears—e.g., fear of being abandoned, left alone, being with others

g. Recurrent statements that something terrible is about to happen—e.g., believes he or she is about to die, have a heart attack

h. Repetitive health complaints—e.g., persistently seeks medical attention, obsessive concern with body functions

i. Repetitive anxious complaints/concerns (non-health related) e.g., persistently seeks attention/reassurance regarding schedules, meals, laundry, clothing, relationship issues

SLEEP-CYCLE ISSUES

j. Unpleasant mood in morning

k. Insomnia/change in usual sleep pattern

SAD, APATHETIC, ANXIOUS APPEARANCE

l. Sad, pained, worried facial expressions—e.g., furrowed brows

m. Crying, tearfulness

n. Repetitive physical movements—e.g., pacing, hand wringing, restlessness, fidgeting, picking

LOSS OF INTEREST

o. Withdrawal from activities of interest—e.g., no interest in long standing activities or being with family/friends

p. Reduced social interaction

E2.	**MOOD PERSIS-TENCE**	One or more indicators of depressed, sad or anxious mood were not easily altered by attempts to "cheer up", console, or reassure the resident over last 7 days 0. No mood indicators 1. Indicators present, easily altered 2. Indicators present, not easily altered

MDS 2.0 PPS July 2002

Resident Identifier _____

Numeric Identifier _____

E4. BEHAVIORAL SYMPTOMS

(A) *Behavioral symptom frequency in last 7 days*

0. Behavior not exhibited in last 7 days
1. Behavior of this type occurred 1 to 3 days in last 7 days
2. Behavior of this type occurred 4 to 6 days, but less than daily
3. Behavior of this type occurred daily

(B) *Behavioral symptom alterability in last 7 days*

0. Behavior not present OR behavior was easily altered
1. Behavior was not easily altered

	(A)	(B)
a. WANDERING (moved with no rational purpose, seemingly oblivious to needs or safety)		
b. VERBALLY ABUSIVE BEHAVIORAL SYMPTOMS (others were threatened, screamed at, cursed at)		
c. PHYSICALLY ABUSIVE BEHAVIORAL SYMPTOMS (others were hit, shoved, scratched, sexually abused)		
d. SOCIALLY INAPPROPRIATE/DISRUPTIVE BEHAVIORAL SYMPTOMS (made disruptive sounds, noisiness, screaming, self-abusive acts, sexual behavior or disrobing in public, smeared/threw food/feces, hoarding, rummaged through others' belongings)		
e. RESISTS CARE (resisted taking medications/injections, ADL assistance, or eating)		

G1. (A) ADL SELF-PERFORMANCE—(Code for resident's PERFORMANCE OVER ALL SHIFTS during last 7 days—Not including setup)

0. INDEPENDENT—No help or oversight —OR— Help/oversight provided only 1 or 2 times during last 7 days
1. SUPERVISION—Oversight, encouragement or cueing provided 3 or more times during last 7 days —OR— Supervision (3 or more times) plus physical assistance provided only 1 or 2 times during last 7 days
2. LIMITED ASSISTANCE—Resident highly involved in activity; received physical help in guided maneuvering of limbs or other nonweight bearing assistance 3 or more times —OR—More help provided only 1 or 2 times during last 7 days
3. EXTENSIVE ASSISTANCE—While resident performed part of activity, over last 7-day period, help of following type(s) provided 3 or more times:
   —Weight-bearing support
   — Full staff performance during part (but not all) of last 7 days
4. TOTAL DEPENDENCE—Full staff performance of activity during entire 7 days
8. ACTIVITY DID NOT OCCUR during entire 7 days

(B) ADL SUPPORT PROVIDED—(Code for MOST SUPPORT PROVIDED OVER ALL SHIFTS during last 7 days; code regardless of resident's self-performance classification)

0. No setup or physical help from staff
1. Setup help only
2. One person physical assist
3. Two+ persons physical assist
8. ADL activity itself did not occur during entire 7 days

		(A) SELF-PERF	(B) SUPPORT
a. BED MOBILITY	How resident moves to and from lying position, turns side to side, and positions body while in bed		
b. TRANSFER	How resident moves between surfaces—to/from: bed, chair, wheelchair, standing position (EXCLUDE to/from bath/toilet)		
c. WALK IN ROOM	How resident walks between locations in his/her room		
d. WALK IN CORRIDOR	How resident walks in corridor on unit		
e. LOCOMOTION ON UNIT	How resident moves between locations in his/her room and adjacent corridor on same floor. If in wheelchair, self-sufficiency once in chair		
f. LOCOMOTION OFF UNIT	How resident moves to and returns from off unit locations (e.g., areas set aside for dining, activities, or treatments). If facility has only one floor, how resident moves to and from distant areas on the floor. If in wheelchair, self-sufficiency once in chair		
g. DRESSING	How resident puts on, fastens, and takes off all items of **clothing**, including donning/removing prosthesis		
h. EATING	How resident eats and drinks (regardless of skill). Includes intake of nourishment by other means (e.g., tube feeding, total parenteral nutrition)		
i. TOILET USE	How resident uses the toilet room (or commode, bedpan, urinal); transfer on/off toilet, cleanses, changes pad, manages ostomy or catheter, adjusts clothes		
j. PERSONAL HYGIENE	How resident maintains personal hygiene, including combing hair, brushing teeth, shaving, applying makeup, washing/drying face, hands, and perineum (EXCLUDE baths and showers)		

G2. BATHING

How resident takes full-body bath/shower, sponge bath, and transfers in/out of tub/shower (EXCLUDE washing of back and hair.) *Code for most dependent in self-performance.*

(A) BATHING SELF PERFORMANCE codes appear below

0. Independent—No help provided
1. Supervision—Oversight help only
2. Physical help limited to transfer only
3. Physical help in part of bathing activity
4. Total dependence
8. Activity itself did not occur during entire 7 days

	(A)

G3. TEST FOR BALANCE (see training manual)

(Code for ability during test in the *last 7 days*)
0. Maintained position as required in test
1. Unsteady, but able to rebalance self without physical support
2. Partial physical support during test; or stands (sits) but does not follow directions for test
3. Not able to attempt test without physical help

a. Balance while standing	
b. Balance while sitting—position, trunk control	

G4. FUNCTIONAL LIMITATION IN RANGE OF MOTION

(Code for limitations during *last 7 days* that interfered with daily functions or placed residents at risk of injury)

(A) RANGE OF MOTION
0. No limitation
1. Limitation on one side
2. Limitation on both sides

(B) VOLUNTARY MOVEMENT
0. No loss
1. Partial loss
2. Full loss

	(A)	(B)
a. Neck		
b. Arm—Including shoulder or elbow		
c. Hand—Including wrist or fingers		
d. Leg—Including hip or knee		
e. Foot—Including ankle or toes		
f. Other limitation or loss		

G5. MODES OF LOCOMOTION

(Check if applied during *last 7 days*)

b. Wheeled self	

G6. MODES OF TRANSFER

(Check all that apply during *last 7 days*)

a. Bedfast all or most of time	
b. Bed rails used for bed mobility or transfer	

G7. TASK SEGMENTATION

Some or all of ADL activities were broken into subtasks during **last 7 days** so that resident could perform them
0. No   1. Yes

H1. CONTINENCE SELF-CONTROL CATEGORIES

(Code for resident's *PERFORMANCE OVER ALL SHIFTS*)

0. CONTINENT—Complete control [includes use of indwelling urinary catheter or ostomy device that does not leak urine or stool]
1. USUALLY CONTINENT—BLADDER, incontinent episodes once a week or less; BOWEL, less than weekly
2. OCCASIONALLY INCONTINENT—BLADDER, 2 or more times a week but not daily; BOWEL, once a week
3. FREQUENTLY INCONTINENT—BLADDER, tended to be incontinent daily, but some control present (e.g., on day shift); BOWEL, 2-3 times a week
4. INCONTINENT—Had inadequate control BLADDER, multiple daily episodes; BOWEL, all (or almost all) of the time

a. BOWEL CONTINENCE	Control of bowel movement, with appliance or bowel continence programs, if employed	
b. BLADDER CONTINENCE	Control of urinary bladder function (if dribbles, volume insufficient to soak through underpants), with appliances (e.g., foley) or continence programs, if employed	

H2. BOWEL ELIMINATION PATTERN

c. Diarrhea	
d. Fecal impaction	

H3. APPLIANCES AND PROGRAMS

a. Any scheduled toileting plan	**d.** Indwelling catheter	
b. Bladder retraining program	**i.** Ostomy present	
c. External (condom) catheter		

For Section I : check only those diseases that have a relationship to current ADL status, cognitive status, mood and behavior status, medical treatments, nursing monitoring, or risk of death. (Do not list inactive diagnoses)

I1. DISEASES

a. Diabetes melitus		**v.** Hemiplegia/Hemiparesis	
d. Arteriosclerotic heart disease (ASHD)		**w.** Multiple sclerosis	
f. Congestive heart failure		**x.** Paraplegia	
j. Peripheral vascular disease		**z.** Quadriplegia	
		ee. Depression	
m. Hip fracture		**ff.** Manic depressive (bipolar disease)	
r. Aphasia		**gg.** Schizophrenia	
s. Cerebral palsy		**hh.** Asthma	
t. Cerebrovascular accident (stroke)		**ii.** Emphysema/COPD	

I2. INFECTIONS

(If none apply, CHECK the NONE OF ABOVE box)

a. Antibiotic resistant infection (e.g. Methicillin resistant staph)		**g.** Septicemia	
b. Clostridium difficile (c. diff.)		**h.** Sexually transmitted diseases	
c. Conjunctivitis		**i.** Tuberculosis	
d. HIV infection		**j.** Urinary tract infection in **last 30 days**	
e. Pneumonia		**k.** Viral hepatitis	
f. Respiratory infection		**l.** Wound infection	
		m. NONE OF ABOVE	

Resident Identifier _____ Numeric Identifier _____

I3.	**OTHER CURRENT DIAGNOSES AND ICD-9 CODES**	a. _____ | | | • | b. _____ | | | • |
J1.	**PROBLEM CONDITIONS**	(*Check all problems present in* **last 7 days** *unless other time frame is indicated*)

J1. PROBLEM CONDITIONS

INDICATORS OF FLUID STATUS

a. Weight gain or loss of 3 or more pounds within a 7-day period

b. Inability to lie flat due to shortness of breath

c. Dehydrated; output exceeds input

d. Insufficient fluid; did **NOT** consume all/almost all liquids provided during **last 3 days**

OTHER

e. Delusions

g. Edema

h. Fever

i. Hallucinations

j. Internal bleeding

k. Recurrent lung aspirations in **last 90 days**

l. Shortness of breath

n. Unsteady gait

o. Vomiting

J2. PAIN SYMPTOMS (*Code the* **highest level of pain** *present in the* **last 7 days**)

a. **FREQUENCY** with which resident complains or shows evidence of pain

0. No pain (*skip to J4*)
1. Pain less than daily
2. Pain daily

b. **INTENSITY** of pain
1. Mild pain
2. Moderate pain
3. Times when pain is horrible or excruciating

J4. ACCIDENTS (*Check all that apply*)

a. Fell in **past 30 days**
b. Fell in **past 31-180 days**
c. Hip fracture in **last 180 days**
d. Other fracture in **last 180 days**
e. NONE OF ABOVE

J5. STABILITY OF CONDITIONS

a. Conditions/diseases make resident's cognitive, ADL, mood or behavior patterns unstable—(fluctuating, precarious, or deteriorating)
b. Resident experiencing an acute episode or a flare-up of a recurrent or chronic problem
c. End-stage disease, 6 or fewer months to live
d. NONE OF ABOVE

K1. ORAL PROBLEMS

a. Chewing problem
b. Swallowing problem

K2. HEIGHT AND WEIGHT

Record (a.) **height in inches** and (b.) **weight in pounds**. Base weight on most recent measure in **last 30 days**; measure weight consistently in accord with standard facility practice—e.g., in a.m. after voiding, before meal, with shoes off, and in nightclothes

a. HT (in.)   b. WT (lb.)

K3. WEIGHT CHANGE

a. **Weight loss**—5 % or more in **last 30 days**; or 10 % or more in **last 180 days**
0. No   1. Yes
b. **Weight gain**—5 % or more in **last 30 days**; or 10 % or more in **last 180 days**
0. No   1. Yes

K5. NUTRITIONAL APPROACHES (*Check all that apply in last 7 days*)

a. Parenteral/IV
b. Feeding tube
h. On a planned weight change program

K6. PARENTERAL OR ENTERAL INTAKE (*Skip to Section M if neither 5a nor 5b is checked*)

a. Code the proportion of **total calories** the resident received through parenteral or tube feedings in the **last 7 days**
0. None
1. 1% to 25%
2. 26% to 50%
3. 51% to 75%
4. 76% to 100%

b. Code the average **fluid intake** per day by IV or tube in **last 7 days**
0. None
1. 1 to 500 cc/day
2. 501 to 1000 cc/day
3. 1001 to 1500 cc/day
4. 1501 to 2000 cc/day
5. 2001 or more cc/day

M1. ULCERS (Due to any cause)

(Record the number of ulcers at each ulcer stage—regardless of cause. If none present at a stage, record "0" (zero). Code all that apply during last 7 days. Code 9 = 9 or more.) *[Requires full body exam.]*

Number at Stage

a. Stage 1. A persistent area of skin redness (without a break in the skin) that does not disappear when pressure is relieved.
b. Stage 2. A partial thickness loss of skin layers that presents clinically as an abrasion, blister, or shallow crater.
c. Stage 3. A full thickness of skin is lost, exposing the subcutaneous tissues - presents as a deep crater with or without undermining adjacent tissue.
d. Stage 4. A full thickness of skin and subcutaneous tissue is lost, exposing muscle or bone.

M2. TYPE OF ULCER (*For each type of ulcer, code for the highest stage in the last 7 days using scale in item M1—i.e., 0=none; stages 1, 2, 3, 4*)

a. Pressure ulcer—any lesion caused by pressure resulting in damage of underlying tissue
b. Stasis ulcer—open lesion caused by poor circulation in the lower extremities

M3. HISTORY OF RESOLVED ULCERS

Resident had an ulcer that was resolved or cured in **LAST 90 DAYS**
0. No   1. Yes

M4. OTHER SKIN PROBLEMS OR LESIONS PRESENT (*Check all that apply during last 7 days*)

a. Abrasions, bruises
b. Burns (second or third degree)
c. Open lesions other than ulcers, rashes, cuts (e.g., cancer lesions)
d. Rashes—e.g., intertrigo, eczema, drug rash, heat rash, herpes zoster
e. Skin desensitized to pain or pressure
f. Skin tears or cuts (other than surgery)
g. Surgical wounds
h. NONE OF ABOVE

M5. SKIN TREATMENTS (*Check all that apply during last 7 days*)

a. Pressure relieving device(s) for chair
b. Pressure relieving device(s) for bed
c. Turning/repositioning program
d. Nutrition or hydration intervention to manage skin problems
e. Ulcer care
f. Surgical wound care
g. Application of dressings (with or without topical medications) other than to feet
h. Application of ointments/medications (other than to feet)
i. Other preventative or protective skin care (other than to feet)
j. NONE OF ABOVE

M6. FOOT PROBLEMS AND CARE (*Check all that apply during last 7 days*)

a. Resident has one or more foot problems—e.g., corns, callouses, bunions, hammer toes, overlapping toes, pain, structural problems
b. Infection of the foot—e.g., cellulitis, purulent drainage
c. Open lesions on the foot
d. Nails/calluses trimmed during **last 90 days**
e. Received preventative or protective foot care (e.g., used special shoes, inserts, pads, toe separators)
f. Application of dressing (with or without topical medications)
g. NONE OF ABOVE

N1. TIME AWAKE (*Check appropriate time periods over last 7 days*)
Resident awake all or most of time (i.e., naps no more than one hour per time period) in the:
a. Morning   c. Evening
b. Afternoon   d. NONE OF ABOVE

(If resident is comatose, skip to Section O)

N2. AVERAGE TIME INVOLVED IN ACTIVITIES (*When awake and not receiving treatments or ADL care*)
0. Most—more than 2/3 of time   2. Little—less than 1/3 of time
1. Some—from 1/3 to 2/3 of time   3. None

O1. NUMBER OF MEDICATIONS (*Record the number of different medications used in the last 7 days; enter "0" if none used*)

O3. INJECTIONS (*Record the number of DAYS injections of any type received during the last 7 days; enter "0" if none used*)

O4. DAYS RECEIVED THE FOLLOWING MEDICATION (*Record the number of DAYS during last 7 days; enter "0" if not used. Note—enter "1" for long-acting meds used less than weekly*)
a. Antipsychotic   d. Hypnotic
b. Antianxiety   e. Diuretic
c. Antidepressant

P1. SPECIAL TREATMENTS, PROCEDURES, AND PROGRAMS

a. SPECIAL CARE—Check treatments or programs received during **the last 14 days**

TREATMENTS
a. Chemotherapy
b. Dialysis
c. IV medication
d. Intake/output
e. Monitoring acute medical condition
f. Ostomy care
g. Oxygen therapy
h. Radiation
i. Suctioning
j. Tracheostomy care
k. Transfusions
l. Ventilator or respirator

PROGRAMS
m. Alcohol/drug treatment program
n. Alzheimer's/dementia special care unit
o. Hospice care
p. Pediatric unit
q. Respite care
r. Training in skills required to return to the community (e.g., taking medications, house work, shopping, transportation, ADLs)
s. NONE OF THE ABOVE

Resident Identifier _____

Numeric Identifier _____

P1.	SPECIAL TREAT-MENTS, PROCE-DURES, AND PROGRAMS	**b. THERAPIES** - *Record the number of days and total minutes each of the following therapies was administered (for at least 15 minutes a day) in the **last 7 calendar days** (Enter 0 if none or less than 15 min. daily)* **[Note — count only post admission therapies]** (A) = # of days administered for **15 minutes or more** (B) = total # of minutes provided in **last 7 days**		
			DAYS **(A)**	**MIN** **(B)**
		a. Speech - language pathology and audiology services		
		b. Occupational therapy		
		c. Physical therapy		
		d. Respiratory therapy		
		e. Psychological therapy (by any licensed mental health professional)		

P3.	NURSING REHABILITA-TION/ RESTOR-ATIVE CARE	*Record the NUMBER OF DAYS each of the following rehabilitation or restorative techniques or practices was **provided to the residents for more than or equal to 15 minutes per day in the last 7 days** (ENTER 0 if none or less than 15 min. daily.)*		
		a. Range of motion (passive)		f. Walking
		b. Range of motion (active)		g. Dressing or grooming
		c. Splint or brace assistance		h. Eating or swallowing
		TRAINING AND SKILL PRACTICE IN:		i. Amputation/prosthesis care
		d. Bed mobility		j. Communication
		e. Transfer		k. Other

P4.	DEVICES AND RESTRAINTS	*Use the following codes for **last 7 days**:*	
		0. Not used	
		1. Used less than daily	
		2. Used daily	
		Bed rails	
		a. —Full bed rails on all open sides of bed	
		b. —Other types of side rails used (e.g., half rail, one side)	
		c. Trunk restraint	
		d. Limb restraint	
		e. Chair prevents rising	

P7.	PHYSICIAN VISITS	In the **LAST 14 DAYS** (or since admission if less than 14 days in facility) how many days has the physician (or authorized assistant or practitioner) examined the resident? *(Enter 0 if none)*

P8.	PHYSICIAN ORDERS	In the **LAST 14 DAYS** (or since admission if less than 14 days in facility) how many days has the physician (or authorized assistant or practitioner) changed the resident's orders? *Do not include order renewals without change. (Enter 0 if none)*	

Q1.	DISCHARGE POTENTIAL	**a.** Resident expresses/indicates preference to return to the community 0. No 1. Yes	
		c. Stay projected to be of a short duration—discharge projected **within 90 days** (do not include expected discharge due to death) 0. No 2. Within 31-90 days 1. Within 30 days 3. Discharge status uncertain	

Q2.	OVERALL CHANGE IN CARE NEEDS	Resident's overall level of self sufficiency has changed significantly as compared to status of **90 days ago** (or since last assessment if less than 90 days) 0. No change 1. Improved—receives 2. Deteriorated—receives fewer supports, needs more support less restrictive level of care	

R2. SIGNATURE OF PERSON COORDINATING THE ASSESSMENT:

a. Signature of RN Assessment Coordinator (sign on above line)
b. Date RN Assessment Coordinator signed as complete

Month		Day		Year

T1.	SPECIAL TREATMENTS AND PROCE-DURES	*Skip unless this is a Medicare 5 day or Medicare readmission/return assessment*	
		b. ORDERED THERAPIES—Has physician ordered any of the following therapies to begin in FIRST 14 days of stay—physical therapy, occupational therapy, or speech pathology service? 0. No 1. Yes	
		c. Through day15, provide an estimate of the number of days when at least 1 therapy service can be expected to have been delivered.	
		d. Through day15, provide an estimate of the number of therapy minutes (across the therapies) that can be expected to be delivered.	

T3.	CASE MIX GROUP	Medicare				State			

MDS 2.0 PPS July 2002

Outcome and Assessment Information Set (OASIS-B1)

Outcome and Assessment Information Set (OASIS-B1)

START OF CARE VERSION
(also used for Resumption of Care Following Inpatient Stay)

Items to be Used at this Time Point--- **M0080-M0825**

CLINICAL RECORD ITEMS

(M0080) Discipline of Person Completing Assessment:

☐ 1-RN ☐ 2-PT ☐ 3-SLP/ST ☐ 4-OT

(M0090) Date Assessment Completed: __ __ / __ __ / __ __ __ __
month   day   year

(M0100) This Assessment is Currently Being Completed for the Following Reason:

Start/Resumption of Care
☐ 1 – Start of care—further visits planned
☐ 3 – Resumption of care (after inpatient stay)

DEMOGRAPHICS AND PATIENT HISTORY

(M0175) From which of the following **Inpatient Facilities** was the patient discharged <u>during the past 14 days</u>? **(Mark all that apply.)**

☐ 1 - Hospital
☐ 2 - Rehabilitation facility
☐ 3 - Skilled nursing facility
☐ 4 - Other nursing home
☐ 5 - Other (specify) _____
☐ NA - Patient was not discharged from an inpatient facility **[If NA, go to *M0200*]**

(M0180) Inpatient Discharge Date (most recent):

__ __ / __ __ / __ __ __ __
month   day   year

☐ UK - Unknown

(M0190) Inpatient Diagnoses and ICD-9-CM code categories (three digits required; five digits optional) <u>for only those conditions treated during an inpatient facility stay within the last 14 days</u> (no surgical or V-codes):

Inpatient Facility Diagnosis	ICD-9-CM
a. _____	(__ __ __ . __ __)
b. _____	(__ __ __ . __ __)

Effective 10/1/2003
List each Inpatient Diagnosis and ICD-9-CM code at the level of highest specificity for only those conditions treated during an inpatient stay within the last 14 days (no surgical, E-codes, or V-codes):

Inpatient Facility Diagnosis	ICD-9-CM
a. _____	(__ __ __ . __ __)
b. _____	(__ __ __ . __ __)

(M0200) Medical or Treatment Regimen Change Within Past 14 Days: Has this patient experienced a change in medical or treatment regimen (e.g., medication, treatment, or service change due to new or additional diagnosis, etc.) within the last 14 days?

☐ 0 - No   **[If No, go to *M0220*]**
☐ 1 - Yes

(M0210) List the patient's **Medical Diagnoses** and ICD-9-CM code categories (three digits required; five digits optional) <u>for those conditions requiring changed medical or treatment regimen</u> (no surgical or V-codes):

Changed Medical Regimen Diagnosis	ICD-9-CM
a. _____	(__ __ __ . __ __)
b. _____	(__ __ __ . __ __)
c. _____	(__ __ __ . __ __)
d. _____	(__ __ __ . __ __)

Effective 10/1/2003

List the patient's Medical Diagnoses and ICD-9-CM codes at the level of highest specificity for those conditions requiring changed medical or treatment regimen (no surgical, E-codes, or V-codes):

Changed Medical Regimen Diagnosis	ICD-9-CM
a. _____	(__ __ __ . __ __)
b. _____	(__ __ __ . __ __)
c. _____	(__ __ __ . __ __)
d. _____	(__ __ __ . __ __)

(M0220) Conditions Prior to Medical or Treatment Regimen Change or Inpatient Stay Within Past 14 Days: If this patient experienced an inpatient facility discharge or change in medical or treatment regimen within the past 14 days, indicate any conditions which existed <u>prior to</u> the inpatient stay or change in medical or treatment regimen. **(Mark all that apply.)**

☐ 1 - Urinary incontinence
☐ 2 - Indwelling/suprapubic catheter
☐ 3 - Intractable pain
☐ 4 - Impaired decision-making
☐ 5 - Disruptive or socially inappropriate behavior
☐ 6 - Memory loss to the extent that supervision required
☐ 7 - None of the above
☐ NA - No inpatient facility discharge <u>and</u> no change in medical or treatment regimen in past 14 days
☐ UK - Unknown

(M0230/M0240) Diagnoses and Severity Index: List each medical diagnosis or problem for which the patient is receiving home care and ICD-9-CM code category (three digits required; five digits optional – no surgical or V-codes) and rate them using the following severity index. (Choose one value that represents the most severe rating appropriate for each diagnosis.) ICD-9-CM sequencing requirements must be followed if multiple coding is indicated for any diagnoses.

Effective 10/1/2003

List each diagnosis and ICD-9-CM code at the level of highest specificity (no surgical codes) for which the patient is receiving home care. Rate each condition using the following severity index. (Choose one value that represents the most severe rating appropriate for each diagnosis.) E-codes (for M0240 only) or V-codes (for M0230 or M0240) may be used. ICD-9-CM sequencing requirements must be followed if multiple coding is indicated for any diagnoses. If a V-code is reported in place of a case mix diagnosis, then M0245 Payment Diagnosis should be completed. Case mix diagnosis is a primary or first secondary diagnosis that determines the Medicare PPS case mix group.

Severity Rating
0 - Asymptomatic, no treatment needed at this time
1 - Symptoms well controlled with current therapy
2 - Symptoms controlled with difficulty, affecting daily functioning; patient needs ongoing monitoring
3 - Symptoms poorly controlled, patient needs frequent adjustment in treatment and dose monitoring
4 - Symptoms poorly controlled, history of rehospitalizations

(M0230) Primary Diagnosis	ICD-9-CM	Severity Rating
a. _____	(___ ___ ___ . ___ ___)	☐ 0 ☐ 1 ☐ 2 ☐ 3 ☐ 4

(M0240) Other Diagnoses	ICD-9-CM	Severity Rating
b. _____	(___ ___ ___ . ___ ___)	☐ 0 ☐ 1 ☐ 2 ☐ 3 ☐ 4
c. _____	(___ ___ ___ . ___ ___)	☐ 0 ☐ 1 ☐ 2 ☐ 3 ☐ 4
d. _____	(___ ___ ___ . ___ ___)	☐ 0 ☐ 1 ☐ 2 ☐ 3 ☐ 4
e. _____	(___ ___ ___ . ___ ___)	☐ 0 ☐ 1 ☐ 2 ☐ 3 ☐ 4
f. _____	(___ ___ ___ . ___ ___)	☐ 0 ☐ 1 ☐ 2 ☐ 3 ☐ 4

Effective 10/1/2003

(M0245) Payment Diagnosis (optional): If a V-code was reported in M0230 in place of a case mix diagnosis, list the primary diagnosis and ICD-9-CM code, determined in accordance with OASIS requirements in effect before October 1, 2003--no V-codes, E-codes, or surgical codes allowed. ICD-9-CM sequencing requirements must be followed. Complete both lines (a) and (b) if the case mix diagnosis is a manifestation code or in other situations where multiple coding is indicated for the primary diagnosis; otherwise, complete line (a) only.

(M0245) Primary Diagnosis	ICD-9-CM
a. _____	(___ ___ ___ . ___ ___)

(M0245) First Secondary Diagnosis	ICD-9-CM
b. _____	(___ ___ ___ . ___ ___)

(M0250) Therapies the patient receives <u>at home</u>: **(Mark all that apply.)**

☐ 1 - Intravenous or infusion therapy (excludes TPN)
☐ 2 - Parenteral nutrition (TPN or lipids)
☐ 3 - Enteral nutrition (nasogastric, gastrostomy, jejunostomy, or any other artificial entry into the alimentary canal)
☐ 4 - None of the above

(M0260) Overall Prognosis: BEST description of patient's overall prognosis for <u>recovery from this episode of illness</u>.

☐ 0 - Poor: little or no recovery is expected and/or further decline is imminent
☐ 1 - Good/Fair: partial to full recovery is expected
☐ UK - Unknown

(M0270) Rehabilitative Prognosis: BEST description of patient's prognosis for <u>functional status</u>.

☐ 0 - Guarded: minimal improvement in functional status is expected; decline is possible
☐ 1 - Good: marked improvement in functional status is expected
☐ UK - Unknown

(M0280) Life Expectancy: (Physician documentation is not required.)

☐ 0 - Life expectancy is greater than 6 months
☐ 1 - Life expectancy is 6 months or fewer

(M0290) **High Risk Factors** characterizing this patient: **(Mark all that apply.)**

- ☐ 1 - Heavy smoking
- ☐ 2 - Obesity
- ☐ 3 - Alcohol dependency
- ☐ 4 - Drug dependency
- ☐ 5 - None of the above
- ☐ UK - Unknown

LIVING ARRANGEMENTS

(M0300) **Current Residence:**

- ☐ 1 - Patient's owned or rented residence (house, apartment, or mobile home owned or rented by patient/couple/significant other)
- ☐ 2 - Family member's residence
- ☐ 3 - Boarding home or rented room
- ☐ 4 - Board and care or assisted living facility
- ☐ 5 - Other (specify) _____

(M0340) **Patient Lives With: (Mark all that apply.)**

- ☐ 1 - Lives alone
- ☐ 2 - With spouse or significant other
- ☐ 3 - With other family member
- ☐ 4 - With a friend
- ☐ 5 - With paid help (other than home care agency staff)
- ☐ 6 - With other than above

SUPPORTIVE ASSISTANCE

(M0350) **Assisting Person(s) Other than Home Care Agency Staff: (Mark all that apply.)**

- ☐ 1 - Relatives, friends, or neighbors living outside the home
- ☐ 2 - Person residing in the home (EXCLUDING paid help)
- ☐ 3 - Paid help
- ☐ 4 - None of the above **[If None of the above, go to *M0390*]**
- ☐ UK - Unknown **[If Unknown, go to *M0390*]**

(M0360) **Primary Caregiver** taking <u>lead</u> responsibility for providing or managing the patient's care, providing the most frequent assistance, etc. (other than home care agency staff):

- ☐ 0 - No one person **[If No one person, go to *M0390*]**
- ☐ 1 - Spouse or significant other
- ☐ 2 - Daughter or son
- ☐ 3 - Other family member
- ☐ 4 - Friend or neighbor or community or church member
- ☐ 5 - Paid help
- ☐ UK - Unknown **[If Unknown, go to *M0390*]**

(M0370) **How Often** does the patient receive assistance from the primary caregiver?

- ☐ 1 - Several times during day and night
- ☐ 2 - Several times during day
- ☐ 3 - Once daily
- ☐ 4 - Three or more times per week
- ☐ 5 - One to two times per week
- ☐ 6 - Less often than weekly
- ☐ UK - Unknown

(M0380) Type of Primary Caregiver Assistance: (Mark all that apply.)

☐   1 -   ADL assistance (e.g., bathing, dressing, toileting, bowel/bladder, eating/feeding)
☐   2 -   IADL assistance (e.g., meds, meals, housekeeping, laundry, telephone, shopping, finances)
☐   3 -   Environmental support (housing, home maintenance)
☐   4 -   Psychosocial support (socialization, companionship, recreation)
☐   5 -   Advocates or facilitates patient's participation in appropriate medical care
☐   6 -   Financial agent, power of attorney, or conservator of finance
☐   7 -   Health care agent, conservator of person, or medical power of attorney
☐ UK -   Unknown

SENSORY STATUS

(M0390) Vision with corrective lenses if the patient usually wears them:

☐   0 -   Normal vision: sees adequately in most situations; can see medication labels, newsprint.
☐   1 -   Partially impaired: cannot see medication labels or newsprint, but <u>can</u> see obstacles in path, and the surrounding layout; can count fingers at arm's length.
☐   2 -   Severely impaired: cannot locate objects without hearing or touching them <u>or</u> patient nonresponsive.

(M0400) Hearing and Ability to Understand Spoken Language in patient's own language (with hearing aids if the patient usually uses them):

☐   0 -   No observable impairment. Able to hear and understand complex or detailed instructions and extended or abstract conversation.
☐   1 -   With minimal difficulty, able to hear and understand most multi-step instructions and ordinary conversation. May need occasional repetition, extra time, or louder voice.
☐   2 -   Has moderate difficulty hearing and understanding simple, one-step instructions and brief conversation; needs frequent prompting or assistance.
☐   3 -   Has severe difficulty hearing and understanding simple greetings and short comments. Requires multiple repetitions, restatements, demonstrations, additional time.
☐   4 -   <u>Unable</u> to hear and understand familiar words or common expressions consistently, <u>or</u> patient nonresponsive.

(M0410) Speech and Oral (Verbal) Expression of Language (in patient's own language):

☐   0 -   Expresses complex ideas, feelings, and needs clearly, completely, and easily in all situations with no observable impairment.
☐   1 -   Minimal difficulty in expressing ideas and needs (may take extra time; makes occasional errors in word choice, grammar or speech intelligibility; needs minimal prompting or assistance).
☐   2 -   Expresses simple ideas or needs with moderate difficulty (needs prompting or assistance, errors in word choice, organization or speech intelligibility). Speaks in phrases or short sentences.
☐   3 -   Has severe difficulty expressing basic ideas or needs and requires maximal assistance or guessing by listener. Speech limited to single words or short phrases.
☐   4 -   <u>Unable</u> to express basic needs even with maximal prompting or assistance but is not comatose or unresponsive (e.g., speech is nonsensical or unintelligible).
☐   5 -   Patient nonresponsive or unable to speak.

(M0420) Frequency of Pain interfering with patient's activity or movement:

☐   0 -   Patient has no pain or pain does not interfere with activity or movement
☐   1 -   Less often than daily
☐   2 -   Daily, but not constantly
☐   3 -   All of the time

(M0430) Intractable Pain: Is the patient experiencing pain that is <u>not easily relieved</u>, occurs at least daily, and affects the patient's sleep, appetite, physical or emotional energy, concentration, personal relationships, emotions, or ability or desire to perform physical activity?

☐   0 - No
☐   1 - Yes

INTEGUMENTARY STATUS

(M0440) Does this patient have a **Skin Lesion** or an **Open Wound**? This excludes "OSTOMIES."

- ☐   0 -   No **[If No, go to M0490]**
- ☐   1 -   Yes

(M0445) Does this patient have a **Pressure Ulcer**?

- ☐   0 -   No **[If No, go to M0468]**
- ☐   1 -   Yes

(M0450)   **Current Number of Pressure Ulcers at Each Stage:** (Circle one response for each stage.)

	Pressure Ulcer Stages	Number of Pressure Ulcers				
a)	Stage 1: Nonblanchable erythema of intact skin; the heralding of skin ulceration. In darker-pigmented skin, warmth, edema, hardness, or discolored skin may be indicators.	0	1	2	3	4 or more
b)	Stage 2: Partial thickness skin loss involving epidermis and/or dermis. The ulcer is superficial and presents clinically as an abrasion, blister, or shallow crater.	0	1	2	3	4 or more
c)	Stage 3: Full-thickness skin loss involving damage or necrosis of subcutaneous tissue which may extend down to, but not through, underlying fascia. The ulcer presents clinically as a deep crater with or without undermining of adjacent tissue.	0	1	2	3	4 or more
d)	Stage 4: Full-thickness skin loss with extensive destruction, tissue necrosis, or damage to muscle, bone, or supporting structures (e.g., tendon, joint capsule, etc.)	0	1	2	3	4 or more
e)	In addition to the above, is there at least one pressure ulcer that cannot be observed due to the presence of eschar or a nonremovable dressing, including casts? ☐ 0 - No ☐ 1 - Yes					

(M0460)   **Stage of Most Problematic (Observable) Pressure Ulcer:**

- ☐   1 -   Stage 1
- ☐   2 -   Stage 2
- ☐   3 -   Stage 3
- ☐   4 -   Stage 4
- ☐ NA -   No observable pressure ulcer

(M0464)   **Status of Most Problematic (Observable) Pressure Ulcer:**

- ☐   1 -   Fully granulating
- ☐   2 -   Early/partial granulation
- ☐   3 -   Not healing
- ☐ NA -   No observable pressure ulcer

(M0468) Does this patient have a **Stasis Ulcer**?

- ☐   0 -   No **[If No, go to M0482]**
- ☐   1 -   Yes

(M0470)   **Current Number of Observable Stasis Ulcer(s):**

- ☐   0 -   Zero
- ☐   1 -   One
- ☐   2 -   Two
- ☐   3 -   Three
- ☐   4 -   Four or more

(M0474) Does this patient have at least one **Stasis Ulcer that Cannot be Observed** due to the presence of a nonremovable dressing?

☐   0 - No
☐   1 - Yes

(M0476) **Status of Most Problematic (Observable) Stasis Ulcer:**

☐   1 - Fully granulating
☐   2 - Early/partial granulation
☐   3 - Not healing
☐ NA - No observable stasis ulcer

(M0482) Does this patient have a **Surgical Wound?**

☐   0 - No **[If No, go to *M0490*]**
☐   1 - Yes

(M0484) **Current Number of (Observable) Surgical Wounds:** (If a wound is partially closed but has <u>more</u> than one opening, consider each opening as a separate wound.)

☐   0 - Zero
☐   1 - One
☐   2 - Two
☐   3 - Three
☐   4 - Four or more

(M0486) Does this patient have at least one **Surgical Wound that Cannot be Observed** due to the presence of a nonremovable dressing?

☐   0 - No
☐   1 - Yes

(M0488) **Status of Most Problematic (Observable) Surgical Wound:**

☐   1 - Fully granulating
☐   2 - Early/partial granulation
☐   3 - Not healing
☐ NA - No observable surgical wound

RESPIRATORY STATUS

(M0490) When is the patient dyspneic or noticeably **Short of Breath?**

☐   0 - Never, patient is not short of breath
☐   1 - When walking more than 20 feet, climbing stairs
☐   2 - With moderate exertion (e.g., while dressing, using commode or bedpan, walking distances less than 20 feet)
☐   3 - With minimal exertion (e.g., while eating, talking, or performing other ADLs) or with agitation
☐   4 - At rest (during day or night)

(M0500) **Respiratory Treatments** utilized at home: **(Mark all that apply.)**

☐   1 - Oxygen (intermittent or continuous)
☐   2 - Ventilator (continually or at night)
☐   3 - Continuous positive airway pressure
☐   4 - None of the above

ELIMINATION STATUS

(M0510) Has this patient been treated for a **Urinary Tract Infection** in the past 14 days?

☐   0 - No
☐   1 - Yes
☐   NA - Patient on prophylactic treatment
☐   UK - Unknown

(M0520) Urinary Incontinence or Urinary Catheter Presence:

☐   0 - No incontinence or catheter (includes anuria or ostomy for urinary drainage) **[If No, go to *M0540*]**
☐   1 - Patient is incontinent
☐   2 - Patient requires a urinary catheter (i.e., external, indwelling, intermittent, suprapubic) **[Go to *M0540*]**

(M0530) When does Urinary Incontinence occur?

☐   0 - Timed-voiding defers incontinence
☐   1 - During the night only
☐   2 - During the day and night

(M0540) Bowel Incontinence Frequency:

☐   0 - Very rarely or never has bowel incontinence
☐   1 - Less than once weekly
☐   2 - One to three times weekly
☐   3 - Four to six times weekly
☐   4 - On a daily basis
☐   5 - More often than once daily
☐   NA - Patient has ostomy for bowel elimination
☐   UK - Unknown

(M0550) Ostomy for Bowel Elimination: Does this patient have an ostomy for bowel elimination that (within the last 14 days): a) was related to an inpatient facility stay, or b) necessitated a change in medical or treatment regimen?

☐   0 - Patient does not have an ostomy for bowel elimination.
☐   1 - Patient's ostomy was not related to an inpatient stay and did not necessitate change in medical or treatment regimen.
☐   2 - The ostomy was related to an inpatient stay or did necessitate change in medical or treatment regimen.

NEURO/EMOTIONAL/BEHAVIORAL STATUS

(M0560) Cognitive Functioning: (Patient's current level of alertness, orientation, comprehension, concentration, and immediate memory for simple commands.)

☐   0 - Alert/oriented, able to focus and shift attention, comprehends and recalls task directions independently.
☐   1 - Requires prompting (cuing, repetition, reminders) only under stressful or unfamiliar conditions.
☐   2 - Requires assistance and some direction in specific situations (e.g., on all tasks involving shifting of attention), or consistently requires low stimulus environment due to distractibility.
☐   3 - Requires considerable assistance in routine situations. Is not alert and oriented or is unable to shift attention and recall directions more than half the time.
☐   4 - Totally dependent due to disturbances such as constant disorientation, coma, persistent vegetative state, or delirium.

(M0570) When Confused (Reported or Observed):

- ☐   0 -   Never
- ☐   1 -   In new or complex situations only
- ☐   2 -   On awakening or at night only
- ☐   3 -   During the day and evening, but not constantly
- ☐   4 -   Constantly
- ☐   NA -   Patient nonresponsive

(M0580) When Anxious (Reported or Observed):

- ☐   0 -   None of the time
- ☐   1 -   Less often than daily
- ☐   2 -   Daily, but not constantly
- ☐   3 -   All of the time
- ☐   NA -   Patient nonresponsive

(M0590) Depressive Feelings Reported or Observed in Patient: (Mark all that apply.)

- ☐   1 -   Depressed mood (e.g., feeling sad, tearful)
- ☐   2 -   Sense of failure or self reproach
- ☐   3 -   Hopelessness
- ☐   4 -   Recurrent thoughts of death
- ☐   5 -   Thoughts of suicide
- ☐   6 -   None of the above feelings observed or reported

(M0610) Behaviors Demonstrated <u>at Least Once a Week</u> (Reported or Observed): (Mark all that apply.)

- ☐   1 -   Memory deficit: failure to recognize familiar persons/places, inability to recall events of past 24 hours, significant memory loss so that supervision is required
- ☐   2 -   Impaired decision-making: failure to perform usual ADLs or IADLs, inability to appropriately stop activities, jeopardizes safety through actions
- ☐   3 -   Verbal disruption: yelling, threatening, excessive profanity, sexual references, etc.
- ☐   4 -   Physical aggression: aggressive or combative to self and others (e.g., hits self, throws objects, punches, dangerous maneuvers with wheelchair or other objects)
- ☐   5 -   Disruptive, infantile, or socially inappropriate behavior (**excludes** verbal actions)
- ☐   6 -   Delusional, hallucinatory, or paranoid behavior
- ☐   7 -   None of the above behaviors demonstrated

(M0620) Frequency of Behavior Problems (Reported or Observed) (e.g., wandering episodes, self abuse, verbal disruption, physical aggression, etc.):

- ☐   0 -   Never
- ☐   1 -   Less than once a month
- ☐   2 -   Once a month
- ☐   3 -   Several times each month
- ☐   4 -   Several times a week
- ☐   5 -   At least daily

(M0630) Is this patient receiving Psychiatric Nursing Services at home provided by a qualified psychiatric nurse?

- ☐   0 -   No
- ☐   1 -   Yes

ADL/IADLs

> For M0640-M0800, complete the "Current" column for all patients. For these same items, complete the "Prior" column only at start of care and at resumption of care; mark the level that corresponds to the patient's condition 14 days prior to start of care date (M0030) or resumption of care date (M0032). In all cases, record what the patient is *able to do*.

(M0640) Grooming: Ability to tend to personal hygiene needs (i.e., washing face and hands, hair care, shaving or make up, teeth or denture care, fingernail care).

Prior Current
- ☐ ☐ 0 - Able to groom self unaided, with or without the use of assistive devices or adapted methods.
- ☐ ☐ 1 - Grooming utensils must be placed within reach before able to complete grooming activities.
- ☐ ☐ 2 - Someone must assist the patient to groom self.
- ☐ ☐ 3 - Patient depends entirely upon someone else for grooming needs.
- ☐   UK - Unknown

(M0650) Ability to Dress <u>Upper</u> Body (with or without dressing aids) including undergarments, pullovers, front-opening shirts and blouses, managing zippers, buttons, and snaps:

Prior Current
- ☐ ☐ 0 - Able to get clothes out of closets and drawers, put them on and remove them from the upper body without assistance.
- ☐ ☐ 1 - Able to dress upper body without assistance if clothing is laid out or handed to the patient.
- ☐ ☐ 2 - Someone must help the patient put on upper body clothing.
- ☐ ☐ 3 - Patient depends entirely upon another person to dress the upper body.
- ☐   UK - Unknown

(M0660) Ability to Dress <u>Lower</u> Body (with or without dressing aids) including undergarments, slacks, socks or nylons, shoes:

Prior Current
- ☐ ☐ 0 - Able to obtain, put on, and remove clothing and shoes without assistance.
- ☐ ☐ 1 - Able to dress lower body without assistance if clothing and shoes are laid out or handed to the patient.
- ☐ ☐ 2 - Someone must help the patient put on undergarments, slacks, socks or nylons, and shoes.
- ☐ ☐ 3 - Patient depends entirely upon another person to dress lower body.
- ☐   UK - Unknown

(M0670) Bathing: Ability to wash entire body. **<u>Excludes</u> grooming (washing face and hands only).**

Prior Current
- ☐ ☐ 0 - Able to bathe self in <u>shower or tub</u> independently.
- ☐ ☐ 1 - With the use of devices, is able to bathe self in shower or tub independently.
- ☐ ☐ 2 - Able to bathe in shower or tub with the assistance of another person:
  (a) for intermittent supervision or encouragement or reminders, <u>OR</u>
  (b) to get in and out of the shower or tub, <u>OR</u>
  (c) for washing difficult to reach areas.
- ☐ ☐ 3 - Participates in bathing self in shower or tub, <u>but</u> requires presence of another person throughout the bath for assistance or supervision.
- ☐ ☐ 4 - <u>Unable</u> to use the shower or tub and is bathed in <u>bed or bedside chair</u>.
- ☐ ☐ 5 - Unable to effectively participate in bathing and is totally bathed by another person.
- ☐   UK - Unknown

(M0680) Toileting: Ability to get to and from the toilet or bedside commode.

Prior   Current
☐   ☐   0 -   Able to get to and from the toilet independently with or without a device.
☐   ☐   1 -   When reminded, assisted, or supervised by another person, able to get to and from the toilet.
☐   ☐   2 -   Unable to get to and from the toilet but is able to use a bedside commode (with or without assistance).
☐   ☐   3 -   Unable to get to and from the toilet or bedside commode but is able to use a bedpan/urinal independently.
☐   ☐   4 -   Is totally dependent in toileting.
☐   UK -   Unknown

(M0690) Transferring: Ability to move from bed to chair, on and off toilet or commode, into and out of tub or shower, and ability to turn and position self in bed if patient is bedfast.

Prior Current
☐   ☐   0 -   Able to independently transfer.
☐   ☐   1 -   Transfers with minimal human assistance or with use of an assistive device.
☐   ☐   2 -   Unable to transfer self but is able to bear weight and pivot during the transfer process.
☐   ☐   3 -   Unable to transfer self and is unable to bear weight or pivot when transferred by another person.
☐   ☐   4 -   Bedfast, unable to transfer but is able to turn and position self in bed.
☐   ☐   5 -   Bedfast, unable to transfer and is unable to turn and position self.
☐   UK -   Unknown

(M0700) Ambulation/Locomotion: Ability to SAFELY walk, once in a standing position, or use a wheelchair, once in a seated position, on a variety of surfaces.

Prior Current
☐   ☐   0 -   Able to independently walk on even and uneven surfaces and climb stairs with or without railings (i.e., needs no human assistance or assistive device).
☐   ☐   1 -   Requires use of a device (e.g., cane, walker) to walk alone or requires human supervision or assistance to negotiate stairs or steps or uneven surfaces.
☐   ☐   2 -   Able to walk only with the supervision or assistance of another person at all times.
☐   ☐   3 -   Chairfast, unable to ambulate but is able to wheel self independently.
☐   ☐   4 -   Chairfast, unable to ambulate and is unable to wheel self.
☐   ☐   5 -   Bedfast, unable to ambulate or be up in a chair.
☐   UK -   Unknown

(M0710) Feeding or Eating: Ability to feed self meals and snacks. **Note: This refers only to the process of eating, chewing, and swallowing, not preparing the food to be eaten.**

Prior Current
☐   ☐   0 -   Able to independently feed self.
☐   ☐   1 -   Able to feed self independently but requires:
             (a) meal set-up; OR
             (b) intermittent assistance or supervision from another person; OR
             (c) a liquid, pureed or ground meat diet.
☐   ☐   2 -   Unable to feed self and must be assisted or supervised throughout the meal/snack.
☐   ☐   3 -   Able to take in nutrients orally and receives supplemental nutrients through a nasogastric tube or gastrostomy.
☐   ☐   4 -   Unable to take in nutrients orally and is fed nutrients through a nasogastric tube or gastrostomy.
☐   ☐   5 -   Unable to take in nutrients orally or by tube feeding.
☐   UK -   Unknown

(M0720) Planning and Preparing Light Meals (e.g., cereal, sandwich) or reheat delivered meals:

Prior Current
☐   ☐   0 - (a) Able to independently plan and prepare all light meals for self or reheat delivered meals; <u>OR</u>
              (b) Is physically, cognitively, and mentally able to prepare light meals on a regular basis but has
                  not routinely performed light meal preparation in the past (i.e., prior to this home care
                  admission).
☐   ☐   1 - <u>Unable</u> to prepare light meals on a regular basis due to physical, cognitive, or mental limitations.
☐   ☐   2 - Unable to prepare any light meals or reheat any delivered meals.
☐   UK - Unknown

(M0730) Transportation: Physical and mental ability to <u>safely</u> use a car, taxi, or public transportation (bus, train,
          subway).

Prior Current
☐   ☐   0 - Able to independently drive a regular or adapted car; <u>OR</u> uses a regular or handicap-accessible
              public bus.
☐   ☐   1 - Able to ride in a car only when driven by another person; <u>OR</u> able to use a bus or handicap van
              only when assisted or accompanied by another person.
☐   ☐   2 - <u>Unable</u> to ride in a car, taxi, bus, or van, and requires transportation by ambulance.
☐   UK - Unknown

(M0740) Laundry: Ability to do own laundry -- to carry laundry to and from washing machine, to use washer and
          dryer, to wash small items by hand.

Prior Current
☐   ☐   0 - (a) Able to independently take care of all laundry tasks; <u>OR</u>
              (b) Physically, cognitively, and mentally able to do laundry and access facilities, <u>but</u> has not
                  routinely performed laundry tasks in the past (i.e., prior to this home care admission).
☐   ☐   1 - Able to do only light laundry, such as minor hand wash or light washer loads. Due to physical,
              cognitive, or mental limitations, needs assistance with heavy laundry such as carrying large loads
              of laundry.
☐   ☐   2 - <u>Unable</u> to do any laundry due to physical limitation or needs continual supervision and assistance
              due to cognitive or mental limitation.
☐   UK - Unknown

(M0750) Housekeeping: Ability to safely and effectively perform light housekeeping and heavier cleaning tasks.

Prior Current
☐   ☐   0 - (a) Able to independently perform all housekeeping tasks; <u>OR</u>
              (b) Physically, cognitively, and mentally able to perform <u>all</u> housekeeping tasks but has not
                  routinely participated in housekeeping tasks in the past (i.e., prior to this home care
                  admission).
☐   ☐   1 - Able to perform only <u>light</u> housekeeping (e.g., dusting, wiping kitchen counters) tasks
              independently.
☐   ☐   2 - Able to perform housekeeping tasks with intermittent assistance or supervision from another
              person.
☐   ☐   3 - <u>Unable</u> to consistently perform any housekeeping tasks unless assisted by another person
              throughout the process.
☐   ☐   4 - Unable to effectively participate in any housekeeping tasks.
☐   UK - Unknown

(M0760) Shopping: Ability to plan for, select, and purchase items in a store and to carry them home or arrange delivery.

Prior Current

☐ ☐ 0 - (a) Able to plan for shopping needs and independently perform shopping tasks, including carrying packages; <u>OR</u>
    (b) Physically, cognitively, and mentally able to take care of shopping, but has not done shopping in the past (i.e., prior to this home care admission).

☐ ☐ 1 - Able to go shopping, but needs some assistance:
    (a) By self is able to do only light shopping and carry small packages, but needs someone to do occasional major shopping; <u>OR</u>
    (b) <u>Unable</u> to go shopping alone, but can go with someone to assist.

☐ ☐ 2 - <u>Unable</u> to go shopping, but is able to identify items needed, place orders, and arrange home delivery.

☐ ☐ 3 - Needs someone to do all shopping and errands.

☐   UK - Unknown

(M0770) Ability to Use Telephone: Ability to answer the phone, dial numbers, and <u>effectively</u> use the telephone to communicate.

Prior Current

☐ ☐ 0 - Able to dial numbers and answer calls appropriately and as desired.

☐ ☐ 1 - Able to use a specially adapted telephone (i.e., large numbers on the dial, teletype phone for the deaf) and call essential numbers.

☐ ☐ 2 - Able to answer the telephone and carry on a normal conversation but has difficulty with placing calls.

☐ ☐ 3 - Able to answer the telephone only some of the time or is able to carry on only a limited conversation.

☐ ☐ 4 - <u>Unable</u> to answer the telephone at all but can listen if assisted with equipment.

☐ ☐ 5 - Totally unable to use the telephone.

☐ ☐ NA - Patient does not have a telephone.

☐   UK - Unknown

MEDICATIONS

(M0780) Management of Oral Medications: <u>Patient's ability</u> to prepare and take <u>all</u> prescribed oral medications reliably and safely, including administration of the correct dosage at the appropriate times/intervals. <u>Excludes</u> injectable and IV medications. (NOTE: This refers to ability, not compliance or willingness.)

Prior Current

☐ ☐ 0 - Able to independently take the correct oral medication(s) and proper dosage(s) at the correct times.

☐ ☐ 1 - Able to take medication(s) at the correct times if:
    (a) individual dosages are prepared in advance by another person; <u>OR</u>
    (b) given daily reminders; <u>OR</u>
    (c) someone develops a drug diary or chart.

☐ ☐ 2 - <u>Unable</u> to take medication unless administered by someone else.

☐ ☐ NA - No oral medications prescribed.

☐   UK - Unknown

(M0790) Management of Inhalant/Mist Medications: <u>Patient's ability</u> to prepare and take <u>all</u> prescribed inhalant/mist medications (nebulizers, metered dose devices) reliably and safely, including administration of the correct dosage at the appropriate times/intervals. **Excludes all other forms of medication (oral tablets, injectable and IV medications).**

<u>Prior</u> <u>Current</u>

☐ ☐ 0 - Able to independently take the correct medication and proper dosage at the correct times.

☐ ☐ 1 - Able to take medication at the correct times if:
    (a) individual dosages are prepared in advance by another person, <u>OR</u>
    (b) given daily reminders.

☐ ☐ 2 - <u>Unable</u> to take medication unless administered by someone else.

☐ ☐ NA - No inhalant/mist medications prescribed.

☐   UK - Unknown

(M0800) Management of Injectable Medications: <u>Patient's ability</u> to prepare and take <u>all</u> prescribed injectable medications reliably and safely, including administration of correct dosage at the appropriate times/intervals. **Excludes IV medications.**

<u>Prior</u> <u>Current</u>

☐ ☐ 0 - Able to independently take the correct medication and proper dosage at the correct times.

☐ ☐ 1 - Able to take injectable medication at correct times if:
    (a) individual syringes are prepared in advance by another person, <u>OR</u>
    (b) given daily reminders.

☐ ☐ 2 - <u>Unable</u> to take injectable medications unless administered by someone else.

☐ ☐ NA - No injectable medications prescribed.

☐   UK - Unknown

EQUIPMENT MANAGEMENT

(M0810) Patient Management of Equipment (includes <u>ONLY</u> oxygen, IV/infusion therapy, enteral/parenteral nutrition equipment or supplies): <u>Patient's ability</u> to set up, monitor and change equipment reliably and safely, add appropriate fluids or medication, clean/store/dispose of equipment or supplies using proper technique. **(NOTE: This refers to ability, not compliance or willingness.)**

☐ 0 - Patient manages all tasks related to equipment completely independently.

☐ 1 - If someone else sets up equipment (i.e., fills portable oxygen tank, provides patient with prepared solutions), patient is able to manage all other aspects of equipment.

☐ 2 - Patient requires considerable assistance from another person to manage equipment, but independently completes portions of the task.

☐ 3 - Patient is only able to monitor equipment (e.g., liter flow, fluid in bag) and must call someone else to manage the equipment.

☐ 4 - Patient is completely dependent on someone else to manage all equipment.

☐ NA - No equipment of this type used in care **[If NA, go to *M0825*]**

(M0820) Caregiver Management of Equipment (includes <u>ONLY</u> oxygen, IV/infusion equipment, enteral/parenteral nutrition, ventilator therapy equipment or supplies): <u>Caregiver's ability</u> to set up, monitor, and change equipment reliably and safely, add appropriate fluids or medication, clean/store/dispose of equipment or supplies using proper technique. **(NOTE: This refers to ability, not compliance or willingness.)**

☐ 0 - Caregiver manages all tasks related to equipment completely independently.

☐ 1 - If someone else sets up equipment, caregiver is able to manage all other aspects.

☐ 2 - Caregiver requires considerable assistance from another person to manage equipment, but independently completes significant portions of task.

☐ 3 - Caregiver is only able to complete small portions of task (e.g., administer nebulizer treatment, clean/store/dispose of equipment or supplies).

☐ 4 - Caregiver is completely dependent on someone else to manage all equipment.

☐ NA - No caregiver

☐ UK - Unknown

THERAPY NEED

(M0825) Therapy Need: Does the care plan of the Medicare payment period for which this assessment will define a case mix group indicate a need for therapy (physical, occupational, or speech therapy) that meets the threshold for a Medicare high-therapy case mix group?

☐   0 -   No

☐   1 -   Yes

☐ NA -   Not applicable

Advanced Practice Nurse Legislation

Summary of Advanced Practice Nurse (APN) Legal Authority for Scope of Practice*

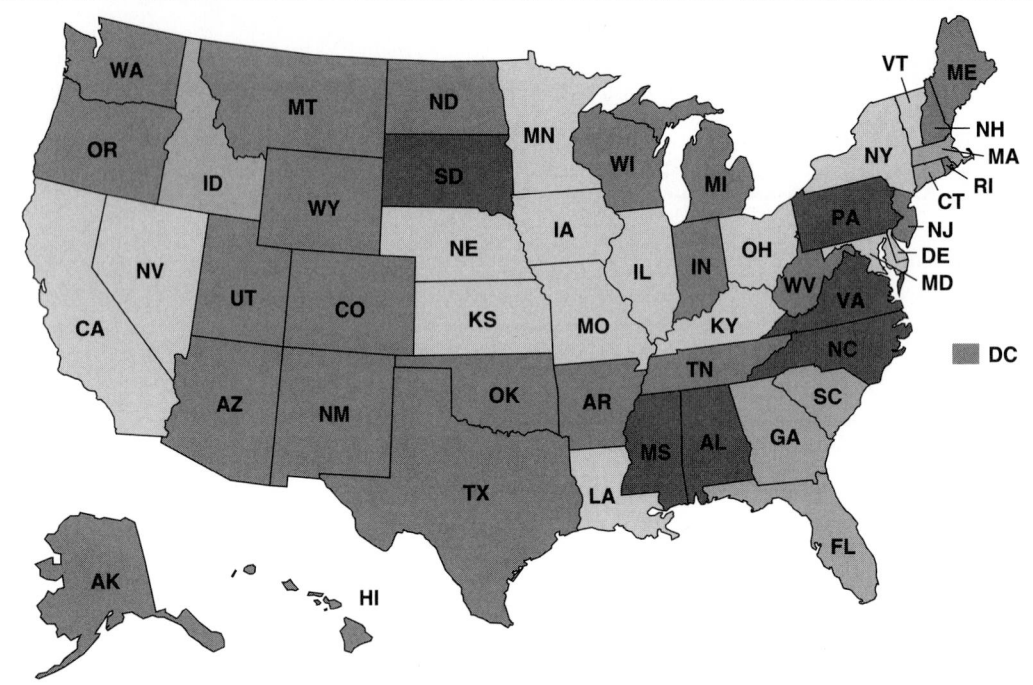

States with nurse practitioner** title protection; the board of nursing has sole authority in scope of practice, with no statutory or regulatory requirements for physician collaboration, direction, or supervision: **AK, AR, AZ, CO, DC, HI, IA, KS, KY, ME, MI, MT, ND, NH, NJ, NM, OK, OR, RI, TN, TX, UT, WA,WI WV, WY**

States with nurse practitioner** title protection; the board of nursing has sole authority in scope of practice, but scope of practice has a requirement for physician supervision: **CT, FL, GA, ID, MA, SC**

States with nurse practitioner** title protection, but the scope of practice is authorized by the board of nursing and the board of medicine: **AL, MS, NC, PA, SD, VA**

States with nurse practitioner** title protection; the board of nursing has sole authority in scope of practice, but scope of practice has a requirement for physician collaboration: **CT, DE, IL, IN, LA, MD, MN, MO, NE†, NV, NY, OH, PA, VT**

[Washington, D.C. is included as a state in this table.]

KEY: * This table provides a state-by-state summary of the degree of independence for all aspects of the NP scope of practice including diagnosing and treating (except prescribing). See table: Summary of APN Legislation: Prescriptive Authority for a state-by-state analysis of the degree of independence for the prescriptive authority aspect of the NP scope of practice.

** The information may apply to other APNs (clinical nurse specialists, nurse midwives, and nurse anesthetists). See State Survey for details.

† State with APRN Board

SOURCE: PEARSON L: FIFTEENTH ANNUAL LEGISLATIVE UPDATE, *THE NURSE PRACTITIONER* 28(1): 26-58, JANUARY 2003.

Summary of Advanced Practice Nurse (APN) Legislation: Prescriptive Authority*

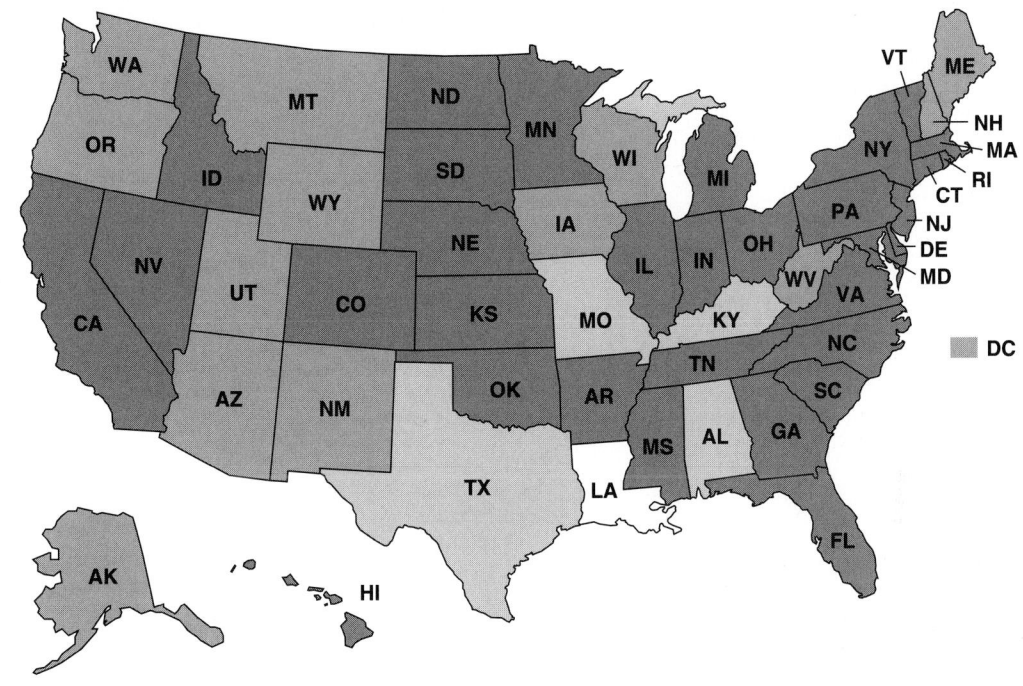

States where nurse practitioners** can prescribe (including controlled substances) independent of any required physician involvement in prescriptive authority: **AK, AZ, DC, IA, ME, MT, NH, NM, OR, UT†, WA, WI, WY**

States where nurse practitioners** can prescribe (excluding controlled substances) with some degree of physician involvement or delegation of prescription writing: **AL, FL, KY, MO, TX**

States where nurse practitioners† can prescribe (including controlled substances) with some degree of physician involvement or delegation of prescription writing: **AR, CA, CO, CT, DE, GA‡, HI, ID, IL, IN, KS, MA, MD, MN, MS, MI, NC, ND, NE, NJ, NV, NY, OH, OK, PA, RI, SC†, SD, TN, VA, VT, WV**

All states: Nurse practitioners** may receive and/or dispense drug samples based on authorized scope of practice, rules and regulations, or statutes.

[Washington, D.C. is included as a state in this table.]

KEY: * This table provides a state-by-state analysis of the prescriptive authority. For analysis of other aspect of the NP scope of practice (including diagnosing and treating), see table: Summary of APN Legislation: Legal Authority for Scope of Practice

** The information may apply to other APNs (clinical nurse specialists, nurse midwives, and nurse anesthetists). See State Survey for details.

† Schedule IV and/or V controlled substance only.

‡ Nurse practitioners do not have written prescribing or dispensing authority; the process falls under delegated medical authority.

Index

Page numbers followed by f indicate figures;
t, tables; and b, boxes.